T0177467

OXFORD HANDBOOK OF

Endocrinology and Diabetes

Published and forthcoming Oxford Medical Handbooks

OXFORD HANDBOOK OF
Endocrinology and Diabetes

FOURTH EDITION

EDITED BY

Katharine Owen

Associate Professor of Diabetes and Honorary Consultant
Physician, Oxford Centre for Diabetes, Endocrinology and
Metabolism, Radcliffe Department of Medicine, University of
Oxford, Oxford, UK

Helen Turner

Consultant in Endocrinology, Oxford Centre for Diabetes,
Endocrinology and Metabolism, Oxford University Hospitals
NHS Trust, Churchill Hospital, Oxford, UK

John Wass

Professor of Endocrinology, University of Oxford, Oxford, UK

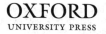

OXFORD
UNIVERSITY PRESS

OXFORD
UNIVERSITY PRESS

Great Clarendon Street, Oxford, OX2 6DP,
United Kingdom

Oxford University Press is a department of the University of Oxford.
It furthers the University's objective of excellence in research, scholarship,
and education by publishing worldwide. Oxford is a registered trade mark of
Oxford University Press in the UK and in certain other countries

© Oxford University Press 2022

The moral rights of the authors have been asserted

First Edition published in 2002
Second Edition published in 2009
Third Edition published in 2014
Fourth Edition published in 2022

Impression: 2

Published in the United States of America by Oxford University Press
198 Madison Avenue, New York, NY 10016, United States of America

British Library Cataloguing in Publication Data
Data available

Library of Congress Control Number: 2021944933

ISBN 978–0–19–885189–9

DOI: 10.1093/med/9780198851899.001.0001

Printed in China by
C&C Offset Printing Co. Ltd.

Foreword

For someone who loves endocrinology, it is a great pleasure to read and use the Oxford Handbook in day-to-day clinical practice. The editors have tried to make an accessible, succinct, comprehensive, and up-to-date text, laid out to be readable and readily assimilable. It aims to cover all endocrine and diabetes occasions, common and less common, dealing with the background science, guidelines on investigation, and advice on treatment. It is written by internationally highly acknowledged experts for trainees, consultants who may have the occasional memory lapse, nurses, and those in primary care with whom we are increasingly sharing joined-up management.

This Handbook is special, as it presents a global appreciation of endocrinology, describing clinical pathways and medications which are primarily based on, and used in, the European experience, while where possible also medical therapy in countries with limited medical resources is addressed.

It is remarkable how much has changed since the first publication in 2002, as well as since the third edition in 2014. New genetic and metabolic mechanisms of disease, new and improved imaging techniques, new drugs, and complications thereof, and thus new management, are all covered in this new edition. In doing this, the editors have sought to include many of the recent guidelines which summarize new evidence in the significantly updated references that are given.

In the new edition, topic sections have been included on transitional endocrinology and diabetes, and newly recognized conditions such as IgG4 disease. The sections on fertility and transgender issues have been extensively updated to encompass new developments. There is also a new chapter on medicolegal issues engendered by some of the complaints within our specialty. This includes governance issues such as consent, duty of confidentiality, and safe driving advice. The nursing section has also been expanded to include more practical advice about travel, fasting, updated glucocorticoid advice, and psychological challenges which face our patients. There is also a discussion on nurse-led clinics which are an important newer addition to our specialty and which can not only increase the quality of care given to our patients, but also increase throughput, in a specialty where outpatient numbers are going up over and above those in general medicine.

The diabetes section has also been carefully reviewed to encompass changes in technology (continuous glucose monitoring/glucose monitoring/closed-loop), new treatments, including immunotherapy for type 1 diabetes and an update on new treatments in type 2 diabetes, and their link to cardiovascular outcomes.

The section on genetics has been updated with guidance on screening, as well as a practical overview of genetic screening for the non-geneticist.

In both the endocrinology and diabetes sections, advice has been included on difficult clinical decisions, tricky issues, and clinical pearls in the relevant sections. Lastly, a publication from 2021 would not be complete without a COVID-19 section, which has been added in the form of website links.

The Editors have to be congratulated in providing a beautiful and most readable new edition of this now classic, internationally highly rated handbook. This 'Herculean' task has resulted in a handbook that presents a science and knowledge base for this specialty which greatly helps to maintain high standards of care of our patients.

Steven WJ Lamberts
Erasmus University Rotterdam
Professor of Medicine
Past President of the European Society for Endocrinology

Preface

Endocrinology and diabetes remain among the most fascinating of special-ties with a very broad range of causation, presentation, and management. We have the ability in our specialty to radically change the quality and quan-tity of life, often within a few days of starting treatment.

Editing the Oxford Handbook has been huge fun and challenging. We have tried to make an accessible, succinct, comprehensive, and up-to-date text, laid out to be readable and readily assimilable. It aims to cover all endocrine and diabetes occasions, common and less common, dealing with the background science, guidelines on investigation, and advice on treat-ment. It is written by experts for trainees, consultants who may have the occasional memory lapse, nurses, and those in primary care with whom we are increasingly sharing joined-up management.

It is remarkable how much has changed since the last edition. New gen-etic and metabolic mechanisms of disease, new and improved imaging tech-niques, new drugs, and complications thereof, and thus new management, are all covered in this edition. In doing this, we have sought to include many of the recent guidelines which summarize new evidence in the significantly updated references that are given.

In the new topics, we have included sections on transitional endocrin-ology and diabetes, newly recognized conditions such as IgG4 disease. The sections on fertility and transgender issues have been extensively up-dated to encompass new developments. There is also a new chapter on medicolegal issues engendered by some of the complaints within our spe-cialty. This includes governance issues such as consent, duty of confidenti-ality, and safe driving advice. The nursing section has also been expanded to include more practical advice about travel, fasting, updated glucocorticoid advice, and psychological challenges which face our patients. There is also a discussion on nurse-led clinics which are an important newer edition to our specialty and which not only can increase the quality of care given to our patients, but also can increase throughput, in a specialty where outpatient numbers are going up over and above those in general medicine.

The diabetes section has also been carefully reviewed to encompass changes in technology (continuous glucose monitoring/glucose moni-toring/closed-loop), new treatments including immunotherapy for type 1 diabetes and an update on new treatments for type 2 diabetes, and their link to cardiovascular outcomes.

The section on genetics has been updated with guidance on screening, as well as a practical overview of genetic screening for the non-geneticist.

In both sections, we have included advice on difficult clinical decisions, tricky issues, and clinical pearls in the relevant sections. Lastly, a publication from 2021 would not be complete without a COVID-19 section, which we have added in the form of website links.

We are very indebted to our excellent authors who have worked diligently to keep the publication on track. We hope that this publication will help to improve the science and knowledge base in our specialty in order to maintain high standards of care for our patients.

JW, KO, HT
February 2021

Contents

Contributors

Ali Abbara
NIHR Clinician Scientist/Clinical Senior Lecturer, Imperial College London at Hammersmith Campus, London, UK

Ramzi Ajjan
Professor of Metabolic Medicine, Leeds Institute of Cardiovascular and Metabolic Medicine, University of Leeds and Leeds Teaching Hospitals Trust, Leeds, UK

Rachel Besser
Consultant in Paediatric Endocrinology, Oxford Children's Hospital, John Radcliffe; Oxford University Hospitals NHS Foundation Trust, Oxford, UK

Karin Bradley
Consultant Endocrinologist, University Hospitals Bristol NHS Foundation Trust, Bristol, UK

Antonia Brooke
Clinical Lead Endocrine, Diabetes, and Metabolic Medicine, Royal Devon and Exeter Hospital NHS Foundation Trust, Exeter, UK

Jodie Buckingham
Lead Podiatrist, Oxford Centre for Diabetes, Endocrinology and Metabolism (OCDEM), Oxford University Hospitals Foundation Trust, Oxford, UK

Pratik Choudhary
Professor of Diabetes, Leicester Diabetes Centre, University of Leicester, Leicester, UK

Melanie Davies
Consultant Gynaecologist, Reproductive Medicine Unit, University College London Hospitals, London, UK

Ketan Dhatariya
Consultant, Diabetes and Endocrinology/Honorary Professor, Norfolk and Norwich University Hospitals, and Norwich Medical School, University of East Anglia, Norwich, UK

Waljit Dhillo
Professor of Endocrinology and Metabolism, Imperial College London at Hammersmith Campus, London, UK

Patrick Divilly
Diabetes Clinical Research Fellow, Diabetes Research Group, Weston Education Centre, London, UK

Richard Eastell
Professor of Bone Metabolism, University of Sheffield, Northern General Hospital, Sheffield, UK

Iona Galloway
Endocrine Fellow, Beaumont Hospital/RCSI Medical School, Dublin, Ireland

Neil Gittoes
Consultant and Honorary Professor of Endocrinology, Queen Elizabeth Hospital and University of Birmingham, Birmingham, UK

Helena Gleeson
Consultant Endocrinologist, Queen Elizabeth Hospital, Birmingham, UK

Emile Hendriks
University Lecturer and Honorary Consultant in Paediatric Endocrinology, University of Cambridge, Cambridge, UK

Claire Higham
Consultant Endocrinologist, Christie Hospital NHS Foundation Trust, Manchester, UK

Kagabo Hirwa
Specialist Trainee Registrar, Diabetes and Endocrinology, University Hospitals Plymouth NHS Trust, Plymouth, UK

Channa Jayasena
Reader in Reproductive Endocrinology, Imperial College London Faculty of Medicine, Hammersmith Hospital, London, UK

Niki Karavitaki
Senior Clinical Lecturer in Endocrinology and Honorary Consultant Endocrinologist, Institute of Metabolism and Systems Research, University of Birmingham and Queen Elizabeth Hospital, Birmingham, UK

Fredrik Karpe
Professor of Metabolic Medicine, Oxford Centre for Diabetes, Endocrinology and Metabolism (OCDEM), University of Oxford, Oxford, UK

Márta Korbonits
Professor of Endocrinology and Metabolism, Barts and the London School of Medicine, Queen Mary University of London, London, UK

Alex Lewis
Specialist Registrar, Christie Hospital NHS Foundation Trust, Manchester, UK

Alistair Lumb
Consultant in Diabetes and Acute General Medicine, Oxford Centre for Diabetes, Endocrinology and Metabolism (OCDEM), Oxford University Hospitals Foundation Trust, Churchill Hospital, Oxford, UK

Anne Marland
Endocrine Lead Nurse, Oxford Centre for Diabetes, Endocrinology and Metabolism (OCDEM), Oxford University Hospitals Foundation Trust, Churchill Hospital, Oxford, UK

Andrew McGovern
Academic Clinical Fellow, Royal Devon and Exeter Hospital, Exeter, UK

Phillip Monaghan
Consultant Clinical Scientist, The Christie Pathology Partnership, The Christie NHS Foundation Trust, Manchester, UK

Helen Murphy
Professor of Medicine (Diabetes and Antenatal Care), University of East Anglia, Norwich Research Park, Norwich, UK

Paul Newey
Senior Lecturer in Endocrinology, Ninewells Hospital & Medical School, University of Dundee, Dundee, UK

Ken Ong
Professor of Paediatric Epidemiology and Paediatric Endocrinologist, University of Cambridge, Cambridge, UK

Katherine Owen
Associate Professor of Diabetes and Honorary Consultant Physician, Oxford Centre for Diabetes, Endocrinology and Metabolism (OCDEM), Radcliffe Department of Medicine, University of Oxford, Oxford, UK

Ana Pokrajac
Consultant in Diabetes and Endocrinology, West Hertfordshire Hospitals NHS Trust, Watford, UK

Peter Scanlon
Ophthalmologist and Associate Professor, Department of Neuroscience, University of Oxford, John Radcliffe Hospital, Oxford, UK

Rebecca Scott
Obstetric Physician and Specialist Registrar in Diabetes and Endocrinology, Imperial College Healthcare NHS Trust, London, UK

Leighton Seal
Consultant and Honorary Reader in Diabetes and Endocrinology, St George's University Hospitals NHS Foundation Trust and St George's Hospital Medical School, London, UK

Mike Tadman
Senior Clinical Nurse Specialist in Neuroendocrine Tumours, Oxford University Hospitals Foundation Trust, Churchill Hospital, Oxford, UK

Solomon Tesfaye
Consultant Endocrinologist and Honorary Professor of Diabetic Medicine at the University of Sheffield, Sheffield Teaching Hospitals, Royal Hallamshire Hospital, Sheffield, UK

Gaya Thanabalasingham
Consultant in Diabetes and Acute General Medicine, Oxford Centre for Diabetes, Endocrinology and Metabolism (OCDEM), Oxford University Hospitals Foundation Trust, Churchill Hospital, Oxford, UK

Chris Thompson
Professor of Endocrinology, Beaumont Hospital/RCSI Medical School, Dublin, Ireland

Layla Thurston
Clinical Research Fellow, Imperial College London at Hammersmith Campus, London, UK

Jeremy Tomlinson
Professor of Metabolic Endocrinology, Oxford Centre for Diabetes, Endocrinology and Metabolism (OCDEM), Churchill Hospital, University of Oxford, Oxford, UK

Peter Trainer
Consultant Endocrinologist, The Christie NHS Foundation Trust, Manchester, UK

Helen Turner
Consultant in Endocrinology, Oxford Centre for Diabetes, Endocrinology and Metabolism (OCDEM), Oxford University Hospitals NHS Trust, Churchill Hospital, Oxford, UK

Mark Vanderpump
Consultant Physician and Endocrinologist, OneWelbeck Endocrinology, London, UK

John Wass
Professor of Endocrinology, University of Oxford, Oxford, UK

John Wilding
Professor of Medicine and Honorary Consultant Physician, Clinical Sciences Centre, Aintree University Hospital, Liverpool, UK

Catherine Williamson
Professor of Women's Health and Honorary Consultant in Obstetric Medicine, King's College London, London, UK

Symbols and abbreviations

➲	cross-reference
🖰	website
~	approximately
↑	increased
↓	decreased
↔	normal
→	leads to
1°	primary
2°	secondary
α	alpha
β	beta
δ	delta
γ	gamma
κ	kappa
%	per cent
♀	female
♂	male
+ve	positive
−ve	negative
=	equal to
≡	equivalent to
<	less than
>	more than
≤	less than or equal to
≥	greater than or equal to
°C	degree Celsius
£	pound Sterling
®	registered trademark
►	important
<>	warning
AAS	androgenic anabolic steroid
ACA	adrenocortical adenoma
ACC	adrenocortical carcinoma
ACE	angiotensin-converting enzyme
ACEI	angiotensin-converting enzyme inhibitor
aCGH	array comparative genomic hybridization
ACLY	adenosine triphosphate citrate lyase
ACMG	American College of Medical Genetics and Genomics
ACR	albumin:creatinine ratio
ACTH	adrenocorticotrophic hormone
AD	autosomal dominant
ADA	American Diabetes Association
ADH	antidiuretic hormone; autosomal dominant hypocalcaemia
ADI	adipsic diabetes insipidus
aFP	alpha fetoprotein
AGE	advanced glycation end-product
AGHDA	Adult Growth Hormone Deficiency Assessment (score)
AHC	adrenal hypoplasia congenita
AI	adrenal insufficiency
AIDS	acquired immune deficiency syndrome
AIH	amiodarone-induced hypothyroidism
AIMAH	ACTH-independent macronodular adrenal hyperplasia
AIP	aryl hydrocarbon receptor interacting protein
AIT	amiodarone-induced thyrotoxicosis
AITD	autoimmune thyroid disease
ALL	acute lymphoblastic leukaemia
ALP	alkaline phosphatase
ALT	alanine transaminase
a.m.	ante meridiem (before noon)
AME	apparent mineralocorticoid excess
AMH	anti-Müllerian hormone
AMN	adrenomyeloneuropathy
AMP	adenosine monophosphate
AN	autonomic neuropathy
ANCA	antineutrophil cytoplasmic antibody
ANP	advanced nurse practitioner
aPCA	adrenal phaeochromocytoma
apo	apoprotein
APS	autoimmune polyglandular syndrome; artificial pancreas system
AR	autosomal recessive
ART	assisted reproductive technique
AST	aspartate transaminase
ATA	American Thyroid Association
ATD	antithyroid drug

ATDT	antithyroid drug therapy
ATP	adenosine triphosphate
AVP	arginine vasopressin
AVS	adrenal vein sampling
BAM	bile acid malabsorption
bd	bis in die (twice daily)
BMD	bone mineral density
BMI	body mass index
BMT	bone marrow transplantation
BP	blood pressure
bpm	beat per minute
Ca	calcium
CAH	congenital adrenal hyperplasia
cAMP	cyclic adenosine monophosphate
CASR	calcium-sensing receptor
CBG	cortisol-binding globulin
CCF	congestive cardiac failure
CDKI	cyclin-dependent kinase inhibitor
CEA	carcinoembryonic antigen
CF	cystic fibrosis
CFS	chronic fatigue syndrome
CGH	comparative genomic hybridization
CGM	continuous glucose monitoring
cGMP	cyclic guanosine monophosphate
cGy	centigray
CHD	coronary heart disease
CHH	congenital hypogonadotrophic hypogonadism
CHO	carbohydrate
CK	creatine kinase
CKD	chronic kidney disease
CLA	cutaneous lichen amyloidosis
CLAH	congenital lipoid adrenal hyperplasia
cm	centimetre
CMV	cytomegalovirus
CNC	Carney complex
CNS	central nervous system
COCP	combined oral contraceptive pill
COPD	chronic obstructive pulmonary disease
COVID-19	coronavirus disease
CPA	cyproterone acetate
CPI	checkpoint inhibitor
CPK	creatine phosphokinase
CPRD	Clinical Practice Research Datalink
Cr	creatinine

CRF	chronic renal failure
CRH	corticotrophin-releasing hormone
CRP	C-reactive protein
CSF	cerebrospinal fluid
CSII	continuous subcutaneous insulin infusion
CSMO	'clinically significant' diabetic macular oedema
CSW	cerebral salt wasting
CT	computed tomography
CTLA-4	cytotoxic T lymphocyte antigen-4
CVA	cerebrovascular accident
CVD	cardiovascular disease
CVOT	cardiovascular outcome trial
CVP	central venous pressure
CXR	chest X-ray
4D	four-dimensional
DCCT	Diabetes Control and Complications Trial
DCT	distal convoluted tubule
DD	disc diameter
ddPCR	digital polymerase chain reaction
DHEA	dehydroepiandrostenedione
DHEAS	dehydroepiandrostenedione sulphate
DHT	dihydrotestosterone
DI	diabetes insipidus
DIT	di-iodotyrosine
DKA	diabetic ketoacidosis
dL	decilitre
DM	diabetes mellitus
DMSA	dimercaptosuccinic acid
DN	diabetic neuropathy
DNA	deoxyribonucleic acid
DOC	deoxycorticosterone
DPN	diabetic peripheral neuropathy
DPP-IV	dipeptidyl peptidase IV
DR	diabetic retinopathy
DRS	Diabetic Retinopathy Study
DSD	disorders of sexual differentiation; disorder of sex development
DSN	diabetes specialist nurse
DTC	differentiated thyroid cancer
DVA	Driver and Vehicle Agency
DVLA	Driver and Vehicle Licensing Agency
DVT	deep vein thrombosis
DXA	dual-energy absorptiometry

E2	oestradiol
EASD	European Association for the Study of Diabetes
ECF	extracellular fluid
ECG	electrocardiogram
EDC	endocrine disrupting chemical
EDTA	ethylenediaminetetraacetic acid
EE2	ethinylestradiol
EEG	electroencephalogram
eFPGL	extra-adrenal functional paraganglioma
eGFR	estimated glomerular filtration rate
ELST	endolymphatic sac tumour
EM	electron microscopy
EMA	European Medicines Agency
ENaC	epithelial sodium channel
ENETS	European Neuroendocrine Tumor Society
ENT	ear, nose, and throat
EOSS	Edmonton Obesity Staging System
EPO	erythropoietin
ER	(o)estrogen receptor
ERT	(o)estrogen replacement therapy
ESC	European Society of Cardiology
ESN	endocrine specialist nurse
ESR	erythrocyte sedimentation rate
FSRD	end-stage renal disease
ESRF	end-stage renal failure
ETDRS	Early Treatment of Diabetic Retinopathy Study
EUA	examination under anaesthesia
EU-AIR	European Adrenal Insufficiency Registry
FAI	free androgen index
FAZ	foveal avascular zone
FBC	full blood count
FCH	familial combined hyperlipidaemia
FCS	familial chylomicronaemia syndrome
FDA	Food and Drug Administration
FDG	fluorodeoxyglucose
FGD	familial glucocorticoid deficiency
FGF	fibroblast growth factor
FGFR1	fibroblast growth factor receptor 1
FH	familial hypercholesterolaemia
FHA	functional hypothalamic amenorrhoea

FHH	familial hypocalciuric hypercalcaemia
FIH	familial isolated hypoparathyroidism
FIHP	familial isolated hyperparathyroidism
FIPA	familial isolated pituitary adenoma
FISH	fluorescence in situ hybridization
FMTC	familial medullary thyroid carcinoma
FNA	fine needle aspiration
FNAC	fine needle aspiration cytology
FPG	fasting plasma glucose
FRIII	fixed-rate intravenous insulin infusion
FSH	follicle-stimulating hormone
FT_3	free tri-iodothyronine
FT_4	free thyroxine
FTC	follicular thyroid carcinoma
FTO	fat mass and obesity associated
FU	fluorouracil
g	gram
^{68}Ga	gallium-68
GAD	glutamic acid decarboxylase
GAG	glycosaminoglycan
GBM	glomerular basement membrane
GBq	giga becquerel
GC	glucocorticoid
GCK	glucokinase
GCS	Glasgow Coma Scale
gCSF	granulocyte colony-stimulating factor
GDF15	growth differentiation factor
GDM	gestational diabetes mellitus
GEP	gastroenteropancreatic
GFR	glomerular filtration rate
GGT	gamma glutamyl transferase
GH	growth hormone
GHD	growth hormone deficiency
GHDC	growth hormone day curve
GHRH	growth hormone-releasing hormone
GI	gastrointestinal
GIP	gastric inhibitory polypeptide
GK	glycerol kinase
GLP-1	glucagon-like peptide-1
GLUT4	glucose transporter type 4
GnRH	gonadotrophin-releasing hormone

GO	Graves' orbitopathy	HNF	hepatocyte nuclear factor
GO-QOL	Graves' Ophthalmopathy Quality of Life	HNPGL	head and neck paraganglioma
GP	general practitioner	HP	hypothalamus/pituitary
GPCR	G-protein-coupled receptor	HPA	hypothalamic–pituitary–adrenal
GRA	glucocorticoid-remediable aldosteronism	HPO	hypothalamic–pituitary–ovarian
		HPT	hypothalamo–pituitary–thyroid
GRS	genetic risk score	HPT-JT	hyperparathyroidism jaw tumour (syndrome)
GTN	glyceryl trinitrate		
GTT	glucose tolerance test	HPV	human papillomavirus
GWAS	genome-wide association studies	HRT	hormone replacement therapy
Gy	gray	HSCT	haematopoietic stem cell transplantation
h	hour		
HA	hypothalamic amenorrhoea	11β-HSD2	11β-hydroxysteroid dehydrogenase type 2
HAART	highly active antiretroviral therapy		
		HSG	hysterosalpingography
Hb	haemoglobin	5-HT2B	5-hydroxytryptamine 2B
HbA1c	glycated haemoglobin	HTLV-1	human T lymphotropic virus type 1
hCG	human chorionic gonadotrophin		
HCl	hydrochloric acid	HU	Hounsfield unit
HCL	hybrid closed loop	HVFT	fibrous variant of Hashimoto's thyroiditis
Hct	haematocrit		
HD	Hirschsprung's disease	HyCoSy	hysterosalpingo contrast sonography
HDL	high-density lipoprotein		
HDL-C	high-density lipoprotein cholesterol	Hz	hertz
		IADPSG	International Association of Diabetes and Pregnancy Study Groups
HDU	high dependency unit		
HEEADDSS	Home, Education and employment, Exercise and eating, Activity and peers, Drugs, Depression, Sexuality and sexual health, Sleep, Safety		
		ICA	islet cell antibodies
		ICSI	intracytoplasmic sperm injection
		IDDM	insulin-dependent diabetes mellitus
HELLP	haemolysis, elevated liver enzymes, and low platelet		
		IDL	intermediate-density lipoprotein
HERS	Heart and Oestrogen-Progestin Replacement Study	IFCC	International Federation of Clinical Chemistry
		IFG	impaired fasting glycaemia
HFEA	Human Fertilisation and Embryology Authority	Ig	immunoglobulin
		IGF	insulin-like growth factor
hGH	human growth hormone	IGFBP3	insulin-like growth factor-binding protein 3
HH	hypogonadotrophic hypogonadism		
		IGF-1R	insulin-like growth factor-1 receptor
HHS	hyperglycaemic hyperosmolar state		
		IGT	impaired glucose tolerance
5-HIAA	5-hydroxindoleacetic acid	IHD	ischaemic heart disease
HIF	hypoxia-inducible factor	IHH	idiopathic hypogonadotropic hypogonadism
HIV	human immunodeficiency virus		
HLA	human leucocyte antigen	IM	intramuscular
hMG	human menopausal gonadotrophin	IMRT	intensity-modulated radiotherapy
		IPSS	inferior petrosal sinus sampling
HMG CoA	3-hydroxy-3-methylglutaryl coenzyme A	IQ	intelligence quotient
		IRMA	intraretinal microvascular abnormality

IRT	immune reconstitution therapy
ITT	insulin tolerance test
ITU	intensive treatment unit
IU	international unit
IUGR	intrauterine growth restriction
IUI	intrauterine insemination
IV	intravenous
IVC	inferior vena cava
IVF	in vitro fertilization
IVII	intravenous insulin infusion
J	joule
K+	potassium ion
kb	kilobase
kcal	kilocalorie
kDa	kilodalton
kg	kilogram
KPD	ketosis-prone diabetes
L	litre
LADA	latent autoimmune diabetes of adulthood
LCAT	lecithin:cholesterol acyltransferase
LCCSCT	large cell calcifying Sertoli cell tumour
LDL	low-density lipoprotein
LDL-C	LDL cholesterol
LDLR	LDL receptor
LFT	liver function test
LH	luteinizing hormone
LHRH	luteinizing hormone-releasing hormone
LMWH	low-molecular weight heparin
LOH	loss of heterozygosity
Lpa	lipoprotein a
LPL	lipoprotein lipase
LSCS	lower-segment Caesarean section
LVEF	left ventricular ejection fraction
LVH	left ventricular hypertrophy
m	metre
M	molar
MAI	Mycobacterium avium cellulare
MAOI	monoamine oxidase inhibitor
MAPK	mitogen-activated protein kinase
MBq	mega becquerel
MC	mineralocorticoid
MCA	Medicines Control Agency
MC1R	melanocortin 1 receptor
MC4R	melanocortin 4 receptor
MDI	multiple-dose injection

MDT	multidisciplinary team
MEN	multiple endocrine neoplasia
mg	milligram
Mg	magnesium
MGMT	O-6-methylguanine DNA methyltransferase
mGy	milligray
MHC	major histocompatibility complex
MHRA	Medicines and Healthcare Products Regulatory Agency
MI	myocardial infarction
MIBG	metaiodobenzylguanidine
min	minute
MIT	monoiodotyrosine
mIU	milli international unit
MJ	megajoule
mL	millilitre
MLPA	multiplex ligation-dependent probe amplification
mm	millimetre
mmHg	millimetre of mercury
mmol	millimole
MODY	maturity-onset diabetes of the young
mOsm	milliosmole
MPH	mid-parental height
MPNST	malignant peripheral nerve sheath tumour
MRAP	MC2R accessory protein
MRI	magnetic resonance imaging
mRNA	messenger ribonucleic acid
MS	mass spectrometry
MSH	melanocyte-stimulating hormone
MSU	midstream urine
MTC	medullary thyroid carcinoma
mTESE	microdissection testicular sperm extraction
mTOR	mammalian target of rapamycin
mU	milliunit
Na	sodium
NaCl	sodium chloride
NAFLD	non-alcoholic fatty liver disease
NASH	non-alcoholic steatohepatitis
NDA	National Diabetes Audit
NEFA	non-esterified fatty acid
NET	neuroendocrine tumour
NF	neurofibromatosis
NFA	non-functioning pituitary adenoma
NFPA	non-functioning pituitary adenoma

ng	nanogram
NG	nasogastric
NGS	next-generation sequencing
NHS	National Health Service
NICE	National Institute for Health and Care Excellence
NIDDM	non-insulin-dependent diabetes mellitus
NIFTP	non-invasive follicular thyroid neoplasm with papillary-like nuclear features
NIH	National Institutes of Health
NIPD	non-invasive prenatal genetic diagnosis
NIPT	non-invasive prenatal genetic testing
NIS	sodium/iodide symporter
NMC	Nursing and Midwifery Council
nmol	nanomole
NPHPT	normocalcaemic primary hyperparathyroidism
NSAID	non-steroidal anti-inflammatory drug
NTI	non-thyroidal illness
NT-proBNP	N-terminal pro B-type natriuretic peptide
NVD	new vessels on the disc
NVE	new vessels elsewhere
O_2	oxygen
OA	osteoarthritis
OCP	oral contraceptive pill
od	omne in die (once daily)
OGTT	oral glucose tolerance test
OHA	oral hypoglycaemic agent
25OHD	25-hydroxyvitamin D
1,25(OH)$_2$D	1,25-dihydroxyvitamin D
17OHP	17-hydroxyprogesterone
OHSS	ovarian hyperstimulation syndrome
OR	odds ratio
PAI	plasminogen activator inhibitor
PAK	pancreas after kidney
PAR-Q	Physical Activity Readiness Questionnaire
PBC	primary biliary cirrhosis
PCC	phaeochromocytoma
PCOS	polycystic ovary syndrome
PCSK9	proprotein convertase subtilisin/kexin 9
PD-1	programmed death 1
PDE	phosphodiesterase

PD-L1	programme death ligand 1
PDR	proliferative diabetic retinopathy
PE	pulmonary embolism
PED	performance-enhancing drug
PEG	polyethylene glycol
PERT	pancreatic enzyme replacement therapy
PET	positron emission tomography
pg	picogram
PGD	prenatal/preimplantation genetic diagnosis
PGL	paraganglioma
PHPT	primary hyperparathyroidism
PI	protease inhibitor
PID	pelvic inflammatory disease
PIH	pregnancy-induced hypertension
PitNET	pituitary neuroendocrine tumour
PKA	protein kinase A
p.m.	post meridiem (after noon)
PMC	papillary microcarcinoma of the thyroid
pmol	picomole
PMS	psammomatous melanotic schwannoma
PNDM	permanent neonatal diabetes mellitus
pNET	pancreatic neuroendocrine tumour
PNMT	phenylethanolamine-N-methyltransferase
PO	per os (orally)
PO$_4$	phosphate
POEMS	progressive polyneuropathy, organomegaly, endocrinopathy, M-protein, and skin change
POF	premature ovarian failure
POI	premature ovarian insufficiency
POMC	pro-opiomelanocortin
POME	pulmonary oil microembolism
POP	progesterone-only pill
PPAR	peroxisome proliferator-activated receptor
PPGL	phaeochromocytoma/paraganglioma
PPI	proton pump inhibitor
PPNAD	primary pigmented nodular adrenocortical disease
PPT	post-partum thyroiditis
PR	per rectum
PRA	plasma renin activity

PRH	postprandial reactive hypoglycaemia		SDH	succinate dehydrogenase
PRL	prolactin		SDHx	succinate dehydrogenase enzyme complex
PRRT	peptide receptor radionuclide therapy		SERM	selective (o)estrogen receptor modulator
PSA	prostate-specific antigen		SGA	small-for-gestational age
PTA	pancreas transplantation alone		SGLT2	sodium–glucose cotransporter 2
PTC	papillary thyroid carcinoma		SH	severe hypoglycaemia
PTH	parathyroid hormone		SHBG	sex hormone-binding globulin
PTHrP	parathyroid hormone-related peptide		SIAD	syndrome of inappropriate
PTU	propylthiouracil		SIADH	syndrome of inappropriate antidiuretic hormone
PVD	peripheral vascular disease		SLE	systemic lupus erythematosus
QCT	quantitative computed tomography		SNP	single nucleotide polymorphism
qds	quarter die sumendus (four times daily)		SNRI	serotonin–noradrenaline reuptake inhibitor
QoL	quality of life		SNV	single-nucleotide variant
QTc	corrected QT interval		SPECT	single-photon emission computed tomography
RAA	renin–angiotensin–aldosterone		SPK	simultaneous pancreas kidney (transplant)
RAI	radioactive iodine		SSA	somatostatin analogue
RANK	receptor activator of nuclear factor kappa-B		SSRI	selective serotonin reuptake inhibitor
RANKL	receptor activator of nuclear factor kappa-B		SST	short Synacthen® test
RAS	renin–angiotensin system		StAR	steroidogenic acute regulatory protein
RCAD	renal cysts and diabetes (syndrome)		STED	sight-threatening diabetic eye disease
RCC	renal cell carcinoma		STI	sexually transmitted infection
RCN	Royal College of Nursing		SU	sulfonylurea
RCPCH	Royal College of Paediatrics and Child Health		T_3	tri-iodothyronine
RCT	randomized controlled trial		T_4	thyroxine
RECIST	response evaluation criteria in solid tumours		TART	testicular adrenal rest tissue
RED-S	relative energy deficiency in sport		TB	tuberculosis
RFA	radiofrequency ablation		TBG	thyroid-binding globulin
rhGH	recombinant human growth hormone		TBI	traumatic brain injury
			TBPA	T_4-binding prealbumin
RNA	ribonucleic acid		TC	total cholesterol
RR	relative risk		TCA	tricyclic antidepressant
RRT	renal replacement therapy		TDD	total daily dose
rT_3	reverse T_3		T1DM	type 1 diabetes mellitus
RTH	resistance to thyroid hormone		T2DM	type 2 diabetes mellitus
RTK	receptor tyrosine kinase		tds	ter die sumendus (three times daily)
s	second		TENS	transcutaneous electrical nerve stimulation
SARS-Cov-2	severe acute respiratory syndrome coronavirus 2		TERT	telomerase reverse transcriptase
SC	subcutaneous		TFT	thyroid function test
SD	standard deviation		Tg	thyroglobulin

TG	triglyceride	UKPDS	United Kingdom Prospective Diabetes Study
TgAb	thyroglobulin antibody	US	ultrasound
TGF	transforming growth factor	USA	United States of America
TIND	treatment-induced neuropathy of diabetes	USP8	ubiquitin-specific peptidase 8
TI-RADS	thyroid imaging, reporting, and data system	V	volt
TK	tyrosine kinase	VA	visual acuity
TKI	tyrosine kinase inhibitor	VDDR	vitamin D-dependent rickets
TNDM	transient neonatal diabetes mellitus	VEGF	vascular endothelial growth factor
TNF	tumour necrosis factor	VHL	von Hippel–Lindau
TPO	thyroid peroxidase	VIP	vasoactive intestinal polypeptide
TPOAb	antithyroid peroxidase antibody	VLCFA	very long-chain fatty acid
TPP	thyrotoxic periodic paralysis	VLDL	very low-density lipoprotein
TR	thyroid hormone receptor	VMA	vanillylmandelic acid
TRAb	thyroid-stimulating hormone receptor antibody	VRIII	variable-rate intravenous insulin infusion
TRE	thyroid hormone response element	vs	versus
		VTE	venous thromboembolism
TRH	thyrotropin-releasing hormone	VUS	variant of uncertain significance
tRNA	transfer ribonucleic acid	WBS	whole-body scan
TSA	transsphenoidal approach	WES	whole-exome sequencing
TSH	thyroid-stimulating hormone	WGS	whole-genome sequencing
TTR	transthyretin	WHI	Women's Health Initiative
TZD	thiazolidinedione	WHO	World Health Organization
U	unit	w/v	weight by volume
U&E	urea and electrolytes	XLAG	X-linked acrogigantism
UFC	urinary free cortisol	XLR	X-linked recessive
UK	United Kingdom	ZES	Zollinger–Ellison syndrome
		ZnT8	zinc transporter 8

Table 1.1 Disordered thyroid hormone–protein interactions

	Serum total T_4 and T_3	Free T_4 and T_3
Primary abnormality in TBG		
↑ concentration	↑	Normal
↓ concentration	↓	Normal
Primary disorder of thyroid function		
Hyperthyroidism	↑	↑
Hypothyroidism	↓	↓

Table 1.2 Circumstances associated with altered concentration of TBG

↑ TBG	↓ TBG
Pregnancy	Androgens
Newborn state	Large doses of glucocorticoids (GCs); Cushing's syndrome
Oral contraceptive pill and other sources of oestrogens	Chronic liver disease
Tamoxifen	Severe systemic illness
Hepatitis A; chronic active hepatitis	Active acromegaly
Biliary cirrhosis	Nephrotic syndrome
Acute intermittent porphyria	Genetically determined
Genetically determined	Drugs, e.g. phenytoin (see also Table 1.4)

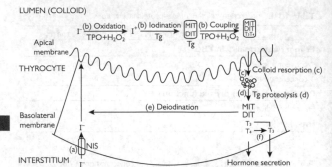

Fig. 1.1 Thyroid hormone biosynthesis. Iodine is transported via NIS located in the basal membrane of follicular thyrocytes (a). Iodine is organified onto tyrosyl residues in Tg at the apical membrane, requiring the presence of TPO, first to produce MIT and then DIT (b). TPO links two DITs to form T_4, and MIT and DIT to form small amounts of T_3 and rT_3 (b). Once formed, thyroid hormone is stored in the colloid as part of the structure of Tg (b). After TSH stimulation, Tg enters the thyroid cell from colloid (c). It is cleaved by endopeptidases in lysosomes (d), thus allowing thyroid hormone to be released into the circulation, mostly in the form of levothyroxine (e). H_2O_2, hydrogen peroxide.

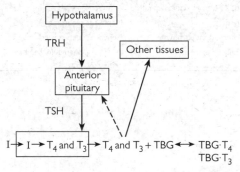

Fig. 1.2 Regulation of thyroid function. Solid arrows indicate stimulation; broken arrow indicates inhibitory influence. I, iodine; T_3, tri-iodothyronine; T_4, thyroxine; TBG, thyroid-binding globulin; TRH, thyrotropin-releasing hormone; TSH, thyroid-stimulating hormone.

Molecular action of thyroid hormone

- T_3 is the active form of thyroid hormone and binds to thyroid hormone receptors (TRs) in target cell nuclei to initiate a range of physiological effects, including cellular differentiation, postnatal development, and metabolic homeostasis. The actions of thyroid hormone are mediated by two genes (*TRα, TRβ*), which encode three nuclear receptor subtypes with differing tissue expression (TRα1: central nervous system (CNS), cardiac and skeletal muscle; TRβ1: liver and kidney; TRβ2: pituitary and hypothalamus).

- Both T_4 and T_3 enter the cell via active transport mediated by monocarboxylate transporter-8 and other proteins. Three iodothyronine deiodinases (D1–3) regulate T_3 availability to target cells. The D1 enzyme in the kidney and liver is generally considered to be responsible for the production of the majority of circulating T_3. Although serum T_3 concentrations are maintained constant by the negative feedback actions of the HPT axis, the intracellular thyroid status may vary as a result of differential action of deiodinases. In the hypothalamus and pituitary, 5′-deiodination of T_4 by D2 results in the generation of T_3, whereas 5′-deiodination by the D3 enzyme irreversibly inactivates T_4 and T_3, resulting in the production of the metabolites rT_3 and T_2. Thus, the relative activities of D2 and D3 enzymes in T_3 target cells regulate the availability of the active hormone T_3 to the nucleus and ultimately determine the saturation of the nuclear TR (see Fig. 1.3).

- TRs belong to the nuclear hormone receptor superfamily and function as ligand-inducible transcription factors. They are expressed in virtually all tissues and involved in many physiological processes in response to T_3 binding. TRα and TRβ receptors bind to specific DNA thyroid hormone response elements (TREs) located in the promoter regions of T_3-responsive target genes and mediate the actions of T_3.

- Unliganded TR (unoccupied TR, ApoTR) inhibits basal transcription of T_3 target genes by interacting preferentially with co-repressor proteins, leading to repression of gene transcription. Upon T_3 binding, the liganded TR undergoes conformational change and reverses histone deacetylation associated with basal repression. Subsequent recruitment of a large transcription factor complex, known as vitamin D receptor interacting protein/TR-associated protein (DRIP/TRAP), leads to binding and stabilization of ribonucleic acid (RNA) polymerase II and hormone-dependent activation of transcription.

- The roles of TRα and TRβ have been shown to be tissue-specific. For example, TRα mediates important T_3 actions during heart, bone, and intestinal development and controls basal heart rate and thermoregulation in adults, while TRβ mediates T_3 action in the liver and is responsible for regulation of the HPT axis.

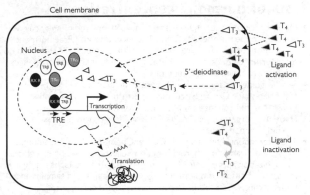

Fig. 1.3 Thyroid hormone action.

Abnormalities of development

- Remnants of the thyroglossal duct may be found in any position along the course of the tract of its descent:
  - In the tongue, it is referred to as the '*lingual thyroid*'.
  - *Thyroglossal cysts* may be visible as midline swellings in the neck.
  - *Thyroglossal fistula* develops as an opening in the middle of the neck.
  - As thyroglossal nodules *or*
  - The '*pyramidal lobe*', a structure contiguous with the thyroid isthmus which extends upwards.
- The gland can descend too far down to reach the anterior mediastinum.
- Congenital hypothyroidism may result from failure of the thyroid to develop (agenesis).

Further reading

Luongo C, et al. (2019). Deiodinases and their intricate role in thyroid hormone homeostasis. *Nat Rev Endocrinol* **15**, 479–88.

Tests of hormone concentration

- Highly specific and sensitive chemiluminescent and radioimmunoassays are used to measure serum T_4 and T_3 concentrations.[1] Free hormone concentrations usually correlate better with the metabolic state than do total hormone concentrations because they are unaffected by changes in binding protein concentration or affinity.
- See UK guidelines for the use of thyroid function tests (TFTs) (Association for Clinical Biochemistry, British Thyroid Association, British Thyroid Foundation, ℘ https://www.british-thyroid-association.org/sandbox/bta2016/uk_guidelines_for_the_use_of_thyroid_function_tests.pdf).
- The International Federation of Clinical Chemistry (IFCC) Committee for Standardization of Thyroid Function Tests have developed a global harmonization approach for FT_4 and TSH measurements, based on a multiassay method comparison study with clinical serum samples and target setting with a robust factor analysis method.[2,3]

References

1. Favresse J, et al. (2018). Interferences with thyroid function immunoassays: clinical implications and detection algorithm. *Endocr Rev* **39**, 830–50.
2. De Grande LAC, et al. (2017). Standardization of free thyroxine measurements allows the adoption of a more uniform reference interval. *Clin Chem* **63**, 1642–52.
3. Thienpont LM, et al. (2017). Harmonization of serum thyroid-stimulating hormone measurements paves the way for the adoption of a more uniform reference interval. *Clin Chem* **63**, 1248–60.

Tests of homeostatic control

(See Table 1.3.)

- Serum TSH concentration is used as 1st line in the diagnosis of 1°
  hypothyroidism and hyperthyroidism. The test is misleading in patients
  with 2° thyroid dysfunction due to hypothalamic/pituitary disease,
  including TSH-secreting pituitary adenoma (see ➔ Anterior pituitary
  hormone replacement, p. 144), recent treatment for thyrotoxicosis
  (TSH may remain suppressed, even when thyroid hormone
  concentrations have normalized), non-thyroidal illness (NTI), TSH assay
  interference, resistance to thyroid hormone (RTH), and disorders of
  thyroid hormone transport or metabolism.
- The TRH stimulation test, which can be used to assess the functional
  state of the TSH secretory mechanism, is now rarely used to diagnose
  1° thyroid disease since it has been superseded by sensitive TSH assays.
  Its main use is in the differential diagnosis of elevated TSH in the setting
  of elevated thyroid hormone levels and the differential diagnosis of
  RTH (see Box 1.1) and TSH-secreting pituitary adenoma.

In interpreting results of TFTs, the effects of drugs that the patient might be
on should be borne in mind. Table 1.4 lists the influence of drugs on TFTs.
Table 1.5 sets out some examples of atypical TFTs.

Table 1.3 Thyroid hormone concentrations in various thyroid abnormalities

Condition	TSH	Free T_4	Free T_3
1° hyperthyroidism	Undetectable	↑↑	↑
T_3 toxicosis	Undetectable	Normal	↑↑
Subclinical hyperthyroidism	↓	Normal	Normal
2° hyperthyroidism (TSHoma)	↑ or normal	↑	↑
Thyroid hormone resistance	↑ or normal	↑	↑
1° hypothyroidism	↑	↓	↓ or normal
Subclinical hypothyroidism	↑	Normal	Normal
2° hypothyroidism	↓ or normal	↓	↓ or normal

- Knowledge of HPT axis physiology, the factors governing thyroid
  hormone action at a tissue/cellular level, and the different patterns
  of TFTs that may be encountered in clinical practice is central to
  establishing the correct diagnosis when clinical features and TFT results
  appear discordant/incongruous.
- Reappraisal of the clinical context and exclusion of confounding
  intercurrent illness or medication usage, coupled with reassessment of
  thyroid status, are the 1st step to resolving such cases.
- Targeted investigation to definitively exclude assay interference may
  require specialist laboratory input. It may be helpful to send specimens
  to different labs to use a different assay.

Table 1.4 Influence of drugs on thyroid function tests

Metabolic process	↑	↓
TSH secretion	Amiodarone (transiently; becomes normal after 2–3 months), sertraline, St John's wort (*Hypericum*)	GCs, dopamine agonists, phenytoin, dopamine, octreotide, paroxetine
T_4 synthesis/release	Iodide, amiodarone, interferon alfa, lithium	Iodide, amiodarone, interferon alfa, lithium, tyrosine kinase inhibitors (TKIs)
Binding proteins	Oestrogen, clofibrate, heroin	GCs, androgens, phenytoin, carbamazepine
T_4 metabolism	Anticonvulsants, rifampicin	
T_4/T_3 binding in serum	Heparin	Salicylates, furosemide, mefenamic acid

Table 1.5 Atypical thyroid function tests

Test	Possible cause
Suppressed TSH and normal FT_4	T_3 toxicosis (~5% of thyrotoxicosis)
Suppressed TSH and normal FT_4 and free T_3 (FT_3)	Subclinical hyperthyroidism Recovery from thyrotoxicosis Excess thyroxine replacement NTI
Detectable TSH and elevated FT_4 and FT_3	TSH-secreting pituitary tumour Thyroid hormone resistance Heterophile antibodies, leading to spurious measurements of FT_4 and FT_3 Thyroxine replacement therapy (including poor compliance)
Elevated FT_4 and FT_3, and suppressed TSH	Biotin
Elevated FT_4 and low-normal FT_3, normal TSH	Amiodarone
Elevated free T_4 and T_3	Heparin
Suppressed or normal TSH, and low-normal FT_4 and FT_3	NTI Central hypothyroidism Isolated TSH deficiency

- Genetic and acquired disorders of the HPT axis are rare but should be considered if all other steps have failed to identify a cause for anomalous/discordant TFTs.
- Ingestion of 5–10 mg of biotin can cause spurious results in thyroid test assays.[1] Biotin will cause falsely ↓ values in immunometric assays used to measure TSH, and falsely ↑ values in competitive binding assays used to measure T_4, T_3, and TRAbs. These biochemical findings suggest a diagnosis of Graves' disease; however, discontinuation of biotin supplements results in resolution of the biochemical abnormalities. Thyroid tests should be repeated at least 2 days after discontinuation of biotin supplements.
- In heparin-treated subjects, serum non-esterified fatty acid (NEFA) concentrations may increase markedly as a consequence of heparin-induced activation of endothelial lipoprotein lipase *in vivo*, leading to increased NEFA generation *in vitro* during sample storage or incubation. In the presence of normal serum albumin concentrations, NEFA concentrations >2–3mmol/L exceed normal serum binding capacity, resulting in direct competition for T_4 and T_3 binding sites on TBG either by NEFAs themselves or as a result of displacement of other ligands from the albumin sites that normally limit their free concentration. This artefact is more pronounced in hypertriglyceridaemia and hypoalbuminaemia, and with laboratory methods that require long incubation periods. Even very low-dose intravenous (IV) heparin (equivalent to that used to maintain the patency of an indwelling cannula) and subcutaneous (SC) low-molecular weight heparin (LMWH) prophylaxis can lead to ↑ FT_4 (and FT_3). The heparin effect has been observed with a variety of assay platforms, including equilibrium dialysis, ultracentrifugation, and direct immunoassay.

References

1. Kummer S, et al. (2016). Biotin treatment mimicking Graves' disease. *N Engl J Med* **375**, 704–6.

Further reading

Cambridge Addenbrooke's Hospital Endocrine Laboratory. Service Supra-Regional Assay Service. ℘ http://www.sas-centre.org/centres/hormones/Cambridge/html

Koulouri O, et al. (2013). Pitfalls in the measurement and interpretation of thyroid function tests. *Best Pract Res Clin Endocrinol Metab* **27**, 745–62.

Rare genetic disorders of thyroid hormone metabolism

- RTH is caused by heterozygous mutations in *TR*β (see Box 1.1).

> ### Box 1.1 Thyroid hormone resistance (RTH)
> - Rare syndrome (incidence 1:40,000) characterized by reduced responsiveness to elevated circulating levels of FT_4 and FT_3, non-suppressed serum TSH, and intact TSH responsiveness to TRH.
> - Clinical features, apart from goitre, are usually absent but may include short stature, hyperactivity, attention deficits, learning disability, and goitre.
> - Associated with *TR*β gene defects, and identification by gene sequencing can confirm diagnosis in 80–85%.
> - Differential diagnosis includes TSH-secreting pituitary tumour (see ➜ Thyrotrophinomas, pp. 200–1).
> - Most cases require no treatment. If needed, it is usually β-adrenergic blockers to ameliorate some of the tissue effects of raised thyroid hormone levels.

- Inactivating mutations in *TR*α have now been identified which are associated with growth retardation, macrocephaly, delayed closure of fontanel, delayed motor and mental milestones in childhood, constipation, mild normocytic anaemia, and excessive skin tags in adulthood. TFTs may show normal TSH with normal/↓ FT_4, ↑ FT_3, and ↓ rT_3 levels. Beneficial effects of levothyroxine have been described.[1]
- Allan–Herndon–Dudley syndrome is an X-linked disorder of childhood onset with psychomotor retardation, including speech and developmental delay and spastic quadriplegia, caused by defects in the *MCT8* (*SLC16A2*) gene encoding a membrane transporter. In addition to neurological abnormalities, ♂ patients have ↑ FT_3, ↓ FT_4, and normal TSH levels. Triac, a T_3 analogue, has been shown to be of clinical benefit.
- The deiodinase enzymes are part of a larger family of 25 human proteins containing selenocysteine. A multisystem selenoprotein deficiency disorder has been identified, manifested by growth retardation in childhood and ♂ infertility, skeletal myopathy, photosensitivity, and hearing loss in adults. TFTs show ↑ FT_4, normal/↓ FT_3, and normal TSH levels due to functional D2 deficiencies.

References

1. Moran C, Chatterjee K (2015). Resistance to thyroid hormone due to defective thyroid receptor alpha. *Best Pract Res Clin Endocrinol Metab* **29**, 647–57.

Antibody screen

Raised serum concentrations of thyroid antibodies (antithyroid peroxidase (microsomal) (TPOAb) and anti-thyroglobulin (TgAb)) correlate with the presence of focal thyroiditis in thyroid tissue obtained by biopsy and at autopsy from patients with no evidence of hypothyroidism during life. Early postmortem studies confirmed histological evidence of chronic autoimmune thyroiditis in 27% of adult ♀, with a rise in frequency over 50 years, and 7% of adult ♂, and diffuse changes in 5% of ♀ and 1% of ♂. Patients with hypothyroidism caused by either atrophic or goitrous autoimmune thyroiditis usually have high serum concentrations of these same antibodies. These antibodies also are often detected in serum of patients with Graves' disease and other thyroid diseases, but the concentrations are usually lower. There is considerable variation in the frequency and distribution of antithyroid antibodies because of variations in techniques of detection, definition of abnormal titres, and inherent differences in the populations tested.

A significant proportion of subjects in the community have asymptomatic chronic autoimmune thyroiditis of whom a substantial proportion have subclinical hypothyroidism. The percentage of subjects with high serum TPOAb and TgAb concentrations increase with age in both ♂ and ♀, and high concentrations were more prevalent in ♀ than in ♂, and less prevalent in blacks than in other ethnic groups. A hypoechoic ultrasound (US) pattern may precede TPOAb positivity in autoimmune thyroid disease (AITD), and TPOAb may not be detected in >20% of individuals with US evidence of thyroid autoimmunity (see Table 1.6).

Table 1.6 Antithyroid antibodies and thyroid disease

Condition	Anti-TPO	Anti-Tg	TRAb
Graves' disease	70–80%	30–50%	70–100% (stimulating)
Autoimmune hypothyroidism	95%	60%	10–20% (blocking)

NB. TRAbs may be stimulatory or inhibitory. Heterophile antibodies present in patient sera may cause abnormal interference, causing abnormally low or high values of FT_4 and FT_3, and can be removed with absorption tubes.

Screening for thyroid disease

Controversy exists as to whether healthy adults living in an area of iodine sufficiency benefit from screening for thyroid disease (see Box 1.2). The benefit from a screening programme must outweigh the physical and psychological harm caused by the test, diagnostic procedures, and treatment. The prevalence of unsuspected overt thyroid disease is low, but a substantial proportion of subjects tested will have evidence of thyroid dysfunction, with ~10% with subclinical hypothyroidism and 1% with subclinical hyperthyroidism. No appropriately powered prospective, randomized controlled, double-blinded interventional trial of either levothyroxine therapy for subclinical hypothyroidism or antithyroid therapy for subclinical hyperthyroidism exists.[1,2]

Box 1.2 Recommendations for screening for thyroid dysfunction in an iodine-replete community

- Screening in ♀ <50 and in ♂ is not warranted in view of the relatively low point prevalence of unsuspected overt thyroid dysfunction.
- Case finding in ♀ during menopause or during visits to a 1° care physician with non-specific symptoms is justified due to the high prevalence of subclinical hypothyroidism.
- If ↑ serum TSH is found at screening, then measurement should be repeated 2 months later, together with FT_4 measurement, after excluding NTI, drugs, etc.
- Treatment with levothyroxine is recommended if serum TSH is >10mU/L, irrespective of whether FT_4 is low.
- Subjects with serum TSH between 5 and 10mU/L and normal FT_4 are at ↑ risk of developing hypothyroidism, and repeat measurement of serum TSH is warranted at least every 3 years, if not annually.
- If suppressed serum TSH is found at screening, it should be remeasured 2 months later, and if it is still suppressed, FT_3 should be measured.
- After levothyroxine replacement is initiated, for whatever indication, long-term follow-up with at least an annual measurement of serum TSH is required.

The following categories of patients should be screened for thyroid disease:

- The value of screening for congenital hypothyroidism in heel-prick blood specimens is unquestioned (1:2000 newborns).
- There is no consensus on whether healthy pregnant ♀ should be screened for thyroid disorders or post-partum thyroiditis, although it has been shown to be cost-effective in analytical models.
- Patients with a goitre, atrial fibrillation, and hyperlipidaemia. Subfertility and osteoporosis.
- Annual review of people with diabetes mellitus (DM) appears cost-effective.

- ♀ with type 1 diabetes mellitus (T1DM) in the 1st trimester of pregnancy and post-delivery (because of 3-fold increase in incidence of post-partum thyroid dysfunction in such patients) (see ➡ Post-partum thyroid dysfunction, p. 477).[3,4,5]
- Periodic (6-monthly) assessments in patients receiving amiodarone, lithium, and interferon-alfa, and within 3 months of initiation of immune checkpoint inhibitor therapy.
- ♀ with past history of post-partum thyroiditis.
- Annual check of thyroid function in people with Down's syndrome, Turner syndrome, and autoimmune Addison's disease[6] and following head and neck irradiation, in view of the high prevalence of hypothyroidism in such patients.
- All patients with hyperthyroidism who receive ablative treatment should be followed indefinitely for the development of hypothyroidism beginning 4–8 weeks after treatment, and then at 3-monthly intervals for 1 year and annually thereafter.
- Among patients hospitalized for acute illness, testing should be limited, but with a high index of clinical suspicion and with an awareness of the difficulties in interpreting TFTs in the presence of acute illness.
- ♀ with thyroid autoantibodies—8× risk of developing hypothyroidism over 20 years, compared to antibody −ve controls.
- ♀ with thyroid autoantibodies and isolated elevated TSH—38× risk of developing hypothyroidism, with 4% annual risk of overt hypothyroidism.
- Maternal thyroid antibodies are associated with recurrent miscarriage and preterm birth.[4] Levothyroxine in euthyroid ♀ with TPOAbs did not increase the rate of live births.[7]

References

1. Taylor PN, et al. (2010). Global epidemiology of hyperthyroidism and hypothyroidism. Nat Rev Endocrinol **14**, 301–16.
2. Rugge JB, et al. (2015). Screening and treatment of thyroid dysfunction: an evidence review for the U.S. Preventive services task force. Ann Intern Med **162**, 35–45.
3. Biondi B, et al. (2019). Thyroid dysfunction and diabetes mellitus: two closely associated disorders. Endocr Rev **40**, 789–824.
4. De Leo S, Pearce EN (2018). Autoimmune thyroid disease during pregnancy. Lancet Diabetes Endocrinol **6**, 575–86.
5. Dosiou C, et al. (2012). Cost-effectiveness of universal and risk-based screening for autoimmune thyroid disease in pregnant women. J Clin Endocrinol Metab **97**, 1536–46.
6. Fallahi P, et al. (2016). The association of other autoimmune diseases in patients with autoimmune thyroiditis: review of the literature and report of a large series of patients. Autoimmun Rev **15**, 1125–8.
7. Dhillon-Smith RK, et al. (2019). Levothyroxine in women with thyroid peroxidase antibodies before conception. N Engl J Med **380**, 1316–25.

Scintiscanning

Permits localization of sites of accumulation of radioiodine or sodium pertechnetate (^{99m}Tc), which gives information about the activity of the iodine trap by the NIS.

- After IV pertechnetate, imaging and uptake measurements are obtained within 10–20 minutes, rather than hours or days, as is the case with radioiodine. The percentage uptake is usually in the range of 1.5–3.5%.
- Oral ^{123}I has a clinically useful half-life of 13 hours and can be used in routine diagnostic scans or whole-body scans (WBS) at 24–48 hours with high-quality images at low radiation dose, providing quantitative information in imaging residual thyroid and functioning metastases after thyroidectomy in thyroid cancer.
- Oral ^{131}I, with a half-life of 8 days, is used for WBS 5–10 days post-therapeutic ^{131}I but provides lower-quality imaging and has a higher dose of radiation.

Thyroid isotope imaging can be used:

- To define areas of ↑ or ↓ function within the thyroid (see Table 1.7), which occasionally helps in cases of uncertainty as to the cause of the thyrotoxicosis.
- To distinguish between Graves' disease and thyroiditis (autoimmune or viral—de Quervain's thyroiditis).
- To detect retrosternal goitre.
- To detect ectopic thyroid tissue.

Factors that can alter thyroid imaging

- Agents which influence thyroid uptake, including intake of high-iodine foods and supplements such as kelp (seaweed).
- Drugs containing iodine such as amiodarone.
- Recent use of radiographic contrast dyes that can potentially interfere with the interpretation of the scan.

Table 1.7 Radionuclide scanning (scintigram) in thyroid disease

Condition	Scan appearance
Graves' hyperthyroidism	Enlarged gland
	Homogeneous radionucleotide uptake
Thyroiditis (e.g. de Quervain's or autoimmune)	Low or absent uptake
Toxic nodule	A solitary area of high uptake
Thyrotoxicosis factitia	Depressed thyroid uptake
Thyroid cancer	Successful ^{131}I uptake by tumour tissue requires an adequate level of TSH, achieved by giving recombinant TSH injection or stopping T_3 replacement 10 days before scanning

Ultrasound scanning

Provides an accurate indication of thyroid size and assesses if focal or diffuse thyroid disease.

- US is useful for differentiating cystic nodules from solid ones, whether a nodule is solitary or part of a multinodular process, and sequential scanning can assess changes in size over time. It is not routinely indicated in a patient with a goitre.
- In Hashimoto's thyroiditis and Graves' disease, the lymphocytic infiltration and damage to tissue architecture result in a variable decrease in echogenicity.
- Colour Doppler imaging shows ↑ blood flow in Graves' disease, while in Hashimoto's thyroiditis, vascularization may be either moderately ↑ or nearly completely absent.
- de Quervain's thyroiditis is characterized by multiple ill-defined hypoechoic areas.
- US is useful for differentiating cystic nodules from solid ones, whether a nodule is solitary or part of a multinodular process, and sequential scanning can assess changes in size over time. It is not routinely indicated in a patient with a goitre.

When performed by an experienced sonographer, it can be used to distinguish between benign and malignant disease. A few well-defined ultrasonographic prognostic finding are recognized:[1,2]

- Benign lesion: simple cyst (fluid collection with thin, regular margins), spongiform nodule, and mostly cystic nodule (>80%) containing colloid fluid (comet tail signs) with regular margins devoid of vascular signals.
- Suspicious for thyroid cancer: hypoechoic, microcalcifications (<2mm in diameter are observed in ~60% of malignant nodules, but in <2% of benign lesions), irregular margins, central vascularity, taller-than-wide shape, incomplete halo, extension beyond capsule, and suspicious lymphadenopathy.
- Calcification is a prominent feature of medullary carcinoma of the thyroid.
- Elastographic stiffness is reported to have a high sensitivity for malignancy with a negative predictive value.
- Radiologists should use US classification (U1, normal; U2, benign; U3, indeterminate/equivocal; U4, suspicious; and U5, malignant) for the prediction of malignancy which helps to determine whether a fine needle aspiration (FNA) biopsy should be performed.[1]

Thyroid imaging, reporting, and data system (TI-RADS)

(See Fig. 1.4.)

References

1. Perros P, et al. (2014). Guidelines for the management of thyroid cancer. *Clin Endocrinol* **81**(Suppl 1), 1–122.
2. Haugen BR, et al. (2016). 2015 American Thyroid Association Management Guidelines for adult patients with thyroid nodules and differentiated thyroid cancer. *Thyroid* **26**, 1–133.

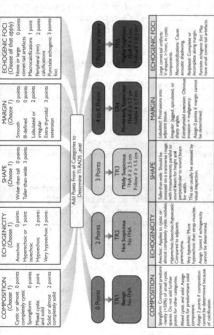

Fig. 1.4 Chart showing five categories on the basis of the American College of Radiology thyroid imaging, reporting, and data system (TI-RADS) lexicon, TR levels, and criteria for FNA or follow-up US. Explanatory notes appear at the bottom. TI-RADS recommendation:

0 points = TR1: benign, no FNA required.

2 points = TR2: non-suspicious, no FNA required.

3 points = TR3: mildly suspicious, FNA if ≥2.5cm, follow if ≥1.5cm at 1, 3, and 5 years.

4–6 points = TR4: moderately suspicious, FNA if ≥1.5cm, follow if >1cm at 1, 2, 3, and 5 years.

≥7 points = TR5: highly suspicious, FNA if ≥1cm, follow if ≥0.5cm annually for 5 years.

Reprinted from Tessler et al. ACR thyroid imaging, Reporting and Data System (TI-RADS): White paper of the ACR TI-RADS committee. J Am Coll Radiol 2017, with permission from Elsevier.

Fine needle aspiration cytology

- US-guided fine needle aspiration cytology (FNAC) is a valuable and cost-effective preoperative investigation for thyroid nodules (see Table 1.8). The results can reassure that a nodule is benign, triage patients for diagnostic surgery, or provide a definite diagnosis of some thyroid malignancies, enabling one-stage therapeutic surgery.
- It is performed in an outpatient setting. One to two aspirations are carried out at different sites for each suspicious nodule. Cytologic findings are *satisfactory* or *diagnostic* in ~85% of specimens and *non-diagnostic* in the remainder.
- Drawbacks of FNAC include the rates of inadequate/unsatisfactory samples; inability to distinguish between non-neoplastic, benign, and malignant follicular lesions; and difficulty in detecting follicular variant of papillary thyroid carcinoma.
- US appearances that are indicative of a benign nodule (U1–U2) should be regarded as reassuring, not requiring FNAC unless the patient has a statistically high risk of malignancy.
- Non-palpable nodules (discovered incidentally during other imaging procedures) have the same risk of malignancy as palpable nodules of similar size. US-guided FNAC can be performed for non-palpable nodules and nodules that are technically difficult to aspirate using palpation methods alone such as predominantly cystic or posteriorly located nodules. In patients with large nodules (>4cm), US-guided FNAC directed at several areas within the nodule may reduce the risk of a false −ve biopsy.
- It is impossible to differentiate between benign and malignant follicular neoplasm using FNAC. Therefore, surgical excision of a follicular neoplasm is usually indicated (see ➔ Follicular thyroid carcinoma, p. 112).
- An FNAC which initially yields benign cytology (Thy2) should be repeated if there is any clinical suspicion of malignancy and/or when the US is indeterminate or suspicious.
- There is a false −ve rate for benign (Thy2) cytology results (usually <3%).
- Malignancy can also be found in nodules with Thy1 cytology (up to 5%), especially if the lesion is cystic.
- When there is clinical suspicion of malignancy and/or indeterminate or suspicious US features, and an unsatisfactory FNAC (Thy1) is obtained, repeat FNAC is mandatory.
- When there is discordance between the level of clinical suspicion, FNAC, or US appearances, management should be discussed in the thyroid cancer multidisciplinary team (MDT).
- The Thy numerical diagnostic categories should be used, in addition to a full text report (see Table 1.9).
- In selected cases, and in an MDT context, molecular testing of FNAC material may be helpful in deciding whether diagnostic or therapeutic surgery should be undertaken.
- Use of BRAF, RAS, RET/PTC, and PAX8/PPARγ testing[1] shows promise in the diagnosis and treatment of patients with nodular thyroid disease and thyroid cancer. Experience remains limited and no test has perfect sensitivity and specificity, and there remain limitations in the data supporting their routine use.[1,2]

Table 1.8 Diagnostic features of FNAC

Feature	Range (%)	Mean value (%)
Accuracy	85–100	95
Specificity	72–100	92
Sensitivity	65–98	83
False −ve	1–11	5

Table 1.9 Diagnostic categories from FNAC

Category		Action
Thy1	Non-diagnostic. Insufficient epithelial cells	US assessment ± repeat sampling.
Thy1c	Cyst fluid with insufficient colloid and epithelial cells	Correlate with clinical and US findings
Thy2	Non-neoplastic	Correlate with clinical and US findings
Thy3a	Atypical features present, but not enough to place into any of the other categories	Further US ± repeat FNAC. Discussion at thyroid cancer MDT
Thy3f	Suspected follicular neoplasm. Histological possibilities include a hyperplastic nodule, follicular adenoma or follicular carcinoma, and follicular variant of papillary carcinoma	Diagnostic hemithyroidectomy, with completion thyroidectomy if malignant (10–40% risk of malignancy in Thy3 nodules)
Thy4	Suspicious of malignancy, e.g. papillary, medullary, or anaplastic carcinoma/ lymphoma	Diagnostic hemithyroidectomy (70% risk of malignancy)
Thy5	Diagnosis of malignancy	Surgical excision for differentiated thyroid cancer (>98% risk of malignancy). Radiotherapy/chemotherapy for anaplastic thyroid cancer, lymphoma/metastases

References

1. Xing M, et al. (2013). Progress in molecular-based management of differentiated thyroid cancer. *Lancet* **381**, 1058–69.
2. Nikiforov YE (2017). Role of molecular markers in thyroid nodule management: then and now. *Endocr Pract* **23**, 979–88.

Computed tomography

- Computed tomography (CT) is useful in the evaluation of retrosternal and retrotracheal extension of an enlarged thyroid.
- Compression of the trachea and displacement of the major vessels can be identified with CT of the superior mediastinum.
- It can demonstrate the extent of intrathoracic extension of thyroid malignancy and infiltration of adjacent structures such as the carotid artery, internal jugular vein, trachea, oesophagus, and regional lymph nodes.

Further reading

Kim DW, Jung SJ, Baek HJ (2015). Computed tomography features of benign and malignant solid thyroid nodules. *Acta Radiol* **56**, 1196–202.

Positron emission tomography

- Up to 20% of thyroid incidentalomas found on positron emission tomography (PET) scans may be malignant and usually require US-guided FNAC. However, overall survival may be poor because of the prognosis associated with underlying malignancy, which must be considered before investigation and certainly before aggressive treatment. Active surveillance can be considered in this group of patients.[1,2]
- ^{18}F-fluorodeoxyglucose (FDG)-PET/CT is a useful technique for imaging dedifferentiation of metastatic thyroid cancer and is also valuable for risk stratification and prediction of survival in high-risk thyroid cancer patients.
- Recurrent thyroid cancer that is FDG avid-positive on FDG PET scanning is unlikely to respond to even high-dose radioiodine therapy.
- [124]I PET/CT is more sensitive in detecting metastatic thyroid cancer than γ camera imaging with [131]I.

References

1. Abdel-Halim CN, *et al.* (2019). Risk of malignancy in FDG-avid thyroid incidentalomas on PET/CT: a prospective study. *World J Surg* **43**, 2454–8.
2. Chung SR, *et al.* (2018). Thyroid incidentalomas detected on 18F-fluorideoxyglucose positron emission tomography with computed tomography: malignant risk stratification and management plan. *Thyroid* **28**, 762–8.

Further reading

Pattison DA, *et al.* (2018). 18F-FDG-avid thyroid incidentalomas: the importance of contextual interpretation. *J Nucl Med* **59**, 749–55.
Russ G, *et al.* (2014). Thyroid incidentalomas: epidemiology, risk stratification with ultrasound and workup. *Eur Thyroid J* **3**, 154–63.

Additional laboratory investigations

Haematological tests

- Long-standing thyrotoxicosis may be associated with *normochromic anaemia*, and occasionally *mild neutropenia* and *lymphocytosis*, and rarely *thrombocytopenia*.
- In hypothyroidism, a macrocytosis is typical, although concurrent vitamin B12 deficiency should be considered.
- There may also be a *microcytic anaemia* due to menorrhagia and impaired iron utilization.

Biochemical tests

- *Alkaline phosphatase* (ALP) may be elevated in thyrotoxicosis.
- Mild *hypercalcaemia* occasionally occurs in thyrotoxicosis and reflects ↑ bone resorption. *Hypercalciuria* is commoner.
- In a hypothyroid patient, *hyponatraemia* may be due to reduced renal tubular water loss or, less commonly, due to coexisting cortisol deficiency.
- In hypothyroidism, *creatinine* kinase is often raised and the lipid profile altered with ↑ low-density lipoprotein cholesterol (LDL-C).

Endocrine tests

- In untreated hypothyroidism, there may be inadequate responses to provocative testing of the hypothalamic–pituitary–adrenal (HPA) axis.
- In hypothyroidism, serum prolactin (PRL) may be elevated because ↑ TRH leads to ↑ PRL secretion (may be partly responsible for ↓ fertility in young women with hypothyroidism).
- In thyrotoxicosis, there is an increase in sex *hormone-binding globulin* (SHBG) and a complex interaction with sex steroid hormone metabolism, resulting in changes in levels of androgens and oestrogens. The net physiological result is an increase in *oestrogenic* activity, with *gynaecomastia* and a decrease in libido in ♂ presenting with thyrotoxicosis.

Non-thyroidal illness (sick euthyroid syndrome)

- Multiple mechanisms have been identified to contribute to the development of sick euthyroid syndrome, including alterations in iodothyronine deiodinases, TSH secretion, thyroid hormone binding to plasma protein, transport of thyroid hormone in peripheral tissues, and TRr activity.
- Sick euthyroid syndrome appears to be a complex mix of physiologic adaptation and pathologic response to acute illness. The underlying cause for these alterations has not yet been elucidated.
- Biochemistry:
  - $\downarrow T_4$ and T_3.
  - Inappropriately normal/$\downarrow$ TSH.
- Tissue thyroid hormone concentrations are very low.
- Context—starvation.
  - Severe illness, e.g. ITU, severe infections, renal failure, cardiac failure, liver failure, end-stage malignancy.
- Treatment of euthyroid sick syndrome with thyroid hormone to restore normal serum thyroid hormone levels in an effort to improve disease prognosis and outcomes continues to be a focus of many clinical studies
- However, thyroxine replacement is not indicated because there is no evidence that treatment provides benefit or is safe.
- Pitfalls with TFTs in NTI are shown in Box 1.3.

> **Box 1.3 Pitfalls with thyroid function tests in non-thyroidal illness**
>
> - TSH suppressed in hospitalized patients with acute illness.
> - Dopamine and steroids may suppress TSH, e.g. in critically ill patients.
> - TSH increase during recovery from acute illness.
> - TSH may fall during 1st trimester of pregnancy (human chorionic gonadotrophin (hCG)).
> - TSH inhibited by SC octreotide.
> - Anorexia nervosa is associated with low TSH and FT_4.
> - Heterophilic antibodies, including rheumatoid factor, may falsely elevate TSH.
> - Adrenal insufficiency (AI) may be associated with raised TSH which reverses on treatment with GCs.
> - Heparin leads to $\uparrow FT_4$ and no change in TSH.

Further reading

Fliers E, et al. (2015). Thyroid function in critically ill patients. *Lancet Diabetes Endocrinol* **3**, 816–25.
Lee S, Farwell AP (2016). Euthyroid sick syndrome. *Compr Physiol* **15**, 1071–80.

Atypical clinical situations

- *Thyrotoxicosis factitia* (usually unprescribed intake of exogenous thyroid hormone in non-thyroid disease):
  - No thyroid enlargement.
  - ↑ FT$_4$ and suppressed TSH.
  - Depressed thyroid uptake on scintigraphy.
  - ↓ Tg differentiates from thyroiditis (which shows depressed uptake on scintigraphy, but ↑ Tg) and all other causes of elevated thyroid hormones.
- *Struma ovarii* (ovarian teratoma containing hyperfunctioning thyroid tissue):
  - No thyroid enlargement.
  - Depressed thyroid uptake on scintigraphy.
  - Body scan after radioiodine confirms diagnosis.
- *Trophoblast tumours.* hCG has structural homology with TSH and leads to thyroid gland stimulation and usually mild thyrotoxicosis.
- *Hyperemesis gravidarum.* TFTs may be abnormal with suppressed TSH (see ➲ Thyrotoxicosis in pregnancy, pp. 50–4).
- *Choriocarcinoma of the testes* may be associated with gynaecomastia and thyrotoxicosis—measure hCG.

Thyrotoxicosis—aetiology

Epidemiology

- Ten times commoner in ♀ than in ♂ in the UK.
- Prevalence is ~2% of the ♀ population.
- Annual incidence is three cases per 1000 ♀.

Definition of thyrotoxicosis and hyperthyroidism

- The term *thyrotoxicosis* denotes the clinical, physiological, and biochemical findings that result when the tissues are exposed to excess thyroid hormone. It can arise in a variety of ways (see Table 1.10). It is essential to establish a specific diagnosis, as this determines therapy choices and provides important information for the patient regarding prognosis.
- The term *hyperthyroidism* should be used to denote only those conditions in which hyperfunction of the thyroid leads to thyrotoxicosis.

Genetics of autoimmune thyroid disease[1]

- AITD consists of Graves' disease, Hashimoto's thyroiditis, atrophic autoimmune hypothyroidism, post-partum thyroiditis, and Graves' orbitopathy (GO) that appear to share a common genetic predisposition.
- There is a ♂ preponderance, and sex steroids appear to play an important role.
- Twin studies show ↑ concordance (20–40%) for Graves' disease and autoimmune hypothyroidism in monozygotic, compared to dizygotic, twins.
- It is estimated that genetic factors account for ~70% of the susceptibility for Graves' disease.
- Sibling studies indicate that sisters and children of ♂ with Graves' disease have a 5–8% risk of developing Graves' disease or autoimmune hypothyroidism.
- On the background of a genetic predisposition, environmental factors are thought to contribute to the development of disease.
- A number of interacting susceptibility genes are thought to play a role in the development of disease—a complex genetic trait. Data emphasize the complex nature of genetic susceptibility and the likely interplay of environmental factors.
- *CTLA-4* (cytotoxic T lymphocyte antigen-4) is associated with Graves' disease in Caucasian populations. In particular, the CT60 allele has a prevalence of 60% in the general population but is also the allele most highly associated with Graves' disease.
- Association of major histocompatibility complex (MHC) loci with Graves' disease has been demonstrated in some populations, but not in others. HLA DR3 is associated with Graves' disease in whites. HLA-DQA1*0501 is associated in some populations, especially for men. However, the overall contribution of *MHC* genes to Graves' disease has been estimated to be only 10–20% of the inherited susceptibility.
- There is evidence of ↑ risks associated with polymorphisms of intron 1 in the TSH receptor gene and the Tg gene.

Table 1.10 Classification of the aetiology of thyrotoxicosis

Associated with hyperthyroidism	
Excessive thyroid stimulation	Graves's disease, Hashitoxicosis
	Pituitary thyrotroph adenoma
	Pituitary thyroid hormone resistance syndrome (excess TSH) (see ➜ Secondary hyperthyroidism, pp. 58–9)
	Trophoblastic tumours producing hCG with thyrotrophic activity
Thyroid nodules with autonomous function	Toxic solitary nodule, toxic multinodular goitre
	Very rarely, thyroid cancer

Not associated with hyperthyroidism	
Thyroid inflammation	Silent and post-partum thyroiditis, subacute (de Quervain's) thyroiditis
	Drug-induced thyroiditis (amiodarone, interferon-alfa, lithium, TKIs, immunotherapy)
Exogenous thyroid hormones	Overtreatment with thyroid hormone
	Thyrotoxicosis factitia (thyroxine use in non-thyroidal disease)
Ectopic thyroid tissue	Metastatic thyroid carcinoma
	Struma ovarii (teratoma containing functional thyroid tissue)

Thyrotoxicosis in COVID-19

Early studies[2] have shown preliminary evidence that coronavirus disease (COVID-19) may affect thyroid function, or severe acute respiratory syndrome coronavirus 2 (SARS-CoV-2) may act directly on thyroid cells. Data suggest a high risk of thyrotoxicosis in parallel with the systemic immune reaction induced by infection.

References

1. Brix TH, Hegedüs L (2011). Twins as a tool for evaluating the influence of genetic susceptibility in thyroid autoimmunity. *Ann Endocrinol (Paris)* **72**, 103–7.
2. Lania A, et al. (2020). Thyrotoxicosis in patients with COVID-19: the THYRCOV study. *Eur J Endocrinol* **183**, 381–7.

Further reading

Marino M, et al. (2015). Role of genetic and non-genetic factors in the etiology of Graves' disease. *J Endocrinol Invest* **38**, 283–94.

Manifestations of hyperthyroidism

(See Box 1.4.)

Box 1.4 Manifestations of hyperthyroidism (all forms)

Symptoms
- Hyperactivity, irritability, altered mood, insomnia.
- Heat intolerance, ↑ sweating.
- Palpitations.
- Fatigue, weakness.
- Dyspnoea.
- Weight loss with ↑ appetite (weight gain in 10% of patients).
- Pruritus.
- ↑ stool frequency.
- Thirst and polyuria.
- Oligomenorrhoea or amenorrhoea, loss of libido, erectile dysfunction (50% of men may have sexual dysfunction).

Signs
- Sinus tachycardia, atrial fibrillation.
- Fine tremor, hyperkinesia, hyperreflexia.
- Warm, moist skin.
- Palmar erythema, onycholysis.
- Hair loss.
- Muscle weakness and wasting.
- Congestive (high-output) heart failure, chorea, periodic paralysis (primarily in Asian ♂), psychosis (rare).

Investigation of thyrotoxicosis

(See Table 1.11.)
- TFTs—↑ FT_4 and suppressed TSH (↑ FT_3 in T_3 toxicosis).
  - TRAbs[1] (see Table 1.6). The 2nd- and 3rd-generation TRAb assays have >95% sensitivity and specificity for the diagnosis of Graves' disease and have improved the utility of TRAb to predict relapse. TRAb levels decline with antithyroid drug (ATD) therapy and after thyroidectomy. Levels increase for a year following radioiodine therapy, with a gradual fall thereafter. TRAb ≥5IU/L in pregnant ♀ with current or previously treated Graves' disease is associated with ↑ risk of fetal and neonatal thyrotoxicosis, and hence close monitoring is needed. TRAb levels parallel the course of GO, and elevated TRAb is an indication for steroid prophylaxis to prevent progression of orbitopathy with radioiodine therapy.
  - Radionucleotide thyroid scan if diagnosis uncertain (see ➔ Ultrasound scanning, p. 20), but now seldom required, unless radioiodine is planned.

Manifestations of Graves' disease[2,3,4]

(In addition to those in Box 1.4)
- Diffuse goitre with bruit.
- Orbitopathy (see ➔ Graves' orbitopathy, pp. 60–2).
  - A feeling of grittiness and discomfort in the eye.
  - Retrobulbar pressure or pain, eyelid lag or retraction.

- Periorbital oedema, chemosis,>Combination scleral injection.*
- Exophthalmos (proptosis).*
- Extraocular muscle dysfunction.*
- Exposure keratitis.*
- Optic neuropathy.*
- Localized dermopathy (pretibial myxoedema; see ➔ Graves' dermopathy, p. 68).
- Lymphoid hyperplasia.
- Thyroid acropachy (see ➔ Thyroid acropachy, p. 68).

Table 1.11 Tests which help to differentiate different causes of thyrotoxicosis

Cause	Thyroid iodine uptake	TPO antibodies	TRAbs	Tg
Graves' disease	↑	Usually +ve	+	↑
Toxic nodular goitre	↑	−	−	↑
TSH-secreting pituitary adenoma	↑	−	−	↑
Hyperemesis gravidarum	↑	−	−	↑
Trophoblastic tumour	↑	−	−	↑
de Quervain's thyroiditis	↓	−	−	↑
Drugs, e.g. amiodarone	↓	Usually −ve	−	↑
Struma ovarii	↓	−	−	↑
Thyrotoxicosis factitia	↓	−	−	↓

Conditions associated with Graves' disease[5]

- T1DM.
- Addison's disease.
- Vitiligo.
- Pernicious anaemia.
- Alopecia areata.
- Myasthenia gravis.
- Coeliac disease (4.5%).
- Other autoimmune disorders associated with the HLA-DR3 haplotype.

References

1. Hesarghatta Shyamasunder A, Abraham P (2017). Measuring TSH receptor antibody to influence treatment choices in Graves' disease. *Clin Endocrinol (Oxf)* **86**, 652–7.
2. Gilbert J (2017). Thyrotoxicosis: investigation and management. *Clin Med (Lond)* **17**, 274–7.
3. De Leo S, et al. (2016). Hyperthyroidism. *Lancet* **388**, 906–18.
4. Burch HB, Cooper DS (2015). Management of Graves' disease: a review. *JAMA* **314**, 2544–54.
5. Ferrari SM, et al. (2019). The association of other autoimmune diseases in patients with Graves' disease (with or without ophthalmopathy): review of the literature and report of a large series. *Autoimmun Rev* **18**, 287–92.

* Combination of these suggests congestive ophthalmopathy. Urgent action necessary if: corneal ulceration, congestive ophthalmopathy, or optic neuropathy (see ➔ Graves' orbitopathy, pp. 60–2).

Medical treatment

In general, the standard policy in Europe is to offer a course of ATD first. However, recent National Institute for Health and Care Excellence (NICE) guidance has recommended early consideration of radioactive iodine (RAI) (% https://cks.nice.org.uk/topics/hyperthyroidism/).

In the United States (USA), radioiodine is more likely to be offered as 1st-line treatment. Regardless of the method of treatment, early and effective control of hyperthyroidism among patients with Graves' disease is associated with improved survival, compared with less effective control. Rapid and sustained control of hyperthyroidism should be prioritized in the management of Graves' disease, and early definitive treatment with radioiodine should be offered to patients who are unlikely to achieve remission with ATD alone.

Aims and principles of medical treatment

- To induce remission in Graves' disease.
- Monitor for relapse off treatment, initially 6- to 8-weekly for 6 months, then 6-monthly for 2 years, and then annually thereafter or sooner if symptoms return.
- For relapse, consider definitive treatment, such as radioiodine or surgery. A 2nd course of ATD rarely results in remission.

Choice of drugs—thionamides

- *Carbimazole*, which can be given as a once-daily (od) dose, is usually the drug of 1st choice in the UK. Carbimazole is converted to methimazole by cleavage of a carboxyl side chain on 1st liver passage. It has a lower rate of side effects when compared with PTU (14% vs 52%).
- *PTU* should never be used as a 1st-line agent in either children or adults, with the possible exceptions of pregnant women and patients with life-threatening thyrotoxicosis. PTU use should be restricted to circumstances when neither surgery nor RAI is a treatment option in a patient who has developed a side effect (not agranulocytosis) to carbimazole and ATD therapy is needed.
- During the 1st trimester of pregnancy, PTU is preferred because of the association of carbimazole with aplasia cutis.

Action of thionamides

- Thyroid hormone synthesis is inhibited by blockade of the action of TPO.
- Thionamides are especially actively accumulated in thyrotoxic tissue.
- PTU also inhibits deiodinase type 1 activity and thus may have advantages when given at high doses in severe thyrotoxicosis.

Dose and effectiveness

- Carbimazole 5mg is roughly equivalent to 50mg of PTU. PTU has a theoretical advantage of inhibiting the conversion of T_4 to T_3, and T_3 levels decline more rapidly after starting the drug.

- Thirty to 40% of patients treated with an ATD remain euthyroid 10 years after discontinuation of therapy. If hyperthyroidism recurs after treatment with an ATD, there is little chance that a 2nd course of treatment will result in permanent remission. Young patients, smokers, and those with large goitres, ophthalmopathy, or high serum concentrations of TRAb at the time of diagnosis are unlikely to have permanent remission.
- β-*adrenergic antagonists*. Propranolol 20–80mg 3× daily. Considerable relief from symptoms, such as anxiety, tremor, and palpitations, may be gained in the initial 4–8 weeks of treatment, before euthyroidism is achieved.

Atrial fibrillation

Should, if present, convert to sinus rhythm if no structural cardiac abnormality on echocardiography—otherwise, cardiovert after 4 months euthyroid. Consider use of aspirin or warfarin according to usual guidelines.

Side effects

- ATDs are generally well tolerated. Uncommonly, patients may complain of gastrointestinal (GI) symptoms or an alteration in their sense of taste and smell.
- Agranulocytosis represents a potentially fatal, but rare side effect of ATD, occurring in 0.1–0.5% of patients. It is less frequent with carbimazole than with PTU, and because cross-reactivity of this reaction has been reported, one drug should never be substituted for the other after this reaction has been diagnosed. Agranulocytosis usually occurs within the first 3 months after initiation of therapy (97% within the first 6 months, especially on higher doses), but cases have been documented (less frequently) a long time after starting treatment. Treatment with granulocyte colony-stimulating factor (gCSF) can be helpful.
- As agranulocytosis occurs very suddenly and is potentially fatal, routine monitoring of full blood count (FBC) is thought to be of little use. Patients typically present with fever and evidence of infection, usually in the oropharynx, and *each patient should therefore receive written instructions to discontinue the medication and contact their doctor for a blood count, should this situation arise.*
- Neutrophil dyscrasias occur more frequently in ♂ and are more often fatal in the elderly.
- Much commoner are the allergic-type reactions of rash, urticaria, and arthralgia, which occur in 1–5% of patients taking these drugs. These side effects are often mild and do not usually necessitate drug withdrawal, although one ATD may be substituted for another in the expectation that the 2nd agent may be taken without side effects.
- Thionamides may cause cholestatic jaundice, and elevated serum aminotransaminases have been reported, as has fulminant hepatic failure.
- The frequency of PTU-related severe liver damage is ~0.1% in adults, of whom 10% will develop liver failure resulting in liver transplantation or death (1:10,000 incidence). Data for children suggest that the risk of drug-induced liver failure may be greater for children than for adults (1:1000 incidence).

- In addition to agranulocytosis warning, Medicines Control Agency (MCA) advise warning patients about the following:
  - Carbimazole is associated with an ↑ risk of congenital malformations when used during pregnancy, especially in the 1st trimester and at high doses (daily dose of 15mg or more).
    ○ Women of childbearing potential should use effective contraception during treatment with carbimazole. It should only be considered in pregnancy after a thorough benefit–risk assessment and at the lowest effective dose without additional administration of thyroid hormones—close maternal, fetal, and neonatal monitoring is recommended.
  - Cases of acute pancreatitis have been reported during treatment with carbimazole. It should be stopped immediately and permanently if acute pancreatitis occurs.
    ○ Carbimazole should not be used in patients with a history of acute pancreatitis associated with previous treatment—re-exposure may result in life-threatening acute pancreatitis with ↓ time to onset.
- All patients should be given written and verbal warnings about the potential side effects of thionamides.
- Rarely, antineutrophil cytoplasmic antibody (ANCA) −ve vasculitis develops with PTU therapy. It may cause arthralgia, skin lesions, glomerulonephritis, fever, and alveolar haemorrhage. Skin lesions include ulcers. Biopsy reveals vasculitis. PTU should be stopped and steroids may be needed.

Treatment regimen

Two alternative regimens are used for Graves' disease: dose titration and block and replace.

Dose titration regime
- The 1° aim is to achieve a euthyroid state with relatively high drug doses and then to maintain euthyroidism with a low stable dose. The dose of carbimazole or PTU is titrated according to the TFTs performed every 4–8 weeks, aiming for serum FT_4 in the normal range and detectable TSH. High serum TSH indicates the need for a dose reduction. TSH may remain suppressed for some weeks after normalization of thyroid hormone levels.
- The typical starting dose of carbimazole is 20–30mg/day. Higher doses (40–60mg) may be indicated in severe cases with very high levels of FT_4.
- This regimen has a lower rate of side effects than the block-and-replace regimen.

The treatment is continued for 18 months, as this appears to represent the length of therapy which is generally optimal in producing the remission rate of up to 40% at 5 years after discontinuing therapy.
- Relapses are most likely to occur within the 1st year and may be more likely in the presence of a large goitre, orbitopathy, current smokers, and high T_4 level at the time of diagnosis, or in the presence of TRAb at the end of treatment. ♂ have a higher recurrence rate than ♀.
- Patients with multinodular goitres (and thyroid nodules) and thyrotoxicosis always relapse on cessation of antithyroid medication, and definitive treatment with radioiodine or surgery is usually advised. Long-term thionamide therapy at low dose is also an option, particularly for the elderly.

Block-and-replace regimen
- After achieving a euthyroid state on carbimazole alone, carbimazole at a dose of 40mg daily, together with levothyroxine at a dose of 100 micrograms, can be prescribed. This is usually continued for 6 months.
- The main advantages are fewer hospital visits for checks of thyroid function and a shorter duration of treatment.
- Most patients achieve a euthyroid state within 4–6 weeks of carbimazole therapy.
- During treatment, FT_4 values are measured 4 weeks after starting levothyroxine and the dose of levothyroxine altered, if necessary, in 25-microgram increments to maintain FT_4 in the normal range. Most patients do not require any dose adjustment.
- The remission rate of the block-and-replace regimen is similar to carbimazole alone, but side effects are commoner.[1]

Risk of relapse and TRAb
- Relapses are most likely to occur within the 1st year with either treatment regimen:
  - TRAb level >12IU/L at diagnosis of Graves' disease is associated with 60% risk of relapse at 2 years and 84% at 4 years. Prediction of risk of relapse improves further to >90% with TRAb >7.5IU/L at 12 months or >3.85IU/L at cessation of ATD therapy.
  - Elevated TRAb favours definitive treatment (radioiodine or thyroidectomy), depending on the presence or absence of moderate to severe GO.
  - Patients with persistently high TRAb at 12–18 months can continue ATD treatment, repeating the TRAb measurement after an additional 12 months, or opt for therapy with radioiodine or thyroidectomy.
  - If the patient relapses after completing a course of ATD, definitive treatment is recommended; however, continued long-term low-dose ATD therapy can be considered.

References
1. Okosieme OE, et al. (2019). Primary therapy of Graves' disease and cardiovascular morbidity and mortality: a linked-record cohort study. *Lancet Diabetes Endocrinol* **7**, 278–87.

Further reading
Abraham P, et al. (2010). Antithyroid drug regimen for treating Graves' hyperthyroidism. *Cochrane Database Syst Rev* **1**, CD003420.

Andersen SL (2014). Relapse following antithyroid drug therapy for Graves' hyperthyroidism. *Curr Opin Endocrinol Diabetes Obes* **21**, 415–21.

Boelaert K, et al. (2013). Comparison of mortality in hyperthyroidism during periods of treatment with thionamides and after radioiodine. *J Clin Endocrinol Metab* **98**, 1869–82.

Kahaly GJ, et al. (2018). 2018 European Thyroid Association Guideline for the management of Graves' hyperthyroidism. *Eur Thyroid J* **7**, 167–86.

Ross DS, et al. (2016). 2016 American Thyroid Association guidelines for diagnosis and management of hyperthyroidism and other causes of thyrotoxicosis. *Thyroid* **26**, 1343–421.

Smith TJ, Hegedüs L (2016). Graves' disease. *N Engl J Med* **375**, 1552–65.

Radioiodine treatment

(See Table 1.12.)

Indications

- Definitive treatment of multinodular goitre or adenoma.
- Relapsed Graves' disease.[1,2,3]

Contraindications

- Young children because of the potential risk of thyroid carcinogenesis.
- Pregnant and lactating ♀. (Avoid conception for at least 6 months following RAI.)
- Situations where it is clear that the safety of other people cannot be guaranteed.
- GO. There is some evidence that orbitopathy may worsen after administration of radioiodine, especially in smokers. In cases of moderate to severe ophthalmopathy, radioiodine may be avoided. Alternatively, steroid cover in a dose of 40mg prednisolone should be administered on the day of administering radioiodine, 30mg daily for the next 2 weeks, 20mg daily for the following 2 weeks, reducing to zero over subsequent 3 weeks. Lower steroid doses, e.g. starting with 20mg, may be effective. It is essential that euthyroidism is closely maintained following radioiodine to avoid worsening of ophthalmopathy. TRAb levels parallel the course of orbitopathy, and elevated TRAb is an indication for steroid prophylaxis to prevent progression of orbitopathy with radioiodine therapy.

Caveats

- Control of the disease may not occur for a period of weeks or a few months.
- More than one treatment may be needed in some patients, depending on the dose given; 15% require a 2nd dose and a few patients require a 3rd dose. The 2nd dose should be considered only at least 6 months after the 1st dose.
- Compounds that contain iodine, such as amiodarone, block iodine uptake for a period of several months following cessation of therapy; iodine uptake measurements may be helpful in this instance in determining the activity required and the timing of radioiodine therapy.
- ♀ of childbearing age should avoid pregnancy for a minimum of 6 months following RAI ablation.
- ♂ should avoid fathering children for 4 months after radiation.
- The prevalence of hypothyroidism is over 80% at 25 years and continues to increase thereafter.

Side effects

Rare.

- Anterior neck pain caused by radiation-induced thyroiditis (1%).
- Transient rise (72h) in thyroid hormone levels which may exacerbate heart failure, if present. This aspect needs consideration in elderly patients.

Table 1.12 Recommended activity of radioiodine

Aetiology	Comments	Guide dose (MBq)
Graves' disease	1st presentation; no significant eye disease	400–600
	Moderate goitre (40–50g)	
Toxic multinodular goitre in older person	Mild heart failure; atrial fibrillation or other concomitant disease, e.g. cancer	500–800
Toxic adenoma	Usually mild hyperthyroidism	500
Severe Graves' disease with GO	Postpone RAI until eye disease stable	
	Prednisolone 40mg to be administered at same time as radioiodine and for further 4–6 weeks (see ➲ Contraindications, p. 38)	500–800
Ablation therapy	Severe accompanying medical condition such as heart failure; atrial fibrillation or other concurrent medical disorders (e.g. psychosis)	500–800

Data taken from The Use of Radioiodine in Benign Thyroid Disease. Royal College of Physicians, 2007.

Hypothyroidism after radioiodine

- After radioiodine administration, ATDs may be recommenced. The ATDs should be withdrawn gradually, guided by a 6- to 8-weekly TFT. Early post-radioiodine hypothyroidism may be transient. TSH should be monitored initially, then annually after radioiodine to determine late hypothyroidism.
- In patients treated for autonomous toxic nodules, the incidence of hypothyroidism is lower since the toxic nodule takes up radioiodine while the surrounding tissue will recover normal function once the hyperthyroidism is controlled.
- Morbidity and mortality are not ↑ if euthyroid on levothyroxine therapy

Cancer risk after radioiodine therapy[4,5,6]

In a recently published study of radioiodine-treated patients with hyperthyroidism, greater organ-absorbed doses appeared to be modestly positively associated with a risk of death from solid cancer, including breast cancer. Additional studies are needed on the risks and advantages of all major treatment options available to patients with hyperthyroidism. However, there is no consistent evidence that radioiodine for hyperthyroidism increases the overall risk of malignancy or thyroid cancer.

Clinical guidelines

The recommendation is to administer enough RAI to achieve correct hyperthyroidism with the acceptance of hypothyroidism.

Instructions to patients before treatment

Discontinue ATDs 2–7 days before radioiodine administration since their effects last for 24h or more, although PTU has a prolonged radioprotective effect. ATDs may be recommenced 3–7 days after RAI administration without significantly affecting the delivered radiation dose.

Administration of radioiodine

(See Table 1.13.)

- Radioactive ^{131}I is administered orally (PO) as a capsule or a drink.
- There is no universal agreement regarding the optimal dose.
- A dose of 400–800MBq should be sufficient to cure hyperthyroidism in 90%.
- Most patients are treated with 400–600MBq as the 1st dose, and 600–800MBq if thyrotoxicosis persists 6–12 months after the 1st dose.

Outcomes of radioiodine treatment

- In general, 50–70% of patients have restored normal thyroid function within 6–8 weeks of receiving radioiodine. Shrinkage of goitre occurs but is slower.
- The cumulative incidence of hypothyroidism in patients with Graves' disease and toxic multinodular goitre at 1, 10, and 25 years is 24% vs 4%, 59% vs 15%, and 82% vs 32%, respectively.[7]

Instructions to patients after treatment

Precautions for patients following treatment with radioiodine are summarized in Table 1.13.

References

1. Ross DS (2011). Radioiodine therapy for hyperthyroidism. *N Engl J Med* **364**, 542–50.
2. Bonnema SJ, Hegedüs L (2012). Radioiodine therapy in benign thyroid diseases. *Endocr Rev* **33**, 920–80.
3. Ma C, *et al.* (2016). Radioiodine therapy versus antithyroid medications for Graves' disease. *Cochrane Database Syst Rev* **2**, CD010094.
4. Metso S, *et al.* (2007). Increased cardiovascular and cancer mortality after radioiodine treatment for hyperthyroidism. *J Clin Endocrinol Metab* **92**, 2190–6.
5. Kitahara CM, *et al.* (2019). Association of radioactive iodine treatment with cancer mortality in patients with hyperthyroidism. *JAMA Intern Med* **179**, 1034–42.
6. Ron E, *et al.* (1998). Cancer mortality following treatment for adult hyperthyroidism. Cooperative Thyrotoxicosis Therapy Follow-up Study Group. *JAMA* **280**, 347–55.
7. Metso S, *et al.* (2004). Long-term follow-up study of radioiodine treatment of hyperthyroidism. *Clin Endocrinol (Oxf)* **61**, 641–8.

Table 1.13 Number of days to apply caution after radioiodine

Precaution	Administered activity of ^{131}I MBq			
	≤200	≤400	≤600	≤800
Avoid journeys on public transport >1h	0	0	0	6
Avoid places of entertainment or close contact with other people (duration 3h)	1	5	8	11
Stay off work when travelling alone by private transport and work does not involve close contact with other people	0	0	0	0
Stay off work which involves prolonged contact with other people at a distance of 1m, e.g. bank cashier	8	13	16	18
Stay off work which involves close contact with other people, including pregnant ♀ or children, work of a radiosensitive nature, or commercial food production	11	17	20	22
Avoid non-essential close contact (<1m) with children, teenagers, and pregnant women within the family	16*	22*	25*	27*
Avoid non-essential close contact and sleeping with another person	4	9	13	15

* These times need to be extended if the child concerned is young and needs a lot of close contact.

NB. These apply only in the UK; they are less stringent in the USA.

Surgery

Total thyroidectomy is now considered the operation of choice because of the risk of relapse with partial thyroidectomy.[1] All such patients go home on levothyroxine (see Box 1.3).

Indications

- Documented suspicious or malignant thyroid nodule by FNAC.
- Pregnant ♀ who are not adequately controlled by ATDs or in whom serious allergic reactions develop while being treated medically. Thyroidectomy is usually performed in the 2nd trimester.
- Patients:
  - Who reject or fear exposure to radiation.
  - With poor compliance to medical treatment.
  - In whom rapid control of symptoms is desired, e.g. for fertility.
  - Who develop serious allergic reactions while being treated medically with ATD.
  - With severe manifestations of orbitopathy, as total or near-total thyroidectomy may improve eye manifestations (avoiding post-operative hypothyroidism with early use of adequate levothyroxine).[1]
  - With relapsed Graves' disease.
  - With local compressive symptoms which may not improve rapidly with radioiodine, whereas operation removes these symptoms in most patients.
  - With large thyroid glands and relatively low radioiodine uptake.

References

1. Ross DS, et al. (2016). 2016 American Thyroid Association Guidelines for diagnosis and management of hyperthyroidism and other causes of yhyrotoxicosis. *Thyroid* **26**, 1343–421.

Further reading

Doran HE, et al. (2012). Questionable safety of thyroid surgery with same day discharge. *Ann R Coll Surg Engl* **94**, 543–7.

Farooq MS, et al. (2017). Patterns, timing and consequences of post-thyroidectomy haemorrhage. *Ann R Coll Surg Engl* **99**, 60–2.

Liu ZW, et al. (2015). Thyroid surgery for Graves' disease and Graves' ophthalmopathy. *Cochrane Database Syst Rev* **11**, CD010576.

Preparation for surgery

- ATDs should be used preoperatively to achieve euthyroidism.
- Propranolol may be added to achieve β-blockade, especially in those patients where surgery must be performed sooner than achieving euthyroid state.
- Potassium iodide, 60mg 3× daily (tds), can be used during the preoperative period to prevent unwanted liberation of thyroid hormones during surgery. Preoperatively, it should be given for 10 days. Operating later than this can be associated with exacerbation of thyrotoxicosis, as the thyroid escapes from the inhibitory effect of the iodide. In practice, it is rarely needed, as good control of thyrotoxicosis can be achieved with ATDs in the majority of patients.
- In patients who appear to be non-compliant with ATDs and remain thyrotoxic prior to surgery, it may be necessary to admit them as inpatient for supervised administration of high-dose ATDs, together with β-blockade, and measurement of FT_4 and FT_3 twice weekly. There is a risk of thyroid crisis or storm if a patient undergoes operation when thyrotoxic. Most patients can be rendered euthyroid within 2–4 weeks, and potassium iodide can be administered to coincide with the timing of surgery.
- Additional measures are as for thyroid storm.
- Check vocal function by indirect laryngoscopy.
- Ensure vitamin D-replete.

(For complications, see Table 1.14.)

Post-surgery

- Risk of haemorrhage, the majority within 4–6 hours but may occur up to 72h, deep to the strap muscles leading to airway compression. Watch for stridor, respiratory difficulties, and wound swelling. Treat by evacuating the haematoma. Clip removers and artery forceps should be available on the ward.
- Recurrent laryngeal nerve damage is permanent in 1% and transient in 5%. Patient's voice is often husky for about 3 weeks. Speech therapy may be necessary if persists.
- Monitor calcium (Ca). Transient hypoparathyroidism is normally evident within 7 days (for treatment, see ➲ Hypoparathyroidism, p. 530).

Table 1.14 Complications of thyroidectomy

Immediate	Late
• Recurrent laryngeal nerve damage (permanent in 1% and transient in 5%)	• Hypothyroidism
• Hypoparathyroidism (permanent in 10% and transient in 20%)	• Keloid formation
• Transient hypothyroidism if partial	
• Permanent hypothyroidism if total	
• Thyroid crisis	
• Local haemorrhage in first 24–48h	
• Wound infection	

Thyroid crisis (storm)

Thyroid crisis represents a rare, but life-threatening exacerbation of the manifestations of thyrotoxicosis. It should be promptly recognized since the condition is associated with significant mortality (30–50%, depending on series).[1] Precipitating causes of a thyroid crisis in hyperthyroid patients include:

- Acute infection.
- Diabetic ketoacidosis (DKA), hypoglycaemia, and hyperosmolar coma.
- Undergoing thyroidal or non-thyroidal surgery or radioiodine treatment.
- Withdrawal or non-compliance with ATD therapy.
- Pulmonary embolism (PE) or vascular events.
- No obvious cause in 20–25%.

Thyroid crisis should be considered as a clinical diagnosis in a very sick patient if there is:

- Recent history suggestive of thyrotoxicosis.
- Acute stressful precipitating factor such as surgery or trauma.
- History of previous thyroid treatment.

Laboratory investigations

- Routine haematology may indicate leucocytosis, which is well recognized in thyrotoxicosis, even in the absence of infection.
- The biochemical screen may reveal raised ALP and mild hypercalcaemia.
- TFTs and thyroid antibodies should be requested, although treatment should not be delayed while awaiting the results.
- The levels of thyroid hormones will be raised but may not be grossly elevated, and are usually within the range of uncomplicated thyrotoxicosis.

Diagnostic parameters

(See Box 1.5.)
- $\uparrow$ FT$_3$ or FT$_4$
- CNS manifestations, including agitation, delirium, somnolence, convulsion, and coma.
- Non-CNS manifestations, including fever (>38°C), tachycardia (>130/min), congestive cardiac failure (CCF)/pulmonary oedema, and GI and hepatic (nausea, vomiting, diarrhoea, jaundice).
- Definite diagnosis if elevated thyroid hormones and: (1) any CNS symptom and one or more non-CNS symptom; or (2) three or more non-CNS symptoms.

Treatment

General supportive therapy
- The patient is best managed in an intensive care unit where close attention can be paid to the cardiorespiratory status, fluid balance, and cooling.
- Standard antiarrhythmic drugs can be used, including digoxin (usually in higher than normal dose) after correction for hypokalaemia.

If anticoagulation is indicated because of atrial fibrillation, then it must be remembered that thyrotoxic patients are very sensitive to warfarin.

- Chlorpromazine (50–100mg intramuscularly (IM)) can be used to treat agitation and because of its effect in inhibiting central thermoregulation, it may be useful in treating the hyperpyrexia.
- Identify precipitating factors.
- Broad-spectrum antibiotics should be given if infection is suspected.

Box 1.5 Clinical signs suggestive of a thyroid storm
- Alteration in mental status.
- High fever.
- Tachycardia or tachyarrhythmias.
- Severe clinical hyperthyroid signs.
- Vomiting, jaundice, and diarrhoea.
- Multisystem decompensation: cardiac failure, respiratory distress, congestive hepatomegaly, dehydration, and prerenal failure.
- Not all patients have a goitre.

Specific treatment
- To inhibit thyroid hormone synthesis completely:
  - PTU 600mg–1g loading, then 200–300mg 4-hourly via nasogastric (NG) tube or per rectum (PR). PTU is preferred because of its ability to block T_4 to T_3 conversion in peripheral tissues. There are no clinical data comparing PTU and carbimazole in this situation. ATDs should be commenced first.
- To inhibit thyroid hormone release:
  - Potassium iodide, 60mg via NG tube 6-hourly, 6h *after* starting PTU, will inhibit thyroid hormone release.
  - Alternatives are Lugol's solution 8–10 drops every 6–8h, ipodate 0.5 3g/day, and lithium 300mg 6-hourly.
- β-adrenergic blocking agents are essential in the management to control tachycardia, tremor, and other adrenergic manifestations.
- Propranolol 1–2mg IV boluses every 10–15min until stable, then 160–320mg/day in divided doses or as an infusion 2–5mg/h.
- Calcium channel blockers can be tried in patients with known bronchospastic disease where β-blockade is contraindicated.
- Prevention of peripheral conversion of T_4 to T_3 with high doses of GCs such as dexamethasone 2mg 6-hourly, prednisolone 60mg daily, or hydrocortisone 100mg 8-hourly.
- Plasmapheresis and peritoneal dialysis may be effective in cases resistant to the usual pharmacological measures.
- Colestyramine (3g tds) reduces enterohepatic circulation of thyroid hormones and may help improve thyrotoxicosis.
- Consider definitive therapy with RAI or thyroidectomy.

References

1. Satoh T, *et al.* (2016). 2016 Guidelines for the management of thyroid storm from The Japan Thyroid Association and Japan Endocrine Society (first edition). *Endocr J* **63**, 1025–64.

Subclinical hyperthyroidism

(See Box 1.6.)

- Values of thyroid hormones should be repeated to exclude NTI.
- Subclinical hyperthyroidism is defined as low serum TSH concentration in patients with normal levels of T_4 and T_3. Subtle symptoms and signs of thyrotoxicosis may be present.
- Prevalence of 3%.
- Classified as endogenous in patients with thyroid hormone production associated with nodular thyroid disease or underlying Graves' disease, and as exogenous in those with low or undetectable serum TSH concentrations as a result of treatment with levothyroxine.
  - Recent meta-analyses, including those based on large prospective cohort studies, indicate that subclinical hyperthyroidism is associated with ↑ risk of coronary heart disease (CHD) mortality, incident atrial fibrillation, heart failure, fractures, and excess mortality in patients with serum TSH levels <0.1mIU/L.[1,2]
  - Subclinical hyperthyroidism might be associated with an elevated risk of dementia.[3] Available data are limited, and additional large, high-quality studies are needed.
  - Among adults, subclinical hyperthyroidism was associated with ↑ femoral neck bone loss, potentially contributing to ↑ fracture risk.
  - Despite the absence of randomized prospective trials, there is evidence that treatment is indicated in patients older than 65 years to potentially avoid these serious cardiovascular events, fractures, and the risk of progression to overt hyperthyroidism.
  - Treatment could be considered in patients older than 65 years with TSH levels of 0.1–0.39mIU/L because of their ↑ risk of atrial fibrillation, and might also be reasonable in younger (<65 years) symptomatic patients because of the risk of progression, especially in the presence of symptoms and/or underlying risk factors or comorbidity.
  - There are no data to support treating subclinical hyperthyroidism in younger asymptomatic patients with serum TSH levels of 0.1–0.39mIU/L. These patients should be followed without treatment due to the low risk of progression to overt hyperthyroidism and the weaker evidence for adverse health outcomes.
- Treatment options include long-term, low-dose ATD therapy or ablative therapy with radioiodine.
- In patients with exogenous subclinical hyperthyroidism, the dose of levothyroxine should be reduced, if possible, excluding those with prior thyroid cancer in whom TSH suppression may be required. The dose of levothyroxine used for treating hypothyroidism may be reduced if the patient develops:
  - New atrial fibrillation, angina, or cardiac failure.
  - Accelerated bone loss.
  - Borderline high serum T_3 concentration.

Box 1.6 Indications to treat subclinical hyperthyroidism

- Age >65 years and TSH <0.1mIU/L.
- Age >65 years and TSH 0.1–0.39mIU/L if cardiovascular risk factors.
- Age <65 years and TSH <0.1mIU/L if symptoms and confirmed thyroid disease, e.g. Graves' disease or toxic nodular goitre.
- Atrial fibrillation.
- Low bone density.

Natural history of subclinical hyperthyroidism[4]

- Reversion to euthyroidism 76% is TSH 0.1–0.4, 12.5% if <0.1.
- Stable at 7 years 50% TSH 0.1–0.4, 37.5% TSH <0.1.
- Overt hyperthyroidism 0% TSH 0.1–0.4 at 7 years, 3.1% TSH <0.1 at 7 years.

References

1. Biondi B, et al. (2015). The 2015 European Thyroid Association guidelines on diagnosis and treatment of endogenous subclinical hyperthyroidism. *Eur Thyroid J* **4**, 149–63.
2. Collet TH, et al. (2012). Subclinical hyperthyroidism and the risk of coronary heart disease and mortality. *Arch Intern Med* **172**, 799–809.
3. Floriani C, et al. (2018). Subclinical thyroid dysfunction and cardiovascular diseases: 2016 update. *Eur Heart J* **39**, 503–7.
4. Mitchell AL, Pearce SH (2016). Subclinical hyperthyroidism: first do no harm. *Clin Endocrinol* **85** 15–16.

Further reading

Rieben C, et al. (2016). Subclinical thyroid dysfunction and the risk of cognitive decline: a meta-analysis of prospective cohort studies. *J Clin Endocrinol Metab* **101**, 4945–54.

Williams GR, Bassett JHD (2018). Thyroid diseases and bone health. *Endocrinol Invest* **41**, 99–109.

Wirth CD, et al. (2014). Subclinical thyroid dysfunction and the risk for fractures: a systematic review and meta-analysis. *Ann Intern Med* **161**, 189–99.

Thyrotoxic periodic paralysis (TPP)

- A rare complication of hyperthyroidism characterized by acute, reversible episodes of muscle weakness and hypokalaemia.
- Often precipitated by heavy exercise or high-carbohydrate meals and is most commonly described in young Asian men aged 20–40 years.
- Although the pathogenesis remains unclear, the recurrent paralytic muscle weakness is caused by hypokalaemia resulting from a shift of potassium (K^+) into the intracellular space without a total K^+ deficit.
- Clinical features of TPP and the factors precipitating the acute paralysis episodes are similar to those of familial periodic paralysis associated with hypokalaemia which is an autosomal dominant (AD) channelopathy commoner in Caucasians.
- Recurrent episodes of painless muscle weakness.
- Duration from minutes to days.
- Flaccid paralysis, usually spreading from the legs proximally.
- Symptoms usually improve within 2–4h; full resolution in 24–48h.
- Although rare, early treatment of TPP is necessary to avoid reversible, but potentially life-threatening complications such as cardiac arrhythmias and respiratory failure.
- Symptoms and signs of thyrotoxicosis may be subtle in TPP, so the diagnosis requires an awareness of precipitants and clinical features, with recognition of biochemical and electrocardiogram (ECG) abnormalities.
- Improves as thyrotoxicosis treated.
- Treatment doses of potassium chloride required to recover from paralysis need to be minimized to avoid rebound hyperkalaemia.
- Non-selective β-blockers can prevent paradoxical hypokalaemia associated with hyperadrenergic activity.

Further reading

Vanderpump M (2018). Thyrotoxic periodic paralysis. In: Matfin G (ed.) *Endocrine and Metabolic Medical Emergencies: A Clinician's Guide*, 2nd edn. Wiley-Blackwell, Chichester; pp. 296–304.

Thyrotoxicosis in pregnancy

(See also Maternal hyperthyroidism, pp. 472–3 and Table 1.15.)

- Thyrotoxicosis occurs in about 0.2% of pregnancies.
- Graves' disease accounts for 90% of cases.
- Less common causes include toxic adenoma and multinodular goitre, gestational hyperthyroidism (hyperemesis gravidarum), and trophoblastic neoplasia.
- Diagnosis of thyrotoxicosis during pregnancy may be difficult or delayed.
- Physiological changes of pregnancy are similar to those of hyperthyroidism.
- Total T_4 and T_3 are ↑ in pregnancy because of an ↑ TBG level, but with free hormone assays available, this is now rarely a problem.
- Physiological features of normal pregnancy include an increase in basal metabolic rate, cardiac stroke volume, palpitations, and heat intolerance.
- Serum FT_3 concentrations remain within the normal range in most pregnant ♀; serum TSH concentration decreases during the 1st trimester.

Symptoms

- Hyperemesis gravidarum is the classic presentation (one-third is toxic). Tiredness, palpitations, insomnia, heat intolerance, proximal muscle weakness, shortness of breath, and irritability may be other presenting symptoms.
- Thyrotoxicosis may be diagnosed occasionally when the patient presents with pregnancy-induced hypertension (PIH) or congestive heart failure.

Signs

- Failure to gain weight despite good appetite.
- Persistent tachycardia with pulse rate >90bpm at rest.
- Other signs of thyrotoxicosis as described previously.

Natural history of Graves' disease in pregnancy

There is aggravation of symptoms in the 1st half of the pregnancy; amelioration of symptoms in the 2nd half of the pregnancy, and often recurrence of symptoms in the post-partum period.

Transient hyperthyroidism of gestational hyperthyroidism (hyperemesis gravidarum)

- The likely mechanism is a raised β-hCG level.
- β-hCG, luteinizing hormone (LH), follicle-stimulating hormone (FSH), and TSH are glycoprotein hormones that contain a common α subunit and a hormone-specific β subunit. There is an inverse relationship between the serum levels of TSH and hCG, best seen in early pregnancy. There is also structural homology of the TSH and hCG receptors.
- Serum FT_4 concentration may be ↑ and the TSH levels suppressed in ♀ with hyperemesis gravidarum.
- TFTs recover after the resolution of hyperemesis.

- Pregnant ♀ with gestational hyperthyroidism (hyperemesis gravidarum) (which only accounts for two-thirds of hyperemesis) are not usually given ATD treatment, but managed supportively with fluids, antiemetics, and nutritional support.
- There is no ↑ risk of thyrotoxicosis in subsequent pregnancies.
- Can be differentiated from Graves' disease by the absence of a goitre, antithyroid antibodies, or a family history of Graves' disease, a history of other autoimmune phenomena, and a previous history of ophthalmic Graves'.

Management of Graves' disease in the mother

- Aim of treatment is alleviation of thyroid symptoms and normalization of tests in the shortest time. Patients should be seen every 4–8 weeks, and TFTs performed. Serum FT_4 is the best test to follow the response to ATDs. The block-and-replace regimen should not be used, as this will result in fetal hypothyroidism.
- Both PTU (150mg twice daily (bd)) and carbimazole (10–20mg od) are effective in controlling the disease in pregnancy—although current MCA recommendations are to avoid, if possible, and to aim for <15mg/day carbimazole.
- Carbimazole and PTU are associated with urinary system malformation, and PTU with malformations in the face and neck region. Choanal atresia, oesophageal atresia, omphalocele, omphalomesenteric duct anomalies, and aplasia cutis are commoner in carbimazole-exposed children.
- As the birth defects associated with PTU are less severe, PTU is preferred in pregnancy because it is not associated with aplasia cutis and omphalocele, which may be the case for carbimazole. However, in view of concern regarding hepatotoxicity of PTU, particularly in children, it is recommended that PTU should only be prescribed in the 1st trimester (check liver function monthly) and carbimazole thereafter from the 2nd trimester.
- A β-blocker (propranolol 20–40mg 6- to 8-hourly) is effective in controlling the hypermetabolic symptoms but should be used only for a few weeks until symptoms abate.
- The dosage of ATDs is frequently adjusted during the course of the pregnancy; therefore, thyroid tests should be done at 2- to 4-weekly intervals, with the goal of keeping free thyroid hormone levels in the upper third of the reference range.
- Thyroid tests may normalize spontaneously, with the progression of a normal pregnancy as a result of immunological changes.
- The use of iodides and radioiodine is contraindicated in pregnancy.
- Surgery is rarely necessary in pregnancy. It is reserved for patients not responding to ATDs. It is preferable to perform surgery in the 2nd trimester.
- Breastfeeding mothers should be treated with the lowest possible dose of carbimazole (<30mg daily), rather than with PTU, in view of the concern regarding hepatotoxicity. Women should be advised to take it in divided doses after breastfeeding to minimize doses to the baby.

Pre-pregnancy counselling

- Hyperthyroid ♀ who want to conceive should attain euthyroidism before conception since uncontrolled hyperthyroidism is associated with an ↑ risk of miscarriage, PIH, preterm delivery, stillbirth and low birthweight, and congenital abnormalities such as cranial synostosis (see Table 1.15).
- There is no evidence that radioiodine treatment given to the mother (or father) 6 months or more before pregnancy has an adverse effect on the fetus or on an offspring in later life.
- Antithyroid medication requirements usually decrease during gestation; in about 50–60% of patients, the dose may be discontinued in the last few weeks of gestation.
- The risk of recurrent hyperthyroidism should be discussed with the patient.
- The rare occurrence of fetal and neonatal hyperthyroidism should be included during counselling sessions and the diagnosis of Graves' hyperthyroidism conveyed to the obstetrician and neonatologist.

Management of the fetus

- The HPT axis is well developed at 12 weeks' gestation, with significant fetal thyroid hormone production from 20 weeks. Circulating TRAbs in the mother can cross the placenta, and it is these, rather than the thyroid status of the mother, that cause neonatal thyrotoxicosis. The fetal TSH receptor responds to stimulation from maternal TRAbs by 18 weeks' gestation. The risk of hyperthyroidism to the neonate can be assessed by measuring TRAbs in the maternal circulation at the beginning of the 3rd trimester. TgAb and TPOAb have no effect on the fetus.
- Long-term follow-up studies of children whose mothers received either carbimazole or PTU have not shown an ↑ incidence of any physical or psychological defects. The block-and-replace regimen using relatively high doses of carbimazole is contraindicated because the ATDs readily cross the placenta, but replacement T_4 does not, thus potentially rendering the fetus hypothyroid.
- Monitoring the fetal heart rate and growth rates are the standard means whereby fetal thyrotoxicosis may be detected. A rate >160bpm is suspicious of fetal thyrotoxicosis in the 3rd trimester. Fetal thyrotoxicosis may complicate the latter part of the pregnancy of ♀ with Graves' disease, even if they have been treated previously with radioiodine or surgery, since TRAbs may persist. If there is evidence of fetal thyrotoxicosis, the dose of the ATD should be ↑. If this causes maternal hypothyroidism, a small dose of T_4 can be added since, unlike carbimazole, T_4 crosses the placenta less. A paediatrician should be involved to monitor neonatal thyroid function and detect thyrotoxicosis.
- Hypothyroidism in the mother should be avoided because of the potential adverse effect on subsequent cognitive function of the neonate (see Box 1.6).

- If the mother has been treated with carbimazole, post-delivery levels of T_4 may be low and neonatal levels of T_4 may only rise to the thyrotoxic range after a few days. In addition, TSH is usually absent in neonates who subsequently develop thyrotoxicosis. Clinical indicators of neonatal thyrotoxicosis include low birthweight, poor weight gain, tachycardia, and irritability. Carbimazole can be given at a dose of 0.5mg/kg per day and withdrawn after a few weeks after the level of TRAbs declines.

Post-partum thyroiditis

- Defined as a syndrome of post-partum thyrotoxicosis or hypothyroidism in ♀ who were euthyroid during pregnancy.
- Post-partum thyroid dysfunction, which occurs in ♀ with autoimmune thyroid disease, is characterized in one-third by a thyrotoxic phase occurring in the first 3 months post-partum, followed by a hypothyroid phase that occurs 3–6 months after delivery, followed by spontaneous recovery. In the remaining two-thirds, a single-phase pattern or the reverse occurs.
- Five to 7% of ♀ develop biochemical evidence of thyroid dysfunction after delivery. An ↑ incidence is seen in patients with T1DM (25%) and other autoimmune diseases, in the presence of TPOAb, and in the presence of a family history of thyroid disease.
- Hyperthyroidism due to Graves' disease accounts for 10–15% of all cases of post-partum thyrotoxicosis. In the majority of cases, hyperthyroidism occurs later in the post-partum period (>3–6 months) and persists.
- Providing the patient is not breastfeeding, a radioiodine uptake scan can differentiate the two principal causes of autoimmune thyrotoxicosis by demonstrating ↑ uptake in Graves' disease and low uptake in post-partum thyroiditis.
- TRAb assays have >95% sensitivity and specificity for the diagnosis of Graves' disease and significantly lessen the requirement for radioiodine uptake scan imaging.
- Graves' hyperthyroidism should be treated with carbimazole. Thyrotoxic symptoms due to post-partum thyrotoxicosis are managed symptomatically using propranolol.
- One-third of affected ♀ with post-partum thyroiditis develop symptoms of hypothyroidism and may require levothyroxine for 6–12 months. There is an ↑ risk of post-partum mood disorders.
- Histology of the thyroid in the case of post-partum thyroiditis shows lymphocytic infiltration with destructive thyroiditis and predominantly occurs at 16 weeks in ♀ with +ve TPOAb.
- There is an ↑ risk of subsequent permanent hypothyroidism in 25–30%. Patients with a history of post-partum thyroiditis should be followed up with annual serum TSH measurements.

Table 1.15 Potential maternal and fetal complications in uncontrolled hyperthyroidism in pregnancy

Maternal	Fetal
PIH	Hyperthyroidism
Preterm delivery	Neonatal hyperthyroidism
Congestive heart failure	Intrauterine growth retardation
Thyroid storm	Small for gestational age
Miscarriage	Prematurity
Abruptio placentae	Stillbirth
Accidental haemorrhage	Cranial synostosis

Further reading

Alexander EK, et al. (2017). 2017 Guidelines of the American Thyroid Association for the diagnosis and management of thyroid disease during pregnancy and the postpartum. *Thyroid* **27**, 315–89.

Andersen SL, et al. (2016). Antithyroid drug side effects in the population and in pregnancy. *J Clin Endocrinol Metab* **101**, 1606–14.

Cooper DS, Laurberg P (2013). Hyperthyroidism in pregnancy. *Lancet Diabetes Endocrinol* **1**, 238–49.

Kobaly K, Mandel SJ (2019). Hyperthyroidism and pregnancy. *Endocrinol Metab Clin North Am* **48**, 533–45.

Harding KB, et al. (2017). Iodine supplementation for women during the preconception, pregnancy and postpartum period. *Cochrane Database Syst Rev* **3**, CD011761.

Laurberg P, Andersen SL (2015). Antithyroid drug use in pregnancy and birth defects: why some studies find clear associations, and some studies report none. *Thyroid* **25**, 1185–90.

Okosieme OE, et al. (2018). Preconception management of thyroid dysfunction. *Clin Endocrinol (Oxf)* **89**, 269–79.

Spencer L, et al. (2015). Screening and subsequent management for thyroid dysfunction pre-pregnancy and during pregnancy for improving maternal and infant health. *Cochrane Database Syst Rev* **9**, CD011263.

Hyperthyroidism in children

Epidemiology

Thyrotoxicosis is rare before the age of 5 years. Although there is a progressive increase in incidence throughout childhood, it is still rare and accounts for <5% of all cases of Graves' disease.

Clinical features

- Behavioural abnormalities, hyperactivity, and declining school performance may bring the child to medical attention. Features of hyperthyroidism are as described previously.
- Acceleration of linear growth is common in patients increasing in height percentiles on the growth charts. The disease may be part of McCune–Albright syndrome, and café-au-lait pigmentation, precocious puberty, and bony abnormalities should be considered during clinical examination.

Investigations

The cause of thyrotoxicosis in children is nearly always Graves' disease (with +ve TRAb), although thyroiditis and toxic nodules have been described, and a radioiodine scan may be useful if the diagnosis is not clear. Hereditary syndromes of thyroid hormone resistance, often misdiagnosed as Graves' disease, are now being increasingly recognized in children.

Treatment

ATDs represent the initial treatment of choice for thyrotoxic children. Therapy is generally started with carbimazole 250 micrograms/kg (initial dose 10mg/day). Since relapse after withdrawal of ATDs is common, definitive treatment with surgery or radioiodine may be offered. Hepatotoxicity with PTU is a greater risk in children (1:2000, compared with reported 1:10,000 adults). In the past 20 years in the USA, 12 children developed liver failure on PTU (three deaths and six liver transplants). PTU-related hepatotoxicity occurs within 90 days of starting (although cases occurring up to 1 year have been reported) and are not dose-related.

Further reading

Azizi F, Amouzegar A (2018). Management of thyrotoxicosis in children and adolescents: 35 years' experience in 304 patients. *J Pediatr Endocrinol Metab* **31**, 159–65.

De Luca F, Valenzise M (2018). Controversies in the pharmacological treatment of Graves' disease in children. *Expert Rev Clin Pharmacol* **11**, 1113–21.

Léger J, et al. (2018). Graves' disease in children. *Ann Endocrinol (Paris)* **79**, 647–55.

Secondary hyperthyroidism

Elevated serum FT_4 and non-suppressed serum TSH are characteristic of TSH-secreting adenomas or RTH once methodological interference has been excluded (see ➲ Table 1.3).

TSH-secreting pituitary tumours

- Estimated incidence of 1 per million and <1% of all pituitary tumours.
- There are characteristically *elevated* serum free T_4 and T_3 concentrations and *non-suppressed* (inappropriately normal or frankly elevated) serum TSH levels.
- ~25% of TSHomas co-secrete one or more other pituitary hormones; about 15% secrete growth hormone (GH), 10% PRL, and rarely gonadotrophins. ~80% are macroadenomas (>1cm in diameter), and over two-thirds exhibit suprasellar extension or invasion, or both, into adjacent tissues (see ➲ Thyrotrophinomas, pp. 200–1).
- Patients with pure TSHomas present with typical symptoms and signs of thyrotoxicosis and the presence of a usually nodular goitre. Patients may exhibit features of oversecretion of the other pituitary hormones, e.g. PRL or GH. Headaches, visual field defects, menstrual irregularities, amenorrhoea, delayed puberty, and hypogonadotrophic hypogonadism (HH) have also been reported. Careful establishment of the diagnosis is the key to treatment. Inappropriate treatment of such patients with subtotal thyroidectomy or radioiodine administration not only fails to cure the underlying disorder, but may also be associated with subsequent pituitary tumour enlargement and an ↑ risk of invasiveness into adjacent tissues.
- Failure to correctly diagnose TSHomas may result in inappropriate thyroid ablation, which results in a significant increase of pituitary tumour mass. The diagnosis is mainly achieved by measuring TSH suppression after T_3 suppression and TRH stimulation tests. These dynamic tests, together with pituitary imaging and genetic testing, are useful in distinguishing TSHomas from the syndromes of RTH action (see Table 1.16).
- Treatment options are:
  - Transsphenoidal surgery—considered as the definitive therapy.
  - Pituitary radiotherapy, including radiosurgery, if surgical results are unsatisfactory or surgery is contraindicated or not desired—effective in achieving tumour control in the majority of patients.
  - Medical therapy with somatostatin analogues (SSAs) such as octreotide or lanreotide—may be useful preoperatively and suppresses TSH secretion in 80% of the cases.
  - In the past, radiation therapy was used as 2nd-line treatment in patients with residual or recurrent tumour after surgery. However, the availability of SSAs, which can lead to normalization of thyroid function, as well as shrink these tumours, has led to an increase in the role of medical therapy in patients who are not in remission after pituitary surgery. Dopamine agonists have shown some efficacy in the management of these tumours.

Table 1.16 Tests useful in the differential diagnosis of TSHomas and RTH

Test	TSHomas	RTH
Clinical thyrotoxicosis	Present	Usually absent
Family history	Absent	Present
TSH response to TRH	Blunted	Normal
TSH response to liothyronine (100 micrograms/day + β-blockers)	−ve	Partial
SHBG	Elevated	Normal
α subunit	Elevated in 70%	Normal
Pituitary magnetic resonance imaging (MRI)	Tumour—80% macroadenomas	Normal
Fall in TSH on octreotide LAR 20mg/month for 2 months	95%	No change
Analyse *TRβ* gene	Wild-type	Mutation identified in 80%

Further reading

Amlashi FG, Tritos NA (2016). Thyrotropin-secreting pituitary adenomas: epidemiology, diagnosis, and management. *Endocrine* **52**, 427–40.

Beck-Peccoz P, et al. (2013). 2013 European Thyroid Association guidelines for the diagnosis and treatment of thyrotropin-secreting pituitary tumors. *Eur Thyroid J* **2**, 76–82.

Tjörnstrand A, Nyström HF (2017). Diagnosis of endocrine disease. Diagnostic approach to TSH-producing pituitary adenoma. *Eur J Endocrinol* **177**, R183–97.

Graves' orbitopathy

(See European Group on Graves' Orbitopathy, ℳ http://www.eugogo.eu)

- An organ-specific autoimmune disorder characterized by swelling of the extraocular muscles, lymphocytic infiltration, late fibrosis, muscle tethering, and proliferation of orbital fat and connective tissue.
- The volume of both the extraocular muscles and retro-orbital connective and adipose tissue is ↑ due to inflammation and accumulation of hydrophilic glycosaminoglycans (GAGs), principally hyaluronic acid, in these tissues. GAG secretion by fibroblasts is ↑ by activated T-cell cytokines, such as tumour necrosis factor (TNF) α and interferon γ, implying that T-cell activation is an important part of this immunopathology. The accumulation of GAG causes a change in osmotic pressure, which, in turn, leads to fluid accumulation and an increase in pressure within the orbit. These changes displace the eyeball forward and can also interfere with the function of the extrocular muscles and the venous drainage of the orbits.
- Clinically evident in ~20% of patients, but a further 30% may have evidence on imaging. Mostly bilateral, but often asymmetrical, and 15% have unilateral disease.
- Most have mild self-limiting disease, but ~5% (more ♂ and the elderly) have severe disease that threatens sight. The natural history is variable, with spontaneous amelioration in 66%, no change in 20%, and worsening in 14%.
- Incidence higher in ♀ (except for severe disease where equal sex incidence). Prevalence decreasing (? associated with ↓ smoking and earlier detection and treatment of hyperthyroidism).
- Bimodal age distribution in ♀, with peak onsets between 40–44 years and 60–64 years. In ♂, a single peak incidence occurs at 65–69 years.
- There are two stages in the development of the disease, which can be recognized as an active inflammatory (dynamic) stage and a relatively quiescent static stage.
- The appearance of eye disease follows a different time course to thyroid dysfunction, and in a minority, there is a lag period between the presentation of hyperthyroidism and the appearance of eye signs; 85% of patients develop Graves' disease within 18 months of orbitopathy developing (20% preceding, 40% following).
- Five per cent of patients with GO have hypothyroidism, and 5% are euthyroid.
- High levels of TRAb identify high-risk patients.
- Current smokers (>20/day) are more likely to develop orbitopathy.
- Continuing smoking and uncontrolled hyperthyroidism or hypothyroidism moderately worsen GO.
- The role of an endocrinologist during a routine review of Graves' patients is to record accurately the clinical features of Graves' eye disease and to identify ocular emergencies, such as corneal ulceration, congestive ophthalmopathy, and optic neuropathy, which should be referred urgently to an ophthalmologist, preferably in a multidisciplinary clinic setting.

Clinical features

(See Table 1.17.)

- Retraction of eyelids is extremely common in thyroid eye disease. The margin of the upper eyelid normally rests about 2mm below the limbus, and retraction can be suspected if the lid margin is either level with or above the superior limbus, allowing the sclera to be visible. The lower lid normally rests at the inferior limbus, and retraction is suspected when the sclera shows above the lid.
- Proptosis or exophthalmos can result in failure of lid closure, increasing the likelihood of exposure keratitis and the common symptom of gritty eyes. This can be confirmed with fluorescein or Rose Bengal stain. As papilloedema can occur, fundoscopy should be performed. Proptosis may result in periorbital oedema and chemosis because the displaced orbit results in less efficient orbital drainage.
- Persistent visual blurring may indicate optic neuropathy and requires urgent treatment.
- Severe conjunctival pain may indicate corneal ulceration, requiring urgent referral.

Table 1.17 Assessment of severity of Graves' orbitopathy

Ocular involvement	Features
Mild GO	Minor lid retraction (<2mm)
	Mild soft tissue involvement
	Exophthalmos <3mm
	No or transient diplopia
Moderate GO	Mild corneal exposure lid retraction (≥2mm)
	Moderate to severe soft tissue involvement
	Exophthalmos ≥3mm
	Diplopia
Sight-threatening GO	Optic neuropathy
	Corneal breakdown
	Congestive ophthalmopathy

Investigation of proptosis

(See ⌖ http://www.eugogo.eu for details of the 'NOSPECS' classification.) NOSPECS is not always satisfactory for prospective objective assessment of orbital changes, and determining an overall activity score is sometimes more helpful. This is done by assigning 1 point for the presence of each of the following: spontaneous retrobulbar pain, pain on eye movement, eyelid erythema, conjunctival injection, chemosis, swelling of the carbuncle, and eyelid oedema.

- *Documentation using a Hertel ophthalmometer.* The feet of the apparatus are placed against the lateral orbital margin as defined by the zygomatic bones. The marker on the body of the ophthalmometer is then superimposed on the reflection of the contralateral one by adjusting the scale. The position of each cornea can be read off against the reflections on a millimetre scale, as seen in the mirror of the apparatus. A normal result is generally taken as being <20mm (<18mm in Asians, <22mm in Afro-Caribbeans). A reading of 21mm or more is abnormal, and a difference of 2mm between the eyes is suspicious.

- *Soft tissue involvement.* Soft tissue signs and symptoms include conjunctival hyperaemia, chemosis, and foreign body sensation. The soft tissue changes can be 2° to exposure but are often seen in the absence of these aetiological factors.
- *CT or MRI scan of the orbit.* Demonstrates enlargement of the extraocular muscles, and this can be useful in cases of diagnostic difficulty. This is also more accurate for demonstration of proptosis.

Ophthalmoplegia

- Patients may complain of diplopia due to ocular muscle dysfunction caused by either oedema during the early active phase or fibrosis during the later phase. Assessment using a Hess chart may be helpful. Intraoptic pressure may increase on upgaze and result in compression of the globe by a fibrotic inferior rectus muscle. Ocular mobility may be restricted by oedema during the active inflammatory phase or by fibrosis during the fibrotic stage.
- The two commonest findings are defective elevation caused by fibrotic contraction of the inferior rectus muscle and a convergence defect caused by fibrotic contraction of the medial rectus. Disorders of the medial rectus, superior rectus, and lateral rectus muscles produce typical signs of defective adduction, depression, and abduction, respectively.

Examining for possible optic neuropathy

- A history of *poor vision*, a recent or *rapid change in vision*, or *poor colour vision* are reasons for prompt referral.
- A *VA* of <6/18 warrants referral to an ophthalmologist. For *colour vision*, each eye should be evaluated by using a simple 15-plate Ishihara colour vision test. Colour vision is a subtle indicator of optic nerve function. Failure to identify >2 of the plates with either eye is an indication for referral. This is unhelpful in the 8% of ♂ who may be colour-blind.
- *Marcus Gunn pupil.* The 'swinging flashlight' test detects the presence of an *afferent pupillary defect* associated with optic nerve compression.

Medical treatment of Graves' orbitopathy

(See Table 1.18.)

Simple treatment for lid retraction

- Most patients do not require any treatment since clinical signs usually improve with treatment of hyperthyroidism or spontaneously with time (40%).
- Sunglasses help with photophobia and excess tears.
- In patients with significant lid retraction and exposure keratopathy, topical lubricants improve symptoms (surgery to reduce the vertical lid fissures can be considered when euthyroid and eye disease inactive).
- Botulinum toxin injection may reduce persistent upper lid retraction.
- Head elevation during sleep and diuretics may help congestion.

Acute treatment for active orbitopathy threatening sight

- Effectiveness is more likely in those with diplopia at neutral gaze and an inflammatory component to ophthalmoplegia.
- IV GC pulse therapy has the advantage of fewer side effects than high PO doses of prednisolone (e.g. 0.5g methylprednisolone weekly for 6 weeks, followed by 0.25g weekly for 6 weeks, with monitoring of liver function tests (LFTs) ± proton pump inhibitors (PPIs) and a bisphosphonate). GCs at high dose improve orbitopathy in 60–75% of cases.
- The advantage of IV over PO GC therapy was demonstrated in a meta-analysis of four trials. IV GCs were significantly better in reducing clinical activity scores; the advantage was mostly due to improvements in patients with severe orbitopathy. Adverse events were commoner in patients receiving oral therapy, and high doses have been seen to induce liver failure.
- The optimal cumulative dose of methylprednisolone IV appears to be 4.5–5g. Higher doses (up to 8g) can be used for more severe forms. There is an ↑ risk of hepatic necrosis seen at higher doses.[1]
- If high-dose PO prednisolone treatment—give for 2 weeks and then taper gradually.
- Steroid-sparing agents used in long-term therapy include mycophenolate mofetil, azathioprine, methotrexate, and ciclosporin, but there are few data suggesting which is more effective.
- Urgent referral to an ophthalmologist is indicated for any suspicion of optic neuropathy or corneal ulceration. Multidisciplinary clinics are strongly advised.

Orbital radiotherapy

- Indications for lens-sparing orbital radiotherapy are similar to those for high-dose GCs.
- Radiotherapy works by killing retro-orbital T-cells.
- The standard regimen is 20Gy delivered over ten fractions.
- Treatment with both radiotherapy and GCs is more effective than either alone.
- Effectiveness in 60% of cases <40 years.

Other medical therapies

- Selenium may improve symptoms in patients with mild GO, as illustrated by the results of a randomized trial of selenium (100 micrograms bd), pentoxifylline (600 milligrams bd), or placebo in 159 patients. After 6 months of treatment, eyelid aperture (37% vs 12%) and soft tissue signs (43% vs 32%) significantly improved in patients taking selenium vs placebo. Compared with placebo, selenium also significantly improved quality of life (QoL) (both visual functioning and appearance scores), as assessed by the Graves' Ophthalmopathy Quality of Life Questionnaire (GO-QOL). Evaluation at 12 months confirmed the findings at 6 months.[2]

- Rituximab, a monoclonal antibody directed against the B-cell CD20 molecule, induces B-cell depletion. Rituximab induces a fall in TRAb levels and depletion of B-cells in the retro-orbital tissues, not just the periphery. High doses of this antibody may be associated with severe side effects from profound immunosuppression; it is possible that much lower doses may be effective in GO to avoid such effects. Two randomized controlled trials (RCTs) reached seemingly contradictory conclusions—rituximab was not better with respect to the 1° outcome (clinical activity score) than placebo in one trial (which, however, was confounded by rather long GO duration) but was slightly better than IV methylprednisolone pulses in the other (disease flare-ups occurred only in the latter group). On the basis of evidence published so far, rituximab cannot replace IV methylprednisolone pulses but could have a role in corticosteroid-resistant cases.[3]

- Teprotumumab, a human monoclonal antibody inhibitor of IGF-1 receptor (IGF-1R), was more effective than placebo in reducing proptosis (a reduction of 2mm or more in proptosis at week 24) and the clinical activity score in a placebo-controlled RCT of patients with active, moderate to severe ophthalmopathy. In the intention-to-treat population, 29 of 42 patients who received teprotumumab (69%), as compared with 9 of 45 patients who received placebo (20%), had a response at week 24 (P <0.001). Therapeutic effects were rapid; at week 6, a total of 18 of 42 patients in the teprotumumab group (43%) and 2 of 45 patients in the placebo group (4%) had a response (P <0.001). Differences between the groups ↑ at subsequent time points. The only drug-related adverse event was hyperglycaemia in patients with DM.[4]

References

1. Bartalena L, et al. (2016). The 2016 European Thyroid Association/European Group on Graves' Orbitopathy (EUGOGO) Guidelines for the management of Graves' orbitopathy. Eur Thyroid J 5, 9–26.
2. Marcocci C, et al. (2011). Selenium and the course of mild Graves' orbitopathy. N Engl J Med 364, 1920–31.
3. Wiersinga WM (2017). Advances in treatment of active, moderate-to-severe Graves' ophthalmopathy. Lancet Diabetes Endocrinol 5, 134–42.
4. Smith TJ, et al. (2017). Teprotumumab for thyroid-associated ophthalmopathy. N Engl J Med 376, 1748–61.

Surgical treatment of Graves' orbitopathy

(See Table 1.18.)

Shared decision-making is recommended for selecting 2nd-line treatments, including a 2nd course of IV GCs, PO GCs combined with orbital radiotherapy or mycophenolate mofetil, azathioprine, ciclosporin, rituximab, or watchful waiting. Rehabilitative treatment (orbital decompression surgery, squint surgery, or eyelid surgery) is needed in the majority of patients when GO has been conservatively managed and inactivated by immunosuppressive treatment.[1,2,3]

Surgery for decompression

- Orbital decompression may be indicated for urgent treatment of optic neuropathy.
- Posteromedial wall of orbit usually removed.
- Complications include dysmotility of the eye, blindness, orbital cellulitis, cerebrospinal fluid (CSF) leak, cerebral haematoma, obstruction to nasolacrimal flow, and anosmia.

Surgery for strabismus

- Should be performed after any necessary orbital decompression.
- Aims to allow correct binocular vision.
- Is performed when eyes are in a quiescent phase for at least 6 months after active disease.
- Involves alteration, loosening, or tightening of eye muscles, often over several operations, to improve binocular vision.

Eyelid surgery

The final stage of any surgical approach and aims to adjust upper and lower eyelid position to improve comfort and appearance.

Table 1.18 Treatment of Graves' orbitopathy

General measures

- Stop smoking.
- Dark glasses, with eye protection.
- Control thyroid function to maintain strict euthyroidism.
- Prisms for diplopia.
- Consider selenium supplements.

Specific measures

Problem	Treatment
Grittiness	Artificial tears and simple eye ointment
Eyelid retraction	Tape eyelids at night to avoid corneal damage
	Surgery if risk of exposure keratopathy
Proptosis	Head elevation during sleep
	Diuretics
	Systemic steroids
	Radiotherapy
	Orbital decompression
Ophthalmoplegia	Prisms in the acute phase
	Orbital decompression
	Orbital muscle surgery
Optic neuropathy	Systemic steroids
	Radiotherapy
	Orbital decompression

References

1. Zhou X, et al. (2020). Treatment strategies for Graves' ophthalmopathy: a network meta-analysis. *Br J Ophthalmol* **104**, 551–6.
2. Rajendram R, et al. (2018). Combined immunosuppression and radiotherapy in thyroid eye disease (CIRTED): a multicentre, 2 × 2 factorial, double-blind, randomised controlled trial. *Lancet Diabetes Endocrinol* **6**, 299–309.
3. Kahaly GJ, et al. (2018). Mycophenolate plus methylprednisolone versus methylprednisolone alone in active, moderate-to-severe Graves' orbitopathy (MINGO): a randomised, observer-masked, multicentre trial. *Lancet Diabetes Endocrinol* **6**, 287–98.

Further reading

Taylor PN, et al. (2020). New insights into the pathogenesis and nonsurgical management of Graves' orbitopathy. *Nat Rev Endocrinol* **16**, 104–16.

Thyroid dermopathy and acropachy

Graves' dermopathy

- This is a rare complication of Graves' thyrotoxicosis (0.5%). It is usually pretibial in location (99%) and hence called *pretibial myxoedema*.
- Associated with ophthalmopathy (97%) and acropachy (18%).
- It typically appears as raised, discoloured, and indurated lesions on the front or back of the legs or on the dorsum of the feet and has occasionally been described in other areas, including the hands and face.
- The lesions are due to localized accumulation of *GAGs*. It is now recognized that there is a lymphocytic infiltrate. Lesions are characteristically asymptomatic, but they can also be pruritic and tender. They can be very disfiguring.
- *Treatment.* Usually not treated. Potent topical fluorinated steroids, such as fluocinolone acetonide, may be effective (4–8 weeks), not only in the treatment of localized pain and tenderness, but also in some resolution of visible skin signs. Surgery may worsen the condition.
- Twenty-five per cent remit completely; 50% are chronic on no therapy. A beneficial effect of topical steroids on remission rates is unproven.

Thyroid acropachy

- This is the rarest manifestation of Graves' disease.
- It presents as clubbing of the digits and subperiosteal new bone formation. The soft tissue swelling is similar to that seen in localized myxoedema and consists of GAG accumulation.
  - Patients almost inevitably have GO or pretibial myxoedema. If not, an alternative cause of clubbing should be looked for.
- It is typically painless, and there is no effective treatment.

Further reading

Fatourechi V (2012). Thyroid dermopathy and acropachy. *Best Pract Res Clin Endocrinol Metab* **26**, 553–65.

Goitre

- Goitre defines a thyroid enlargement above the gender- and age-specific reference range.
- Goitre can arise from very different pathological conditions and may present with euthyroidism, hypothyroidism, or hyperthyroidism (see Box 1.7 for aetiology).
- The commonest thyroid disease in the community is simple (diffuse) physiological goitre. Ultrasonography results in much higher estimates of goitre prevalence than by physical examination.
- Diffuse goitre declines with age, and the greatest prevalence is in premenopausal ♀, and the ratio of ♀: ♂ is at least 4:1. In the Whickham survey, among ♀, 26% had a goitre; the frequency ranged from 31% in those aged <45 years (mostly diffuse) to 12% in those aged >75 years (who had a higher proportion of nodular goitre).
- Goitre prevalence is an index of the degree of long-standing iodine deficiency but is less sensitive than urinary iodine in the evaluation of a recent change in the status of iodine nutrition. The overall prevalence of goitre in iodine-replete populations is <5%.

> **Box 1.7 Aetiology of goitre**
> - Simple goitre.
> - AITD (Hashimoto's thyroiditis or Graves' disease).
> - Nodular thyroid disease.
> - Endemic (iodine deficiency, dietary origins, e.g. *Brassica* vegetables).
> - Pregnancy.
> - Thyroid cancer.
> - Drug-induced (ATDs, lithium, amiodarone).
> - Thyroiditis syndromes.
> - Thyroid hormone resistance.
> - TSHoma.
> - Acromegaly (IGF-1-dependent).
> - Thyroid hormone biosynthesis defects (mutations in *NIS*, Tg, *TPO*, and *THOX* genes).

Iodine status

- Iodine is an essential component of the thyroid hormones T_4 and T_3 produced by the thyroid gland.
- The ideal dietary allowance of iodine recommended by World Health Organization (WHO) in adults is 150 micrograms of iodine per day, which increases to 250 micrograms per day in pregnancy and lactation.
- Iodine deficiency impairs thyroid hormone production and has adverse effects throughout life, particularly early in life as it impairs cognition and growth.
- Iodine deficiency is recognized as a global problem, with large populations at risk who are living in an environment where the soil has been deprived of iodine. The mountainous regions of Europe, the Northern Indian subcontinent, the extensive mountain ranges of China, the Andean region in South America, and the lesser ranges of Africa are all iodine-deficient.

- Iodine deficiency remains despite efforts to increase iodine intake primarily through the voluntary or mandatory iodization of salt. Recent epidemiological data suggest that iodine deficiency is an emerging issue in industrialized countries such as the UK, previously thought of as iodine-sufficient.
- Iodine supplementation with potassium iodide 150 micrograms daily is recommended preconception and during pregnancy.

Further reading

Harding KB, et al. (2017). Iodine supplementation for women during the preconception, pregnancy and postpartum period. *Cochrane Database Syst Rev* **3**, CD011761.

Vanderpump MP (2017). Epidemiology of iodine deficiency. *Minerva Med* **108**, 116–23.

Thyroid multinodular goitre and solitary adenomas

Background

Nodular thyroid disease denotes the presence of single or multiple palpable or non-palpable nodules within the thyroid gland.

- Prevalence rates range from 5% to 50%, depending on the population studied and the sensitivity of detection methods. Prevalence increases linearly with age, exposure to ionizing radiation, and iodine deficiency.
- Clinically apparent thyroid nodules are evident in ~5% of the UK population.
- Incidence of thyroid nodules is about 4× more in ♀.
- Thyroid nodules always raise the concern of cancer, but <5% are cancerous.

(See Table 1.19 for the aetiology of thyroid nodules.)

Table 1.19 Aetiology of thyroid nodules

Common causes	Uncommon causes
• Colloid nodule	• Granulomatous thyroiditis
• Cyst	• Infections
• Lymphocytic thyroiditis	• Malignancy:
• Benign neoplasms:	• Medullary
• Hürthle cell	• Anaplastic
• Follicular	• Metastatic
• Malignancy:	• Lymphoma
• Papillary	
• Follicular	

Pathology

- Thyroid nodules may be described as *adenomas* if the follicular cell differentiation is enclosed within a capsule, and *adenomatous* when the lesions are circumscribed but not encapsulated.
- The commonest benign thyroid tumours are the nodules of multinodular goitres (colloid nodules) and follicular adenomas. The oncogene changes accounting for these benign thyroid nodules are not well delineated. Multinodular goitres are occasionally familial, which means that the patient has at least one germline mutation. One familial form of non-toxic multinodular goitre has been linked to DNA markers on chromosome 14q, but the aetiologic gene is not known. Follicular adenomas are clonal, and ~25% of sporadic follicular adenomas have a hemizygous deletion of a chromosome region containing *PTEN* (*MMAC1*), the tumour suppressor gene in which germline defects cause Cowden syndrome (see ➲ Cowden syndrome, pp. 670–1).
- Autonomously functioning thyroid adenomas (or nodules) are benign tumours that produce thyroid hormone. Clinically, they present as a single nodule that is hyperfunctioning ('hot') on thyroid radionuclide scan, sometimes causing hyperthyroidism. Many of these tumours are caused by somatic mutations in genes that code for the TSH receptor and the α subunit of guanyl nucleotide stimulatory protein (Gs).

- Activating mutations of the TSH receptor produce constitutive activation of adenylyl cyclase in the absence of TSH. The thyroid follicular cell with this TSH receptor mutation divides and produces thyroid hormone without TSH stimulation, eventually becoming clinically recognized as a hot nodule. Among patients with an autonomously functioning thyroid adenoma, the frequency of TSH receptor mutations in the adenoma varies from ~5% to 80%. Since the mutations are scattered throughout the receptor, studies of the entire receptor are most likely to identify a mutation. In rare families, germline mutations in the TSH receptor cause hereditary hyperthyroidism, initially with a diffuse goitre, but ultimately with a nodular goitre with multiple hot nodules.

Clinical evaluation

- An asymptomatic thyroid mass may be discovered either by a clinician on routine neck palpation or by the patient during self-examination. It is most commonly detected incidentally while imaging for another aetiology.
- History should concentrate on:
  - An enlarging thyroid mass.
  - A previous history of radiation, especially childhood head and neck irradiation.
  - A family history of thyroid cancer.
  - The development of hoarseness or dysphagia.
- Nodules are more likely to be malignant in patients <20 or >60 years.
- Thyroid nodules are commoner in ♀, but more likely to be malignant in ♂.
- The risk of malignancy is similar in a patient with a single or multiple nodules. Thus, a dominant nodule in a multinodular goitre should be evaluated as if it were a single nodule.
- Physical findings suggestive of malignancy include a firm or hard, non-tender nodule, a recent history of enlargement, fixation to adjacent tissue, and the presence of regional lymphadenopathy.
- *Pemberton's sign* is facial erythema and jugular venous distension on raising the arms. It is a sign of superior vena caval obstruction caused by a substernal mass.
- A hot nodule on a radioisotope scan makes malignancy less likely.
- Clinical features that raise suspicion of malignancy include (see Table 1.20):
  - Age (childhood or elderly).
  - Short history of enlarging nodule.
  - Local symptoms, including dysphagia, stridor, or hoarseness.
  - Previous exposure to radiation.
  - +ve family history of thyroid cancer or multiple endocrine neoplasia (MEN) syndrome.
  - Gardner's syndrome (familial large intestinal polyposis).
  - Familial polyposis coli.
  - Cowden syndrome (autosomal dominantly inherited multiple hamartomas and breast, thyroid, and other tumours) (see ➲ Cowden syndrome, pp. 670–1).
  - Lymphadenopathy.
  - History of Hashimoto's disease (↑ incidence of lymphoma).
  - ↑ serum TSH.

Table 1.20 Clinical features indicating malignancy or benignity

Increasing suspicion of malignancy	Favouring a benign goitre
Age <20 or >50 years	Age 20–50 years
Men	Women
Mild hypothyroidism	Hyperthyroidism
Cervical lymphadenopathy	Multinodular goitre without dominant nodule
Firm, hard, irregular, fixed nodule	Soft, smooth, mobile nodule
Family history of thyroid cancer, including men	Family history of benign thyroid nodule or thyroid autoimmunity
History of external neck radiotherapy	Associated pain or tenderness
Dysphagia/hoarseness/stridor	Compression symptoms rare

Investigations
- FNAC (see ➋ Fine needle aspiration cytology, pp. 24–5).
- Serum TSH concentration.
- Respiratory flow loop, especially for a large goitre possibly causing tracheal obstruction.
- CT scan or MRI if there are concerns about retrosternal goitre or tracheal compression.

Treatment
Toxic multinodular goitre or nodule

Antithyroid drugs

ATDs are effective in controlling the hyperthyroidism but are not curative. As the hot nodules are autonomous, the condition will recur after stopping the drugs. Carbimazole is a useful treatment to gain control of the disease in preparation for surgery or as long-term treatment in those patients unwilling to accept radioiodine or surgery.

Radioiodine
- This form of treatment is often considered as 1st choice for definitive treatment. ^{131}I is preferentially accumulated in hot nodules, but not in normal thyroid tissue which, because of the thyrotoxic state, is non-functioning.
- Radioiodine treatment commonly induces a euthyroid state, as the hot nodules are destroyed and the previously non-functioning follicles gradually resume normal function. A dose of 500–800MBq for small to medium, and 600 or 800MBq for medium to large, goitres is recommended.

Surgery
- The aim of surgery is to remove as much of the nodular tissue as possible and, if the goitre is large, to relieve local symptoms. Post-operative follow-up should involve checks of thyroid function.
- Goitre recurrence, although rare, does occasionally occur.

Non-toxic multinodular goitre

Surgery
- The preferred treatment for patients with:
  - Local compression symptoms.
  - Cosmetic disfigurement.
- Solitary nodule with FNAC suspicious of malignancy.

Radioiodine
- Radioiodine may be particularly indicated in elderly patients in whom surgery is not appropriate. It may require admission. Up to 50% shrinkage of goitre mass has been reported in recent studies.
- Hypothyroidism following radioiodine occurs in 20%.

Radiofrequency ablation (RFA)
- US-guided RFA after local anaesthesia is a new technique that has been demonstrated to shrink benign thyroid nodules. In a recent study of 215 patients, there was an early significant reduction of nodule volume at 1 year, lasting up to 5 years. A 67% nodule shrinkage was observed at the end of the observation period. The best response was recorded in nodules below 10mL (79% early reduction and 81% at 5 years). Patients' symptoms were significantly reduced.

Medical treatment
Use of levothyroxine to suppress TSH is associated with a risk of cardiac arrhythmias and bone loss. Levothyroxine is useful only if serum TSH is detectable but is not generally indicated.

Thyroid nodules in pregnant women
- Where necessary, US-guided FNA is needed to exclude malignancy.
- Most thyroid cancers detected during pregnancy will not grow nor pose significant risk during gestation, and thyroid surgery in pregnant ♀ poses higher risks than in non-pregnant ♀.
- If necessary, can be operated upon in 2nd trimester or preferably post-partum.

Further reading
Angell TE, Alexander EK (2019). Thyroid nodules and thyroid cancer in the pregnant woman. *Endocrinol Metab Clin North Am* **48**, 557–67.

Bonnema SJ, et al. (2014). The role of radioiodine therapy in benign nodular goitre. *Best Pract Res Clin Endocrinol Metab* **28**, 619–31.

Deandrea M, et al. (2019). Long-term efficacy of a single session of RFA for benign thyroid nodules: a longitudinal 5-year observational study. *J Clin Endocrinol Metab* **104**, 3751–6.

Ferraz C, Paschke R (2017). Inheritable and sporadic non-autoimmune hyperthyroidism. *Best Pract Res Clin Endocrinol Metab* **31**, 265–75.

Knobel M (2016). Etiopathology, clinical features, and treatment of diffuse and multinodular nontoxic goiters. *J Endocrinol Invest* **39**, 357–73.

Lueblinghoff J, et al. (2011). Shared sporadic and somatic thyrotropin receptor mutations display more active in vitro activities than familial thyrotropin receptor mutations. *Thyroid* **21**, 221–9.

McLeod DS, et al. (2012). Thyrotropin and thyroid cancer diagnosis: a systematic review and dose–response meta-analysis. *J Clin Endocrinol Metab* **97**, 2682–92.

Paschke R, et al. (2012). 2012 European Thyroid Association guidelines for the management of familial and persistent sporadic non-autoimmune hyperthyroidism caused by thyroid-stimulating hormone receptor germline mutations. *Eur Thyroid J* **1**, 142–7.

Thyroiditis

Background

Inflammation of the thyroid gland is characterized by hyperthyroidism due to release of pre-formed hormones. The ↑ concentration of thyroid hormone suppresses serum TSH. RAI uptake is close to nil in all cases when hyperthyroidism is present. The duration of hyperthyroidism is generally 2–3 months and limited by the amount of thyroid hormone present. The ratio of serum $T_3:T_4$ is lower in destructive thyroiditis than in Graves' disease. Hypothyroidism is common after the hyperthyroid phase. In some patients, only the hyperthyroid or hypothyroid phase is noted. Permanent hypothyroidism can complicate some forms of destructive thyroiditis more than others.

In most cases, specific therapy is not necessary during the hyperthyroid phase, although β-adrenergic antagonists can be helpful for those with significant symptoms. GCs may decrease the duration of the clinical syndrome but are rarely necessary in painful or painless subacute thyroiditis. Post-partum thyroiditis is the commonest variant of a painless subacute thyroiditis, occurring in ~5% of all post-partum women in iodine-sufficient areas. The presence of pain in patients with destructive thyroiditis is generally considered an important diagnostic point and is usually post-viral and self-limited with a granulomatous histology. Painless thyroiditis is usually considered to be autoimmune and to require long-term surveillance.

A destructive thyroiditis occurs in a significant number of patients treated with immune checkpoint inhibitors (immunomodularity antibodies) which have substantially improved the prognosis for patients with advanced melanoma and a number of other malignancies.

Overt hypothyroidism caused by autoimmunity has two main forms: *Hashimoto's (goitrous) thyroiditis* and *atrophic thyroiditis* (see Tables 1.21 and 1.22).

Table 1.21 Causes and characteristics of thyroiditis

Cause	Characteristic features
Autoimmune thyroiditis (Hashimoto's)	Grossly lymphocytic and fibrotic hypothyroidism or thyrotoxicosis
Post-partum thyroiditis	Lymphocytic thyroiditis, transient thyrotoxicosis or hypothyroidism
Drug-induced	Iodine excess, amiodarone, lithium, interferon-alfa, TKIs, and immune checkpoint inhibitors
Subacute (de Quervain's)	Thought to be viral in origin, multinuclear giant cells
Riedel's thyroiditis	Extensive fibrosis of the thyroid
Radiation thyroiditis	Radiation injury, transient thyrotoxicosis
Pyogenic (rare)	*Staphylococcus aureus*, streptococci, *Escherichia coli*, tuberculosis, fungal

Table 1.22 Clinical presentation of thyroiditis

Form of thyroiditis	Clinical presentation	Thyroid function
Suppurative (acute)	Painful, tender thyroid, fever	Usually normal
Subacute (de Quervain's)	Painful anterior neck, arthralgia, antecedent upper respiratory tract infection, generalized malaise	Early thyrotoxicosis, occasionally late hypothyroidism
Autoimmune	Hashimoto's: goitre	Usually hypothyroid
	Atrophic: no goitre	Sometimes euthyroid
		Rarely early thyrotoxicosis
Riedel's	Hard, woody consistency of the thyroid	Usually normal

Chronic autoimmune (atrophic or Hashimoto's) thyroiditis

(See Tables 1.21 and 1.22.)

- *Hashimoto's thyroiditis.* Characterized by a painless, variably sized goitre with a rubbery consistency and an irregular surface. The normal follicular structure of the gland is extensively replaced by lymphocytic and plasma cell infiltrates, with the formation of lymphoid germinal centres. The patient may have normal thyroid function or subclinical or overt hypothyroidism. Occasionally, patients present with thyrotoxicosis in association with a thyroid gland that is unusually firm and with high titres of circulating antithyroid antibodies.
- *Atrophic thyroiditis.* Probably indicates end-stage thyroid disease. These patients do not have a goitre and are antibody +ve. Biochemically, the picture is that of frank hypothyroidism.

Investigations

Investigations which are useful in establishing a diagnosis of Hashimoto's thyroiditis include:

- Testing of thyroid function.
- Thyroid antibodies (TgAb +ve in 20–25% and TPOAb in >90%).
- Occasionally, thyroid biopsy to exclude malignancy in patients who present with a goitre and a dominant nodule.

Prognosis

The long-term prognosis of patients with chronic thyroiditis is good because hypothyroidism can be corrected easily with levothyroxine and the goitre is not usually of sufficient size to cause local symptoms. In the atypical situation where Hashimoto's thyroiditis presents with a rapidly enlarging goitre and pain, a short course of prednisolone at a dose of 40mg daily may prove helpful.

Any unusual increase in size of the thyroid in patients known to suffer from Hashimoto's thyroiditis should be investigated with an FNA and, possibly later, a biopsy since there is an association between this condition and thyroid lymphoma (rare, but risk ↑ by a factor of 70).

Other types of thyroiditis

Silent (autoimmune) thyroiditis

Associated with transient thyrotoxicosis or hypothyroidism. A significant percentage of patients have a personal or family history of AITD. It may progress to permanent hypothyroidism. There is depressed radionuclide uptake.

Post-partum thyroiditis

Thyroid dysfunction occurring within the first 6 months post-partum. Clinical features often mild and include goitre, with mood disorder. Prevalence ranges from 5% to 7%. Post-partum thyroiditis (PPT) develops in 40–60% of ♀ who have +ve TPOAb; 25% have hyperthyroid phase, and the remainder only hypothyroid. Most euthyroid in 12 months, but 20–40% permanent hypothyroid in 3–12 years. ↑ rates in T1DM (up to 25%) and previous PPT (42%). Differential includes Graves' disease, and TRAb is useful. Consider screening in high-risk cases.

Chronic fibrosing (Riedel's) thyroiditis

A rare disorder characterized by intense fibrosis of the thyroid gland and surrounding structures, leading to induration of the tissues of the neck. May be associated with mediastinal and retroperitoneal fibrosis, salivary gland fibrosis, sclerosing cholangitis, lacrimal gland fibrosis, and parathyroid gland fibrosis leading to hypoparathyroidism. Excessive numbers of IgG4 +ve plasma cells in clinically diagnostic thyroid histology samples by immunohistochemistry have been demonstrated in some cases. Patients are usually euthyroid. Main differential diagnosis is thyroid neoplasia.

Management

Recognition of certain clinical finding patterns will increase the likelihood of recognizing Riedel's thyroiditis promptly. Local restrictive or infiltrative symptoms out of proportion to a demonstrable mass or simultaneous biochemical deficiencies, especially of Ca, should lead the clinician to consider this diagnosis. Corticosteroids are usually ineffective. Surgery may be required to relieve obstruction and to exclude malignancy. Tamoxifen may be of benefit.

Pyogenic thyroiditis

- Rare. Usually anteceded by a pyogenic infection elsewhere.
  Characterized by tenderness and swelling of the thyroid gland, redness and warmth of the overlying skin, and constitutional signs of infection.
- Piriform sinus infection should be excluded. Excision of tract is preferable to incision and drainage.
- Treatment consists of antibiotic therapy and incision and drainage should a fluctuant area within the thyroid occur.

Subacute thyroiditis (granulomatous, giant cell, or de Quervain's thyroiditis)

- Viral in origin. Symptoms include pronounced asthenia, malaise, pain over the thyroid, or pain referred to the lower jaw, ear, or occiput. Less commonly, the onset is acute, with fever, pain over the thyroid, and symptoms of thyrotoxicosis. Characteristically, signs include exquisite tenderness and nodularity of the thyroid gland. There is characteristically elevated erythrocyte sedimentation rate (ESR)/C-reactive protein (CRP) and depressed radionuclide (^{99m}Tc can be used) uptake. Biochemically, the patient may be initially thyrotoxic, though later the patient may become transiently hypothyroid, and permanent hypothyroidism is reported in 5%.
- In mild cases, non-steroidal anti-inflammatory agents and paracetamol offer symptom relief. In severe cases, GCs (prednisolone 20–40mg/day) are effective. Propranolol can be used to control associated thyrotoxicosis. Treatment can be withdrawn when T_4 returns to normal. Levothyroxine replacement is required if the patient becomes hypothyroid. Treatment with carbimazole or PTU is not indicated.

Drug-induced thyroiditis

Causes
- Amiodarone.
- Lithium.
- Interferon-alfa (15% develop TPOAb and/or thyroid dysfunction).
- Interleukin 2.

Immune checkpoint inhibitors

Cancer cells 'hide' from the immune system by keeping immune cells from recognizing tumour cells. 'Checkpoints' on T-cells act as 'brakes' on their aggressiveness, including programmed death 1 (PD-1) and CTLA-4.
- Ipilimumab and tremelimumab block CTLA-4, allowing activated T-cells to proliferate, which enables targeting of otherwise poorly immunogenic tumour antigens to cancer cells. Effective in metastatic melanoma.
- Pembrolizumab and nivolumab inhibit interaction between PD-1 and its ligands and increase immune response against cancer cells. Effective against non-small cell lung cancer, renal and bladder cancer, and Hodgkin's lymphoma.
- Hypophysitis, thyroid dysfunction, insulin-deficient DM, and 1° AI have been reported. Hypophysitis is particularly associated with anti-CTLA-4 therapy, whereas thyroid dysfunction is particularly associated with anti-PD-1 therapy.
- Associated with transient thyrotoxicosis, transient or permanent hypothyroidism, orbitopathy, painless thyroiditis, and rarely thyroid storm.
- Incidence of 1–6% with ipilimumab, nivolumab, and tremelimumab.
- Hyperthyroidism (9.9%) and hypothyroidism (22%) when ipilimumab and nivolumab combined.
- Incidence of hypothyroidism of 5–7% with pembrolizumab.

- Incidence of side effects of pembrolizumab and nivolumab varies according to the malignancy being treated. In advanced lung cancer, thyroid dysfunction in 10–15% of cases.
- Time of onset 2–4 cycles of therapy but may be delayed.
- Cancer patients who develop thyroid dysfunction following various immune agents have improved prognosis.
- Assess thyroid function and antithyroid antibodies at baseline and commence monitoring at 1 month.

Immune reconstitution therapy (IRT)

Thyroid dysfunction occurs in up to 50% of treated patients as an auto-immune complication of IRT, especially in individuals with multiple sclerosis treated with alemtuzumab, a pan-lymphocyte-depleting drug, with subsequent recovery of immune cell numbers. Less frequently, thyroid dysfunction is triggered by highly active antiretroviral therapy (HAART) in patients infected with human immunodeficiency virus (HIV) or in patients undergoing bone marrow/haematopoietic stem cell transplantation (BMT/HSCT).

- In both alemtuzumab-induced thyroid dysfunction and HIV/HAART patients, the commonest disorder is Graves' disease, followed by hypothyroidism and thyroiditis, and rarely GO is observed in some Graves' disease patients.
- Hypothyroidism is commoner than Graves' disease post-BMT/HSCT, probably as a consequence of the associated radiation damage.
- In alemtuzumab-induced thyroid dysfunction, TRAbs play a major role, and two main aspects distinguish this condition from the spontaneous form:
  - Up to 20% of Graves' disease cases exhibit a fluctuating course, with alternating phases of hyper- and hypothyroidism, due to the coexistence of TRAbs with stimulating and blocking function.
  - TRAbs are also +ve in about 70% of hypothyroid patients, with blocking TRAbs responsible for nearly half of the cases.
- Post-IRT thyroid dysfunction might follow an atypical fluctuating course, necessitating appropriate diagnostic and therapeutic management. Clinical symptoms can take up to 3 months to develop following biochemical thyroid dysfunction. As a result, routine monitoring of thyroid function may mean that biochemical abnormalities are detected in the absence of clinical symptoms.
- If Graves' disease confirmed, commence trial of ATD after 3 months (excluding patients symptomatic and/or high risk) and if fluctuating course, consider block-and-replace.
- Commence levothyroxine if overt hypothyroidism, or subclinical and persistent (>3 months) and/or with symptoms.

Further reading

Chang LS, et al. (2019). Endocrine toxicity of cancer immunotherapy targeting immune checkpoints. *Endocr Rev* **40**, 17–65.

Costelloe SJ, et al. (2010). Thyroid dysfunction in a UK hepatitis C population treated with interferon-alpha and ribavirin combination therapy. *Clin Endocrinol* **73**, 249–56.

Fatourechi MM, et al. (2011). Invasive fibrous thyroiditis (Riedel thyroiditis): the Mayo Clinic experience, 1976–2008. *Thyroid* **21**, 765–72.

Ferrari SM, et al. (2018). Thyroid disorders induced by checkpoint inhibitors. *Rev Endocr Metab Disord* **19**, 325–33.

Hennessey JV (2011). Riedel's thyroiditis: a clinical review. *J Clin Endocrinol Metab* **96**, 3031–41.

Muller I, et al. (2019). 2019 European Thyroid Association guidelines on the management of thyroid dysfunction following immune reconstitution therapy. *Eur Thyroid J* **8**, 173–85.

Paes JE, et al. (2010). Acute bacterial suppurative thyroiditis: a clinical review and expert opinion. *Thyroid* **20**, 247–55.

Tran HA, et al. (2013). Thyroid disease in chronic hepatitis C infection treated with combination interferon-α and ribavirin: management strategies and future perspective. *Endocr Pract* **19**, 292–300.

Hypothyroidism

Background

Hypothyroidism results from a variety of abnormalities that cause insufficient secretion of thyroid hormones (see Table 1.23). The commonest cause is AITD. *Myxoedema* is severe hypothyroidism in which there is accumulation of hydrophilic mucopolysaccharides in the ground substance of the dermis and other tissues, leading to thickening of the facial features and a doughy induration of the skin. (See Box 1.3 for pitfalls with the TFTs in NTI.)

Epidemiology

- High TSH in 7.5% of ♀ and 2.5% of ♂ >65 years, 1.7% overt hypothyroidism, and 13.7% subclinical hypothyroidism (Whickham survey, UK).
- Incidence higher in whites than in Hispanics or African-American populations.
- Incidence higher in areas of high iodine intake.

Clinical picture

Adult

- Insidious, non-specific onset.
- Fatigue, lethargy, constipation, cold intolerance, muscle stiffness, cramps, carpal tunnel syndrome, menorrhagia, later oligo- or amenorrhoea.
- Slowing of intellectual and motor activities.
- ↓ appetite and weight gain.
- Dry skin; hair loss.
- Deep hoarse voice, ↓ VA.
- Obstructive sleep apnoea.

Myxoedema

- Dull, expressionless face, sparse hair, periorbital puffiness, macroglossia.
- Pale, cool skin that feels rough and doughy.
- Enlarged heart (dilation and pericardial effusion).
- Megacolon/intestinal obstruction.
- Cerebellar ataxia.
- Prolonged relaxation phase of deep tendon reflexes.
- Peripheral neuropathy.
- Encephalopathy.
- Hyperlipidaemia.
- Hypercarotenaemia (also caused by hyperlipidaemia, DM, anorexia, and porphyria).
- Psychiatric symptoms, e.g. depression, psychosis.
- Marked respiratory depression with ↑ arterial pCO_2.
- Hyponatraemia from impaired water excretion and disordered regulation of vasopressin secretion.

Myxoedema coma

- Predisposed to by cold exposure, trauma, infection, and administration of CNS depressants.

Table 1.23 Classification of causes of hypothyroidism

	TSH	FT$_4$
Non-goitrous	↑	↓
Post-ablative (radioiodine, surgery)		
Congenital development defect		
Atrophic thyroiditis		
Post-radiation (e.g. for lymphoma)		
Goitrous	↑	↓
Chronic thyroiditis (Hashimoto's thyroiditis)		
Transient, 2–8 weeks (de Quervain's thyroiditis)		
Severe iodine deficiency		
Drug-elicited (amiodarone, aminosalicylic acid, iodides, phenylbutazone, lithium, aminoglutethimide, interferon-alfa, thalidomide, sunitinib, rifampicin, stavudine)		
Haemochromatosis		
Heritable biosynthetic defects		
Maternally transmitted (antithyroid agents, iodides)		
Pituitary	↓	↓
Panhypopituitarism		
Isolated TSH deficiency		
Drugs (bexarotene)		
Hypothalamic	↓	↓
Neoplasm		
Infiltrative (sarcoidosis)		
Congenital defects		
Infection (encephalitis)		
Self-limiting	↑	↓
Following withdrawal of suppressive thyroid therapy		
Subacute thyroiditis and chronic thyroiditis with transient hypothyroidism		
Post-partum thyroiditis		

Subclinical hypothyroidism

- This term is used to denote raised TSH levels in the presence of normal concentrations of free thyroid hormones.
- Treatment may be indicated if the biochemistry is sustained in patients with a past history of radioiodine treatment for thyrotoxicosis or +ve thyroid antibodies as in these situations, progression to overt hypothyroidism is almost inevitable (at least 5% per year of those with +ve TPOAb).
- Two samples should be taken 2–3 months apart to distinguish from NTI.
- The reference range for serum TSH rises with age.
- There is controversy over the advantages of levothyroxine treatment in patients with −ve thyroid antibodies and no previous radioiodine treatment.
- If treatment is not given, follow-up with annual TFTs is important.
- There is no generally accepted consensus of when patients should receive treatment. Some authorities suggest treatment when serum TSH is >10mU/L because of ↑ rate of progression to overt hypothyroidism. Below that, if TSH is raised, treatment is geared to the individual patient.
- ↑ incidence of cardiovascular risk if <65 years old.
- There is some evidence that women with autoimmune thyroiditis are more likely to have an ↑ risk of recurrent miscarriage, although it is not known whether the risk is related to thyroid autoimmunity or to subtle thyroid failure. In this situation, there may be an advantage to giving levothyroxine if TSH is >4mU/L.
- Acceleration of thyroid hormone metabolism during pregnancy can lead to hypothyroidism in women with limited thyroid hormone reserve. If untreated, mild hypothyroidism can lead to subtle impairment of subsequent childhood neuropsychological development. Early correction of maternal hypothyroxinaemia is recommended, aiming to maintain serum TSH in the lower half of the reference range prior to conception, if possible.

Management

- If serum TSH is >10mU/L, then levothyroxine is indicated.
- If serum TSH is mildly ↑ between 4 and 10mU/L and the patient is TPOAb +ve, an annual check of serum TSH is recommended, with commencement of levothyroxine once serum TSH >10mU/L.
- If the patient is thyroid antibody −ve, then ensuring a check of serum TSH every 3–5 years is all that is required.
- If the patient with serum TSH 4–10mU/L has symptoms consistent with hypothyroidism and TSH elevation persists, then a 3-month therapeutic trial of levothyroxine appears justified. If the patient feels improved by therapy, it is reasonable to continue treatment.
- If the patient with serum TSH 4–10mU/L does not have symptoms and the serum TSH level appears stable with +ve TPOAb, the annual risk of progression to overt hypothyroidism is 4% per year, and so an annual serum TSH surveillance strategy is warranted. If TPOAb −ve, then 3-yearly serum TSH surveillance is recommended, with a risk of progression to overt hypothyroidism of 3% per year.

- The exception to the above is in neonates and children, pregnancy, or someone trying to conceive when mildly ↑ serum TSH >4mU/L should always be treated, as it is associated with adverse outcomes for both mother and fetus.
- Levothyroxine treatment for those with serum TSH 4–10mU/L may be justified in subjects <65 years and in those older subjects with documented evidence of heart failure on echocardiography.

Further reading

Cappola AR, et al. (2015). Thyroid function in the euthyroid range and adverse outcomes in older adults. *J Clin Endocrinol Metab* **100**, 1088–96.

Casey BM, et al. (2017). Treatment of subclinical hypothyroidism or hypothyroxinemia in pregnancy. *N Engl J Med* **376**, 815–25.

Maraka S, et al. (2017). Thyroid hormone treatment among pregnant women with subclinical hypothyroidism: US national assessment. *BMJ* **356**, i6865.

Okosieme OE, et al. (2018). Preconception management of thyroid dysfunction. *Clin Endocrinol* **89**, 269–79.

Pearce SH, et al. (2013). 2013 ETA Guideline: management of subclinical hypothyroidism. *Eur Thyroid J* **2**, 215–28.

Rodondi N, et al. (2010). Subclinical hypothyroidism and the risk of coronary heart disease and mortality. *JAMA* **304**, 1365–74.

Stott DJ, et al. (2017). TRUST Study Group: thyroid hormone therapy for older adults with subclinical hypothyroidism. *N Engl J Med* **376**, 2534–44.

Teng W, et al. (2013). Hypothyroidism in pregnancy. *Lancet Diabetes Endocrinol* **1**, 228–37.

Treatment of hypothyroidism

Note that patients in the UK with hypothyroidism are entitled to a medical exemption certificate for prescription charges.

- Thyroid hormone replacement with synthetic levothyroxine remains the treatment of choice in 1° hypothyroidism.
- Levothyroxine with a long half-life enables the patient to take two doses at once if a dose is omitted.
- Normal metabolic state should be restored gradually, as a rapid increase in metabolic rate may precipitate cardiac arrhythmias.
- The average replacement dose is 1.6–1.8 micrograms/kg/day.
- To avoid iatrogenic subclinical disease, fasting ingestion of levothyroxine is best either in the morning or in the evening.
- In the younger patients, start levothyroxine at 50–100 micrograms. In the elderly with a history of ischaemic heart disease (IHD), an initial dose of levothyroxine of 25–50 micrograms can be ↑ by 25-microgram increments at 4-weekly intervals until normal metabolic state and TSH are attained.
- Optimum dose is determined by clinical criteria, with the objective of treatment being to restore serum TSH to the normal range.
- TSH should be checked 6 weeks after any dose change. Once stabilized, serum TSH should be checked on an annual basis.
- For the vast majority of patients on levothyroxine, brand or named supplier prescribing is not considered necessary. The Medicines and Healthcare Products Regulatory Agency (MHRA) have made recommendations to ensure the quality and consistency of levothyroxine tablets that are on the UK market. Rarely, patients may require a specific brand of levothyroxine to be prescribed due to intolerance of generic preparations. Checking excipient contents can be helpful.
- ↑ monitoring of patients with hypothyroidism may demonstrate greater fluctuations in thyroid levels than previously realized, accompanied by a tendency for micromanagement of levothyroxine dosing in 1° care, whether or not this is indicated by a patient's presenting symptoms.
- Symptoms such as lethargy or myalgia may take up to 6 months to fully recover.
- In those patients who remain symptomatic and in whom serum TSH remains towards the upper end of the reference range, it is usual practice for the dose of levothyroxine to be ↑ slightly to target a serum TSH level at the lower end of the reference range (≤2.5mU/L). However, such small changes in serum TSH within the reference range are not associated with improvement in symptoms in randomized clinical trials.
- Patients with iatrogenic hyperthyroidism (serum TSH <0.03 mU/L) have an ↑ risk of arrhythmia and fractures.
- In patients with 2° hypothyroidism, FT_4 is the most useful parameter to follow.
- Dose requirements can increase by 25–50 micrograms in pregnancy due to the increase in TBG. Data have shown that mild maternal hypothyroidism in the 1st trimester is associated with slightly impaired cognitive function in offspring. Thus, it is now recommended to routinely increase levothyroxine dose by 25 micrograms in any ♀ on replacement therapy when she learns she is pregnant.

Controversies in management

1. A normal serum TSH level excludes primary hypothyroidism

- The diagnosis of 1° hypothyroidism is based on clinical features supported by biochemical evidence of elevated serum TSH and low or normal FT_4.
- As the symptoms of hypothyroidism overlap with those of a variety of chronic disease states, 1° hypothyroidism should not be diagnosed on the basis of symptoms alone in individuals with a normal serum TSH level. Such practice may lead to an erroneous label of hypothyroidism in a patient with another condition and will ultimately result in dissatisfaction with levothyroxine therapy.
- UK national audit data suggest that over 10% of those begun on levothyroxine in 1° care initially had a normal serum TSH level.

2. A significant minority of patients on levothyroxine have ongoing symptoms despite 'normal' TFTs

- Non-specific symptoms such as lethargy, 'brain fog', and difficulty with weight management occur in up to 5–10% of treated hypothyroid patients with a serum TSH level within the reference range.
- Symptoms such as tiredness may have been initially misattributed to hypothyroidism (e.g. due to a mood disorder), with relatively minor biochemical abnormalities found coincidentally during diagnostic work-up with blood screening.
- Other explanations include awareness of having a chronic disease, adjustment to being euthyroid—particularly in those recently treated for hyperthyroidism—and autoimmunity. Relative risks of almost all other autoimmune diseases are significantly ↑.
- Screening for other autoimmune diseases is recommended in subjects presenting with new or non-specific symptoms. Other causes include B12 deficiency, consideration of cortisol deficiency, iron deficiency anaemia, chronic fatigue, hypercalcaemia, liver disease, and cardiac disease.

3. Measurement of serum T_3 is of no value in hypothyroidism

- Serum T_3 levels are maintained within the reference range, even in severe hypothyroidism. The measurement of T_3 is not recommended or required for the diagnosis of hypothyroidism or the monitoring of thyroid hormone replacement in known hypothyroidism as its value remains to be ascertained.
- Serum TSH remains the key biochemical indicator of thyroid function reflecting T_4 to T_3 conversion and T_3 action, so pituitary TSH secretion remains the most sensitive indicator of thyroid status.

4. Genetic characterization of type 2 deiodinase gene polymorphism is not indicated

- Limited data suggest that psychological well-being and preference for levothyroxine and liothyronine combination therapy may be influenced by polymorphisms in thyroid hormone pathway genes, specifically in thyroid hormone transporters and deiodinases.
- Genetic characterization according to type 2 deiodinase gene polymorphism status cannot guide the use of combination therapy in hypothyroidism to optimize biochemical and clinical outcomes.

- Genetic testing is not recommended as a guide to selecting therapy. The small effect of the type 2 deiodinase gene variants identified so far that do affect thyroid hormone concentrations suggests that other factors (e.g. yet unidentified genetic variants) may play a far greater role in determining an individual patient's thyroid hormone concentrations.

5. Levothyroxine and liothyronine combination therapy

- Synthetic forms of levothyroxine, available since the 1950s, were introduced without any consideration of the need for RCTs. Porcine thyroid extracts were far from physiological, as the pig thyroid produces T_4 and T_3 in a ratio of 4:1, compared with a ratio of 14:1 in human thyroid.
- Evidence appeared of potential harm from levothyroxine over-replacement, including atrial fibrillation and bone loss, particularly in post-menopausal women.
- More accurate serum TSH measurement meant that patients were prescribed lower doses of levothyroxine than in earlier decades, more closely matched to serum TSH, T_4, and T_3 levels.
- Evidence from controlled trials has shown no added benefit of combined levothyroxine and liothyronine therapy over levothyroxine monotherapy in terms of QoL, mood, or psychometric measures. In general, the clinical trials of combination therapy have not successfully replicated physiological T_4–T_3 production. Although some individuals express a preference for combined therapy, there are limited long-term safety data to support its routine use in practice.
- Specialist referral should be considered in individuals who have unambiguously not benefited from levothyroxine and have been thoroughly evaluated for alternative causes of ill-health.
- Dessicated animal thyroid extracts contain an excessive amount of T_3, not consistent with normal physiology, and are not recommended.
- Combination therapy is not recommended in patients treated for thyroid cancer, pregnancy, patients over the age of 60, or patients of any age with known heart disease, as additional care is required to avoid over-replacement.
- A decision to embark on a 6-month trial of levothyroxine/liothyronine combination therapy in patients who have unambiguously not benefited from levothyroxine alone should be reached following an open and balanced discussion of the uncertain benefits, likely risks of over-replacement, and lack of long-term safety data. Such patients should be supervised by accredited endocrinologists, with documentation of agreement after fully informed and understood discussion.
- It is suggested to start combination therapy in a levothyroxine/liothyronine dose ratio of between 10:1 and 20:1 by weight (levothyroxine od, and the daily liothyronine dose in divided doses). A fixed amount of levothyroxine 50 micrograms can be replaced by liothyronine 10 micrograms bd. Although no specific scoring system exists for reassessment at 6 months, it is recommended that the patient and doctor agree on three symptoms that can be assessed at the start and end of a 6-month trial to determine objective improvement.

Management of myxoedema coma

- Identify and treat concurrent precipitating illness.
- Antibiotic therapy after blood cultures.
- Management of hypothermia by passive external rewarming.
- Manage in intensive treatment unit (ITU) if comatose.
- Give warm, humidified oxygen (O_2) by face mask. Mechanical ventilation needed if hypoventilating.
- Aim for slow rise in core temperature (0.5°C/h).
- Cardiac monitor for supraventricular arrhythmias.
- Correct hyponatraemia (mild fluid restriction), hypotension (cautious volume expansion with crystalloid or whole blood), and hypoglycaemia (glucose administration).
- Monitor rectal temperature, O_2 saturation, BP, central venous pressure (CVP), and urine output hourly.
- Take blood samples for thyroid hormones, TSH, and cortisol before starting treatment. If suspected hypocortisolaemia, administer GCs.
- Thyroid hormone replacement: no consensus has been reached. The following is an accepted regimen:
  - T_4 300–500 micrograms IV or by NG tube as a starting dose, followed by 50–100 micrograms daily until oral medication can be taken.
  - If no improvement within 24–48h, T_3 10 micrograms IV 8-hourly or 25 micrograms IV 8-hourly can be given, in addition to above.
- Give hydrocortisone 50–100mg 6- to 8-hourly in case of cortisol deficiency.

Management of persistently elevated TSH despite levothyroxine replacement

(See Fig. 1.5.)
- As levothyroxine has a narrow therapeutic index, the margin between over- and underdosing can be small.
- Elevated TSH despite levothyroxine replacement is common, most usually due to lack of compliance.
- If TSH still elevated when levothyroxine dose at 1.6 micrograms/kg/day or higher, careful questioning of compliance is needed.
- Levothyroxine should be administered with water on an empty stomach at least 30min before breakfast and avoiding other medications, especially iron supplements and calcium salts.
- Disease states which interfere with levothyroxine absorption include coeliac disease, pernicious anaemia, gastritis, or malabsorption. Rarely, Addison's disease can present as a sudden rise in serum TSH.
- Raised FT_4 and raised serum TSH levels can be seen in a patient poorly compliant with levothyroxine who recommences levothyroxine treatment shortly before a blood test.
- TFTs should be performed at the same time of the day each time, as there is a diurnal variation in serum TSH levels.
- Consider other drugs that may interfere with levothyroxine absorption (see Box 1.8).

- Even after careful consideration of all of these factors, discrimination between an as yet unidentified cause of true thyroxine malabsorption and poor levothyroxine compliance can prove difficult. In these circumstances, a formal thyroxine absorption test may help resolve the issue. Ensure the patient is fasted from midnight, and administer the equivalent of 1.6 × body weight (kg) × 7 micrograms in liquid (preferred) or tablet rounded down to the nearest 50 micrograms, followed immediately by 200mL of water PO. Blood samples for measurement of FT_4, FT_3, and TSH should be collected at 0, 30, 45, 60, 90, 120, 240, and 360min. Continue weekly supervised administration for 6 weeks. TSH normalization confirms poor compliance, and weekly dosing can continue. Inadequate FT_4 rise suggests malabsorption, and no change in TSH requires further investigation into disorders of thyroid hormone metabolism (see Fig. 1.5).

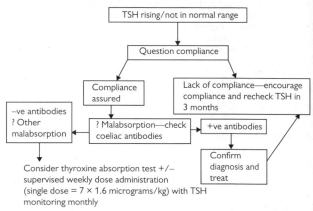

Fig. 1.5 Suggestions for investigations of elevated TSH despite levothyroxine replacement therapy to >1.6 micrograms/kg/day.

Box 1.8 **Interference with absorption of levothyroxine**

- Coeliac disease.
- Drugs: ↑ clearance of thyroxine—rifampicin, phenytoin, phenobarbital, carbamazepine, imatinib; ↓ absorption of thyroxine—calcium salts, ferrous sulfate, aluminum hydroxide, colestyramine, omeprazole, sucralfate, orlistat.
- Atrophic gastritis in *Helicobacter pylori* infection (↓ T_4 by 30%).

Further reading

Chaker L, *et al.* (2017). Hypothyroidism. *Lancet* **390**, 1550–62.

Jonklaas J, *et al.* (2014). Guidelines for the treatment of hypothyroidism: prepared by the American Thyroid Association task force on thyroid hormone replacement. *Thyroid* **24**, 1670–751.

Okosieme O, *et al.* (2016). Management of primary hypothyroidism: statement by the British Thyroid Association Executive Committee. *Clin Endocrinol* **84**, 799–808.

Spencer L, *et al.* (2015). Screening and subsequent management for thyroid dysfunction pre-pregnancy and during pregnancy for improving maternal and infant health. *Cochrane Database Syst Rev* **9**, CD011263.

Surks MI, Boucai L (2010). Age- and race-based serum thyrotropin reference limits. *J Clin Endocrinol Metab* **95**, 496–502.

Wiersinga WM, *et al.* (2012). The use of L-T4 + L-T3 in the treatment hypothyroidism: guidelines of the European Thyroid Association. *Eur Thyroid J* **1**, 55–71.

Congenital hypothyroidism

Incidence is now estimated at 1 in 2000 neonates, which has more than doubled due to more inclusive diagnostic criteria, shifting demographics, and increasing survival of preterm infants. The greatest increase has occurred in mildly affected children.

There is an inverse relationship between age at diagnosis and intelligence quotient (IQ) in later life. In iodine-replete areas, 85% of the cases are due to sporadic developmental defects of the thyroid gland (thyroid dysgenesis), such as arrested migration of the embryonic thyroid (ectopic thyroid) or complete absence of thyroid tissue (athyreosis). The remaining 15% have thyroid dyshormonogenesis defects transmitted by an autosomal recessive (AR) mode of inheritance. Iodine deficiency (urine iodine <25 micrograms per day), particularly in preterm infants, accounts for many cases in Eastern Europe, Asia, and Africa.

Clinical diagnosis occurs in <5% of newborns with hypothyroidism because symptoms and signs are often minimal, so it is not possible to predict which infants are likely to be affected. Without prompt diagnosis and treatment, most affected children gradually develop growth failure, irreversible mental retardation, and a variety of neuropsychological deficits.

Congenital hypothyroidism may be transient or persistent, but the natural history cannot be predicted by the severity at diagnosis. In premature infants, who are especially vulnerable to hypothyroidism, the rise in serum TSH may be delayed and therefore detected only by routine follow-up screening. (See Box 1.9 for clinical features.)

Thyroid hormone dysgenesis

- Caused by inborn errors of thyroid metabolism. The disorders may be AR, indicating single-protein defects.
- Can be caused by inactivation of the TSH receptor or abnormalities of the thyroid transcription factors TTF1, TTF2, and PAX8, or due to defects in iodide transport, organification (peroxidase), coupling, deiodinase, or Tg synthesis.
- In a large proportion of patients with congenital hypothyroidism, the molecular background is unknown.

Pendred's syndrome

Characterized by overt or subclinical hypothyroidism, goitre, and moderate to severe sensorineural hearing impairment. The prevalence varies between 1:15,000 and 1:100,000. There is a partial iodide organification defect detected by ↑ perchlorate discharge. Thyroid hormone synthesis is only mildly impaired and so may not be detected by neonatal thyroid screening.

Laboratory tests

- Neonatal screening by measurement of serum TSH.
- Imaging procedure: ultrasonography or ^{123}I scintigraphy.
- Measurement of serum Tg and low-molecular weight iodopeptides in urine to discriminate between the various types of defects.
- Measurement of neonatal and maternal autoantibodies as an indication of possible transient hypothyroidism.

Box 1.9 Clinical features and congenital hypothyroidism

The following features are late sequelae of congenital hypothyroidism and, with routine screening now available, should never be seen nowadays:

• Physiological jaundice.
• Goitre.
• Hoarse cry, feeding problems, constipation, somnolence.
• Delay in reaching normal milestones of development, short stature.
• Coarse features with protruding tongue, broad flat nose, and widely set eyes.
• Sparse hair and dry skin, protuberant abdomen with umbilical hernia.
• Impaired mental development, retarded bone age.
• Epiphyseal dysgenesis, delayed dentition.

Treatment

Irrespective of the cause of congenital hypothyroidism, early treatment is essential to prevent cerebral damage. Sufficient levothyroxine should be given to maintain serum TSH in the normal range.

Further reading

Cherella CE, Wassner AJ (2017). Congenital hypothyroidism: insights into pathogenesis and treatment. *Int J Pediatr Endocrinol* **2017**, 11

Ford G, LaFranchi SH (2014). Screening for congenital hypothyroidism: a worldwide view of strategies. *Best Pract Res Clin Endocrinol Metab* **28**, 175–87.

Amiodarone and thyroid function

Background

- Amiodarone has a high concentration of iodine (about 37% by weight). It is a benzofuranic derivative, and its structural formula closely resembles that of thyroxine. On a dose of amiodarone between 200 and 600mg daily, 7–21mg of iodine is made available each day. The optimal daily iodine intake is 150–200 micrograms. Amiodarone is distributed in several tissues from where it is slowly released. In one study, the terminal elimination half-life of amiodarone averaged 52.6 days, with a standard deviation of 23.7 days.
- Abnormalities of thyroid function occur in up to 100% of patients (see Table 1.24).
- In the UK and USA, 2% of patients on amiodarone develop thyrotoxicosis (amiodarone-induced thyrotoxicosis (AIT)) and about 13% develop hypothyroidism (amiodarone-induced hypothyroidism (AIH)).
- Patients residing in areas with high iodine intake develop AIH more often than AIT, but AIT occurs more frequently in regions with low iodine intake.
- AIT can present several months after discontinuing the drug because of its long half-life.
- AIH is commoner in ♀ and in patients with thyroid autoantibodies.
- TFTs should be monitored initially prior to commencing therapy and then every 6 months in patients taking amiodarone.
- Other side effects and complications occur (see Table 1.26).
- Dronedarone is a non-iodinated benzofuran derivative with multichannel blocking effects and anti-adrenergic properties. Although it is an antagonist of $TR\alpha1$ and $TR\beta1$ isoforms, it has little impact on thyroid hormones.

Pathogenesis

- The high iodine content of amiodarone may inhibit Tg iodination and thyroid hormone synthesis and release, causing AIH (Wolff–Chaikoff effect), or lead to iodine-induced hyperthyroidism in susceptible individuals (Jod–Basedow phenomenon).
- Amiodarone also inhibits monodeiodination of T_4, thus decreasing T_3 production, and blocks T_3 binding to nuclear receptors.
- Thyrotoxicosis resulting from iodine excess, and therefore ↑ hormone synthesis, in nodular goitres or latent Graves' disease is referred to as *AIT type 1*. Thyrotoxicosis due to a direct toxic effect of amiodarone (thyroiditis) is referred to as *AIT type 2*. Mixed/indefinite forms exist due to both pathogenic mechanisms (see Table 1.25).
- Drug-induced destructive thyroiditis results in leakage of thyroid hormones from damaged follicles into the circulation and, like subacute thyroiditis, can be followed by a transient hypothyroid state before euthyroidism is restored.

Table 1.24 Thyroid function tests in clinically euthyroid patients after administration of amiodarone

Tests	1–3 months	>3 months
FT$_3$	↓	Remains slightly ↓, but within normal range
TSH	Transient increase	Normal
FT$_4$	Modest increase	Slightly ↑, compared to pretreatment values, may be in normal range or slightly ↑
rT$_3$	↑	↑

Table 1.25 Characteristics of AIT (some patients have a mixed form, and classification is not always possible)

	AIT type 1 (10%)	AIT type 2 (90%)
Aetiology	Iodine toxicity	Thyroiditis
Signs of clinical thyroid disease	Yes	No
Goitre	Frequent	Infrequent
Thyroid antibodies	+ve	−ve
Radioiodine uptake	Normal	↓
Tg	Normal or slightly elevated	Very elevated
Late hypothyroidism	No	Possible
Vascularity (Doppler)	↑/normal	Reduced
Subsequent definitive thyroid treatment	Generally yes	No

Diagnosis and treatment

- After chronic administration of amiodarone, a steady state is achieved, typically reflected in mildly ↑ FT$_4$ and ↓ in FT$_3$. Thus, in clinically euthyroid patients on amiodarone, a slightly ↑ T$_4$ level is not indicative of hyperthyroidism, nor is ↓ T$_3$ indicative of hypothyroidism.
- Hypothyroidism is indicated by ↑ TSH, with ↓ FT$_4$. AIH does not require amiodarone withdrawal. Levothyroxine replacement is almost always considered for those with serum TSH >20U/L. If serum TSH is between 5 and 20U/L, the value of levothyroxine replacement can be judged on clinical grounds, such as abnormality of diastolic function, which can be reversible. If serum FT$_4$ is below the reference range, then levothyroxine replacement is usually indicated.
- Hyperthyroidism is indicated by significantly ↑ FT$_4$, together with ↑ FT$_3$ and suppressed serum TSH.
- Discontinuation of amiodarone does not always control the thyrotoxic state because of its long half-life (particularly in the obese) due to its very high volume of distribution and fat solubility.

- Cardiac function may be compromised by propranolol used in combination with amiodarone since this may produce bradycardia and sinus arrest.
- AIT type 1 is best treated with ATDs that may be combined for a few weeks with potassium perchlorate which inhibits iodide uptake by the thyroid gland, reduces intrathyroidal iodine, and renders thionamides more effective. It can be given as a 1g daily dose, together with carbimazole.
- AIT type 2 is best treated with GCs.
- Once euthyroidism has been restored, AIT type 2 patients are followed up without treatment, whereas AIT type 1 patients may require definitive treatment usually with a thyroidectomy.
- Classification into type 1 and type 2 is often difficult. In practice, amiodarone withdrawal is not immediately necessary (see Table 1.25) and most patients are treated at least initially with ATDs ± GCs (see Table 1.27).
- Treatment is outlined in Table 1.28.
- There is often reluctance among endocrinologists to use relatively high-dose GC therapy, particularly in the elderly patient group with significant comorbidities who may often present asymptomatically with a mild, and often self-limiting, disease, but evidence exists that early use of GC therapy is safe and effective in patients with AIT type 2.
- If there is doubt, a regimen of 40mg of carbimazole and 40mg of prednisolone daily for 2 weeks, followed by measurement of serum T_3, is a reasonable initial strategy. If there is a reduction in serum T_3 by >50%, compared to pretreatment levels, then carbimazole is stopped, as the diagnosis of AIT type 2 is suggested. Prednisolone can then be continued in a tapering dose, reducing the course over 2–3 months, according to the clinical and biochemical response. If there is no change in serum T_3 levels following initial treatment, prednisolone can be stopped and carbimazole is continued, as the assumption is that the predominant diagnosis is AIT type 1.
- Radioiodine is not feasible in the short term because of reduced uptake by the thyroid gland, reflecting the iodine load associated with the drug. It may be considered in AIT type 1 after resolution of the iodine load and restoration of adequate radioiodine uptake.
- Surgery remains a very successful form of treatment, with euthyroidism being restored within a matter of days. Achieving preoperative euthyroidism may be difficult and plasmapheresis may be considered. Total thyroidectomy was recently demonstrated to be the therapeutic choice for AIT patients with severe systolic dysfunction, whereas it is not superior to medical therapy in those with normal or mildly reduced left ventricular ejection fraction (LVEF).

Further reading

Bartalena L, et al. (2018). European Thyroid Association (ETA) guidelines for the management of amiodarone associated thyroid dysfunction. *Eur Thyroid J* **7**, 55–66.

Cappellani D, et al. (2020). Comparison between total thyroidectomy and medical therapy for amiodarone-induced thyrotoxicosis. *J Clin Endocrinol Metab* **105**, dgz041.

Eskes SA, et al. (2012). Treatment of amiodarone-induced thyrotoxicosis type 2: a randomized clinical trial. *J Clin Endocrinol Metab* **87**, 499–506.

Han TS, et al. (2009). Benzofuran derivatives and the thyroid. *Clin Endocrinol* **70**, 2–13.

Raghavan RP, et al. (2012). Amiodarone-induced thyrotoxicosis: an overview of UK management. *Clin Endocrinol* **77**, 936–7.

Table 1.26 Side effects and complications of amiodarone therapy

Side effect	Incidence (%)
Corneal microdeposits	100
Anorexia and nausea	80
Photosensitivity, blue/grey skin discoloration	55–75
Ataxia, tremors, peripheral neuropathy	48
Deranged LFTs	25
Abnormal TFTs	14–18
Interstitial pneumonitis	10–13
Cardiac arrhythmias	2–3

Table 1.27 Advantages and disadvantages of amiodarone withdrawal in patients with AIT

Disadvantages	Advantages
Efficient drug for life-threatening arrhythmias	Amiodarone and its metabolites have a long half-life, making an immediate exacerbation of cardiac symptoms unlikely
Cardiac-protective properties: antagonistic effect on β-adrenergic receptors, inhibition of T_4 deiodination, blockade of T_3 binding to thyroid hormone receptors	Greater chance of achieving euthyroidism and delivering definitive thyroid treatment (particularly radioiodine) at an earlier stage
Amiodarone and its metabolites have a long half-life; thus, discontinuation might be useless, at least in the short run	Continuation of the drug in AIT type 2 is associated with delayed restoration of euthyroidism and a higher chance of recurrence

Table 1.28 Treatment of amiodarone-induced thyrotoxicosis

	AIT type 1	AIT type 2
Step 1: aim to restore euthyroidism	Carbimazole up to 40mg/day or PTU 400mg/day, in combination, if necessary, with potassium perchlorate 1g/day for 16–40 days If possible, discontinue amiodarone*	Discontinue amiodarone, if possible* Prednisolone 40mg/day In mixed forms, add carbimazole or PTU, as in AIT type 1
Step 2: definitive treatment	Radioiodine treatment or thyroidectomy	Follow-up for possible spontaneous progression to hypothyroidism

* If amiodarone cannot be withdrawn and medical therapy is unsuccessful, consider total thyroidectomy.

Epidemiology of thyroid cancer

(See Tables 1.29 and 1.30.)

- Clinical presentation of thyroid cancer is usually as a solitary thyroid. Although thyroid nodules are common, thyroid cancers are rare. It accounts for <1% of all cancers, and <0.5% of cancer deaths.
- The four major histological types are papillary, follicular, medullary, and anaplastic, and each displays a different epidemiology.
- The annual incidence of all thyroid cancers ranges between 1 and 10/100,000 population in most countries and is 2–4× more frequent in ♀ than men. Papillary and follicular tumours, which comprise 60–90% of the total, are rare in children and adolescents, but their incidence increases with age in adults.
- Papillary thyroid carcinoma (PTC) is the commonest thyroid malignancy and worldwide constitutes 50–90% of differentiated follicular cell-derived thyroid cancers.
- Papillary thyroid microcarcinomas (diameter <1cm) are found in 4–36% of adult postmortem in population-based studies.
- Most PTC diagnoses occur in patients aged 30–50 years (median age 44 years), and the majority (60–80%) occur in ♀. The increase in incidence of these carcinomas in recent years has been attributed to an improvement in pathological techniques and earlier and ↑ detection of small (subclinical) papillary cancers 2° to more widespread use of neck ultrasonography and FNA of very small thyroid nodules.
- Recent US epidemiological data suggest an annual increase of 3% in the rates of differentiated thyroid cancer (DTC) of all sizes, including tumours >4cm, and an increase in incidence-based mortality between 1974 and 2013 from 0.40 to 0.46/100,000 person-years.
- Follicular thyroid carcinoma (FTC) occurs relatively infrequently, compared to PTC, and accounts for ~15% of all thyroid cancers. There is an ↑ frequency of FTC to PTC (5:1) in iodine-deficient endemic goitre areas. It tends to be a malignancy of older persons, with a peak incidence between ages 40 and 60 years, and is ~3 times commoner in ♀.
- Medullary thyroid carcinoma (MTC) occurs in both sporadic and hereditary forms. The highest incidence of sporadic disease occurs in the 5th decade. Hereditary MTC can be inherited as an AD trait, with a high degree of penetrance associated with MEN type 2 syndrome, or as familial MTC (FMTC) without any other endocrinopathies. It can be diagnosed before clinical presentation by genetic and biochemical screening.
- Anaplastic thyroid cancer is very rare and more frequent in populations with endemic goitre.
- Thyroid lymphoma is also uncommon, constituting ~2% of extranodal lymphomas and occurring predominantly in older women. Up to one-third of patients have a history of goitre, whereas some have established autoimmune thyroiditis and may be taking levothyroxine therapy.

Table 1.29 Classification of thyroid cancer

Cell of origin	Tumour type	Frequency (%)
Differentiated:		
Papillary		>80
Follicular		10
Undifferentiated (anaplastic)		1–5
C cells	Medullary	5–10
Lymphocytes	Lymphoma	1–5

Table 1.30 Comparison of papillary, follicular, and anaplastic carcinomas (Ca) of the thyroid

Characteristic	Papillary Ca	Follicular Ca	Anaplastic Ca
Age at presentation (years)	30–50	40–50	60–80
Spread	Lymphatic	Haematogenous	Haematogenous
Prognosis	Good	Good	Poor
Treatment	Initially: near-total thyroidectomy	Initially: near-total thyroidectomy	Total thyroidectomy with lymph node clearance
	Post-operative TSH suppression	Post-operative TSH suppression	
	High-risk patient: ^{131}I remnant ablation	^{131}I remnant ablation	External beam irradiation and consider chemotherapy
	Post-operative total body radioiodine scan + Tg measurement	Post-operative total body radioiodine scan + Tg measurement	

Aetiology of thyroid cancer

Irradiation

* There does not appear to be a threshold dose of external irradiation for thyroid carcinogenesis; doses of 200–500cGy seem to produce thyroid cancer at a rate of about 0.5%/year.
* There is no evidence that therapeutic or diagnostic ^{131}I administration can induce thyroid cancer, although there is a small increase in death rates from thyroid cancer after ^{131}I. At present, it is unclear whether this is due to an effect of ^{131}I or part of the natural history of the underlying thyroid disease.
* External irradiation at an age <20 years is associated with an ↑ risk of thyroid nodule development and thyroid cancer (most commonly papillary). The radioactive fallout from the Chernobyl nuclear explosion in 1986 resulted in a 4.7-fold increase in thyroid cancer in the regions of Belarus from 1985 to 1993, including a 34-fold increase in children. Children aged <10 years were the most sensitive to radiation-induced carcinogenesis, and the minimal latent period for thyroid cancer development after exposure is as short as 4 years. The vast majority of these cancers were PTCs, many of which have a characteristic solid or solid follicular microscopic appearance.
* The risk is greater for ♀ and when irradiation occurs at a younger age.
* There is a latency of at least 5 years, with maximum risk at 20 years following exposure, though this was not seen following the Chernobyl disaster.

Other environmental factors

Most investigators agree that iodine supplementation has resulted in a decrease in the incidence of FTC.

Molecular alterations in thyroid cancer

* PTCs frequently carry gene mutations and rearrangements that lead to activation of mitogen-activated protein kinase (MAPK) that promotes cell division. Rearrangements of the rearranged tyrosine kinase genes *RET* and *NTRK1*, activating mutations of *BRAF*, and activating mutations of *RAS* are sequential components leading to activation of MAPK. Driver mutations are identified in >95% of cases. The *RAS* mutations are referred to as weak drivers since they do not always predict a malignant phenotype. In contrast, *RET* and *NTRK1* rearrangements, and the activating *BRAF* mutation are strong drivers since their presence almost always predicts a malignant phenotype.
* ~9% of PTCs have both a telomerase reverse transcriptase (*TERT*) gene promoter mutation and one of the driver mutations, and are more aggressive.
* FTCs frequently carry gene mutations that lead to activation of the anaplastic lymphoma kinase (AKT) pathway. *PAX8*/*PPAR-γ-1* rearrangements and mutations of *HRAS*, *NRAS*, and *KRAS* proto-oncogenes are found in FTC and occasionally PTC.

- An indolent variant of a follicular cell-derived neoplasm has been identified, termed non-invasive follicular thyroid neoplasm with papillary-like nuclear features (NIFTP). The most frequent gene mutations are activating *RAS* mutations and, less frequently, activating *BRAF* mutations. More conservative management of these tumours is required and patients can be spared the psychological burden of a cancer diagnosis,
- Anaplastic thyroid cancers and poorly DTCs arise from well-differentiated thyroid carcinomas that originally contained *BRAF* or *RAS* driver mutations and subsequently acquired mutations conferring ↑ aggressiveness. Additional mutations include those in the *TERT* promoter region, *p53*, and *PIK3CA*.
- The use of these and other emerging molecular markers is predicted to improve the diagnosis of malignancy in thyroid nodules, as well as facilitate more individualized operative and post-operative management.

(See Table 1.31.)

Table 1.31 Oncogenes and tumour suppressor genes of thyroid neoplasms

Neoplasm	Genetic abnormalities
Benign neoplasms	
Autonomously functioning thyroid nodules	TSH receptor-activating mutation
	Gs-α mutation decreasing GTPase activity
Follicular adenoma	*RAS* mutations
	RASSF1A promoter hypermethylation
Malignant neoplasms	
PTC	*BRAF (V600E)*-activating mutation
	RET, TRK, ALK, and *BRAF* rearrangements (*RET/PTC*)
	RAS mutations
	TERT promoter mutations
FTC	*PAX8/PPAR-γ-1* fusion
	RAS mutations
	RASSF1A promoter hypermethylation
	TERT promoter mutations
	PIK3CA-activating mutations
Anaplastic thyroid carcinoma	*TP-53* mutations
	CTNNB1-activating mutations
	ALK rearrangements and activating mutations
	Any of the genetic alterations of PTC and FTC
MTC	*RET* gene mutations

Prognostic factors, staging, and risk stratification in differentiated thyroid cancer

The long-term outcome of patients treated effectively for DTC is usually favourable. The overall 10-year survival rate for middle-aged adults with DTC is 80–90%. However, 5–20% of patients develop local or regional recurrences, and 10–15% distant metastases; 9% of patients with a diagnosis of thyroid cancer die of their disease.

Access to a multidisciplinary thyroid team

- The management of DTC and MTC should be the responsibility of a specialist MDT, membership of which will normally be appointed by the regional cancer network.
- The MDT will normally comprise a surgeon, an endocrinologist, and an oncologist (or a nuclear medicine physician), with support from a pathologist, a medical physicist, a biochemist, a radiologist, and a specialist nurse, all with expertise and interest in the management of thyroid cancers. A combined clinic is recommended.
- Patients should be offered full verbal and written information about their condition and treatment, and continuing access to a member of the MDT for guidance and support.

Predictors

Several factors have been shown consistently to be important for predicting death and recurrence in multivariate analyses of large patient cohorts.

Age

The risk of recurrence and death increases with age, particularly after the age of 40 years. Young children, under the age of 10 years, are at higher risk of recurrence than older children or adolescents.

Gender

The ♂ gender is reported as an independent risk factor in some, but not all, studies.

Histology

The prognosis of PTC is better than that of FTC. However, if the confounding effects of age and extent of the tumour at diagnosis are removed, survival rates are comparable. Within the PTC group, poorer prognosis is associated with specific histological types (e.g. tall cell, columnar cell) and the degree of cellular differentiation and vascular invasion. 'Widely invasive' and 'vascular invasion' are features of follicular cancers associated with a poorer prognosis. Poorly differentiated and oncocytic follicular (Hürthle cell) carcinomas are also associated with a poorer outcome.

Tumour extent

The risk of recurrence and mortality correlates with the size of the 1° tumour. Extrathyroidal invasion, lymph node metastases, and distant metastases are all important prognostic factors.

The risk of death from the disease and the risk of recurrence in patients with DTC using a prognostic scoring system enable a more accurate prognosis to be given and appropriate treatment decisions.

Staging systems

Several staging systems have been proposed for DTC.
The most commonly used are:

- TNM: Tumour size, Node metastases, and distant Metastases.
- AMES: Age at presentation, Metastases, Extent, Size of 1° tumour.
- MACIS: Metastases, Age at presentation, Completeness of surgical resection, Invasion (extrathyroidal), Size.
- EORTC: European Organisation for Research and Treatment of Cancer methodology.
- AGES: Age at presentation, Grade of tumour, Extent, Size of 1° tumour.

Any of these systems can be used to assign patients to the high-risk or low-risk group (see Box 1.10) (MACIS is used only for PTC), based on well-established prognostic factors, but TNM and MACIS probably yield the most useful prognostic information and the TNM classification is used extensively for registration and predicts mortality, and is a valuable indicator of overall prognosis (for the latest staging, see ℛ https://www.cancer.net/cancer-types/thyroid-cancer/stages). However, it does not take into account individual responses to treatment, which may alter prognosis, and it does not predict recurrence. (See Online calculator at: ℛ https://www.british-thyroid-association.org/sandbox/bta2016/uk_guidelines_for_the_use_of_thyroid_function_tests.pdf)

Box 1.10 Post-operative stratification for risk of recurrence of DTC

Low-risk patients have the following characteristics:
- No local or distant metastases.
- All macroscopic tumour has been resected, i.e. R0 or R1 resection (pathological definition).
- No tumour invasion of loco-regional tissues or structures.
- The tumour does not have aggressive histology (tall cell or columnar cell PTC, diffuse sclerosing PTC, poorly differentiated elements) or angioinvasion.
Intermediate-risk patients have any of the following characteristics:
- Microscopic invasion of tumour into the perithyroidal soft tissues (T3) at initial surgery.
- Cervical lymph node metastases (N1a or N1b).
- Tumour with aggressive histology (tall cell or columnar cell PTC, diffuse sclerosing PTC, poorly differentiated elements) or angioinvasion.
High-risk patients have any of the following characteristics:
- Extrathyroidal invasion.
- Incomplete macroscopic tumour resection (R2).
- Distant metastases (M1).

Papillary microcarcinoma of the thyroid

- Papillary microcarcinoma of the thyroid (PMC) is defined as a tumour focus of 1.0cm or less in diameter. It is often detected coincidentally on US or following histopathological examination of the thyroid following resection of a multinodular goitre or any thyroid resected.
- No significant difference in the prevalence rates of PMC has been demonstrated between the sexes.
- PMC rarely progresses to clinically apparent thyroid cancer with advancing age.
- PMC can be multifocal.
- Cervical lymph node metastasis from PMC ranges from 4.3% to 18.2%.
- Lymph node metastasis was most often associated with multifocal tumours.
- Although exposure to irradiation increases the likelihood of developing PTC, the tumours will usually be >1.0cm in diameter, and thus not PMC.
- Follow-up studies suggest that PMC is a slow-growing lesion which rarely spreads to distant sites and carries a good prognosis.
- In a study of 2863 patients with PMC (mean tumour size 0.63cm, mean age 50 years, 81% ♀), 66% underwent lobectomy. At median follow-up 5 years after surgery, the rate of recurrence was 1.4%. Recurrence and disease-free survival were similar for those who underwent immediate surgery as for those who delayed surgery.
- Surgery delay/avoidance may benefit some, based on personal convenience/presence of other concurrent health conditions. Younger patients have higher rates of disease progression (up to 46% lifetime probability of progression if diagnosed in 20s).
- Surgical treatment recommendation is ipsilateral lobectomy.
- There is no evidence that targeting TSH below the reference range improves prognosis.

Papillary thyroid carcinoma

Pathology

- Slow-growing, usually non-encapsulated, may spread through the thyroid capsule to structures in the surrounding neck, especially regional lymph nodes. Multifocal in 30% of cases.
- Recognized variants are follicular, papillary, dorsal, columnar cell, tall cell, and diffuse sclerosing.
- *Histology.* The tumour contains complex branching papillae that have a fibrovascular core covered by a single layer of tumour cells.
- Nuclear features include:
  - Large size with a pale-staining, 'ground-glass' appearance (*orphan Annie-eye nucleus*).
  - Deep nuclear grooves.
- The characteristic and pathognomonic cytoplasmic feature is the 'psammoma body' which is a calcified, laminated, basophilic stromal structure.
- It is confined to the neck in over 95% of cases, although 15–20% have local extrathyroidal invasion. Metastases (1–2% of patients) occur via lymphatics to local lymph nodes and, more distantly, to the lungs.
- Several prognostic scoring systems are in use, none of which permits definitive decisions to be made for individual patients.
- Low risk—TNM stage I (under 45, no metastases, tumour size <2cm, who may not need RAI ablation).

Management

Primary treatment—surgery

- Surgery is the 1° mode of therapy for patients with DTC, followed by treatment with thyroid hormone suppressive therapy (most patients) and radioiodine (high-risk and selected intermediate-risk patients).
- Should be performed by an experienced thyroid surgeon at a centre with adequate case load to maintain surgical skills.
- Thyroid lobectomy is recommended for patients with a unifocal PMC and no other risk factors
- Total thyroidectomy is recommended for patients with tumours >4cm in diameter or tumours of any size in association with any of the following characteristics: multifocal disease, bilateral disease, extrathyroidal spread (pT3 and pT4a), familial disease, and those with clinically or radiologically involved nodes and/or distant metastases.
- Central compartment neck dissection is not recommended for patients without clinical or radiological evidence of lymph node involvement, who have all of the following characteristics: classical-type PTC, <45 years, unifocal tumour, <4cm, and no extrathyroidal extension on US.
- Patients with follicular cancer (>4cm tumours) appear to have worse prognosis and should be treated with total thyroidectomy.
- Clinically evident cervical lymph node metastasis is best treated with radical modified neck dissection, with preservation of the sternocleidomastoid muscle, spinal accessory nerve, and internal jugular vein.
- After surgery, the presence or absence of persistent disease and risk for recurrent disease should be assessed in order to determine the need for additional treatment, in particular radioiodine therapy.

Adjuvant therapy—radioiodine therapy

- Radioiodine is administered after thyroidectomy in patients with DIC to ablate residual normal thyroid tissue (remnant ablation), provide adjuvant therapy of subclinical micrometastatic disease, and/or provide treatment of clinically apparent residual or metastatic thyroid cancer.
- The decision to treat with radioiodine depends upon the risk of recurrence/persistent disease.
- Radioiodine is usually administered after total thyroidectomy in high-risk patients and in selected intermediate-risk patients, depending upon specific tumour characteristics (e.g. microscopic invasion into the perithyroidal soft tissue, clinically significant lymph node metastases outside of the thyroid bed, or other higher-risk features).
- In the absence of a proven benefit on either disease-free survival or recurrence, radioiodine ablation is not routinely administered in patients with low-risk disease, especially if unifocal tumours <1cm without other high-risk features or multifocal cancer when all foci are <1cm in the absence of other high-risk features, even in the presence of small-volume regional lymph node metastases (<5 lymph nodes measuring <2mm).
- A WBS done 4–6 months after administration of 150MBq ^{131}I helps to determine the presence of any residual disease. Recent large observational studies show that the recurrence rate among patients who have 1·1GBq radioiodine ablation was not higher than that in those who have 3·7GBq, which favours using low-dose radioiodine for treatment of low-risk DTC. The recurrence risk was not affected by use of recombinant TSH.
- In the presence of metastasis, a dose of ~5.5–7.4GBq radioiodine is used. Recombinant TSH is an alternative to liothyronine cessation. Liothyronine is administered for 4–6 weeks in place of levothyroxine and then omitted for 10 days prior to the scan, allowing TSH to rise. A low-iodine diet for 2 weeks increases the effective specific activity of the administered iodine. The patient should be isolated until residual dose meter readings indicate <30MBq.
- A post-ablation scan should be performed after radioiodine when residual activity levels permit satisfactory imaging (usually 2–10 days). A stimulated Tg and neck US should be performed in preference to a diagnostic ^{131}I WBS between 9 and 12 months from radioiodine ablation therapy.

Adjuvant therapy—levothyroxine suppression

- After initial thyroidectomy, whether or not radioiodine therapy is administered, levothyroxine therapy is required in most patients to prevent hypothyroidism.
- The hypothesis that reduction of serum TSH concentrations to below the normal range decreases morbidity and mortality in all patients with DTC has not been proven.
- For patients with low-risk disease treated with thyroidectomy who have undetectable serum Tg levels (with or without remnant ablation) or who were treated with lobectomy, serum TSH can be maintained between 0.5 and 2.0mU/L. Thyroid hormone treatment may be unnecessary if serum TSH is maintained in this range post-lobectomy.

- For patients with intermediate-risk disease, serum TSH initially can be maintained between 0.1 and 0.5mU/L, and in high-risk disease, serum TSH initially should be <0.1mU/L.
- The risks of overly aggressive levothyroxine therapy include the potential for acceleration of bone loss, atrial fibrillation, and cardiac dysfunction. The dose of levothyroxine should be tailored to the extent of the disease and the likelihood of recurrence.

Thyroglobulin

- A very sensitive marker of recurrence of thyroid cancer.
- Secreted by the thyroid tissue.
- After total thyroidectomy and RAI ablation, the levels of Tg should be <0.27 micrograms/L.
- Measurement of Tg levels could be made difficult in the presence of TgAb, which should be checked.
- Coming off thyroid hormones or giving recombinant TSH increases the sensitivity of Tg to detect recurrence, but this may not affect survival rates.

Recurrent disease/distant metastases

- Patients are followed up with Tg levels. After effective treatment, Tg levels are undetectable. A trend of ↑ Tg values should be investigated with a radioiodine uptake scan.
- The principal indications for a diagnostic WBS after RAI is in cases where measurement of serum Tg is unreliable and where radioiodine uptake was visualized beyond the thyroid bed and neck in the post-ablation scan.
- In the case of recurrence, treatment employs all methods used in 1° and adjuvant therapy:
- Surgery for local metastases.
- Radioactive iodine for those tumours with uptake.
- External radiotherapy is indicated in non-resectable tumours that do not take up ^{131}I. Radiation therapy may be of value in controlling local disease. If thyroidectomy is not possible, it is given alone for palliation.
- Bony and pulmonary metastases (usually osteolytic) may be treated with ^{131}I.
- Unfortunately, only 50% of metastases concentrate ^{131}I.
- Due to the low efficacy of traditional cytotoxic chemotherapies, kinase inhibitors that target either angiogenesis or oncogenic signalling pathways for progressive, locally advanced, or metastatic DTC are now being considered.
- TKIs (e.g. sorafenib, sunitinib, pazopanib, gefitinib) have produced clinical responses and prolonged progression-free survival in randomized trials for advanced metastatic DTC.
- Drugs that inhibit oncogenic mutated kinases, such as BRAF, RET, or TRK, also frequently produce objective responses in DTC, though prolongation of progression-free survival has not yet been demonstrated in randomized trials.

- Selumetinib, a selective MAPK pathway antagonist, allows re-expression of genes responsible for iodine metabolism in radioiodine-refractory DTC, thus permitting restoration of radioiodine uptake (also called 'redifferentiation').
- Side effects that are common to all include hypertension, renal toxicity, bleeding, myelosuppression, arterial thromboembolism, cardiotoxicity, thyroid dysfunction (typically hypothyroidism), cutaneous toxicity, including hand–foot skin reaction, delayed wound healing, hepatotoxicity, and muscle wasting.
- TKIs are usually tumoristatic, rather than tumoricidal. Only one published study has demonstrated that one of these new agents improved overall survival in a specific prespecified subgroup of patients. In view of the significant toxicities, it is important to limit the use of systemic treatments to patients at significant risk of morbidity or mortality due to progressive metastatic disease in whom benefit of therapy is likely to reasonably outweigh the risks and cost. Patients should have a baseline performance status sufficiently functional to tolerate these interventions.

Recombinant TSH

- Avoids morbidity of hypothyroidism during levothyroxine withdrawal.
- Necessary for patients with TSH deficiency (hypopituitarism) and thyroid carcinoma.
- Comparable Tg rise, but slightly reduced ^{131}I scan sensitivity, compared to thyroid hormone withdrawal.
- Give 0.9mg of recombinant TSH on days 1 and 2, and measure Tg on day 5.
- For serum Tg testing, serum Tg should be obtained 72h after the final injection of recombinant TSH.

Follicular thyroid carcinoma

Pathology

- FTC is a neoplasm of the thyroid epithelium that exhibits follicular differentiation and shows capsular or vascular invasion.
- Differentiation of benign follicular adenoma from encapsulated low-grade or minimally invasive tumours can be impossible to diagnose, particularly for the cytopathologist, and surgery is usually necessary for follicular adenoma.
- FTC may be minimally or widely invasive.
- Metastases (15–20% cases) are more likely to be spread by haematogenesis to the lung and bones, and less likely to local lymph nodes.

Hürthle cell carcinoma

- An aggressive and distinct type of follicular tumour, with a poor prognosis because it fails to concentrate [131]I.
- Previously, Hürthle cell carcinoma was considered to be a variant of FTC. Clinically, it often has a clinically similar presentation to FTC (usually asymptomatic thyroid nodule in older patients) and a similar pattern of distant metastases (lung, bone, brain).
- Typical histology characterized by the presence of a cell population of 'oncocytes', but unlike FTC, Hürthle cell carcinoma metastatic foci are often RAI-refractory.
- About 20–30% of patients with Hürthle cell carcinoma have metastatic extension at the time of initial treatment. The most frequent sites of metastases are the lungs and bones, and are associated with significant morbidity and mortality, although some patients with widely metastatic Hürthle cell carcinoma survive for many years with minimal disease progression.
- The specific treatment of metastatic Hürthle cell carcinoma is not well defined. The current approach is aggressive tumour resection locally and at distant sites as it offers the best chance of survival. The multitude and locations of the skeletal lesions often limit the surgical option. For patients with extensive metastatic disease that is not accessible for surgical resection or radiation, systemic therapy may be used.
- TKIs should be considered when patients have symptoms of weight loss, muscle wasting, or fatigue, or other constitutional symptoms attributable to their significant disease burden, when the rate of progression of structural disease is rapid enough that the disease is likely to cause morbidity or when additional metastatic foci are identified.

Treatment

As for PTC (see ➔ Papillary microcarcinoma of the thyroid, p. 106).

Follow-up of DTC

- This should be lifelong—recurrences occur at least to 25 years.
- Follow-up usually involves an annual clinical review, with clinical examination for the presence of suspicious lymph nodes and measurement of serum TSH (to ensure target levels) and Tg.
- Serum Tg should be undetectable in patients with total thyroid ablation. However, detectable levels may be seen for up to 6 months after thyroid ablation. A trend of ↑ Tg level requires investigations with ^{131}I uptake scan (off thyroid hormones or with TSH stimulation) and other imaging modalities such as US of the neck, CT scan of the lungs, or bone scans. TgAb must be checked, as there may be interactions with Tg assays.
- Detectable Tg and absent uptake on radioiodine uptake scan may be due to dedifferentiation of the tumour and failure to take up iodine. In patients with serum Tg >10ng/mL and a negative radioiodine scan, PET imaging is required. Metastatic lesions with high avidity for glucose in PET imaging, measured by elevated standard uptake values, are associated with resistance to radioiodine therapy and worse prognosis.
- Ongoing monitoring strategies are based upon the risk of recurrence and reassessment of response to therapy at each follow-up visit.

Thyroid cancer and pregnancy

- The natural course of thyroid cancer developing during pregnancy does not appear to be different from that in non-pregnant ♀.
- Evaluation should be undertaken with FNAC.
- Lesions <2cm diameter or any lesion appearing after 24 weeks' gestation should be treated with TSH suppression, and further evaluations carried out post-partum.
- If FNAC is diagnostic, operation should be performed at the earliest safe opportunity either during the 2nd trimester or immediately post-partum.
- Pregnancy must be excluded before ^{131}I therapy is administered in women of reproductive age.
- Breastfeeding must be discontinued at least 8 weeks before ^{131}I therapy to avoid breast irradiation and should not be resumed until after a subsequent pregnancy.
- Pregnancy should be avoided for 6 months after any ^{131}I ablation.

Children

(See Box 1.11.)

Box 1.11 Thyroid cancer in children

- Uncommon, with an incidence of 0.2–5 per million per year.
- Over 85% are papillary, but with more aggressive behaviour than in adults (local invasion and distant metastases are commoner).
- An ↑ incidence in children in Belarus and Ukraine has been reported following the Chernobyl nuclear accident in 1986. *RET* oncogene rearrangements are common in these tumours.
- Management is similar to that in adults.
- Various studies report an overall recurrence rate of 0–39%, disease-free survival of 80–93%, and disease-specific mortality of 0–10%.
- Evidence is currently lacking on the independent risks or benefits of RAI or extensive surgery.
- Lifelong follow-up recommended with measurement of serum Tg.

Medullary thyroid carcinoma

(See also → Multiple endocrine neoplasia type 2 (MEN2), pp. 684–5.)
- Accounts for 5–10% of all thyroid cancers.
- MTC is rare, but aggressive. It can be cured only if intrathyroid at diagnosis.
- MTC can be sporadic (75%) or familial (25%), and the two forms are distinguished by *RET* mutation analysis.
- Calcitonin is the specific serum marker; its doubling time is the most important prognostic factor for survival and progression.
- An MDT should care for these patients.

Presentation
- Lump in neck.
- Systemic effects of calcitonin: flushing/diarrhoea.

Diagnosis
- FNAC.
- Comprehensive family history and screening in search for features of MEN type 2 are needed.
- Pathology specimens show immunostaining for calcitonin and staining for amyloid.

Management
- Baseline plasma calcitonin.
- Baseline biochemical investigations for phaeochromocytoma (PCC) and hyperparathyroidism.
- Genetic screening with *RET* mutation analysis in exons 10 and 11; if these are −ve, in exons 13–16.
- Staging with thoracoabdominal CT/MRI.
- MIBG (metaiodobenzylguanidine) and pentavalent ^{99m}Tc DMSA (dimercaptosuccinic acid) scintigraphy may also be used.

Treatment
- Total thyroidectomy and central node dissection are the 1° treatment modality.
- Germline *RET* mutation carriers should ideally undergo thyroidectomy before 5 years of age.

Adjuvant therapy
- Radioiodine and TSH suppression do not play a role.
- External radiotherapy has been shown to be of little benefit.
- Thirty per cent of MTC patients have distant metastases at diagnosis, and when progressing, systemic therapy with vandetanib or cabozantinib should be considered.
- Before starting this treatment, the possibility of using local treatment should be evaluated to delay systemic therapy.
- Therapeutic MIBG may help in some cases.

Follow-up
All patients should have lifelong follow-up at a dedicated regional service.

Anaplastic thyroid cancer and lymphoma

Anaplastic thyroid cancer

- Rare.
- Peak incidence: 7th decade; ♀: ♂ = 1:1.5.
- Characterized by rapid growth of a firm/hard, fixed tumour.
- Often infiltrates local tissue, such as the larynx and great vessels, and so does not move on swallowing. Stridor and obstructive respiratory symptoms are common.
- Aggressive, with poor long-term prognosis—7% 5-year survival rate and a mean survival of 6 months from diagnosis.
- Optimal results occur, following total thyroidectomy. This is usually not possible and external irradiation is used, sometimes in association with chemotherapy.
- Identification of pro-oncogenic targetable alterations shows promise for novel targeted therapeutic approaches.
- The majority of trials to date have consisted of small, single-arm studies and have presented modest results. Only a minority of trials have selected or stratified patients by molecular alterations.
- In *BRAF V600E* mutated anaplastic cancer, dabrafenib/trametinib combination therapy and vemurafenib monotherapy have both demonstrated efficacy.
- Everolimus has shown promising results in patients with PI3K/mTOR/ AKT pathway alterations.

Lymphoma

- Uncommon.
- Almost always associated with AITD (Hashimoto's thyroiditis). Occurs more commonly in ♀ and in patients aged >40 years.
- Characterized by rapid enlargement of the thyroid gland.
- May be limited to the thyroid gland or be part of a more extensive systemic lymphoma (usually non-Hodgkin's lymphoma).
- Treatment with radiotherapy alone or with chemotherapy if more extensive often produces good results.

Further reading

Ahmadi S, et al. (2016). Hürthle cell carcinoma: current perspectives. *Onco Targets Ther* **9**, 6873–84.

Cabanillas ME, et al. (2016). Thyroid cancer. *Lancet* **388**, 2783–95.

Dehbi HM, et al. (2019). Recurrence after low-dose radioiodine ablation and recombinant human thyroid-stimulating hormone for differentiated thyroid cancer (HiLo): long-term results of an open-label, non-inferiority randomised controlled trial. *Lancet Diabetes Endocrinol* **7**, 44–51.

Francis GL, et al. (2015). Management guidelines for children with thyroid nodules and differentiated thyroid cancer. *Thyroid* **25**, 716–59.

Haugen BR, et al. (2016). 2015 American Thyroid Association management guidelines for adult patients with thyroid nodules and differentiated thyroid cancer. The American Thyroid Association Guidelines Task Force on Thyroid Nodules and Differentiated Thyroid Cancer. *Thyroid* **26**, 1–133.

Jeon MJ, et al. (2017). Clinical outcomes after delayed thyroid surgery in patients with papillary thyroid microcarcinoma. *Eur J Endocrinol* **177**, 25–31.

Lim H, et al. (2017). Trends in thyroid cancer incidence and mortality in the United States, 1974–2013. *JAMA* **317**, 1338–48.

Ljubas J, et al. (2019). A systematic review of phase II targeted therapy clinical trials in anaplastic thyroid cancer. *Cancers (Basel)* **11**, 943.

Perros P, et al. (2014). Guidelines for the management of thyroid cancer. *Clin Endocrinol* **81** (Suppl 1), 1–122.

Russ G, *et al.* (2014). Thyroid incidentalomas: epidemiology, risk stratification with ultrasound and workup. *Eur Thyroid J* **3**, 154–63.

Schlumberger M, *et al.* (2018). Outcome after ablation in patients with low-risk thyroid cancer (ESTIMABL1): 5-year follow-up results of a randomised, phase 3, equivalence trial. *Lancet Diabetes Endocrinol* **6**, 618–26.

Tuttle RM, Alzahrani AS (2019). Risk stratification in differentiated thyroid cancer: from detection to final follow-up. *J Clin Endocrinol Metab* **104**, 4087–100.

Tuttle RM, *et al.* (2011). Clinical presentation and clinical outcomes in Chernobyl-related paediatric thyroid cancers: what do we know now? What can we expect in the future? Clin Oncol 23, 268–75.

Viola D, Elisei R (2019). Management of medullary thyroid cancer. *Endocrinol Metab Clin North Am* **48**, 285–301.

Xing M (2019). Genetic-guided risk assessment and management of thyroid cancer. *Endocrinol Metab Clin North Am* **48**, 109–24.

Wells SA Jr, *et al.* (2015). Revised American Thyroid Association guidelines for the management of medullary thyroid carcinoma. *Thyroid* **25**, 567–610.

Suggestions: how do I ... ?

Avoid indiscriminate ultrasound imaging of the thyroid

Although benign thyroid nodules are common, thyroid cancers are rare (annual incidence 2–3 per 100,000 population). Thyroid cancer incidence is reported to have ↑ in part due to ↑ detection of clinically silent papillary microcarcinomas (diameter <1cm) which have been reported in one-third of adults at postmortem. Ultrasonography as a screening tool is too sensitive and will result in unnecessary pursuit of findings which are common and rarely have pathological significance. It may have a place in investigating patients presenting with thyroid nodules to determine whether they are single or multiple, to provide an accurate indication of thyroid size and to differentiate cystic nodules from solid ones. An urgent 2-week referral is required for a thyroid nodule in the young (<18 years) or elderly, with a history of recent increase in size, obstructive symptoms, voice changes, or associated lymphadenopathy.

Hyperthyroidism is not a diagnosis—it is important to establish the cause

Hyperthyroidism commonly results from Graves' disease, toxic multinodular goitre, or toxic nodule. Drug causes include amiodarone, lithium, and ingestion of products containing high iodine loads. Transient causes include viral and silent autoimmune thyroiditis, which cause self-limiting thyrotoxicosis due to release of preformed hormones from a damaged thyroid gland, rather than due to overproduction of thyroid hormones. There are often clues in the history (family history, recent pregnancy, pain and tenderness over the thyroid, drugs) and clinical signs (presence of orbitopathy, diffuse goitre with a bruit, or a nodular goitre). CRP or ESR is elevated in cases of viral thyroiditis. The presence of TRAb is pathognomonic of Graves' disease. Positive TPOAb indicates AITD but are not diagnostic and can be found in both transient autoimmune thyroiditis and persisting hyperthyroidism of Graves' disease.

A 'wait-and-see' approach is reasonable in subclinical hyperthyroidism

Subclinical hyperthyroidism is defined as low serum TSH but normal T_4 and T_3, and has a prevalence of 1%. Elderly people and those with cardiovascular disease (CVD) are at ↑ risk of atrial fibrillation; ↑ bone loss is also reported. If serum TSH is between 0.1 and 0.4mU/L, the risk of progression to overt hyperthyroidism is negligible and there are no significant end-organ effects. But if serum TSH is persistently undetectable (<0.1mU/L), an assessment is needed to establish the aetiology and for possible treatment. For most, adopting a 'wait-and-see' approach is appropriate with checking of thyroid function every 6–12 months. If FT_3 alone is raised, this is termed 'T_3 toxicosis' and should be managed as for overt hyperthyroidism.

Side effects of thionamides

Although generally well tolerated, agranulocytosis is a rare, but potentially fatal side effect, occurring in 0.1–0.5%. As agranulocytosis occurs very suddenly, routine monitoring of FBC is not recommended. It usually occurs within the first 3 months after initiation of therapy (97% within the first 6 months, especially on higher doses), but cases have occurred a long time after starting treatment. Patients present with fever and evidence of infection, usually in the oropharynx. Written instructions should be documented as being given to discontinue the medication and check blood count, should the situation arise. Allergic-type reactions of rash, urticaria, and arthralgia occur in 1–5% and are often mild. In contrast to agranulocytosis, it does not usually necessitate drug withdrawal, as one thionamide may be substituted for another in the expectation that the 2nd agent may be taken without side effects.

Thionamides in pregnancy

Thionamides in low dosage can be given relatively safely, and both PTU and carbimazole are effective. Historically, PTU has been preferred as it is associated with a lower risk of aplasia cutis. However, concern regarding hepatotoxicity of PTU, particularly in children, has led to recommendations that it should only be prescribed preconception and in the 1st trimester, and that carbimazole should be used from the 2nd trimester onwards. The block-and-replace regimen using a thionamide and levothyroxine is contraindicated in pregnant women. Ideally, women should consider definitive treatment of Graves' disease by radioiodine or surgery pre-pregnancy.

Graves' orbitopathy may precede hyperthyroidism

Early symptoms of GO include grittiness, photophobia, lacrimation, swelling and redness of the eyelids and conjunctivae, restriction of eye movements, double or blurred vision, or retro-orbital pain. There may not always be significant exophthalmos. Although usually a clinical diagnosis, TRAb will typically be +ve. GO is present in about 50% of Graves' patients and is severe and potentially sight-threatening in 3–5%. In most cases, GO and hyperthyroidism occur within 18 months of each other, although GO may precede or follow the onset of hyperthyroidism. In ~5%, no evidence of hyperthyroidism is found (dysthyroid eye disease)—and GO can be unilateral. Stopping smoking, controlling thyroid dysfunction, selenium supplements, and eye lubricants are beneficial. Specialist assessment is required to consider MRI if there is diagnostic doubt and to assess whether GCs are required.

Amiodarone-induced thyrotoxicosis

There is often doubt as to whether a patient has AIT type 1 or 2. A regimen of 40mg of carbimazole (or methimazole) and 40mg of prednisone daily for 2 weeks, followed by measurement of serum T_3 levels, is a reasonable initial strategy. A reduction in serum T_3 levels by >50%, compared with pretreatment levels, suggests a diagnosis of AIT type 2, in which case thionamide treatment can be stopped. Prednisone is continued and doses tapered over 2–3 months, according to the patient's clinical and biochemical response. By contrast, if serum T_3 levels do not change following initial treatment, prednisone can be stopped and thionamide treatment continued, as the assumption is that the predominant diagnosis is AIT type 1.

Treat subclinical hypothyroidism if serum TSH >10mU/L or positive thyroid antibodies

Subclinical hypothyroidism is defined as raised serum TSH and normal T_4 and T_3 levels. Treatment is generally advised in patients with +ve thyroid antibodies (usually TPOAb) or serum TSH >10mU/L, as progression to overt hypothyroidism is more likely in such individuals. Younger persons (<65 years old) with cardiovascular risk factors should also be treated, since studies have shown an association between subclinical hypothyroidism and cardiovascular mortality. It is also reasonable to treat those with goitre or symptoms suggesting hypothyroidism—and women who are pregnant or intending conception—because of the potential risk of adverse pregnancy outcomes. If treatment is not advised, monitoring of serum TSH should be carried out 6- to 12-monthly.

Levothyroxine in pregnancy

The dose of levothyroxine should be adjusted to ensure that serum TSH is not higher than 2.5mU/L prior to conception. In treated hypothyroid women, serum TSH may rise during pregnancy and they will require an extra 25–50 micrograms daily during the first 4–8 weeks of pregnancy to maintain serum TSH between 0.5 and 2.5mU/L—especially during the 1st trimester, as the fetus is completely reliant on maternal thyroid status until the 2nd trimester. Women should be advised to increase their dose of levothyroxine by 25 micrograms as soon as their pregnancy is confirmed. Post-delivery, women should usually be advised to decrease the levothyroxine dose to the pre-pregnancy dose.

Websites

American Thyroid Association. https://www.thyroid.org
Association for Multiple Endocrine Neoplasia Disorders. https://www.amend.org.uk
British Association of Endocrine and Thyroid Surgeons. https://www.baets.org.uk/
British Thyroid Association. https://www.british-thyroid-association.org/
British Thyroid Foundation (BTF). https://www.btf-thyroid.org
Butterfly Thyroid Cancer Trust. www.butterfly.org.uk
European Thyroid Association. https://www.eurothyroid.com/
Hormone Health Network. https://www.hormone.org
Parathyroid UK. https://parathyroiduk.org
The UK Iodine Group. https://www.ukiodine.org
Thyroid Eye Disease Charitable Trust. www.tedct.org.uk

Chapter 2

Pituitary

Niki Karavitaki, Chris Thompson, and Iona Galloway

Anatomy and physiology of anterior pituitary gland

Anatomy

The pituitary gland is centrally located at the base of the brain in the sella turcica within the sphenoid bone. It is attached to the hypothalamus by the pituitary stalk and a fine vascular network. The cavernous sinuses are on either side of the sella, lateral and superior to the sphenoid sinuses, and comprise important neurovascular structures, including the cavernous segments of the internal carotid arteries and cranial nerves III, IV, V, and VI. The optic chiasm is located superiorly, separated from the pituitary by the suprasellar cistern and the diaphragma sellae (see Fig. 2.1). The pituitary measures around 13mm transversely, 9mm anteroposteriorly, and 6mm vertically and weighs ~100mg. It increases during pregnancy to almost twice its normal size, and it decreases in the elderly.

The anterior pituitary gland receives most of its blood supply from the hypothalamo-hypophyseal portal system (1° plexus, long portal venous system, and 2° plexus), which originates from the capillary plexus of the median eminence and superior stalk derived from the terminal ramifications of the superior and inferior hypophyseal arteries. This system carries blood and hypophysiotropic hormones down to the stalk. The remainder of the blood supply is through the pituitary capsular vessels originating from the superior hypophyseal arteries. The venous drainage from the anterior pituitary is through the cavernous sinuses into the petrosal sinuses and the internal jugular veins.

Physiology

(See Table 2.1.)

*Prolactin secretion**

Single-chain polypeptide. Pulsatile secretion in a circadian rhythm with around 14 pulses/24h, and a superimposed bimodal 24h pattern of secretion with a nocturnal peak during sleep and a lesser peak in the evening.

*Growth hormone secretion**

Single-chain polypeptide. Pulsatile secretion—usually undetectable in the serum, apart from 5–6 90min pulses/24h that occur more commonly at night. The secretion is modified by age and sex.

LH/FSH secretion

Glycoprotein hormones, with α chain common to LH and FSH (also TSH and hCG), but β chain specific for each hormone. Pulsatile secretion determined by the frequency and amplitude of gonadotrophin-releasing hormone (GnRH) secretion.

Thyroid-stimulating hormone secretion

Glycoprotein with α chain common to LH and FSH (also TSH and hCG), but β chain specific for each hormone. Pulsatile secretion with 9 ± 3 pulses/24h and ↑ amplitude of pulses at night.

---

* Concentrations ↑ with stress: NB. venepuncture.

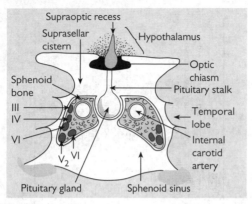

Fig. 2.1 The pituitary gland.

Reproduced from Firth J, Conlon C and Cox T (eds) (2020). *Oxford Textbook of Medicine*, 6th edn. Oxford University Press: Oxford, with permission from Oxford University Press.

Adrenocorticotrophic hormone*

Single-chain polypeptide cleaved from pro-opiomelanocortin (POMC). Circadian rhythm of secretion, beginning to rise from 3 a.m. to a peak before waking in the morning and gradually falling thereafter.

Posterior pituitary

(See ➲ Posterior pituitary, p. 229.)

Table 2.1 Anterior pituitary gland physiology

Cell type (hormone)	% pituitary	+ve regulation	−ve regulation	Targets	Effects
Somatotropes (GH)	45–50	Growth hormone-releasing hormone (GHRH)	IGF-1 and somatostatin	Liver, cartilage, muscle, fat, skin	Linear and somatic growth Metabolism (lipids, proteins, carbohydrates)
Lactotropes (PRL)	15–25 (↑ in pregnancy)	TRH and oestrogen	Dopamine	Breast	Lactation
Gonadotropes (LH/FSH)	10–15	GnRH, oestrogen—late follicular phase of menstrual cycle	Oestrogen Progesterone Testosterone Inhibin (FSH only)	Gonads	Sex steroid production Folliculogenesis and ovulation (♀) Spermatogenesis (♂)
Thyrotropes (TSH)	5–10	TRH	T_4, T_3, somatostatin	Thyroid	Thyroid hormone production
Corticotropes (adrenocorticotrophic hormone (ACTH))	15–20	Corticotrophin-releasing hormone (CRH)	Cortisol	Adrenal gland	GC and dehydroepiandrostenedione (DHEA) production

Reproduced from Drazin and Epstein, *Oxford American Handbook of Endocrinology and Diabetes* (2011), with permission of OUP.

Imaging

Background
- MRI currently provides optimal imaging of the pituitary gland.
- CT scans may still be useful in demonstrating calcification in tumours (e.g. craniopharyngiomas) and hyperostosis in association with meningiomas or evidence of bone destruction.
- Plain skull radiography may show evidence of pituitary fossa enlargement but has been superseded by MRI.

MRI appearances
(See Fig. 2.2.)
- T_1-weighted images demonstrate the CSF as dark grey, and the brain as much whiter. This imaging is useful for demonstrating anatomy clearly. The normal posterior pituitary gland appears bright white (due to neurosecretory granules and phospholipids) on T_1-weighted images, in contrast to the anterior gland which is of the same signal as white matter. The bony landmarks have low signal intensity on MRI, and air in the sphenoid sinus below the fossa shows no signal. Fat in the dorsum sellae may shine white. T_2-weighted images may sometimes be used to characterize haemosiderin and fluid contents of a cyst.
- IV gadolinium compounds are used for contrast enhancement. Because the pituitary and pituitary stalk have no blood–brain barrier, in contrast to the rest of the brain, the normal pituitary gland enhances brightly following gadolinium injection. Contrast enhancement is particularly useful for the demonstration of cavernous sinus involvement and microadenomas.
- The normal pituitary gland has a flat or slightly concave upper surface. In adolescence or pregnancy, the surface may become slightly convex.
- Empty sella syndrome is described in Box 2.1.

Box 2.1 Empty sella syndrome
- Herniation of subarachnoid space within the sella
- Pathogenetic mechanism not well known but may be associated with intracranial hypertension or autoimmune hypophysitis
- Often no clinical implication
- Headache, irregular menses, obesity, visual disturbances
- Endocrinology—high PRL, GH deficiency (GHD) commonest
- MDT assessment essential

Pituitary adenomas
On T_1-weighted images, pituitary adenomas are of lower signal intensity than the remainder of the normal gland. The size and extent of the pituitary adenomas are noted, in addition to the involvement of other structures such as invasion of the cavernous sinus, erosion of the fossa, and relations to the optic chiasm. Larger tumours may show low-intensity areas compatible with necrosis or cystic change, or higher-intensity signal due to haemorrhage. The presence of microadenomas may be difficult to demonstrate. Contrast enhancement, asymmetry of the gland, or stalk position can be helpful in such cases.

Neuroradiological classification
(See ➲ Pituitary carcinoma, pp. 204–5.)

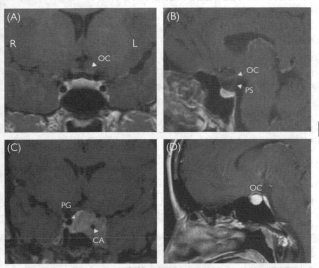

Fig. 2.2 Normal and abnormal pituitary MRI images. (A) Normal coronal, post contrast T_1 image showing optic chiasm (OC). (B) Normal sagittal image showing pituitary stalk (PS) and OC. (C) Pituitary macroadenoma with evidence of pituitary gland (PG) compression, left cavernous sinus invasion, and encroachment of carotid artery (CA). (D) Rathke's cleft cyst—bright T_1 image, consistent with mucinous, proteinaceous, or blood products.

Reproduced from Draznin and Epstein, *Oxford American Handbook of Endocrinology and Diabetes* (2011), with permission of OUP.

Craniopharyngiomas

These appear as intra- and/or suprasellar masses with cystic and/or solid components. A solid lesion appears as iso- or hypointense relative to the brain on precontrast T_1-weighted images, shows enhancement following gadolinium administration, and is usually of mixed hypo- or hyperintensity on T_2-weighted sequences. A cystic element is usually hypointense on T_1-weighted, and hyperintense on T_2-weighted, sequences. Protein, cholesterol, and methaemoglobin may cause high signal on T_1-weighted images. Calcification is present in 45–57%, better visualized by CT or on plain skull X-ray.

Further reading

Bashari WA, *et al.* (2019). Modern imaging of pituitary adenomas. *Best Pract Res Clin Endocrinol Metab* **33**, 101278.
Naidich MJ, Russell EJ (1999). Current approaches to imaging of the sellar region and pituitary. *Endocrinol Metab Clin North Am* **28**, 45.

Pituitary function—dynamic tests: insulin tolerance test (ITT)

Indications
- Assessment of ACTH reserve.
- Assessment of GH reserve.

Physiology
IV insulin is used to induce hypoglycaemia (glucose <2.2mmol/L with signs of glycopenia), which produces a standard stress causing ACTH and GH secretion.

Contraindications
- 9 a.m. serum cortisol <100nmol/L.
- Untreated hypothyroidism.
- Abnormal ECG.
- IHD.
- Seizures.
- Glycogen storage disease.

Note that patients should discontinue oral oestrogen replacement for 6 weeks before the test, as ↑ cortisol-binding globulin (CBG) will make the cortisol results difficult to interpret. Progesterone and transdermal oestrogen may be continued. (See Box 2.2 for procedure.)

Response
- In the presence of inadequate hypoglycaemia (glucose >2.2mmol/L), the test cannot be interpreted.
- A normal cortisol response (peak cortisol depends on the assay used and the most commonly accepted value is >450nmol/L) demonstrates the ability to withstand stress (including major surgery) without requiring GC cover. Subnormal cortisol response requires GC replacement treatment (see ➲ Glucocorticoids, pp. 146–7).
- Severe GHD in adults is diagnosed if peak GH <3 micrograms/L, and in the appropriate clinical situation (see ➲ Growth hormone replacement therapy in adults, pp. 148–9), GH replacement therapy may be recommended. In children, the secretory capacity of GH is higher and a cut-off of 10 micrograms/L is used.

Box 2.2 Insulin intolerance test procedure
- Continued medical surveillance is essential throughout.
- Patient is fasted overnight. Weight is checked.
- Insert cannula. Check basal (time 0) glucose, cortisol, and GH.
- Administer IV soluble insulin 0.15U/kg (occasionally, 0.2–0.3U/kg needed in untreated Cushing's syndrome and acromegaly because of ↑ insulin resistance).
- Measure glucose, GH, and cortisol at 30, 45, 60, 90, and 120min. Repeat insulin dose if a bedside stick test for glucose does not show hypoglycaemia at 45min.
- During the procedure, pulse rate, blood pressure (BP), and manifestations of hypoglycaemia should be recorded.
- The test is terminated if prolonged hypoglycaemia—may need to administer 25mL of 25% glucose and IV 100mg hydrocortisone after sampling for cortisol and GH.
- Ensure the patient eats lunch and has normal glucose before discharge.

Further reading

Fleseriu M, et al. (2016). Hormonal replacement in hypopituitarism in adults: an Endocrine Society Clinical Practice Guideline. J Clin Endocrinol Metab **101**, 3888.

Glucagon test

Indications

- Assessment of ACTH reserve.
- Assessment of GH reserve.

Physiology

Glucagon leads to release of insulin, which then leads to GH and ACTH release. The response may be $2°$ to the drop in glucose seen after the initial rise following glucagon injection or may relate to the nausea induced by glucagon.

Contraindications

- PCC or insulinoma, glycogen storage disease, and severe hypocortisolaemia.
- Often unreliable in patients with DM.
- Note that patients should discontinue oral oestrogen replacement for 6 weeks before the test, as ↑ CBG will make the cortisol results difficult to interpret.

Response

- The normal response is a rise in glucose to a maximum at 90min. The cut-offs for cortisol and GH are those of the ITT.
- This is a less reliable test than the ITT, as 20% of normal individuals may fail to respond.

  (See Box 2.3 for procedure.)

Box 2.3 Glucagon test procedure

The test is performed at 9 a.m. following an overnight fast. Basal GH and cortisol are measured, then 1mg (1.5mg if the patient weighs >90kg) glucagon is administered SC. The injection may cause nausea, abdominal pain, and vomiting. Samples for GH, cortisol, and glucose are checked from 90min, every 30min, until 240min.

GHRH and arginine test

Indications
- Assessment of GH reserve.

Physiology
- GHRH and arginine lead to GH release.

Contraindications
- None.

  (See Box 2.4 for procedure.)

Response
- Normal GH response is >4 micrograms/L, but body mass index (BMI) needs to be taken into account when interpreting the results.
- Can give false normal GH response if GHD is due to hypothalamic damage (e.g. after radiation).

Box 2.4 GHRH and arginine test procedure
- Fast from midnight, and administer GHRH 1g/kg (max 100g) IV, followed by an arginine infusion 0.5g/kg (max 35g) in 100mL of normal saline over 30min from time 0 (9 a.m.). Commonest side effect: flushing.
- Sample for GH at 0, 30, 45, 60, 75, 90, 105, and 120min.

Further reading
Molitch ME, et al. (2011). Evaluation and treatment of adult growth hormone deficiency: an Endocrine Society clinical practice guideline. J Clin Endocrinol Metab **96**, 1587.

ACTH stimulation test

Short Synacthen® test (SST) (tetracosactide test).

Indications
* Assessment of adrenal cortical function.
* Assessment of ACTH reserve.

Physiology

The rationale of its use is that chronic underexposure of the adrenal glands to ACTH (following prolonged corticosteroid therapy or due to hypothalamic–pituitary disease) will result in a blunted cortisol response to exogenously administered ACTH. Furthermore, a lack of cortisol rise following administration of ACTH demonstrates adrenal cortical disease. Prolonged ACTH administration will lead to cortisol secretion in ACTH deficiency, but not in 1° adrenal disease.
(See Box 2.5 for procedure.)

Response

Post-stimulation cortisol should rise to >450nmol/L at 30min (this is the most commonly used accepted cut-off and it is assay-dependent). This is an unreliable test of ACTH reserve within 6 weeks of an insult, e.g. surgery to the pituitary.

> **Box 2.5 ACTH stimulation test procedure**
> * The test can be done at any time of the day; the response is not time-dependent.
> * Synacthen® is administered 250 micrograms IM, and cortisol is measured at 0, 30, and 60min. When this test is used to measure ACTH reserve, only the 0 and 30min values are required. The dose may also be given IV, with identical results.
> * Note that patients should discontinue oestrogen replacement for 6 weeks before the test, as ↑ CBG will make the cortisol results difficult to interpret.

Clomifene test

Indications
- Assessment of gonadotrophin deficiency (e.g. Kallmann syndrome).

Physiology
Clomifene has mixed oestrogen and antioestrogenic effects. The basis of the test is competitive inhibition of oestrogen binding at the hypothalamus and pituitary gland, leading to ↑ LH and FSH after 3 days.

Contraindications
- Avoid in those with liver disease.
- May transiently worsen depression.

  (See Box 2.6 for procedure.)

Response
- The normal response is doubling of gonadotrophins by day 10, usually rising beyond the normal range.
- In hypothalamic or pituitary disease, no gonadotrophin rise is seen. Prepubertal patients may show a fall in gonadotrophins.
- Ovulation is presumed if day 21 progesterone is >30nmol/L.

Box 2.6 Clomifene test procedure
- Advise patient of possible side effects—visual disturbance (peripheral flickering of vision)—and also of possible ovulation in ♀ (contraceptive advice).
- Measure LH and FSH on days 0, 1, 7, and 10. In ♀, measure day 21 progesterone to detect whether ovulation has occurred.
- Administer clomifene 3mg/kg (max 200mg/day) in divided doses for 7 days.

---

hCG test

Indications
- To examine Leydig cell function (see ➲ Evalution of infertility, pp. 446–50).

TRH test

Indications

- Differentiation of pituitary TSH and hypothalamic TRH deficiency.
- Differentiation of TSH-secreting tumour from thyroid hormone resistance (see Table 1.16).

(See Box 2.7 for procedure.)

Response

- Normal response is a rise in TSH by >2mU/L to >3.4mU/L, with a maximum at 20min and lower values at 60min.
- A delayed peak (60min rather than 20min) is typically found in hypothalamic disease.

Box 2.7 TRH test procedure

- Administer TRH 200 micrograms IV to supine patient.
- Measure T_4 and TSH at time 0, and TSH at 20 and 60min.
- Note occasional reports of pituitary tumour haemorrhage. TRH induces a rise in BP.

Hypopituitarism

Definition

Hypopituitarism refers to either partial or complete deficiency of anterior and/or posterior pituitary hormones and may be due to 1° pituitary disease or to hypothalamic pathology which interferes with the hypothalamic control of the pituitary.

Causes

- Sellar and parasellar tumours (e.g. pituitary adenomas, craniopharyngiomas, Rathke's cleft cysts, meningiomas, 2° deposits (e.g. breast, lung), chordomas, gliomas).
- Radiotherapy—pituitary, cranial, nasopharyngeal (>30Gy).
- Pituitary infarction (apoplexy), Sheehan's syndrome.
- Infiltration/inflammation of the pituitary gland (e.g. sarcoidosis, hypophysitis, haemochromatosis, Langerhans cell histiocytosis, Erdheim–Chester disease, Wegener's).
- Empty sella.
- Infection (e.g. tuberculosis (TB), pituitary abscess).
- Medications (e.g. opiates, immune checkpoint inhibitors).
- Traumatic brain injury (TBI).
- Subarachnoid haemorrhage.
- Isolated hypothalamic-releasing hormone deficiency, e.g. Kallmann syndrome due to GnRH deficiency.
- Genetic causes (e.g. Kallmann syndrome, mutations of genes encoding transcription factors, including *HESX1* (homeobox gene expressed in embryonic stem cells 1), *LHX3* (Lim-domain homeobox gene 3), *LHX4* (Lim-domain homeobox gene 4), *PROP-1* (Prophet of Pit1), *POU1F1* (Pou domain, class 1, transcription factor 1)).
- Russell viper envenomation.
- Opiates—prevalence of hypogonadism 63%, hypocortisolism 15%.
- Idiopathic ACTH deficiency, associated with autoimmune disease.

Features

(See Table 2.2.)
- The clinical features depend on the type and degree of the hormonal deficits and the rate of its development, in addition to whether there is intercurrent illness. In the majority of cases, the development of hypopituitarism follows a characteristic order, with secretion of GH, then gonadotrophins being affected first, followed by TSH and ACTH secretion at a later stage. PRL deficiency is rare, except in Sheehan's syndrome associated with failure of lactation. Antidiuretic hormone (ADH) deficiency is virtually unheard of with pituitary adenomas but may be seen rarely with infiltrative disorders and trauma.
- The majority of the clinical features are similar to those occurring when there is target gland insufficiency. There are important differences, e.g. lack of pigmentation and normokalaemia in ACTH deficiency in contrast to ↑ pigmentation and hyperkalaemia (due to aldosterone deficiency) in Addison's disease.

NB. *Houssay phenomenon.* Amelioration of DM in patients with hypopituitarism due to reduction in counter-regulatory hormones.

Apoplexy

Apoplexy refers to infarction of the pituitary gland due to either haemorrhage or ischaemia. It occurs most commonly in patients with pituitary adenomas, usually macroadenomas, but it has also been reported to occur in other pituitary lesions like craniopharyngiomas and Rathke's cleft cysts. Reported predisposing factors include antithrombotic or anticoagulation treatment, arterial hypertension, DM, major surgery, and radiation therapy. It is a medical emergency, and rapid hydrocortisone replacement can be lifesaving.

It may present with a syndrome which is difficult to differentiate from any other intracranial haemorrhage, with sudden-onset headache, vomiting, meningism, visual disturbance, and cranial nerve palsy. The diagnosis is based on the clinical features and pituitary imaging which shows high signal on T_1- and T_2-weighted images a few days after the event (see ⊃ Prolactinomas, pp. 128–9). It should be managed by a pituitary multidisciplinary team (MDT). It has been suggested that early surgery (within 8 days) provides the optimal chance for visual recovery. However, some patients may be managed conservatively, if there are no significant visual or other neurological manifestations.

After apoplexy, pituitary tumour regrowth may occur, so follow-up surveillance is necessary.

Empty sella syndrome

An enlarged pituitary fossa, which may be 1° (due to arachnoid herniation through a congenital diaphragmatic defect) or 2° to surgery, radiotherapy, or pituitary infarction. May be obese. The majority of patients have normal pituitary function, with endocrine abnormalities documented in around 19% of the patients.

Traumatic brain injury

- Associated with subarachnoid haemorrhage and skull base fractures.
- May be seen with moderate to severe head trauma.
- Best assessed 3–6 months after trauma.
- Commonest deficiencies—GH and gonadotrophins.
- Reported prevalence in the chronic phase after TBI shows a wide range, mainly due to differences in the patient groups evaluated, the timing of testing in relation to injury, and tests/criteria applied to diagnose hypopituitarism.

Sheehan's syndrome

Haemorrhagic infarction of the enlarged post-partum pituitary gland causing hypopituitarism, following severe hypotension usually due to blood loss, e.g. post-partum haemorrhage. It can be fatal, and survivors require life replacement therapy. Improvement in obstetric care has made this a rare occurrence in the developed world.

Table 2.2 Main manifestations of hypopituitarism

Hormone deficiency	Clinical features
GH	Adult GHD (see ➲ Investigation of GH deficiency, p. 150)
	↓ energy levels, reduced exercise capacity, reduced lean body mass, impaired psychological well-being, ↑ cardiovascular risk
LH/FSH	Anovulatory cycles, oligo-/amenorrhoea, dyspareunia in ♀
	Erectile dysfunction and testicular atrophy, loss of 2° sexual hair (often after many years), tiredness, reduced muscle mass in ♂
	Reduced libido, infertility, osteoporosis in both sexes
ACTH	As in Addison's disease, except lack of hyperpigmentation, absence of hyperkalaemia (see ➲ Addison's disease title, pp. 292–3)
TSH	As in 1° hypothyroidism (see ➲ Hypothyroidism, p. 84)
PRL	Failure of lactation
ADH	Polyuria and polydipsia

Investigations of hypopituitarism

The aims of investigation of hypopituitarism are to biochemically assess the extent of pituitary hormone deficiency and also to elucidate the cause.

Basal hormone levels

Basal concentrations of the anterior pituitary hormone, as well as the target organ hormone, should be measured, as the pituitary hormones may remain within the normal range despite low levels of target hormone. Measurement of the pituitary hormone alone does not demonstrate that the level is inappropriately low, and the diagnosis may be missed.

* LH and FSH, and testosterone (9 a.m.) or oestradiol.
* TSH and FT4.
* 9 a.m. cortisol and ACTH.
* PRL.
* IGF-1 (NB. May be normal in up to half of GHD, depending on age).

  (See Box 2.8 for dynamic tests.)

Posterior pituitary function

* It is important to assess and replace ACTH deficiency before assessing ADH secretion because ACTH deficiency leads to reduced glomerular filtration rate (GFR) and inability to excrete a water load, which may therefore mask diabetes insipidus (DI).
* Plasma and urine osmolalities are often adequate as baseline measures. However, in patients suspected to have DI, a formal fluid deprivation test should usually be performed (see ⊃ Box 2.32, p. 231).

Investigation of the cause

* Pituitary imaging—MRI ± contrast.
* Investigation of hormonal hypersecretion if a pituitary tumour is demonstrated.
* Investigation of infiltrative disorders (see ⊃ Parasellar inflammatory conditions, pp. 214–15), e.g. serum and CSF angiotensin-converting enzyme (ACE), ferritin, hCG, α fetoprotein (aFP).
* Occasionally, biopsy of a lesion found on imaging is required.

Box 2.8 Dynamic tests

* Dynamic tests, such as the ITT (see ⊃ Pituitary function—dynamic tests: insulin tolerance test (ITT), pp. 130–1), or glucagon test (see ⊃ Glucagon test, p. 132) if the ITT is contraindicated, are used to assess cortisol and GH reserve.
* Some centres use the SST to assess ACTH reserve, using the 0 and 30min values of cortisol (see ⊃ ACTH stimulation test, p. 134). There are few false −ves using this investigation, and it is simpler to perform than the former tests but gives no measure of GH reserve. It is important to note that falsely normal results occur when hypopituitarism is of recent onset because the test relies on the fact that ACTH deficiency causes atrophy of the adrenal cortex, and therefore a delayed response to Synacthen®. Less than 6 weeks of ACTH deficiency may allow a 'normal' adrenal response.

Treatment of hypopituitarism

Treatment involves adequate and appropriate hormone replacement (see ➲ Anterior pituitary hormone replacement, p. 144; ➲ Glucocorticoids, pp. 146–7; and ➲ Growth hormone replacement therapy in adults, pp. 148–9) and management of the underlying cause.

Isolated defects of pituitary hormone secretion

Rarely, patients have isolated insufficiency of one anterior pituitary hormone. The aetiology of these disorders is largely unknown, although loss of hypothalamic control may play a role; an autoimmune pathology has been suggested in some, and genetic mutations in others. Examples include:

- GnRH deficiency (Kallmann syndrome—genetic disorder causing GnRH deficiency ± anosmia).
- Isolated ACTH deficiency.
- *Pit1* gene mutation (leads to isolated GH, PRL, and TSH deficiency).
- *Prop1* gene mutation (leads to isolated GH, PRL, TSH, and gonadotrophin deficiency).

Further reading

Briet C, et al. (2015).. Pituitary apoplexy. *Endocr Rev* **36**, 622–41.

Capatina C, et al. (2015). Management of endocrine disease: pituitary tumour apoplexy. *Eur J Endocrinol* **172**, 179.

Chiloiro S, et al. (2017). Diagnosis of endocrine disease. Primary empty sella: a comprehensive review. *Eur J Endocrinol* **177**, 275.

Fleseriu M, et al. (2016). Hormonal replacement in hypopituitarism in adults: an Endocrine Society Clinical Practice Guideline. *J Clin Endocrinol Metab* **101**, 3888.

Glynn N, Agha A (2019). The frequency and the diagnosis of pituitary dysfunction after traumatic brain injury. *Pituitary* **22**, 249.

Pal A, et al. (2011). Pituitary apoplexy in non-functioning pituitary adenomas: long term follow up is important because of significant numbers of tumour recurrences. *Clin Endocrinol* **75**, 501.

Shivaprasad C, et al. (2019). Delayed hypopituitarism following Russell's viper envenomation: a case series and literature review. *Pituitary* **22**, 4–12.

Tanviverdi F, et al. (2015). Pituitary dysfunction after traumatic brain injury: a clinical and pathophysiological approach. *Endocr Rev* **36**, 305–42.

Anterior pituitary hormone replacement

Background

Anterior pituitary hormone replacement therapy is usually performed by replacing the target hormone rather than the pituitary or hypothalamic hormone that is actually deficient. The exceptions to this are GH replacement (see ➲ Growth hormone replacement therapy in adults, pp. 148–9) and when fertility is desired (see ➲ Management of female infertility, pp. 452–4; ➲ Management of male infertility, p. 456).

(See Table 2.3 for usual doses.) The 2016 Society of Endocrinology guidelines outline interactions between replacement hormones and may be seen in Box 2.9.

Thyroid hormone replacement

This is discussed in the section on 1° hypothyroidism (see ➲ Treatment of hypothyroidism, pp. 88–93).

Monitoring of therapy

- In contrast to replacement in 1° hypothyroidism, the measurement of TSH cannot be used to assess adequacy of replacement in TSH deficiency due to hypothalamo–pituitary disease. Therefore, monitoring of treatment in order to avoid under- and over-replacement should be via both clinical assessment and by measuring FT_4 concentrations, which should be in the middle/upper part of the normal range.
- FT_4 should be monitored before ingestion of daily thyroxine tablets.
- T_4 requirements should be reassessed when additional replacement with other pituitary hormones becomes necessary. Thus, GH therapy, when added, can cause a reduction of FT_4 or unmask previously undiagnosed hypothyroidism.

Sex hormone replacement

(See ➲ Hormone replacement therapy, pp. 392–5; ➲ Androgen replacement therapy, pp. 426–7.)

Oestrogen/testosterone administration is the usual method of replacement, but gonadotrophin therapy is required if fertility is desired (see ➲ Management of male infertility, p. 456; ➲ Gonadotrophins, p. 459).

Table 2.3 Usual doses of hormone replacement therapy

Hydrocortisone	10mg on waking, 5mg at lunchtime, and 5mg early evening or twice-daily regimens with a usual total dose of 15–20mg/day and the highest dose to be taken in the morning at awakening
Levothyroxine	100–150 micrograms/day
GH	0.2–0.6mg/day for adults (0.4–1.0IU)
Oestrogens/ testosterone	Depends on formulation

Box 2.9 Interactions between replacement hormones

Glucocorticoids and GH
- Suggest testing HPA axis functionality before and after starting GH replacement in patients who are not receiving GC replacement and who have demonstrated apparently normal pituitary–adrenal function.

Glucocorticoids and thyroid
- Suggest evaluating patients with CH for AI before starting levothyroxine therapy. If this is not feasible, clinicians should prescribe empiric GC therapy in patients with CH who are starting levothyroxine therapy until there is a definitive evaluation for AI.

Glucocorticoids and oestrogen
- Suggest that when clinicians assess adrenal reserve or the adequacy of HC replacement, they take into consideration that total serum cortisol level can be elevated due to the effects of oestrogen on CBG.

GH and thyroid
- Recommend that clinicians monitor euthyroid patients with GHD who begin GH therapy for the risk of developing CH, and if FT4 levels decrease below the reference range, these patients should begin levothyroxine therapy. CH patients with GHD who are already receiving levothyroxine may require ↑ levothyroxine doses when they begin GH therapy to maintain FT4 levels within target ranges.
- Suggest clinicians treat CH before performing GH stimulation testing because CH may impair the accurate diagnosis of GHD.

Oestrogen and thyroid hormones
- In patients with CH requiring changes in oestrogen therapy, recommend monitoring FT4 levels and adjusting levothyroxine doses to maintain FT4 levels within target ranges.

GH and oestrogen
- Suggest that women on oral oestrogen replacement receive higher GH doses, compared with eugonadal ♀ or ♂.

Glucocorticoids and diabetes insipidus
- Because AI may mask the presence of partial DI, we suggest monitoring for the development of DI after starting GC replacement. Conversely, patients with improved DI without an AI diagnosis should undergo AI testing.

Source: data from Fleseriu M et al (2016) "Hormonal Replacement in Hypopituitarism in Adults: An Endocrine Society Clinical Practice Guideline" *The Journal of Clinical Endocrinology & Metabolism* 101(11): 3888–3921 with permission from Oxford University Press.

Glucocorticoids

Replacement therapy

Patients with ACTH deficiency need GC replacement only and do not require mineralocorticoids (MCs), in contrast to patients with 1° AI (Addison's disease).

The normal production rate of cortisol is 9.9 ± 2.7mg/day. The GC most commonly used for replacement therapy is *hydrocortisone*. It is rapidly absorbed, with a short half-life (90–120min). *Prednisolone* and *dexamethasone* are occasionally used for GC replacement. The longer half-lives of these two drugs make them useful where sustained ACTH suppression is required in, for example, congenital adrenal hyperplasia (CAH). Dexamethasone is useful when monitoring endogenous production, as it is not detected in most cortisol assays. Cortisol acetate was previously used for GC replacement therapy but requires hepatic conversion to active cortisol. More recent approaches for replacement therapy include modified-release hydrocortisone preparations and continuous SC infusion. The GC replacement regimen with the most optimal impact on the metabolic profile, cardiovascular risk factors, bone mineral density, infection rates, risk of adrenal crisis, and QoL remain to be established.

Monitoring of replacement

It is important to avoid over-replacement which is associated with ↑ BP, insulin resistance and impaired glucose metabolism, and reduced bone mineral density (BMD). Under-replacement leads to non-specific symptoms, as seen in Addison's disease (see → Addison's disease, pp. 292–3). As there are no reliable markers to determine the exact GC needs, monitoring of replacement should mainly rely on clinical assessment. Biochemical monitoring with urinary free cortisol (UFC) levels is rarely useful due to wide inter- and intravariability of the measurements. Some centres use plasma cortisol measurements on a hydrocortisone day curve (see Box 2.10). The aim is to keep plasma cortisol between 150 and 300nmol/L, avoiding nadirs of <50nmol/L pre-dose. The day curve is particularly useful for patients with suspected malabsorption or ↑ steroid metabolic clearance. Conventional replacement (20mg hydrocortisone/24h) may overtreat patients with partial ACTH deficiency.

Safety

Patients should be encouraged to wear a MedicAlert, indicating that they are cortisol-deficient, to carry a steroid card, and to keep a vial of parenteral 100mg hydrocortisone and a syringe and needle at home to be administered in emergency situations. Systematic education of patients and family members on sick day rules and management of adrenal crisis is a vital element in the care of these patients.

Equivalent oral glucocorticoid doses

Hydrocortisone 1mg is equivalent to:
- Cortisone acetate 1.5mg.
- Prednisolone 0.2mg.
- Dexamethasone 0.0375mg.
- Prednisolone 4mg ≡ hydrocortisone 20mg ≡ dexamethasone 0.75mg.

Box 2.10 Hydrocortisone day curve

There are various protocols for this test, ranging from a 3-point curve to detect under-replacement (used with 24h UFC to detect over-replacement)—serum cortisol checked at 9 a.m., 12.30 p.m. (before the lunchtime dose), and 5 p.m. (pre-evening dose)—to more frequent sampling to detect over- and under-replacement. This involves serum cortisol at time 0, then administration of the morning dose of hydrocortisone. Plasma cortisol is then checked at 30min, at 1, 2, 3, and 5h (pre-lunchtime dose specimen), and at 7 and 9h (pre-evening dose), followed by samples at 10 and 11h.

- Oral oestrogen therapy should be stopped 6 weeks before the test, as ↑ CBG, leading to higher cortisol values, will make the test uninterpretable.
- This test is only valid for hydrocortisone replacement. Prednisolone or dexamethasone replacement can only be monitored clinically.

Acute/severe intercurrent illness

(See ➡ Intercurrent illness, pp. 304–7.)
- *Mild disease without fever.* No change in GC replacement.
- *Pyrexial illness.* Double replacement dose for duration of fever or until antibiotics are stopped.
- *Vomiting or diarrhoea.* Parenteral therapy 100mg IM (from general practitioner (GP)/trained relative; useful for patient to have vial of hydrocortisone at home with instruction sheet for emergency administration by suitable, trained personnel).
- *Adrenal crisis.* Patients thought to be having an adrenal crisis should be treated promptly with 100mg hydrocortisone by IV or IM injection, followed by 200mg hydrocortisone/24h continuous IV infusion in glucose 5%/24h, or 50mg 6-hourly IM (or IV) and IV fluid (sodium chloride (NaCl) 0.9%).

Further reading

Fleseriu M, *et al.* (2016). Hormonal replacement in hypopituitarism in adults: an Endocrine Society Clinical Practice Guideline. *J Clin Endocrinol Metab* **101**, 3888.

Persani L (2012). Central hypothyroidism: pathogenic, diagnostic and therapeutic challenges. *J Clin Endocrinol Metab* **97**, 3068–78.

Prete A, *et al.* (2020). Prevention of adrenal crisis: cortisol responses to major stress compared to stress dose hydrocortisone delivery. *J Clin Endocrinol Metab* **105**, 2262.

Growth hormone replacement therapy in adults

Background

There is now a considerable amount of evidence that there are significant and specific consequences of GHD in adults and that many of these features improve with GH replacement therapy. GH replacement for adults has now been approved in many countries.

Definition

It is important to differentiate between adult- and childhood-onset GHD.

- Although *childhood-onset* GHD occurs 2° to structural lesions, such as craniopharyngiomas and germinomas, and following treatment, such as cranial irradiation, the commonest cause in childhood is an isolated variable deficiency of GHRH which may resolve in adult life because of maturation of the hypothalamo–somatotroph axis. It is therefore important to retest patients with childhood-onset GHD when linear growth is completed (50% recovery of this group due to, for example, physiological improvement of hypothalamo–pituitary function after puberty, real transient GHD, and false +ve provocative testing).
- *Adult onset.* GHD usually occurs 2° to a structural pituitary or parapituitary condition or due to the effects of surgical treatment or radiotherapy.

Prevalence

- Adult-onset GHD: 1/10,000.
- Adult GHD due to adult- and childhood-onset GHD: 3/10,000.

Benefits of GH replacement

- Improved QoL and psychological well-being.
- Improved exercise capacity.
- ↑ lean body mass and reduced fat mass.
- Prolonged GH replacement therapy (>12–24 months) has been shown to increase BMD.
- There are as yet no outcome studies in terms of cardiovascular mortality. However, GH replacement leads to a reduction in cholesterol, CRP, and inflammatory markers. GH replacement also leads to improved ventricular function and ↑ left ventricular mass.

NICE guidelines for GH replacement

(See ℛ https://www.nice.org.uk/guidance/ta64)

Adult criteria

- Severe GHD—GH <10mU/L.
- Impaired QoL (Adult Growth Hormone Deficiency Assessment (AGHDA) QoL score ≥11).
- Treatment for other pituitary hormone deficiencies.

Reassessment of treatment after 9 months' treatment (3-month dose titration, followed by 6-month therapeutic trial)—GH discontinued if improvement in AGHDA score <7.

Young adults (up to 25 years)
- GH discontinued for 3 months at completion of linear growth (<2cm/ year) and GH status reassessed.
- If severe GHD confirmed, GH continued at adult dose until age 25 years (peak bone mass).
- Age 25 and above—adult criteria apply.

Diagnosis

The diagnosis of GHD depends on appropriate biochemical testing in the presence of an appropriate clinical context. The latter is important because distinguishing 'partial GHD' from physiological causes of reduced GH secretion, such as obesity or ageing, and pathological causes, e.g. hypercortisolaemia in Cushing's syndrome, can be problematic. In these situations, GHD can be diagnosed when there is supportive evidence such as pituitary disease and other anterior pituitary hormone deficiencies.

Who should be tested?

As the features of GHD may be non-specific and biochemical tests can be misleading in certain clinical situations, such as obesity, investigation of GHD should only be performed in the following groups of patients:
- Patients with hypothalamo–pituitary disease (GHD occurs early in hypopituitarism and is almost invariable in patients with other anterior pituitary hormone deficiencies).
- Patients who had childhood-onset GHD.
- Patients who have received cranial irradiation.

Investigation of GH deficiency

Dynamic tests of GH secretion

- The ITT is most widely used test. Peak GH <10mU/L (3 micrograms/L) is diagnostic of severe GHD (see ⮞ Abnormalities in adult GH deficiency, below).
- Alternative tests, if the ITT is contraindicated, include a combination of GHRH (1 microgram/kg) and arginine (0.5g/kg) IV over 30min (see ⮞ GHRH and arginine test, p. 133) or a glucagon test (see ⮞ Glucagon test, p. 132).
- A 2nd confirmatory dynamic biochemical test is recommended, particularly in patients who have suspected isolated GHD.

A single GH dynamic test is sufficient to diagnose GHD in patients with two or three pituitary hormonal defects.

IGF-1

IGF-1 concentrations may remain within the age-matched reference range despite severe GHD in up to 50% of patients, and therefore do not exclude the diagnosis.

Reduced IGF-1 is seen in a number of conditions. (For causes of lowered IGF-1 levels, see Box 2.11.)

Abnormalities in adult GH deficiency

(See Box 2.9.)
- Stimulated GH <10mU/L (3 micrograms/L).
- Low or low-normal IGF-1 (IGF-1 may be normal in up to 50%, depending on age).
- ↓ BMD.
- ↑ insulin resistance.
- Dyslipidaemia (↑ LDL).
- Impaired cardiac function.

Clinical features of GH deficiency

- Impaired well-being.
- Reduced energy and vitality (depressed mood, ↑ social isolation, ↑ anxiety).
- Reduced muscle mass and impaired exercise capacity.
- ↑ central adiposity (↑ waist/hip ratio) and ↑ total body fat.
- ↓ sweating and impaired thermogenesis.
- ↑ cardiovascular risk.
- ↑ fracture risk (osteoporosis).

Box 2.11 Causes of lowered IGF-1 levels

- GHD.
- Malnutrition.
- Poorly controlled DM.
- Hepatic disease.
- Renal disease.
- Severe intercurrent illness.

Treatment of GH deficiency

All patients with GHD should be considered for GH replacement therapy. In particular, patients with impaired QoL, reduced mineral density, an adverse cardiovascular risk profile, and reduced exercise capacity. Currently, GH replacement is offered with daily injections of recombinant human GH. Long-acting forms of GH are also under development and can be administered at weekly intervals.

Dose

(See Table 2.4.)

- Unlike paediatric practice, where GH doses are determined by body weight and surface area, most adult endocrinologists use dose titration, using serial IGF-1 measurements, to increase the dose of GH until the IGF-1 level approaches the middle to upper end of the age-matched IGF-1 reference range. This reduces the likelihood of side effects, mainly related to fluid retention, which were frequently observed in the early studies of GH replacement in adults when doses equivalent to those used in paediatric practice were used.
- The normal production of GH is 200–500 micrograms/day in an adult. Current recommendations are a starting dose of 0.1–0.4mg/day. The maintenance dose is usually 0.2–0.6mg/day. The dose in ♀ is often higher than that for age-matched ♂ (particularly if the ♀ is on oral oestrogens).

Monitoring of treatment

- A clinical examination, looking for reduction in overall body weight (a good response is loss of 3–5kg in 12 months) and reduced waist/hip ratio. BP may be reduced in hypertensive patients because of reduction in peripheral systemic vascular resistance.
- IGF-1 is monitored to avoid over-replacement, aiming to keep values within the age-matched reference range. During dose titration, IGF-1 should be measured every 1–2 months. Once a stable dose is reached, IGF-1 should be checked at least once a year.
- The adverse effects experienced with GH replacement usually resolve with dose reduction and tend to be less frequent with the lower starting doses used in current practice.
- GH treatment may be associated with impairment of insulin sensitivity, and therefore, markers of glycaemia should be monitored every 6 months.
- Lipids should be monitored every 6 months.
- BMD should be monitored every 2 years, particularly in those with ↓ BMD.
- It may be helpful to monitor QoL using a questionnaire such as the AGHDA questionnaire.
- It is recommended that patients receiving GH therapy should remain under the care of an endocrinologist.

Table 2.4 GH starting doses, according to age

Age (years)	Dose (mg/day)
<60	0.2–0.4
>60	0.1–0.2

GH therapy in special situations

- *Pregnancy.* There are currently no data on GH replacement in pregnancy.
- *Critical illness.* There is no good evidence for a beneficial effect of GH replacement during critical illness. Patients should continue GH replacement during non-severe illness, but many endocrinologists would suggest that GH should be discontinued in patients who are severely ill, e.g. those receiving major surgery or on ITU.
- When used in multiple hormone deficiency, adding GH can precipitate adrenal crisis. TFTs should be monitored when adding GH therapy in hypopituitarism

Adverse effects of GH replacement
(See Box 2.12 for contraindications.)
- Sodium (Na) and water retention.
  - Weight gain.
  - Carpal tunnel syndrome.
- Hyperinsulinaemia.
- Arthralgia (possibly due to intra-articular cartilage swelling).
- Myalgia.
- Benign intracranial hypertension (resolves on stopping treatment).
- No data suggest that GH replacement therapy is associated with a risk of pituitary tumour recurrence or risk of 2° malignancies.
- Isolated GHD is not associated with an increase in all-cause mortality.
- The risk of 2nd neoplasm is ↑ with GH treatment in childhood-onset GHD.

Box 2.12 Contraindications to GH replacement
- Active malignancy.
- Benign intracranial hypertension.
- Pre-proliferative/proliferative retinopathy in DM.
- Acute severe/critical illness.
- Renal transplant.
- Prader–Willi (severe obesity, severe respiratory impairment).

Further reading

Carroll PV, et al. (1998). GH deficiency in adulthood and the effects of GH replacement: a review. *J Clin Endocrinol Metab* **83**, 382–95.

Fleseriu M, et al. (2016). Hormonal replacement in hypopituitarism in adults: an Endocrine Society Clinical Practice Guideline. *J Clin Endocrinol Metab* **101**, 3888.

Melmed S (2019). Pathogenesis and diagnosis of growth hormone deficiency in adults. *N Engl J Med* **380**, 2551–62.

Molitch ME, et al. (2011). Endocrine Society. Evaluation and treatment of adult growth hormone deficiency: an Endocrine Society clinical practice guideline. *J Clin Endocrinol Metab* **96**, 1587–609.

Savendahl L, et al. (2020). Long-term mortality after childhood growth hormone treatment: the SAGhE cohort study. *Lancet Diabetes Endocrinol* **8**, 683–92.

Pituitary tumours

Epidemiology

- Pituitary adenomas are the commonest pituitary tumours in adults and constitute 10–15% of 1° brain tumours.
- ~10% of individuals harbour incidental tumours, most commonly microadenomas.
- The incidence of clinically apparent pituitary disease is around 1 in 10,000.
- Pituitary carcinoma is very rare (<0.1% of all tumours) and is most commonly ACTH- or PRL-secreting.

(See Table 2.5.)

Table 2.5 Approximate relative frequencies of pituitary tumours

Tumour type	Mean prevalence (per 100,000)	Annual incidence
Clinically overt pituitary adenomas	72	1–2/100,000
Acromegaly (12%)	9	4 cases/million
Cushing's syndrome (7%)	1	2 cases/million
Non-functioning adenoma (25%)	22	6 cases/million
Prolactinomas (49%)	44	10 cases/million (if hyperprolactinaemia is considered, then higher incidence)
TSHomas (<1%)		

Classification

Size
- Microadenoma <1cm.
- Macroadenoma ≥1cm.

Functional status (clinical or biochemical)
- Prolactinoma 35–40%.
- Non-functioning 30–35%.
- GH (acromegaly) 10–15%.
- ACTH adenoma (Cushing's disease) 5–10%.
- TSH adenoma <5%.

WHO 2017 classification
(See Table 2.6.)

Pathogenesis

The mechanism of pituitary tumourigenesis remains largely unclear. Pituitary adenomas are monoclonal, supporting the theory that there are intrinsic molecular events leading to pituitary tumourigenesis. However, the mutations (e.g. *p53*) found in other tumour types are only rarely found. A role for hormonal factors and, in particular, the hypothalamic hormones in tumour progression is also a suggested hypothesis.

Table 2.6 2017 WHO classification of adenomas

Adenoma type	Morphological variants	Immunostaining	Transcription factors and other cofactors
Lactotroph	Sparsely granulated adenoma	PRL	PIT-1, ERα
	Densely granulated adenoma	PRL	PIT-1, ERα
	Acidophilic stem cell adenoma	PRL, GH	PIT-1, ERα
Somatotroph	Densely granulated adenoma	GH ± PRL ± α-SU Cytokeratin CAM5.2 perinuclear staining	PIT-1
	Sparsely granulated adenoma	GH ± PRL Cytokeratin CAM5.2 Highlights fibrous bodies	PIT-1
	Mammosomatotroph adenoma	GH + PRL (in same cells) ± α-SU	PIT-1, ERα
	Mixed somatotroph–lactotroph adenoma	GH + PRL (in different cells) ± α-SU	PIT-1, ERα
Thyrotroph		β-TSH, α-SU	PIT-1
Corticotroph	Densely granulated adenoma	ACTH	T-PIT
	Sparsely granulated adenoma	ACTH	T-PIT
	Crooke cell adenoma	ACTH Cytokeratin CAM5.2 forming ring-like appearance	T-PIT
Gonadotroph		β-FSH, β-LH, α-SU (various combinations)	SF-1, GATA3, ERα
Null cell	Oncocytic variant	None or focal α-SU	None
Plurihormonal	Plurihormonal Pit-1 +ve adenoma	GH, PRL, β-TSH ± α-SU	PIT-1
	Adenomas with unusual immunohistochemical combinations	Various combinations: ACTH/GH, ACTH/PRL	N/A

Reprinted from Lopes M (2018) "The 2017 World Health Organization classification of tumours of the pituitary gland: a summary" *Acta Neuropathol.* 143(4):521–535 with permission from Springer.

Mortality

Pituitary disease is associated with ↑ mortality, predominantly due to vascular disease. This may be due to oversecretion of GH or ACTH, hormone deficiencies, or excessive replacement (e.g. of hydrocortisone). Radiotherapy of the pituitary is also associated with ↑ mortality (especially cerebrovascular). Craniopharyngioma patients have particularly ↑ mortality.

Further reading

Fernandez A, *et al.* (2010). Prevalence of pituitary adenomas: a community-based, cross-sectional study in Banbury (Oxfordshire, UK). *Clin Endocrinol (Oxf)* **72**, 377.

Fleseriu M, *et al.* (2020). Pituitary society guidance: pituitary disease management and patient care recommendations during the COVID-19 pandemic—an international perspective. *Pituitary* **23**, 327–37.

Lopes MBS (2020). World Health Organization 2017 classification of pituitary tumors. *Endocrinol Metab Clin North Am* **49**, 375.

Molecular mechanisms of pituitary tumour pathogenesis

Genetic landscape of pituitary adenomas

Somatic mutations

- *GNAS*, found in up to 40% of GH-secreting tumours (less in non-Caucasians) and also described in a minority of non-functioning pituitary adenomas (NFAs) and ACTH-secreting tumours.
- *USP8* ((ubiquitin-specific peptidase 8) recurrent somatic gain-of-function mutations have been found in the *USP8* gene in corticotropinomas.

Who to screen

(See Table 13.1.)

Germline mutations

- *MEN1 gene*. Loss of heterozygosity (LOH) at 11q13 had been previously demonstrated in up to 20% of sporadic pituitary tumours; however, the expression of the *MEN1* gene product menin is not downregulated in the majority of sporadic pituitary tumours.
- *MEN-4* (see ➔ Multiple endocrine neoplasia type 4 (MEN4), p. 693). An AD syndrome that results from germline heterozygous loss-of-function mutations in *CDKN1B* or other cyclin-dependent kinase inhibitor genes. Pituitary tumours occur in 37% of reported MEN-4 cases.
- Carney complex (CNC) (see ➔ Carney complex, pp. 666–8.) A rare AD syndrome characterized by skin pigmentation, cardiac myxomas, GH and PRL-secreting pituitary adenomas, and Cushing syndrome from primary pigmented nodular adrenocortical disease (PPNAD). Most often, it is caused by germline mutations in the tumour suppressor gene *PRKAR1A*.
- Familial isolated pituitary adenoma (FIPA). This is an AD disease defined by the presence of pituitary adenomas in two or more family members in the same family, with no other syndromic features. In 90% of FIPA families, the gene responsible for the genetic predisposition is unknown. Heterozygote germline loss-of-function mutations have been identified in the aryl hydrocarbon receptor interacting protein (*AIP*) gene in 10% of FIPA families. Due to incomplete penetrance, this gene has also been identified in apparently sporadic cases (3.6% of unselected sporadic pituitary adenoma patients). Most of the clinically presenting *AIP* mutation +ve patients have somatotroph or somatolactotroph tumours; some 10% have lactotroph tumours and rarely have clinically non-functioning adenomas.
- X-linked acrogigantism (XLAG). This is a rare condition in patients with very early onset of GH excess, usually presenting at a very early age. Disease due to a *de novo* germline or mosaic duplication of the *GRP101* gene, usually within a microduplicated region (Xq23.6) on the X chromosome.
- The association of familial paragangliomas and phaeochromocytomas (PPGL) and pituitary adenomas, called 'the three P association (3PA)', is a rare condition caused by germline *SDHx* mutations.

Further reading

Barry S, Korbonits M (2020). Update on the genetics of pituitary tumors. *Endocrinol Metab Clin North Am* **49**, 433.

Pepe S, *et al.* (2019). Germline and mosaic mutations causing pituitary tumours: genetic and molecular aspects. *J Endocrinol* **240**, R21–45.

Prolactinomas

Epidemiology

- Prolactinomas are the commonest functioning pituitary tumour.
- Postmortem studies show microadenomas in 10% of the population.
- During life, microprolactinomas are commoner than macroprolactinomas, and there is a ♀ preponderance of microprolactinomas.

Pathogenesis

Unknown. Occur in 20% of patients with MEN1 (prolactinomas are the commonest pituitary tumour in MEN1 and may be more aggressive than sporadic prolactinomas). Malignant prolactinomas are very rare.

Clinical features

Hyperprolactinaemia (microadenomas and macroadenomas)
- Galactorrhoea (up to 90% ♀, <10% ♂).
- Disturbed gonadal function in ♀ presents with menstrual disturbance (up to 95%)—amenorrhoea, oligomenorrhoea, or with infertility and reduced libido.
- Disturbed gonadal function in ♂ presents with loss of libido and/ or erectile dysfunction. Presentation with reduced fertility and oligospermia or gynaecomastia is unusual.
- Hyperprolactinaemia is associated with a long-term risk of ↓ BMD.
- Hyperprolactinaemia inhibits GnRH release, leading to ↓ LH secretion. There may be a direct action of PRL on the ovary to interfere with LH and FSH signalling, which inhibits oestradiol and progesterone secretion and also follicle maturation.

Mass effects (macroadenomas only)
- Headaches and visual field defects (usually uni- or bitemporal field defects).
- Hypopituitarism.
- Invasion of the cavernous sinus may lead to cranial nerve palsies and even temporal lobe epilepsy.
- Occasionally, very invasive tumours may erode bone and present with a CSF leak or 2° meningitis.

For causes of hyperprolactinaemia, see Box 2.13.

Box 2.13 Causes of hyperprolactinaemia

- Physiological:
  - Pregnancy.
  - Sexual intercourse.
  - Nipple stimulation/suckling.
  - Neonatal.
  - Stress.
- Pituitary tumour:
  - Prolactinomas.
  - Mixed GH/PRL-secreting tumour.
  - Macroadenoma compressing stalk.
  - Empty sella.
- Hypothalamic disease—mass compressing stalk (craniopharyngioma, meningioma, neurofibromatosis (NF)).
- Infiltration—sarcoidosis, Langerhans cell histiocytosis.
- Stalk section—head injury, surgery.
- Cranial irradiation.
- Drug treatment:
  - Dopamine receptor antagonists—metoclopramide, domperidone.
  - Neuroleptics*—perphenazine, flupentixol, fluphenazine, haloperidol, thioridazine, chlorpromazine, trifluoperazine, risperidone, sulpiride.
  - Antidepressants—tricyclics, selective serotonin reuptake inhibitors (SSRIs), monoamine oxidase inhibitors (MAOIs), sulpiride, amisulpride, imipramine, clomipramine, amitriptyline, pargyline, clorgiline.
  - Cardiovascular drugs—verapamil, methyldopa, reserpine.
  - Opiates.
  - Cocaine.
  - Protease inhibitors (PIs)—e.g. ritonavir, indinavir, zidovudine.
  - Oestrogens.
  - Others—bezafibrate, omeprazole, H_2 antagonists.
- Metabolic:
  - Hypothyroidism—TRH increases PRL.
  - Chronic renal failure (CRF)—reduced PRL clearance.
  - Severe liver disease—disordered hypothalamic regulation.
- Other:
  - Polycystic ovary syndrome (PCOS)—can make differential diagnosis of menstrual problems difficult (PRL raised in 30%).
  - Chest wall lesions—zoster, burns, trauma (stimulation of suckling reflex).
- No cause found:
  - 'Idiopathic' hyperprolactinaemia.

* Quetiapine, clozapine, aripiprazole, and olanzapine are antipsychotics, with little or no effect on PRL (lower binding affinity to D2 receptors).

Investigations of prolactinomas

Serum PRL

- Note that the stress of venepuncture may cause mild hyperprolactinaemia, so 2–3 levels should be checked, preferably through an indwelling cannula after 30min.
- Serum PRL <2000mU/L is suggestive of a tumour—either a microprolactinoma or a non-functioning macroadenoma compressing the pituitary stalk, with loss of dopamine inhibitory tone to the lactotroph and subsequent hyperprolactinaemia. Very rarely, macroprolactinomas may present with PRL <2000mU/L.
- Serum PRL >3000mU/L is diagnostic of a macroprolactinoma.
- *Hook effect.* This occurs where the assay utilizes antibodies recognizing two ends of the molecule. One is used to capture the molecule, and one to label it. If PRL levels are very high, it may be bound by one antibody, but not by the other. Thus, above a certain concentration, the signal will reduce, rather than increase, and very high PRL levels will be spuriously reported as normal or only slightly raised.

Thyroid function and renal function

Hypothyroidism and CRF are causes of hyperprolactinaemia.

Imaging

- *MRI.* Microadenomas usually appear as hypointense lesions within the pituitary on T_1-weighted images. Negative imaging is an indication for contrast enhancement with gadolinium. Stalk deviation or gland asymmetry may also suggest microadenoma.
- Macroadenomas are space-occupying tumours, often associated with bony erosion and/or cavernous sinus invasion.

Macroprolactin ('big' PRL)

Occasionally, aggregate forms (150–170kDa) of PRL are detected in the circulation. Although these are measurable in the PRL assay, they do not interfere with reproductive function. The frequency of detection of macroprolactin depends on the assay used. Typically, there is hyperprolactinaemia with regular ovulatory menstrual cycles. Assays for macroprolactin are available, using polyethylene glycol (PEG) precipitation, where low recovery of PRL demonstrates the presence of macroprolactin, or gel filtration chromatography (gold standard).

Hyperprolactinaemia and drugs

(See Box 2.13.)

Antipsychotic agents are the most likely psychotropic agents to cause hyperprolactinaemia. If dose reduction is not possible or not effective, then MRI to exclude a prolactinoma and treatment of hypogonadism may be indicated. In cases of macroprolactinoma and a history of psychosis, dopamine agonists can be initiated at a low dose with slow dose escalation; the patients will require careful monitoring for the rare complication of worsening of psychosis. Alternative management options include observation, gonadal hormone replacement, and surgery. Where dopamine antagonism is the mechanism of action of the drug, then dopamine agonists may reduce efficacy. Furthermore, antipsychotics may blunt the effect of dopamine agonists on the prolactinoma, and in such cases, aripiprazole, an agent with less of a blocking effect on the D2 receptor, could be considered if appropriate. Drug-induced increases in PRL are usually <3000mU/L.

'Idiopathic' hyperprolactinaemia

When no cause is found following evaluation, as described in → Box 2.13, p. 161, hyperprolactinaemia is designated idiopathic but, in many cases, is likely to be due to a tiny microprolactinoma which is not demonstrable on current imaging techniques. Follow-up of these patients shows that in one-third, PRL levels return to normal; in 10–15%, there is a further increase in PRL, and, in the remainder, PRL levels remain stable.

Prolactinomas after menopause

The clinical phenotype of prolactinomas diagnosed in the post-menopausal period is characterized by dominance of macroadenomas, with frequent supra-/parasellar extension. Headaches and visual deterioration are the most commonly presenting manifestations. In this group of patients, the response of the macroadenomas to dopamine agonists is good, with normal PRL achieved in >90% of the cases.

Treatment of prolactinomas

Aims of therapy

- *Microprolactinomas.* Restoration of gonadal function.
- *Macroprolactinomas.*
- Reduction in tumour size with improvement/resolution of pressure effects (particularly visual disturbances) and prevention of tumour expansion.
- Restoration of gonadal function.
- Although microprolactinomas may expand in size without treatment, the vast majority do not. Therefore, although restoration of gonadal function is usually achieved by lowering PRL levels, ensuring adequate sex hormone replacement is an alternative if the tumour is monitored in size.
- Macroprolactinomas, however, will continue to expand and lead to pressure effects. Definitive treatment of the tumour is therefore usually necessary.

Drug therapy—dopamine agonists

- Dopamine agonist treatment (see ➲ Dopamine agonists, p. 226) leads to suppression of PRL in most patients, with 2° effects of normalization of gonadal function and termination of galactorrhoea. Tumour shrinkage occurs at a variable rate (from 24h to 6–12 months) and extent, and must be carefully monitored. Continued shrinkage may occur for years. Slow chiasmal decompression will correct visual field defect in the majority of patients, and immediate surgical decompression is not necessary. Lack of improvement of visual fields, despite tumour shrinkage, makes improvement with surgery unlikely. Apart from improved gonadal function, hypopituitarism present at presentation does not usually improve and therefore replacement with, for example, GH can commence.
- *Cabergoline* is more effective in normalization of PRL in microprolactinoma (83%, compared with 59% on bromocriptine), with fewer side effects than *bromocriptine*.
- Side effects of cabergoline include psychological manifestations (see Box 2.14).
- Although cabergoline in higher doses used for Parkinson's disease can cause right-sided cardiac fibrosis, there is no evidence for this using the lower doses necessary for control of PRL levels (see Box 2.15).
- Dopamine agonist resistance (see Box 2.16) may occur when there are reduced numbers of D2 receptors.
- Tumour enlargement following initial shrinkage on treatment is usually due to non-compliance. A rare possibility, however, is 2° resistance or malignant transformation.
- In patients with psychosis and macroprolactinoma, oestrogens and surgery should be considered. Higher doses of dopamine agonists may be needed and aripiprazole with less blocking of D2 receptors should be considered. Careful monitoring is essential.

Box 2.14 Dopamine agonists and impulse control disorders
- Include pathological:
  - Hypersexuality.
  - Compulsive shopping.
  - Compulsive eating.
  - Pathological gambling.
- Prevalence ~17%:
  - Hypersexuality commonest, and commoner in men.

Drug therapy—oestrogens

(See Box 2.13.)

Oestrogen replacement, rather than dopamine agonist therapy, may be appropriate in ♀ with idiopathic hyperprolactinaemia or microprolactinomas where fertility and galactorrhoea are not issues. Small short-term series suggest no evidence of tumour enlargement with the commonly used doses of oestrogens. However, monitoring of PRL is important.

Surgery

(See ⬧ Transsphenoidal surgery, p. 218.)
- Since the introduction of dopamine agonist treatment, transsphenoidal surgery is indicated only for patients who are resistant to, or intolerant of, dopamine agonist treatment. The cure rate for macroprolactinomas treated with surgery is poor (30%), and therefore, drug treatment is 1st line in tumours of all size. Occasionally, surgery may be required for patients with CSF leak 2° to an invasive macroprolactinoma. Cure rates for microprolactinomas treated with surgery are >80%, but the risk of hypopituitarism and recurrence of hyperprolactinaemia currently makes this a 2nd-line option.
- Bromocriptine given for >1 month may make the tumour fibrous.
- Surgical management of a CSF leak can be very difficult in patients with very invasive tumours. Tumour shrinkage with dopamine agonists will either precipitate or worsen the leak, with a subsequent risk of meningitis. There is no evidence for the long-term use of prophylactic antibiotics in this group, but patients at risk should be informed of the warning symptoms and advised to seek expert medical attention urgently.

Radiotherapy

(See ⬧ Technique, p. 222.)
- Standard pituitary irradiation leads to slow reduction (over years) of PRL in the majority of patients. While waiting for radiotherapy to be effective, dopamine agonist therapy is continued but should be withdrawn on an annual basis at least to assess if it is still required.
- Radiotherapy is not indicated in the management of patients with microprolactinomas. It is useful in the treatment of macroprolactinomas once the tumour has been shrunken away from the chiasm, only if the tumour is resistant.

Box 2.15 Cabergoline and cardiac valvulopathy
- Cabergoline, but not bromocriptine, is a 5-hydroxytryptamine 2B (5-HT2B) receptor agonist.
- High doses of cabergoline (e.g. 3mg/day for ≥6 months in Parkinson's patients) have been associated with valvular heart disease (aortic, mitral, and tricuspid regurgitations) via a 5-HT2B target effect.
- The risk of cardiac valvulopathy appears to be low in prolactinoma patients on standard doses of cabergoline (<2mg/week).
- All patients should undergo echocardiography before commencing a dopamine agonist.
- Patients taking a dose of cabergoline of ≤2mg/weekly should undergo surveillance echocardiography at 5 years of therapy, whereas those on >2mg/weekly should have annual echocardiography.

Box 2.16 Dopamine agonist resistance
- *Definition*. Failure to normalize PRL. Failure to decrease tumour size to <50%.
- Occurs with 24% of those treated with bromocriptine, 13% with pergolide, and 11% with cabergoline.
- D2 receptors are reduced in number, but in not efficacy.
- Treatment options include switching dopamine agonist, increasing the dose of dopamine agonist, surgery, fertility treatment, or oestrogen replacement (± pituitary radiotherapy) for macroprolactinomas. Temozolomide can be considered in aggressive/malignant prolactinomas.

Prognosis
- The natural history of microprolactinomas is difficult to assess. However, they are a common postmortem incidental finding, and <7% show any increase in tumour size.
- It has been demonstrated that hyperprolactinaemia in approximately one-third of ♀ will resolve, particularly after the menopause or pregnancy. This shows that patients receiving dopamine agonist treatment for microprolactinoma should have treatment withdrawn intermittently to assess the continued requirement for it, and certainly the dose may be titrated downwards over time. After the menopause, dopamine agonist treatment may be stopped, but monitoring of the PRL is needed, as cases with persistent increase in the PRL and tumour enlargement have been reported.
- There are few data on dopamine agonist withdrawal in macroprolactinomas in the absence of definitive treatment (radiotherapy or surgery). There are data suggesting that cautious attempts at dose reduction could be considered after at least 2 years if PRL is normal (on a low maintenance dose of dopamine agonist) and MRI shows no tumour, but it seems that the majority have a recurrence of hyperprolactinaemia (60–80%), but to levels lower than pretreatment values.
- It seems, at present, that there is no increase in the risk of breast cancer.

Management of prolactinomas in pregnancy

(See ➲ Prolactinoma in pregnancy, pp. 484–5.)

Further reading

Barber T, et al. (2011). Recurrence of hyperprolactinaemia following discontinuation of dopamine agonist therapy in patients with prolactinoma occurs commonly especially in macroprolactinoma. *Clin Endocrinol* **75**, 819–24.

Bevan JS, et al. (1992). Dopamine agonists and pituitary tumour shrinkage. *Endocrinol Rev* **13**, 220–40.

Casaneuva FF, et al. (2006). Guidelines of the Pituitary Society for the diagnosis and management of prolactinomas. *Clin Endocrinol* **65**, 265–73.

Dekkers OM, et al. (2011). Recurrence of hyperprolactinaemia after withdrawal of dopamine agonists: systematic review and meta-analysis. *J Clin Endocrinol Metab* **95**, 43–51.

De Sousa S, et al. (2020). Impulse control disorders in dopamine agonist-treated hyperprolactinemia: prevalence and risk factors. *J Clin Endocrinol Metab* **105**, e108–18.

Karavitaki N, et al. (2006). Do the limits of serum prolactin in disconnection hyperprolactinaemia need re-definition? A study of 226 patients with histologically verified non-functioning pituitary macroadenoma. *Clin Endocrinol* **65**, 524–9.

Melmed S, et al. (2011). Diagnosis and treatment of hyperprolactinaemia: an Endocrine Society clinical practice guideline. *J Clin Endocrinol Metab* **96**, 273–88.

Molitch ME (1985). Pregnancy and the hyperprolactinaemic woman. *N Engl J Med* **312**, 1364–70.

Molitch ME (1992). Pathologic hyperprolactinaemia. *Endocrinol Metab Clin North Am* **21**, 877–910.

Molitch ME (2002). Medical management of prolactinomas. *Pituitary* **5**, 55–65.

Molitch ME (2003). Dopamine resistance of prolactinomas. *Pituitary* **6**, 19–27.

Molitch ME (2008). Drugs and prolactin. *Pituitary* **11**, 209–18.

Molitch M (2020). Dopamine agonists and antipsychotics. *Eur J Endocrinol* **183**, C11–13.

Samperi I, et al. (2019). Hyperprolactinaemia. *J Clin Med* **13**, 2203.

Santharam S, et al. (2018). Impact of menopause on outcomes in prolactinomas after dopamine agonist treatment withdrawal. *Clin Endocrinol (Oxf)* **89**, 346.

Steeds R, et al. (2019). Echocardiography and monitoring patients receiving dopamine agonist therapy for hyperprolactinaemia: a joint position statement of the British Society of Echocardiography, the British Heart Valve Society and the Society for Endocrinology. *Clin Endocrinol (Oxf)* **90**, 662–9.

Suliman SGI, et al. (2007). Nonsurgical cerebrospinal fluid rhinorrhea in invasive macroprolactinoma: incidence, radiological, and clinicopathological features. *J Clin Endocrinol Metab* **92**, 3829–35.

Wanatabe S, et al. (2017). Long-term results of cabergoline therapy for macroprolactinomas and analyses of factors associated with remission after withdrawal. *Clin Endocrinol (Oxf)* **86**, 207–13.

Acromegaly

Definition of acromegaly

Acromegaly is the clinical condition resulting from prolonged excessive GH, and hence IGF-1, secretion in adults. GH secretion is characterized by blunting of pulsatile secretion and failure of GH to become undetectable during the 24h day and after glucose, unlike normal controls.

Epidemiology of acromegaly

- Rare. Equal sex distribution. Mean age at diagnosis 49 years.
- Prevalence 40–86 cases/million population. Annual incidence of new cases in the UK is 4/million population.
- Onset is insidious, and there is therefore often a considerable delay between the onset of clinical features and the diagnosis. Most cases are diagnosed at 40–60 years. Typically, acromegaly occurring in an older patient is a milder disease, with lower GH levels and a smaller tumour.
- Women present later, with greater diagnostic delay and a higher prevalence of comorbidities.

Pituitary gigantism

A clinical syndrome resulting from excess GH secretion in children prior to fusion of the epiphyses.

- Rare.
- ↑ growth velocity without premature pubertal manifestations should raise suspicion of pituitary gigantism.
- *Differential diagnosis.* Marfan's syndrome, NF, precocious pubertal disorders, cerebral gigantism (large at birth with accelerated linear growth and disproportionately large extremities—associated normal IGF-1 and GH).
- Arm span > standing height is compatible with eunuchoid features and suggests onset of disease before epiphyseal fusion (pituitary gigantism).
- Genetic screening important (see Table 13.1).

Causes of acromegaly

- *Pituitary adenoma* (>99% of cases). Macroadenomas 60–80%, microadenomas 20–40%. Local invasion is common, but frank carcinomas are very rare.
- *GHRH secretion*:
  - Hypothalamic secretion.
  - Ectopic GHRH, e.g. carcinoid tumour (pancreas, lung) or other neuroendocrine tumours (NETs).
  - Pituitary shows global enlargement. Somatroph hyperplasia seen on histology.
- *Ectopic GH secretion.* Very rare (e.g. pancreatic islet cell tumour, lymphoreticulosis).

Associations of acromegaly

(See also Table 13.1.)

- *MEN1.* Less common than prolactinomas (see ➡ MEN type 1, pp. 674–5).
- *Carney complex.* AD, spotty cutaneous pigmentation, cardiac and other myxomas, and endocrine overactivity, particularly Cushing's syndrome due to nodular adrenal cortical hyperplasia and GH-secreting pituitary tumours in <10% of cases. Mainly due to activating mutations of protein kinase A (see ➡ Carney complex, pp. 666–8).
- *McCune–Albright syndrome* (see ➡ McCune-Albright syndrome, pp. 654–5). Caused by somatic mosaicism for G-stimulatory protein (gsp) mutation.
- *Familial isolated pituitary adenomas:*
  - Existence of two or more cases of acromegaly or gigantism in a family that does not exhibit MEN1 or Carney complex.
  - AD.
  - Most have acromegaly, but acromegaly and prolactinoma families exist as rarely as do NFA families.
  - 10% of cases have a mutation in the *AIP* gene (tumour suppressor gene).
  - Early-onset disease (<30 years).
  - Poor response to SSAs.
  - Take a careful family history, especially in acromegaly patients with a large pituitary tumour presenting below the age of 30 years, and consider screening for *AIP*.
- XLAG:
  - Rare condition in patients with very early onset of GH excess, usually presenting at a very early age due to a *de novo* germline or mosaic duplication of the *GRP101* gene, usually within a microduplicated region (Xq23.6) on the X chromosome.

(See Box 2.17 for causes of macroglossia.)

Box 2.17 Macroglossia—causes

- Acromegaly.
- Hypothyroidism.
- Beckwith–Wiedemann syndrome (macrosomia, visceromegaly)—associated with hypoglycaemia and malignancies.
- Simpson–Golabi–Behmel syndrome (macrosomia and renal skeletal abnormalities).
- Tongue amyloidoses (1° or 2° to myeloma).
- Mucopolysaccharidoses/lysosomal storage disease.
- Focal tongue lesions, e.g. haemorrhage.
- Down's syndrome.
- Hyperinsulinaemia.

Clinical features of acromegaly

The clinical features arise from the effects of excess GH/IGF-1, excess PRL in some (as there is co-secretion of PRL in a minority (30%) of tumours or, rarely, stalk compression), and the tumour mass.

Symptoms

- ↑ sweating—>80% of patients.
- Headaches—independent of tumour effect.
- Tiredness and lethargy.
- Joint pains.
- Change in ring or shoe size.

Signs

- *Facial appearance.* Coarse features, oily skin, frontal bossing, enlarged nose, deep nasolabial furrows, prognathism, and ↑ interdental separation.
- *Deep voice*—laryngeal thickening.
- *Tongue enlargement*—macroglossia (see ⮕ Box 2.17, p. 169).
- *Musculoskeletal changes.* Enlargement of hands and feet, degenerative changes in joints leading to osteoarthritis (OA). Generalized myopathy.
- *Soft tissue swelling.* May lead to entrapment neuropathies such as carpal tunnel syndrome (40% of patients).
- *Goitre and other organomegaly*—liver, heart, kidney.

NB. Fabry's disease causes thickening of the lips.

Complications

- Hypertension (40%).
- Insulin resistance and impaired glucose tolerance (40%)/DM (20%).
- Obstructive sleep apnoea—due to soft tissue swelling in nasopharyngeal region; 74% at baseline, improved in 69% 2.5 years after successful treatment
- ↑ risk of colonic polyps and colonic carcinoma—extent currently considered controversial. Cancer incidence slightly ↑, e.g. thyroid.
- CVD and cerebrovascular disease.
- CCF and possible ↑ prevalence of regurgitant valvular heart disease.
- Higher frequency of vertebral fractures.

Effects of tumour

- Visual field defects.
- Hypopituitarism.

Investigation of acromegaly

(See Box 2.18.)

> **Box 2.18 Growth hormone and IGF-1 measurements in acromegaly**
> - IGF-1 every time.
> - Oral glucose tolerance test (OGTT)—diagnosis and query cure.
> - Random GH and IGF-1 for continued control/cure.
> - If random GH is <1mg/mL and IGF-1 is normal, treatment is effective.

Oral glucose tolerance test

- In acromegaly, there is failure to suppress GH to <0.4 micrograms/L in response to a 75g oral glucose load. In contrast, the normal response is GH suppression to undetectable levels.
- *False +ves.* CRF and chronic liver failure, malnutrition, DM, heroin addiction, adolescence (due to high pubertal GH surges).

Random GH

Not useful in the diagnosis of acromegaly, as although normal healthy subjects have undetectable GH levels throughout the day, there are pulses of GH which are impossible to differentiate from the levels seen in acromegaly.

IGF-1

Useful, in addition to the OGTT, in differentiating patients with acromegaly from normals, as it is almost invariably elevated in acromegaly, except in severe intercurrent illness. It has a long half-life, as it is bound to binding proteins, and reflects the effect of GH on tissues. However, abnormalities of GH secretion may remain while IGF-1 is normal.

MRI

MRI usually demonstrates the tumour (98%) and whether there is extrasellar extension, either suprasellar or into the cavernous sinus.

Pituitary function testing

(See also ➔ Pituitary function—dynamic tests: insulin tolerance test (ITT), pp. 130–1.) Serum PRL should be measured, as some tumours co-secrete both GH and PRL.

Serum calcium

Some patients are hypercalciuric due to ↑ 1,25-dihydroxycholecalciferol, as GH stimulates renal 1α-hydroxylase. There may be an ↑ likelihood of renal stones due to hypercalcaemia as well as hypercalciuria (which occurs in 80%). Rarely, hypercalcaemia may be due to associated MEN1 and hyperparathyroidism.

GHRH

Occasionally, it is not possible to demonstrate a pituitary tumour, or the pituitary gland MRI reveals global enlargement and histology reveals hyperplasia. A serum GHRH, in addition to radiology of the chest and abdomen, may then be indicated to identify the cause, usually a GHRH-secreting carcinoid of the lung or pancreas.

GH day curve

* GH usually taken at 4–5 time points during the day.
* In many centres, this has been replaced by random GH and IGF-1.
* This may be used to assess response to treatment following radiotherapy and also to assess GH suppression on SSAs in order to determine whether an increase in dose is required.
* It does not have a role in the diagnosis of acromegaly, but in acromegaly, GH is detectable in all samples, in contrast to normal. The degree of elevation of GH is relevant to the response to all forms of treatment; the higher the GH level, the less frequent treatment is effective by surgery, drugs, or radiotherapy. (See Box 2.19 for differential diagnosis.)

Note on GH and IGF-I assays

* To improve standardization, it is recommended that the GH reference preparation should be a recombinant 22kDa human GH (hGH); presently, 88/624.
* There is currently no acceptable IGF-1 reference preparation.
* On treatment, not infrequently (around 20%), GH and IGF-1 are discordant.

Box 2.19 Differential diagnosis of elevated GH

* Pain.
* Pregnancy.
* Puberty.
* Adolescence if tall.
* Stress.
* CRF.
* Chronic liver failure.
* Heart failure.
* DM.
* Malnutrition.
* Prolonged fast.
* Severe illness.
* Heroin addiction.

Management of acromegaly

The management strategy depends on the individual patient and also on the tumour size. Lowering of GH is essential in all situations (see Fig. 2.3).

The usual path is transsphenoidal surgery, followed by drugs, followed, if necessary, by radiotherapy.

Transsphenoidal surgery

(See also ➜ Transsphenoidal surgery, p. 218.)
- This is usually the 1st line for treatment in most centres.
- Reported cure rates vary: 40–91% for microadenomas and 10–48% for macroadenomas, depending on surgical expertise (>20 patients per surgeon per year).
- IGF-1 at 3 months and GH + glucose tolerance test (GTT) for GH.
- A GH 48h post-operation will give a valid result.
- Surgical debulking of a large macroadenoma should be undertaken, even if cure is not expected, because this lowers GH levels and improves the cure rate with subsequent SSAs.

Tumour recurrence following surgery

This is defined as tumour regrowth and increase in GH levels, leading to active acromegaly, following post-operative normalization of GH levels. Using the definition of post-operative cure as mean GH <1.0 micrograms/L, the reported recurrence rate is low (6% at 5 years).

Radiotherapy

(See also ➜ Technique, p. 222.)
- This is usually reserved for patients following unsuccessful transsphenoidal surgery and drug treatment, and only occasionally is it used as 1° therapy. The largest fall in GH occurs during the first 2 years, but GH continues to fall after this. However, normalization of mean GH may take several years and during this time, adjunctive medical treatment (usually with cabergoline, SSAs, or pegvisomant) is required. With a starting mean GH >25 micrograms/L, it takes, on average, 6 years to achieve mean GH <2.5 micrograms/L, compared with 4 years with a starting mean GH <25 micrograms/L.
- After radiotherapy, SSAs should be withdrawn on an annual basis to measure IGF-I and GH, to assess progress and identify when mean GH is within acceptable limits and therefore radiotherapy has been effective and SSA treatment is no longer required.
- Radiotherapy can induce GH deficiency which may need GH therapy.
- Stereotactic radiotherapy and radiosurgery are increasingly utilized in some centres, and initial data for tumour control are encouraging, although long-term data are lacking.

Definition of cure

- Controlled disease is most recently defined as random GH <1 micrograms/L or nadir GH <0.4 micrograms/L on GTT + normal age-related IGF-1.

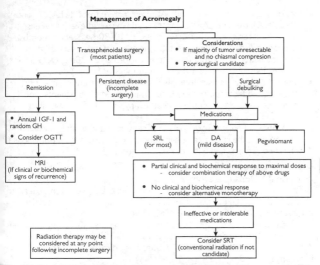

Fig. 2.3 Treatment considerations in the approach to a patient with acromegaly. This approach refers to management of a patient with a pituitary adenoma. DA, dopamine agonist; OGTT, oral glucose tolerance test.

Reprinted from Katznelson L et al (2014) "Acromegaly: An Endocrine Society Clinical Practice Guideline" JCEM 99(1):3933–3951, with permission from Oxford University Press.

Colonic polyps and acromegaly

- ↑ incidence of *colonic polyps and colonic carcinoma* has been reported by many groups. Both retrospective and prospective studies have demonstrated that 9–39% of acromegalic patients studied have colonic polyps and 0–5% have been shown to have colonic carcinoma.
- *Mechanism*. IGF-1 and/or GH are implicated, as both may stimulate colonic mucosal turnover. However, some studies have failed to demonstrate a direct relationship between serum levels and polyps/carcinoma.
- *Importance*. Patients with acromegaly are probably at slightly ↑ risk and therefore need screening for polyps. All patients aged >40 years should have routine colonoscopy at diagnosis, and those with polyps or persistently active acromegaly should receive 5-yearly repeat colonoscopy.

Drug treatment

Somatostatin analogues

(See also ➲ Somatostatin analogues, pp. 226–8.)

- SSAs lead to normal IGF-1 in 17–35%.
- Acute response to these drugs can be assessed by measuring GH at hourly intervals for 6h, following the injection of 50–100 micrograms of octreotide SC. This predicts long-term response.

- Depot preparations—lanreotide Autogel® and octreotide LAR®—are available. Octreotide LAR® 20mg IM is administered every 4 weeks, with dose alterations either down or up to 10–30mg every 3 months. Lanreotide Autogel® 90mg (deep SC) is administered every 28 days, with dose alteration either down to 60mg or up to 120mg every 3 months. Patients can be taught to self-administer lanreotide.
- These drugs may be used as 1° therapy where the tumour does not cause mass effects and surgery is contraindicated or in patients who have received surgery and/or radiotherapy who still have elevated mean GH.
- Pasireotide stimulates somatostatin receptors 2 and 5, and treatment may increase the response rate in patients with acromegaly, but glucose tolerance declines and patients may develop DM.

Dopamine agonists

(See also ➔ Dopamine agonists, p. 226.)

These drugs do lead to lowering of GH levels but, very rarely, lead to normalization of GH or IGF-1 (<30%). They may be helpful, particularly if there is coexistent secretion of PRL, and, in these cases, there may be significant tumour shrinkage. Cabergoline has been shown to be more effective than bromocriptine and may lead to IGF-1 normalization in up to 30%. A lower pretreatment IGF-1 favours a good response. The usual dose in acromegaly is 3mg/week

GH receptor antagonists (pegvisomant)

(See ➔ Growth hormone receptor antagonist, p. 228.)

Indicated for SSA non-responders. LFTs should be monitored 6-weekly for 6 months. MRI of the pituitary is indicated 6-monthly in case of pituitary enlargement (5%). Therapy may be continued with octreotide or lanreotide to decrease the frequency of pegvisomant injections (e.g. pegvisomant 10mg daily and lanreotide). Normalization of IGF-1 in >90% of patients is reported if a sufficient dose is used. More data on the effect on tumour size are required, as GH rises during treatment. GH levels cannot therefore be used to guide treatment, and IGF-1 is used to monitor therapy. Occasional anaphylaxis has been reported.

Upcoming treatment for acromegaly

(See Box 2.20.)

Box 2.20 Upcoming treatments for acromegaly

- PO octreotide.
- Antisense oligomers targeting GH receptor.
- Temozolomide (see also aggressive GH-secreting tumours).

Mortality data of acromegaly

- Mortality in untreated patients is double that in the normal population.
- Major causes include cardiovascular, cerebrovascular, and respiratory disease. More effective treatment has now ↑ life expectancy.

Further reading

Alexopoulou O, et al. (2008). Divergence between growth hormone and insulin-like growth factor-I concentrations in the follow-up of acromegaly. *J Clin Endocrinol Metab* **93**, 1324–30.

Bevan JS, et al. (2002). Primary medical therapy for acromegaly: an open, prospective, multicenter study of the effects of subcutaneous and intramuscular slow-release ocreotide on growth hormone, insulin-like growth factor-I, and tumor size. *J Clin Endocrinol Metab* **87**, 4554–63.

Boyce AM (2020). Fibrous dysplasia/McCune-Albright syndrome: a rare, mosaic disease of $G\alpha$ s activation. *Endocr Rev* **41**, 345–70.

Chahal HS, et al. (2011). AIP mutation in pituitary adenomas in the 18th century and today. *N Engl J Med* **364**, 43–50.

Daly AF, et al. (2007). Aryl hydrocarbon receptor-interacting protein gene mutations in familial isolated pituitary adenomas: analysis in 73 families. *J Clin Endocrinol Metab* **92**, 1891–6.

Dekkers OM, et al. (2008). Mortality in acromegaly: a metaanalysis. *J Clin Endocrinol Metab* **93**, 61–7.

Dal J, et al. (2018). Cancer incidence in patients with acromegaly: a cohort study and meta-analysis of the literature. *J Clin Endocrinol Metab* **103**, 2182–8.

Jenkins PJ, et al. (2006). Conventional pituitary irradiation is effective in lowering serum growth hormone and insulin-like growth factor-I in patients with acromegaly. *J Clin Endocrinol Metab* **91**, 1239–45.

Karavitaki N, et al. (2008). Surgical debulking of pituitary macroadenomas causing acromegaly improves control by lanreotide. *Clin Endocrinol (Oxf)* **68**, 970–5.

Katznelson L, et al.; Endocrine Society (2014). Acromegaly: an Endocrine Society clinical practice guideline. *J Clin Endocrinol Metab.* **99**, 3933.

Lavrentaki A, et al. (2017). Epidemiology of acromegaly: review of population studies. *Pituitary* **20**, 4–9.

Melmed S (2006). Medical progress: acromegaly. *N Engl J Med* **55**, 2558–73.

Orme SM, et al. (1998). Mortality and cancer incidence in acromegaly: a retrospective cohort study. *J Clin Endocrinol Metab* **83**, 2730–4.

Sandret L, et al. (2011). Place of cabergoline in acromegaly: a meta-analysis. *J Clin Endocrinol Metab* **96**, 1322–5.

Sims-Williams HP, et al. (2019). Radiosurgery as primary management for acromegaly. *Clin Endocrinol* **90**, 114–21.

Terzolo M, et al. (2020). Thyroid and colorectal cancer screening in acromegaly patients: should it be different from that in the general population? *Eur J Endocrinol* 183, d1–13.

Trainer PJ, et al. (2000). Treatment of acromegaly with the growth hormone-receptor antagonist pegvisomant. *N Engl J Med* **342**, 1171–7.

Wass JAH (ed.) (2009). *Acromegaly.* BioScientifica, Bristol.

Definition of Cushing's disease

Cushing's syndrome is an illness resulting from excess cortisol secretion, which has a high mortality if left untreated. There are several causes of hypercortisolaemia which must be differentiated, and the commonest cause is iatrogenic (oral, inhaled, or topical steroids). It is important to decide whether the patient has true Cushing's syndrome, rather than pseudo-Cushing's associated with depression or alcoholism. Secondly, ACTH-dependent Cushing's must be differentiated from ACTH-independent disease (usually due to an adrenal adenoma or, rarely, carcinoma; see ➔ Adrenal Cushing's syndrome, pp. 270–1). Once a diagnosis of ACTH-dependent disease has been established, it is important to differentiate between pituitary-dependent (Cushing's disease) and ectopic secretion.

Epidemiology
- Rare; annual incidence ~2/million.
- Commoner in ♀ (♀:♂, 3–15:1).
- Age—most commonly, 20–40 years.

Pathophysiology
- The vast majority of Cushing's syndrome is due to a pituitary ACTH-secreting corticotroph microadenoma. The underlying aetiology is ill understood. *USP8* driver mutations in a significant number.
- Occasionally, corticotroph adenomas reach larger sizes (macroadenomas) and rarely become invasive or malignant. The tumours typically maintain some responsiveness to the usual feedback control factors that influence the normal corticotroph (e.g. high doses of GCs and CRH). However, this may be lost and the tumours become fully autonomous, particularly in Nelson's syndrome.
- NB. Crooke's hyaline change is a fibrillary appearance seen in the non-tumourous corticotroph associated with elevated cortisol levels from any cause.

For causes of Cushing's syndrome, see Box 2.21.

> ### Box 2.21 Causes of Cushing's syndrome
> - Pseudo-Cushing's syndrome:
>   - Alcoholism <1%.
>   - Severe depression 1%.
> - ACTH-dependent:
>   - Pituitary adenoma 68% (Cushing's disease).
>   - Ectopic CRH/ACTH secretion ~12%.
> - ACTH-independent:
>   - Adrenal adenoma 10%.
>   - Adrenal carcinoma 8%.
>   - Nodular (macro- or micro-) hyperplasia 1%.
>   - Carney complex (see ➔ Carney complex, pp. 666–8).
> - Exogenous steroids, including skin creams, oral steroids, inhaled steroids, and joint steroids, e.g. clobetasol.

Clinical features of Cushing's disease

The features of Cushing's syndrome are progressive and may be present for several years prior to diagnosis (>3). A particular difficulty may occur in a patient with cyclical Cushing's where the features and biochemical manifestations appear and disappear with variable periodicity. Features may not always be florid, and clinical suspicion should be high.

- *Facial appearance*—round plethoric complexion, acne and hirsutism, thinning of scalp hair.
- *Weight gain*—truncal obesity, buffalo hump, supraclavicular fat pads.
- *Skin*—thin and fragile due to loss of SC tissue, purple striae on abdomen, breasts, thighs, and axillae (in contrast to silver, healed post-partum striae), easy bruising, tinea versicolor, occasionally pigmentation due to ACTH.
- Proximal *muscle weakness*.
- *Mood disturbance*—labile, depression, insomnia, psychosis.
- *Menstrual disturbance*.
- *Low libido and impotence*.
- There is a high incidence of venous thromboembolism (VTE) (careful during surgery).
- Overall mortality greater than that of general population (by a factor of 6).
- *Growth arrest* in children.

Associated features

- Hypertension (>50%) due to MC effects of cortisol (cortisol overwhelms the renal enzyme 11β-hydroxysteroid dehydrogenase protecting the MC receptor from cortisol). Cortisol may also increase angiotensinogen levels.
- Impaired glucose tolerance (IGT)/DM (30%).
- Osteopenia and osteoporosis (leading to fractures of spine and ribs).
- Vascular disease due to metabolic syndrome.
- Susceptibility to infections.

Investigations of Cushing's disease

Does the patient have Cushing's syndrome?

Outpatient tests

- *2–3× 24h UFC.* This test can be useful for outpatient screening—however, the false −ve rate of 5–10% means that it should not be used alone. (Fenofibrate, carbamazepine, and digoxin may lead to false +ves, depending on the assay, and reduced GFR <30mL/min may lead to false −ves.) In children: correct for body surface area. Mild elevation occurs in pseudo-Cushing's and normal pregnancy.
- *Overnight dexamethasone suppression test.* Administration of 1mg dexamethasone at midnight is followed by a serum cortisol measurement at 9 a.m. Cortisol <50nmol/L makes Cushing's unlikely. (NB. False +ves with poor dexamethasone absorption or hepatic enzyme induction.) The false −ve value is 2% in normal individuals but rises to <20% in obese or hospitalized patients.
- If both the above tests are normal, Cushing's syndrome is unlikely.

Inpatient tests

- *Midnight cortisol.* Loss of circadian rhythm of cortisol secretion is seen in Cushing's syndrome, and this is demonstrated by measuring serum cortisol at midnight (patient must be asleep for this test to be valid and ideally after 48h as an inpatient). In normal subjects, the cortisol level at this time is at a nadir (<50nmol/L), but in patients with Cushing's syndrome, it is elevated. Late-night salivary cortisol can also be used, particularly in those with possible cyclical Cushing's (see Box 2.22).
- *Low-dose dexamethasone suppression test.* Administration of 0.5mg dexamethasone 6-hourly (30 micrograms/kg/day) for 48h at 9 a.m., 3 p.m., 9 p.m., and 3 a.m. should lead to complete suppression of cortisol to <50nmol/L in normal subjects. Serum cortisol is measured at time 0 and 48h (day 2).
- Interfering conditions should be considered with all dexamethasone testing: ↓ dexamethasone absorption, hepatic enzyme inducers (e.g. phenytoin, carbamazepine, and rifampicin), and ↑ CBG.

Pseudo-Cushing's

- Pseudo-Cushing's can be present in patients with neuropsychiatric disorders, PCOS, obesity, alcohol abuse, and eating disorders.
- Patients with pseudo-Cushing's syndrome will also show loss of diurnal rhythm and lack of low-dose suppressibility. Treatment of any condition that may lead to pseudo-Cushing's is important as it can reverse the hormonal abnormalities. Alcoholics return to normal cortisol secretory dynamics after a few days' abstinence in hospital. Severe depression can be more difficult to differentiate, particularly since this may be a feature of Cushing's syndrome itself.
- Typically, patients with pseudo-Cushing's show a normal cortisol rise with hypoglycaemia (tested using ITT), whereas patients with true Cushing's syndrome show a blunted rise. However, this is not 100% reliable, as up to 20% of patients with Cushing's syndrome (especially those with cyclical disease) show a normal cortisol rise with hypoglycaemia.

> **Box 2.22 Cyclical Cushing's**
>
> A small group of patients with Cushing's syndrome have alternating normal and abnormal cortisol levels on an irregular basis. All causes of Cushing's syndrome may be associated with cyclical secretion of cortisol. Clearly, the results of dynamic testing can only be interpreted when the disease is shown to be active (elevated urinary cortisol secretion and loss of normal circadian rhythm and suppressibility on dexamethasone).

- Midnight blood cortisol has been proposed to differentiate from Cushing's syndrome using various cut-offs. The value of late-night salivary cortisol needs to be validated in this setting.
- The combined dexamethasone suppression test–CRH test (0.5mg dexamethasone 6-hourly for 48h, starting at 12 p.m., followed by ovine CRH 1 microgram/kg IV at 8 a.m.) (2h after last dose of dexamethasone) may be helpful, as patients with pseudo-Cushing's are thought to be under chronic CRH stimulation, thus showing a blunted response to CRH after dexamethasone suppression (cortisol 15min after CRH >38nmol/L in Cushing's and <38nmol/L in pseudo-Cushing's).
- IV desmopressin 10 micrograms increases ACTH in 80–90% of patients with Cushing's, but rarely in those with pseudo-Cushing's.
- No screening tests are fully capable of distinguishing all cases of Cushing's syndrome from normal individuals/pseudo-Cushing's (see Table 2.7). In challenging cases, treating the associated condition and close follow-up for detecting progress of possible Cushing's is needed.

What is the underlying cause?

ACTH
(See Table 2.8.)
- Once the presence of Cushing's syndrome has been confirmed, serum basal ACTH should be measured to differentiate between ACTH-dependent and ACTH-independent aetiologies (see Fig. 2.4). ACTH may not be fully suppressed in some adrenal causes of Cushing's.
- Basal ACTH is, however, of very little value in differentiating between pituitary-dependent Cushing's syndrome and ectopic Cushing's syndrome, as there is considerable overlap between the two groups, although patients with ectopic disease tend to have higher ACTH levels (see Fig. 2.4).

Serum potassium
A rapidly spun potassium is a useful discriminatory test, as hypokalaemia <3.2mmol/L is found in almost 100% of patients with ectopic secretion of ACTH, but in <10% of patients with pituitary-dependent disease.

High-dose dexamethasone suppression test
The high-dose dexamethasone suppression test is performed in an identical way to the low-dose test, but with 2mg doses of dexamethasone (120 micrograms/kg/day). In Cushing's disease, cortisol falls by >50% of the basal value. In ectopic disease, there is no suppression. However, ~10% of cases of ectopic disease, particularly those due to carcinoid tumours, show >50% suppression, and 10% of patients with Cushing's disease do not suppress.

Table 2.7 Screening tests for Cushing's syndrome

Test	False +ves	False −ves	Sensitivity
24h UFC	1%	5–10%	95%
Overnight 1mg	2% normal	2%	
Midnight cortisol	?	0	100%
Low-dose dexamethasone suppression test	<2%	2%	98%

Table 2.8 Investigations of ACTH-dependent Cushing's syndrome

Test	Pituitary-dependent disease (% with this finding)	Ectopic disease (% with this finding)
Serum potassium <3.2mmol/L	10	100
Suppression of basal cortisol to >50% on high-dose dexamethasone suppression test	90	10
Exaggerated rise in cortisol on CRH test	95	<1

Reproduced from Besser M and Thorner GM (1994). *Clinical Endocrinology*, 2nd edn. Mosby. Copyright Elsevier, with permission.

Corticotrophin-releasing hormone test
(See Fig. 2.5.)

The administration of 100 micrograms of CRH IV (side effects: transient flushing; very rarely, apoplexy reported) leads to an exaggerated rise in cortisol (14–20%) and ACTH (35–50%) in 95% of patients with pituitary-dependent Cushing's syndrome. There are occasional reports of patients with ectopic disease who show a similar response.

Inferior petrosal sinus sampling
(See Fig. 2.6.)

- Bilateral simultaneous inferior petrosal sinus sampling with measurement of ACTH centrally and in the periphery in the basal state and following stimulation with IV CRH (100 micrograms) allows differentiation between pituitary-dependent and ectopic disease. A central:peripheral ratio of >2 prior to CRH is very suggestive of pituitary-dependent disease, and >3 following CRH gives a diagnostic accuracy approaching 90–95% for pituitary-dependent disease. The test should be performed when cortisol levels are elevated.
- The accurate lateralization of a tumour using the results from inferior petrosal sinus sampling (IPSS) is difficult, as differences in blood flow and catheter placement, etc. will affect the results.
- Brainstem vascular events and deep vein thrombosis (DVT) are rare complications.

Pituitary imaging
- MRI, following gadolinium enhancement which significantly increases the pickup rate, localizes corticotroph adenomas in up to 80% of cases. However, it should be remembered that at least 10% of the normal population harbour microadenomas, and therefore, biochemical investigation of these patients is essential, as a patient with an ectopic source to Cushing's syndrome may have a pituitary 'incidentaloma'.
- C-methionine PET may aid detection of ACTH-secreting tumours.

Other pituitary function
- Hypercortisolism suppresses the thyroidal, gonadal, and GH axes, leading to lowered levels of TSH and thyroid hormones, as well as reduced gonadotrophins, gonadal steroids, and GH.

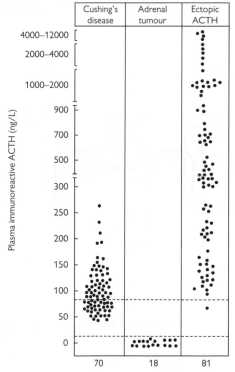

Fig. 2.4 Plasma ACTH levels (9 a.m.) in patients with pituitary-dependent Cushing's disease, adrenal tumours, and ectopic ACTH secretion.

Reproduced from Besser M and Thorner GM (1994). *Clinical Endocrinology*, 2nd edn. Mosby. Copyright Elsevier, with permission.

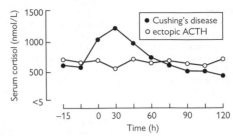

Fig. 2.5 CRH test in pituitary-dependent and ectopic disease. In the patient with pituitary-dependent disease, the characteristic marked plasma cortisol rise after an IV bolus of 100 micrograms of CRH is seen. Serum cortisol levels are unaltered in the patient with ectopic ACTH secretion.

Reproduced from Besser M and Thorner GM (1994). *Clinical Endocrinology*, 2nd edn. Mosby. Copyright Elsevier, with permission.

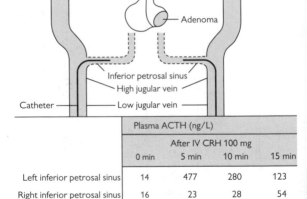

	Plasma ACTH (ng/L)			
		After IV CRH 100 mg		
	0 min	5 min	10 min	15 min
Left inferior petrosal sinus	14	477	280	123
Right inferior petrosal sinus	16	23	28	54
Simultaneous peripheral vein	17	19	25	32

Fig. 2.6 Simultaneous bilateral inferior petrosal sinus and peripheral vein sampling for ACTH. The ratio of >3 between the left central and peripheral vein confirms a diagnosis of Cushing's disease.

Reproduced from Besser M and Thorner GM (1994). *Clinical Endocrinology*, 2nd edn. Mosby. Copyright Elsevier, with permission.

Treatment of Cushing's disease

Transsphenoidal surgery

(See also ❸ Transsphenoidal surgery, p. 218.)

- This is the 1st-line option in most cases. Selective adenomectomy gives the greatest chance of remission, with a reported remission rate of up to 90% by skilled surgical hands. However, strict criteria of a post-operative cortisol level of <50nmol/L lead to lower remission rates, but much lower recurrence rates (<10%, compared with up to 50% in those with detectable post-operative cortisol). This should be the current definition of successful surgery, as the long-term outcome is significantly better in this group of patients.
- Delayed normalization (1–2 months) of cortisol after surgery can occur.
- Complications of surgery may be higher in these patients, as their preoperative general status and the condition of the tissues are poorer than other patients who are referred for surgery.
- Cushing's is associated with a hypercoagulable state, with ↑ cardiovascular thrombotic risks (estimated 1.5–2.5%).
- Some centres use anticoagulation perioperatively.
- Risk of relapse lasts for at least 10 years and is higher in Cushing's disease than for acromegaly (around 13% vs 6% at 5 years).

Pituitary radiotherapy

(See ❸ Pituitary radiotherapy, p. 222.) This is usually administered as 2nd-line treatment, following unsuccessful transsphenoidal surgery. As control of cortisol levels may take months to years, medical treatment to control cortisol levels, while waiting for cortisol levels to fall, is essential. A more rapid response to radiotherapy is seen in childhood. Stereotactic radio-therapy has also been shown to have encouraging results in terms of remission, but longer-term data are required.

Adrenalectomy

- This used to be the favoured form of treatment. It successfully controls cortisol hypersecretion in the majority of patients. Occasionally, a remnant is left and leads to recurrent hypercortisolaemia.
- Nelson's syndrome may occur in up to 60% of patients (the reported prevalence is affected by the diagnostic criteria and the duration of follow-up) (see Box 2.23). Data as to whether the administration of prophylactic radiotherapy ↓ the likelihood of this complication remain controversial. Careful follow-up of these patients is therefore essential to allow prompt treatment of the tumour. These tumours are associated with marked increase in ACTH, and associated pigmentation is common. Loss of normal responsiveness to GCs is characteristic, and therefore, biochemical monitoring should be performed at 6-monthly intervals for the first 3 years and annually thereafter (by measuring basal ACTH and rechecking it 1h and 2h after the morning dose of GC (ACTH curve)). Pituitary MRI is recommended 6 months after bilateral adrenalectomy and then yearly. If ACTH remains low after the initial 3 years, the imaging frequency can be extended to every other year.

- Bilateral adrenalectomy may still be indicated when pituitary surgery, radiotherapy, and medical treatment have failed to control the disease. It is also helpful in Cushing's syndrome due to ectopic disease when the ectopic source remains elusive or inoperable. Laparoscopic surgery minimizes morbidity and complications.

Box 2.23 Nelson's syndrome

- Occurs in patients with Cushing's disease, following bilateral adrenalectomy.
- Hyperpigmentation and an enlarging pituitary tumour, associated with markedly elevated ACTH levels.
- Early rise in ACTH within 2–3 years of adrenalectomy is predictive. At 10 years, 38% show progression.
- MRI and ACTH monitoring are important in the long term and should be initiated 6 months after adrenalectomy.
- Lack of suppression of ACTH after administration of GC to, for example, 200ng/mL is used in some centres.
- Treatment: surgery and radiotherapy (alone or in combination) are the main approaches offering tumour control in a significant number of cases. With observation alone, 10-year tumour progression free-survival is 51%. Pasireotide has also been used, but its value in establishing tumour control needs to be assessed.

Peri- and post-operative management following transsphenoidal surgery for Cushing's disease

- Perioperative hydrocortisone replacement is given in the standard way, as it is assumed that the patient will become cortisol-deficient after successful removal of the tumour.
- After 3–4 days, the evening steroid replacement is omitted and 9 a.m. cortisol and ACTH checked the following day and 24h later after withholding steroids. Undetectable cortisol (<50nmol/L) is suggestive of remission, and GC replacement is commenced. If this is not achieved, further management decisions are individualized, depending on post-operative cortisol levels, imaging features of the tumour, and surgical expertise.
- Antithrombotic prophylaxis should be considered, as Cushing's is associated with a hypercoagulable state which is further ↑ post-surgery.

Medical treatment

(See Table 2.9.)

- This is indicated during preoperative preparation of patients or while awaiting radiotherapy to be effective or if surgery or radiotherapy are contraindicated.
- Antithrombotic prophylaxis should be considered, as active disease is associated with an ↑ risk of thromboembolism.
- Inhibitors of steroidogenesis: *metyrapone* is usually used 1st line, but *ketoconazole* should be used as 1st line in children, as it is unassociated with ↑ adrenal metabolites. There is also a suggestion that ketoconazole may have a direct action on the corticotroph, as well as lower cortisol secretion.

- A disadvantage of these agents inhibiting steroidogenesis is the need to increase the dose to maintain control, as ACTH secretion will increase as cortisol concentrations decrease.
- Steroidogenesis inhibitors may be used with a GC replacement regimen to completely inhibit cortisol or with an aim for *partial* inhibition of cortisol production.
- The dose of these drugs needs to be titrated against the cortisol results from a day curve (cortisol usually taken at 9 a.m., 12 noon, 3 p.m., 6 p.m.), aiming for a mean cortisol of 150–300nmol/L, as this approximates the normal production rate.
- Response rates for drugs that reduce ACTH/CRH synthesis/release, e.g. somatostatin agonists (pasireotide affecting SSTR5 and 2), bromocriptine, valproate, and cyproheptadine, are variable. Pasireotide improves urinary cortisol to normal in about 30%, but carbohydrate tolerance may worsen (40%).
- Successful treatment (surgery or radiotherapy) of Cushing's disease leads to cortisol deficiency, and therefore, GC replacement therapy is essential. In addition, patients who have undergone bilateral adrenalectomy require fludrocortisone. These patients should all receive instructions for intercurrent illness and carry a MedicAlert bracelet and a steroid card.
- Cabergoline (1.5–3.0mg weekly): 20–25% may respond.

Newer treatments for Cushing's syndrome

- Levoketoconazole (less hepatotoxic).
- Osilodrostat (inhibits 11β-hydroxylase).
- Relacorilant (GC receptor antagonist.

Table 2.9 Drug treatment of Cushing's syndrome

Drug	Dose	Action	Side effects
Metyrapone	1–6g/day (usually given in four divided doses)	11β-hydroxylase inhibitor	Nausea ↑ androgenic and MC precursors lead to hirsutism and hypertension
Ketoconazole	400–1600mg/day given 6–8h 1st line in children	Direct inhibitor of P450 enzymes at several different sites	Abnormalities of liver function (usually reversible 1 in 15,000) Gynaecomastia
	NB. Avoid if taking H$_2$ antagonists, as acid required to metabolize active compound	Needs gastric acid for absorption Monitor LFTs MHRA warning—assess LFTs pretreatment weekly, then monthly; discontinue if climb	↓ testosterone Irregular menses Not effective with PPIs

Drug	Dose	Action	Side effects
Mitotane (o-p-DDD)	4–12g/day (begin at 0.5–1g/day and gradually increase dose)	Inhibits steroidogenesis at the side chain cleavage, 11- and 18-hydroxylase, and 3β-hydroxysteroid dehydrogenase Adrenolytic Half-life 18–159 days	Nausea and vomiting Cerebellar disturbance Somnolence Hypercholesterolaemia NB. May increase clearance of steroids—replacement dosage may need to be ↑ ↑ liver enzymes ↑ lipids NB. May be teratogenic. Avoid if fertility desired Avoid concurrent spironolactone—interferes with action
Aminoglute thimide	0.5–2.0g/day	Inhibits 10% steroidogenesis at side chain cleavage enzyme (see ➌ Calcium and bone physiology, pp. 500–1)	Rash 10% ↓ T₄ ↑ hepatic enzymes
Mifepristone	400–1000mg	GC antagonist	Amenorrhoea Hypokalaemia (progesterone and androgen receptor antagonist)
Etomidate	0.3mg/kg/h Useful when parenteral treatment is required	Inhibits side chain cleavage and 11β-hydroxylase	Need steroid replacement with this dose
Pasireotide	900micrograms daily 25% get normal 24h urinary cortisol	Binds SSTR5 and 2	Nearly 50% need glucose-lowering medications because of insulin suppression

Follow-up of Cushing's disease

Successful treatment for Cushing's disease leads to a cortisol that is undetectable (<50nmol/L) following surgery. (This is due to total suppression of cortisol production from the normal pituitary corticotrophs in Cushing's disease.) An undetectable post-operative cortisol level leads to a significantly higher chance of long-term remission, compared to patients who have higher post-operative cortisol levels or whose suppression recovers early.

- The aim of follow-up is to:
  - Detect recurrent Cushing's.
  - Optimize the management of morbidities related with the previous exposure to cortisol excess.
- After successful surgery, the adrenals are suppressed.
- Therefore, patients need to have regular assessment of cortisol production off GC replacement. When cortisol is detectable following surgery, recurrent disease must be excluded (low-dose dexamethasone suppression). If recurrence is excluded, it is then important to document the adequacy of the stress response once weaned off GC replacement (ITT or SST).

Prognosis of Cushing's disease

- Untreated disease leads to ~30–50% mortality at 5 years, owing to vascular disease and ↑ susceptibility to infections.
- Treated Cushing's syndrome has a good prognosis. Patients who have an undetectable post-operative cortisol level are very unlikely to recur (0–20%).
- Although the physical features and severe psychological disorders associated with Cushing's improve or resolve within weeks or months of successful treatment, more subtle mood disturbances may persist for longer. Adults may also have impaired cognitive function. In addition, it is likely that there is an ↑ cardiovascular risk.
- Osteoporosis will usually resolve in children but may not improve significantly in older patients. BMD therefore requires monitoring and may need specific treatment. *Alendronic acid* has been shown to be effective therapy, leading to improved BMD in patients with Cushing's syndrome and osteoporosis.
- Hypertension has been shown to resolve in 80%, and DM in up to 70%.
- Recent data suggest that mortality, even with successful treatment of Cushing's, is ↑ significantly.

Cushing's syndrome in children

In a series of 59 patients aged 4–20 years, the following factors were found.

Causes

- Pituitary-dependent disease 85%.
- Adrenal disease 10%.
- Ectopic ACTH secretion 5%.

Initial presentation

- Excessive weight gain 90%.
- Growth retardation 83%.

Below the age of 5 years, adrenal causes are common. In neonates and young children, McCune–Albright syndrome should be considered, whereas in late childhood and early adolescence, ACTH independence may suggest Carney complex (see also ➔ Carney complex, pp. 666–8).

Treatment

- Transsphenoidal surgery is used as 1st-line therapy in pituitary-dependent Cushing's in children as in adults and is usually successful.
- Radiotherapy cures up to 85% of children, and this may be considered 1st line in some patients. Ketoconazole is the preferred medical therapy in this age group, as it is not associated with ↑ adrenal androgens.
- Long-term management of children with Cushing's syndrome requires careful attention to growth, as growth failure is a very common presentation of this condition. Post-operatively or after radiotherapy, GH therapy may restore growth and final height to normal.

Further reading

Clayton RN, et al. (2016). Mortality in patients with Cushing's disease more than 10 years after remission: a multicentre, multinational, retrospective cohort study. Lancet Diabetes Endocrinol **4**, 569–76.

Coelho MC, et al. (2015). Adverse effects of glucocorticoids: coagulopathy. Eur J Endocrinol **173**, M11–21.

Daniel E, et al. (2015). Effectiveness of metyrapone in treating Cushing's syndrome: a retrospective multicenter study in 195 patients. J Clin Endocrinol Metab **100**, 4146–54.

Feelders RA, et al. (2019). Advances in the medical treatment of Cushing's syndrome. Lancet Diabetes Endocrinol **7**, 300–12.

Fleseriu M, et al. (2019). Efficacy and safety of levoketoconazole in the treatment of endogenous Cushing's syndrome (SONICS): a phase 3, multicentre, open-label, single-arm trial. Lancet Diabetes Endocrinol **7**, 855–65.

Florez JC, et al. (2013). Ectopic ACTH syndrome. N Engl J Med **368**, 2116–36.

Fountas A, Karavitaki N (2020). Nelson's syndrome: an update. Endocrinol Metab Clin North Am **49**, 413–32.

Fountas A, et al. (2020). Outcomes of patients with Nelson's syndrome after primary treatment: a multicenter study from 13 UK pituitary centers. J Clin Endocrinol Metab **105**, 1527–37.

Isidori AM, et al. (2006). The ectopic adrenocorticotropin syndrome: clinical features, diagnosis, management, and long-term follow-up. J Clin Endocrinol Metab **91**, 371–7.

Magiakou MA, et al. (1994). Cushing's syndrome in children and adolescents. N Engl J Med **331**, 629–36.

Newell-Price J, et al. (2002). Optimal response criteria for the human CRH test in the differential diagnosis of ACTH-dependent Cushing's syndrome. J Clin Endocrinol Metab **87**, 1640–5.

Newell-Price J, et al. (1998). The diagnosis and differential diagnosis of Cushing's syndrome and pseudo-Cushing's states. Endocrinol Rev **19**, 647–72.

Nieman LK, et al. (2008). The diagnosis of Cushing's syndrome. An Endocrine Society clinical practice guideline. J Clin Endocrinol Metab **93**, 1526–40.

Nieman LK, et al.; Endocrine Society (2015). Treatment of Cushing's syndrome: an Endocrine Society clinical practice guideline. *J Clin Endocrinol Metab* **100**, 2807–31.

Ntali G, et al. (2013). Mortality in Cushing's syndrome: systematic analysis of a large series with prolonged follow-up. *Eur J Endocrinol* **169**, 715–23.

Pivonello R, et al. (2015). The treatment of Cushing's disease. *Endocr Rev* **36**, 385–486.

Preda VA, et al. (2012). Etomidate in the management of hypercortisolaemia in Cushing's syndrome: a review. *Eur J Endocrinol* **167**, 137–43.

Storr HL, Savage MO (2015). Management of endocrine disease: Paediatric Cushing's disease. *Eur J Endocrinol* **173**, R35–45.

van der Pas R, et al. (2013). Hypercoagulability in Cushing's syndrome: prevalence, pathogenesis and treatment. *Clin Endocrinol* **78**, 481–8.

Non-functioning pituitary tumours

Background

These pituitary tumours are unassociated with clinical syndromes of anterior pituitary hormone excess.

Epidemiology

- NFAs are the commonest pituitary macroadenoma. They represent around 28% of all pituitary tumours.
- There is an equal sex distribution, and the majority of cases present in patients aged >50 years.
- Around 50% enlarge, if left untreated, at 5 years.

Pathology

For pathological classification, see Table 2.6.

- Tumour behaviour is variable, with some tumours behaving in a very indolent, slow-growing manner and others invading the sphenoid and cavernous sinus.

Clinical features

Mass effects

- Visual field defects (uni- or bitemporal quadrantanopia or hemianopia).
- Headache.
- Ophthalmoplegia (cranial nerves III, IV, and VI—rarely).
- Optic atrophy (rarely, following long-term optic nerve compression).
- Apoplexy (rarely).

Hypopituitarism

(See also ➔ Hypopituitarism, pp. 138–9.)

Incidental finding

- An NFA may be detected on the basis of imaging performed for other reasons.

Investigations

- *Pituitary imaging*. MRI/CT demonstrates the tumour and/or invasion into the cavernous sinus or supraoptic recess.
- *Visual assessment*. Visual fields are abnormal in up to two-thirds of cases.
- *PRL*. Essential to exclude a PRL-secreting macroadenoma (see ➔ Investigations of prolactinomas, p. 162).
- Mild elevation (<3000mU/L; usually 2000mU/L) may occur 2° to stalk compression.
- *Pituitary function*. Assessment for hypopituitarism (see ➔ Pituitary function—dynamic tests: insulin tolerance test (ITT), pp. 130–1.)

Management

Surgery

(Aspects of pituitary surgery are also covered in ➔ Surgical treatment of pituitary tumours, pp. 218–20.)

- The initial definitive management in virtually every case causing visual deterioration is surgical. This removes mass effects and may lead to some recovery of pituitary function (12%). The majority of patients can be operated on successfully via the transsphenoidal route.

- Close follow-up is necessary (yearly initially) after surgery, as tumour regrowth can only be detected using pituitary imaging and visual field assessment.

Radiotherapy
- The use of post-operative radiotherapy remains controversial. Some centres advocate its use for every patient following surgery; others reserve its use for those patients who have had particularly invasive or aggressive tumours removed or those with a significant amount of residual tumour remaining (e.g. in the cavernous sinus).
- The regrowth rate at 10 years without radiotherapy approaches 45%, and there are no good predictive factors for determining which tumours will regrow. However, administration of post-operative radiotherapy reduces this regrowth rate to <10%. As discussed in ➔ Complications of pituitary radiotherapy, p. 224, however, there are sequelae to radiotherapy—with a significant long-term risk of hypopituitarism and a possible ↑ risk of visual deterioration and neoplasia in the field of radiation.

Medical treatment
- Unlike the case for GH- and PRL-secreting tumours, medical therapy for NFAs is usually unhelpful, although there are some data suggesting that dopamine agonist treatment is associated with reduced rates of residual tumour enlargement after transsphenoidal surgery.
- Hormone replacement therapy (HRT) is required to treat any hypopituitarism (see ➔ Anterior pituitary hormone replacement, p. 144).
- Visual field defects at diagnosis may improve following surgery in the majority, and improvement may continue for around a year following tumour debulking.

Prediction of regrowth of NFAs?
No markers that provide certainty. However, the following have been suggested as useful markers to raise suspicion of aggressive behaviour:
- Younger age.
- Preoperative cavernous sinus invasion and post-operative extrasellar residual tumour .
- Biochemical markers for NFAs?
  - The majority of patients lack a hormone marker—despite approximately half immunostaining positively for gonadotrophins and containing secretory granules at the electron microscopy (EM) level.
  - A minority of patients have elevated circulating FSH/LH levels (see ➔ Gonadotrophinomas, p. 198).
  - Silent corticotroph adenomas do not have a higher incidence of recurrence than NFAs.

Follow-up
(See Table 2.10.)
- Patients who have not received post-operative irradiation require careful, long-term follow-up with serial pituitary imaging and visual field assessment. The optimal protocol is still not known, but an accepted practice is to image in the first 3 months following surgery, and then reimage annually for 5 years, and biannually thereafter. Tumour recurrence has been reported at up to 15 years following surgery and

therefore, follow-up needs to be long term. The amount of post-operative tumour remnant predicates recurrence risk. Thus, with an empty sella post-operatively, the 10-year recurrence is around 6%. With an intrasellar remnant, it is 50%, and with an extrasellar remnant 90%.

- After radiotherapy, annual visual fields are checked in case of development of new field defects. If these occur, MRI is necessary.

Table 2.10 Follow-up of non-functioning pituitary adenomas

Post-operative assessment of NFA	
Immediately	Cortisol—replace if <500nmol/L
6 weeks	Pituitary function: • T₄/TSH • PRL • GH/IGF-1 • Cortisol—Synacthen® + ITT if necessary • LH/FSH, testosterone/oestradiol • Osmolarities
Replace	Hydrocortisone, thyroxine, gonadal steroids, GH, dehydroepiandrostenedione (DHEA)
3 months	MRI pituitary Consider radiotherapy
Yearly	MRI if no radiotherapy at least to 5 years

Prognosis

Patients with NFAs have a good prognosis once the diagnosis and appropriate treatment, including replacement of hormone deficiency, are performed. The main concern is the risk of tumour regrowth, with subsequent visual failure. As mentioned earlier, administration of radiotherapy, although not without potential complications itself, significantly reduces this risk. Non-irradiated patients require very close follow-up in order to detect regrowth and perform repeat surgery or administer radiotherapy.

Current treatment protocols offer normal or near-normal QoL in patients with NFAs, although mortality is ↑ and mainly attributed to circulatory, respiratory, and infectious causes. Extent of tumour removal, radiotherapy, and tumour recurrence are not predictors of mortality.

Further reading

Batista RL, et al. (2019). Cabergoline in the management of residual nonfunctioning pituitary adenoma: a single-center, open-label, 2-year randomized clinical trial. *Am J Clin Oncol* **42**, 221–7.

Capatina C, et al. (2013). Current treatment protocols can offer a normal or near-normal quality of life in the majority of patients with non-functioning pituitary adenomas. *Clin Endocrinol (Oxf)* **78**, 86–93.

Dekkers OM, et al. (2008). Treatment and follow-up of nonfunctioning pituitary macroadenomas. *J Clin Endocrinol Metab* **93**, 3717–26.

Karavitaki N, et al. (2007). What is the natural history of nonoperated nonfunctioning pituitary adenomas? *Clin Endocrinol (Oxf)* **67**, 938–43.

Karavitaki N, et al. (2006). Do the limits of serum prolactin in disconnection hyperprolactinaemia need re-definition? A study of 226 patients with histologically verified non-functioning pituitary macroadenoma. *Clin Endocrinol (Oxf)* **65**, 524–9.

Minniti G, *et al*. (2018). Management of nonfunctioning pituitary tumors: radiotherapy. *Pituitary* **21**, 154–61.

Ntali G, *et al*. (2016). Mortality in patients with non-functioning pituitary adenoma is increased: systematic analysis of 546 cases with long follow-up. *Eur J Endocrinol* **174**, 137–45.

Ntali G, Wass JA (2018). Epidemiology, clinical presentation and diagnosis of non-functioning pituitary adenomas. *Pituitary* **21**, 111–18.

Reddy R, *et al*. (2011). Can we ever stop imaging in surgically treated and radiotherapy-naive patients with non-functioning pituitary adenoma? Eur J Endocrinol 165, 739–74.

Tampourlou M, *et al*. (2018). Mortality in patients with non-functioning pituitary adenoma. *Pituitary* **21**, 203–7.

Tampourlou M, *et al*. (2017). Outcome of nonfunctioning pituitary adenomas that regrow after primary treatment: a study from two large UK centers. *J Clin Endocrinol Metab* **102**, 1889–97.

Gonadotrophinomas

Background

These are tumours that arise from the gonadotroph cells of the pituitary gland and produce FSH, LH, or the α subunit. They are often indistinguishable from other NFAs, as they are usually silent and unassociated with excess detectable secretion of LH and FSH, although studies demonstrate gonadotrophin/α subunit secretion *in vitro*. Occasionally, however, these tumours do produce detectable excess hormone *in vivo*.

Clinical features

- Gonadotrophinomas present in the same manner as other non-functioning pituitary tumours, with mass effects and hypopituitarism (see ➋ Hypopituitarism, pp. 138–9).
- The rare FSH-secreting gonadotrophinomas may lead to macro-orchidism in ♂.
- May cause ovarian hyperstimulation in premenopausal ♀.

Investigations

The secretion of FSH and LH from these tumours is usually undetectable in the plasma. Occasionally, elevated FSH and, more rarely, LH are measured. This finding is often ignored, particularly in post-menopausal ♀.

Management

These tumours are managed as non-functioning tumours. The potential advantage of FSH/LH secretion from a functioning gonadotrophinoma is that it provides a biochemical marker of the presence of tumour for follow-up.

Further reading

Ntali G, *et al.* (2014). Clinical review: functioning gonadotroph adenomas. *J Clin Endocrinol Metab* **99**, 4423–33.

Thyrotrophinomas

Epidemiology

These are rare tumours, comprising ~1% of all pituitary tumours. The diagnosis may be delayed because the significance of an unsuppressed TSH in the presence of elevated free thyroid hormone concentrations may be missed. Approximately one-third of cases in the literature have received treatment directed at the thyroid in the form of radioiodine treatment or surgery before diagnosis. Unlike 1° hyperthyroidism, thyrotrophinomas are equally common in ♂ and ♀; 5% are associated with MEN1.

Tumour biology and behaviour

- The majority are macroadenomas (90%) and secrete only TSH, often with the α subunit in addition, but some co-secrete GH (55%) and/or PRL (15%).
- The pathogenesis of thyrotoxicosis in the presence of normal TSH levels is poorly understood, but there are reports of secretion of TSH with ↑ bioactivity, possibly due to changes in post-translational hormone glycosylation.
- The observation that prior thyroid ablation is associated with deleterious effects on the size of the tumour suggests some feedback control and is similar to the aggressive tumours seen in Nelson's syndrome after bilateral adrenalectomy has been performed for Cushing's disease. Thyrotropin-secreting pituitary carcinoma has been very rarely reported.
- Five per cent are associated with MEN1.

Clinical features

(See ➌ Manifestations of hyperthyroidism, pp. 32–3.)
- Clinical features of *hyperthyroidism* are usually present but often milder than expected, given the level of thyroid hormones. In mixed tumours, hyperthyroidism may be overshadowed by features of *acromegaly*.
- *Mass effects.* Visual field defects and hypopituitarism.

Investigations

(See also Tables 1.3 and 1.4.)
- *TSH is inappropriately normal or elevated.* The range of TSH that has been described is <1–568mU/L, and one-third of untreated patients had TSH in the normal range. There is no correlation between TSH and T_4.
- *Free thyroid hormones.* Elevated in 65% of patients.
- *α subunit (raised in 65%).* Typically, patients have an ↑ α subunit:TSH molar ratio (>1) (81%).
- *Other anterior pituitary hormone levels.* PRL and/or GH may be elevated in mixed tumours (an OGTT may be indicated to exclude acromegaly).
- *SHBG.* Elevated into the hyperthyroid range.
- *TRH test.* Absent TSH response to stimulation with TRH (useful to differentiate TSH-secreting tumours from thyroid hormone resistance where the TSH response is normal or exaggerated).
- *T_3 suppression test* (lack of suppression of TSH following 100 micrograms/day for 10 days).

- *Thyroid antibodies.* In contrast to Graves' disease, the incidence of thyroid antibodies is similar to that in the general population.
- *Pituitary imaging.* MRI scan will demonstrate a pituitary tumour (macroadenoma) in the majority of cases (90%).

Causes of elevated FT₄ in the presence of an inappropriately unsuppressed TSH

(See also Tables 1.3.)
- TSH-secreting tumour.
- Thyroid hormone resistance.
- Amiodarone therapy.
- Inherited abnormalities of thyroid-binding proteins.

Management

Medical treatment

Somatostatin analogues

- Medical treatment with the somatostatin agonists octreotide and lanreotide is successful in the majority of patients in suppressing TSH secretion and leading to tumour shrinkage. In one study, octreotide reduced TSH secretion in almost all patients treated and normalized thyroid hormone levels in 73% of patients. There was partial tumour shrinkage in 40%.
- Drug therapy is useful in the preoperative preparation of these patients to ensure that they are fit for general anaesthesia and also while waiting for radiotherapy to be effective.

Surgery

- Surgery leads to cure in approximately one-third of patients, as judged by apparent complete removal of tumour mass and normalization of thyroid hormone levels, with another third improved with normal thyroid hormone levels but incomplete removal of the adenoma.
- Microadenomas are cured in higher proportions.

Radiotherapy

Radiotherapy is useful, following unsuccessful surgery, and leads to a gradual (over years) reduction in TSH.

Antithyroid medication

Treatment with ATDs has been associated with ↑ TSH in ~60% of patients reported. It should be avoided, if possible, and the more appropriate somatostatin agonist therapy utilized.

Further reading

Beck-Peccoz P, et al. (1996). Thyrotropin-secreting pituitary tumours. *Endocr Rev* **17**, 610–38.
Chanson P, et al. (1993). Octreotide therapy for thyroid stimulating hormone-secreting pituitary adenomas. *Ann Intern Med* **119**, 236–40.

Pituitary incidentalomas

Definition

The term incidentaloma refers to an incidentally detected lesion that is un-associated with hormonal hyper- or hyposecretion and has a benign natural history.

The increasingly frequent detection of these lesions with technological improvements and more widespread use of sophisticated imaging have led to a management challenge—which, if any, lesions need investigation and/or treatment, and what is the optimal follow-up strategy (if required at all)?

Epidemiology

- Autopsy studies have shown that 10–20% of pituitary glands unsuspected of having pituitary disease harbour pituitary adenomas. Approximately half of the tumours stain for PRL, and the remainder is −ve on immunostaining.
- Imaging studies using MRI demonstrate pituitary microadenomas in ~10% of normal volunteers.
- Incidentally detected macroadenomas have been reported when imaging has been performed for other reasons. However, these are not true incidentalomas, as they are often associated with visual field defects and/or hypopituitarism.
- Clinically significant pituitary tumours are present in about 1 in 1000 patients.

Natural history

Incidentally detected microadenomas are very unlikely (<10%) to increase in size, whereas larger incidentally detected meso- and macroadenomas are more likely (40–50%) to enlarge at 5 years. Thus, conservative manage-ment in selected patients may be appropriate for microadenomas which are incidentally detected, as long as careful follow-up imaging is in place and patients are truly asymptomatic. Macroadenomas should be treated, if clinically indicated.

Clinical features

By definition, a patient with an incidentaloma should be asymptomatic. Any patient who has an incidentally detected tumour should have a neuro-ophthalmology assessment and a clinical review to ensure that this is not the initial presentation of Cushing's syndrome, acromegaly, or a prolactinoma.

Investigations

- Aims:
  - Exclude any hormone hypersecretion from the tumour.
  - Detect hypopituitarism.
- Investigation of hypersecretion of hormones should include measurement of PRL and IGF-1 and an OGTT if acromegaly is suspected, 24h UFC and overnight dexamethasone suppression test, TFTs, and FSH, LH, and gonadal hormones.
- Others suggest that this approach is unnecessary, but with limited data, most endocrinologists would perform investigations as above.

Management

- Extrasellar macroadenomas compressing the optic chiasm (incidentally detected but, by definition, not true incidentalomas) require definitive treatment.
- Tumours with excess hormone secretion require definitive treatment.
- Mass <1cm diameter—repeat MRI at 1, 2, and 5 years.
- Mass >1cm diameter, not compressing or abutting the optic chiasm—repeat MRI at 6 months, and 1, 2, and 5 years; if during this period, the tumour remains stable, the interval of imaging is individualized. For lesions abutting the optic chiasm, surgery could be also considered at the time of detection (given the high probability of enlargement).

Further reading

Fernando A, et al. (2010). Prevalence of pituitary adenomas: a community-based cross-sectional study in Banbury, Oxfordshire (UK). *Clin Endocrinol* **72**, 377–82.

Freda PU, et al. (2011). Pituitary incidentaloma: an Endocrine Society clinical practice guideline. *Clin Endocrinol Metab*. **96**, 894–904.

Huang W, Molitch ME (2018). Management of nonfunctioning pituitary adenomas (NFAs): observation. *Pituitary* **21**, 162–7.

Karavitaki N, et al. (2007). What is the natural history of nonoperated non-functioning pituitary adenomas? Clin Endocrinol (Oxf) 67, 938–43.

Molitch ME (1997). Pituitary incidentalomas. *Endocrinol Metab Clin North Am* **26**, 725–40.

Pituitary carcinoma

Definition

Pituitary carcinoma is defined as a 1° adenohypophyseal neoplasm with craniospinal and/or distant systemic metastases (see Table 2.11 for types).

Epidemiology

These are extremely rare tumours.

Pathology and pathogenesis

- The initial tumours and subsequent carcinomas show higher proliferation indices than the majority of pituitary adenomas. They are also likely to demonstrate p53 positivity and have an ↑ mitotic index. However, histology is unable to reliably distinguish between benign invasive pituitary adenomas and carcinomas.
- The aetiology of these tumours is unknown. Metastatic spread outside the CNS is via lymphatic and vascular routes, while intra-CNS spread is via local invasion and tumour seeding.

Features

Virtually all pituitary carcinomas initially present as invasive pituitary macroadenomas. After a variable interval of time (mean 6.5 years), the majority present with local recurrence. There is a tendency to systemic (liver, lymph nodes, lungs, and bones), rather than craniospinal, metastases, but metastases do not usually predominate in the clinical picture.

Treatment

Treatment involves surgery, radiotherapy, and medical treatment. As mass effects often predominate, initial debulking surgery may provide relief. It may need to be repeated to maintain local control. Some advocate a transsphenoidal route as less likely to disseminate tumour.

Radiotherapy or medical treatment provides palliation only. Radiotherapy has been reported to be successful, in some cases, in controlling growth and occasionally leading to regression. Stereotactic radiosurgery may play a role. Medical treatment with dopamine agonists for malignant prolactinomas and acromegaly has been reported, with varying results. Many pituitary carcinomas are dedifferentiated and therefore escape from control. Temozolomide has also been used (see ➲ Temozolomide, p. 228) and may provide some benefit in some cases. The anti-vascular endothelial growth factor (VEGF) bevacizumab and peptide R radionucleotide therapy have been used. Various chemotherapy regimes have been reported, with occasional success (e.g. fluorouracil and folinic acid or cisplatin, procarbazine, lomustine, everolimus, and vincristine).

Prognosis

Most patients die within a year of diagnosis.

Table 2.11 Types of pituitary carcinoma

Type	Proportion of reported cases (%)
PRL	30
ACTH	28
GH	2
Non-functioning	30

NB. Many 'non-functioning' carcinomas were reported prior to routine measurement of PRL or routine immunostaining, and therefore, the true incidence of PRL-producing carcinomas may be higher.

Further reading

Kaltsas GA, Grossman AB (1998). Malignant pituitary tumours. *Pituitary* **1**, 69–81.

McCormack AI, et al. (2011). Aggressive pituitary tumours: the role of temozolomide and the assessment of MGMT status. *Eur J Clin Invest* **41**, 1133–48.

McCormack A, et al. (2018). Treatment of aggressive pituitary tumours and carcinomas: results of a European Society of Endocrinology (ESE) survey 2016. *Eur J Endocrinol* **178**, 265–76.

Pernicone PJ, et al. (1997). Pituitary carcinoma. *Cancer* **79**, 804–12.

Raverot G, et al. (2018). European Society of Endocrinology Clinical Practice Guidelines for the management of aggressive pituitary tumours and carcinomas. *Eur J Endocrinol* **178**, G1–24.

Pituitary metastases

Incidence

Autopsy series 0.1–28%; <1% found at transsphenoidal surgery.

Epidemiology

Equal sex distribution. Age >60 (occasionally younger).

Features

In recently published series, DI is not present in all cases and only anterior hypopituitarism may be present. Cranial nerve defects are less common. Often difficult to differentiate neuroradiologically from other pituitary mass lesions (adenoma, cyst, or inflammatory pituitary mass). Many do not have symptoms, as features of end-stage malignancy predominate. Disconnection hyperprolactinaemia may be a feature, and very rare cases of endocrine hyperfunction related to metastasis within a 1° adenoma have been reported (see Box 2.24).

> **Box 2.24 Primary tumours associated with pituitary metastases**
> * Breast.
> * Lung.
> * GI.
> * Prostate.
> * Kidney.
>
> Breast and lung 1° tumours account for two-thirds of pituitary metastases.

Diagnosis

Histology is required to confirm.

Treatment

* Of 1° tumour where possible.
* Management of endocrine symptoms.
* Decompression may be indicated for visual dysfunction.

Prognosis

Median survival 11 months.

Further reading

Lithgow K, et al. (2020). Pituitary metastases: presentation and outcomes from a pituitary center over the last decade. *Pituitary* **23**, 25865.

Craniopharyngiomas and perisellar cysts

(See Box 2.25 for Rathke's cleft cysts.)

Prevalence and epidemiology
- 0.065/1000.
- Any age; only 50% present in childhood (<16 years).

Pathology
- Tumour arising from squamous epithelial remnants of craniopharyngeal duct.
- Histology may be either adamantinomatous or papillary.
- *BRAF V600E* mutations have been detected in the papillary subtype, and β-*catenin* mutations in adamantinomatous craniopharyngiomas.
- Cyst formation and calcification are common.
- Benign tumour, although infiltrates surrounding structures.

Features
- Raised intracranial pressure.
- Visual disturbance.
- Hypothalamo–pituitary disturbance (obesity, sleep disorders, thirst disorders, temperature dysregulation).
- Growth failure in children.
- Precocious puberty and tall stature are less common.
- Anterior and posterior pituitary failure, including DI.
- Weight gain.

Other perisellar cysts
- Arachnoid.
- Epidermoid.
- Dermoid.

Investigations
- MRI/CT (CT may be helpful to evaluate bony erosion and calcification).
- Visual field assessment.
- Anterior and posterior pituitary assessment (see ⊃ Pituitary function—dynamic tests: insulin tolerance test (ITT), pp. 130–1; ⊃ Further investigations, p. 232).

Management
(See Fig. 2.7.)
- Surgery.
- Gross total removal is the aim of treatment, as this is associated with a significantly lower recurrence rate. This may be via a transfrontal or a transsphenoidal route. If total removal cannot be safely achieved, adjuvant radiotherapy is beneficial in reducing recurrence. In cases with hypothalamic involvement, conservative surgery with partial removal, followed by radiotherapy, is considered the preferred management options.
- Restoration of pituitary hormone deficiencies is extremely unlikely following surgery.
- Cystic lesions may be treated with biopsy and aspiration alone, although radiotherapy reduces the likelihood of reaccumulation.
- Radiotherapy.

- Drug treatment.
- Recent data on *BRAF* mutations in the papillary subtype are promising for the use of BRAF inhibitors.

Prognosis

- Craniopharyngiomas are associated with ↓ survival (up to 5× the mortality of the general population).
- Recurrence following initial treatment may present early or several decades following initial treatment. Childhood- and adult-onset lesions behave similarly.

Box 2.25 Rathke's cleft cysts

Epidemiology

In routine autopsies, they are encountered in 13–33% of normal pituitary glands

- In routine autopsies, they are encountered in 13–33% of normal pituitary glands.
- There is a ♀ preponderance.

In routine autopsies, they are encountered in 13–33% of normal pituitary glands.

Pathology

Derived from the remnants of Rathke's pouch, lined by epithelial cells (ciliated cuboidal/columnar epithelium, compared with squamous for craniopharyngiomas), and filled with fluid.

Features

Usually asymptomatic, although may present with headache and amenorrhoea and, rarely, hypopituitarism and hydrocephalus.

Endocrine disturbance

Anterior pituitary hormone deficits at presentation vary widely between 19% and 81% depending on the number of the affected reported axes and the diagnostic tests used

Anterior pituitary hormone deficits at presentation vary widely between 19% and 81%, depending on the number of affected reported axes and the diagnostic tests used. Hypogonadism is the most frequently reported hormonal manifestation.

Investigation

- CT/MRI—variable enhancement.

Management

- Decompression if symptomatic.
- Recurrence after surgery is not as rare as originally thought (48% at 4 years).

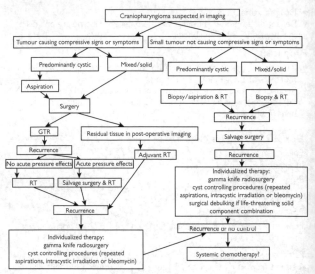

Fig. 2.7 Treatment algorithm for craniopharyngiomas.

Reproduced with permission from Karavitaki N, Cudlip S, Adams CB, Wass JA (2006). Craniopharyngiomas. *Endocr Rev* 27 (4), pp.371–97. Epub 2006 Mar 16, copyright 2006, The Endocrine Society.

Further reading

Karavitaki N, *et al.* (2006). Craniopharyngiomas. *Endocr Rev* **27**, 371–93.

Trifanescu R, *et al.* (2011). Outcome in surgically treated Rathke's cleft cysts: long-term monitoring needed. *Eur J Endocrinol* **165**, 33–7.

Trifanescu R, *et al.* (2012). Rathke's cleft cysts. *Clin Endocrinol (Oxf)* **76**, 51–60.

Alexandraki KI, *et al.* (2020). The medical therapy of craniopharyngiomas: the way ahead. *J Clin Endocrinol Metab* **104**, 5751–64.

Karavitaki N (2014). Management of craniopharyngiomas. *J Endocrinol Invest* **37**, 219–28.

Thompson CJ, *et al.* (2019). Management of hypothalamic disease in patients with craniopharyngioma. *Clin Endocrinol (Oxf)* **90**, 506–16.

Parasellar tumours

Meningiomas

- Suprasellar meningiomas arise from the tuberculum sellae or the chiasmal sulcus.
- Usually present with a chiasmal syndrome where loss of VA occurs in one eye, followed by reduced VA in the other eye.
- Differentiation from a 1° pituitary tumour can be difficult where there is downward extension into the sella.
- MRI is the imaging of choice. T_1-weighted images demonstrate meningiomas as isodense with grey matter and hypointense with respect to pituitary tissue, with marked enhancement after gadolinium.
- Cerebral angiography also demonstrates a tumour blush.
- Management is surgical and may also be complicated by haemorrhage, as these are often very vascular tumours. They are relatively radioresistant, but inoperable or partially removed tumours may respond. As they are slow-growing, a conservative approach with regular imaging may be appropriate.
- Associations include type 2 NF (see ➔ Neurofibromatosis, pp. 658–60).

Clivus chordomas

- Rare. Arise from embryonic crest cells of the notochord.
- May present with cranial nerve palsies (III, VI, IX, X) or pyramidal tract dysfunction.
- Anterior and posterior pituitary hypofunction is reported.
- Often invasive and relentlessly progressive.
- Treatment is surgical, followed by radiotherapy in some cases, although they are relatively radioresistant. Data on radiosurgery are not yet available, but this may be considered.

Hamartomas

- Non-neoplastic overgrowth of neurones and glial cells.
- Rare. May present with seizures—typically gelastic (laughing).
- May release GnRH leading to precocious puberty or, very rarely, GHRH leading to disorders of growth or acromegaly.
- Appear as homogeneous, isointense with grey matter, pedunculated or sessile non-enhancing tumours on T_1-weighted MRI scans.

Management

Tumours do not enlarge, and therefore, treatment is of endocrine consequences—most commonly, precocious puberty.

Ependymomas

- Intracranial ependymomas typically affect children and adolescents.
- Pituitary insufficiency may follow craniospinal irradiation.
- Occasionally, 3rd ventricle tumours may interfere with hypothalamic function.

- Parasellar germ cell turnover:
  - 5% of 1° CNS tumours.
  - Suprasellar or pineal or both.
  - Present with DI, ↓ growth velocity or hypopituitarism ± visual defects, and Parinaud's syndrome (upgaze palsy, convergence retraction nystagmus, and pupillary hyporeflexia).
  - Measures tumour markers in CSF and blood (hCG and aFP).
  - Staging—local or disseminated.
  - Sensitive to radiation and chemotherapy.

Further reading

Graillon T, et al. (2020). Parsellar meningiomas. *Neuroendocrinology* **110**, 780–96.

MacDonald SM, et al. (2016). Case 32-2016. A 20-year-old man with gynecomastia. *N Engl J Med* **375**, 1567–79.

Stacchiotti S, Sommer J; Chordoma Global Consensus Group (2015). Building a global consensus approach to chordoma: a position paper from the medical and patient community. *Lancet Oncol* **16**, e71–83.

Whittle IR, et al. (2004). Meningiomas. *Lancet* **363**, 1535–43.

Parasellar inflammatory conditions

Neurosarcoidosis

The pituitary and hypothalamus may be affected by meningeal disease. Most patients with hypothalamic sarcoidosis also have involvement outside the CNS.

Features

Hypopituitarism and DI, in addition to hypothalamic syndrome of absent thirst, somnolence, and hyperphagia.

Investigations

- Serum and CSF ACE may be raised.
- CSF examination may reveal a pleocytosis, oligoclonal bands, and low glucose.
- MRI may demonstrate additional enhancement, e.g. meningeal.
- Gallium scan may reveal ↑ uptake in lacrimal and salivary glands.

Management

- High doses of GC (60–80mg prednisolone) for initial treatment. Subsequent treatment with 40mg/day is often required for several months. Pulsed methylprednisolone may also be useful. Steroid-sparing agents, such as azathioprine, may be helpful.
- Management of hormonal deficiency can be very difficult, particularly in the context of absent thirst and poor memory.

Langerhans cell histiocytosis

- >50% of cases occur in children.
- Its pathogenesis is not clearly defined. However, the identification of a distinctive clonal component, along with a tumour-associated mutation, suggests that this is a neoplastic, rather than reactive, disease.
- Most frequent endocrine abnormalities are DI (up to 55% of cases) and growth retardation due to hypothalamic infiltration by Langerhans cells or involvement of the meninges adjacent to the pituitary. Rarely, hyperprolactinaemia and panhypopituitarism develop. Anterior pituitary hormone deficiency is not always associated with DI. In adults, DI may precede the bone and soft tissue abnormalities, making diagnosis difficult.

Management

The role of radiotherapy is controversial, with some workers reporting improvement and others questioning the efficacy. If radiotherapy is used, rapid institution of treatment appears to be important (within 10 days of diagnosis). High-dose GCs can lead to transient improvement, but chemotherapy does not alter the course of DI, although it may lead to temporary regression of lesions.

Wegener's granulomatosis

- Systemic vasculitis, affecting mainly 30- to 50-year olds.
- Necrotizing vasculitis, affecting the lungs and kidneys in 85% (cavitating nodule infiltrates).
- Pituitary involvement 1%.
- Present with DI and hyperprolactinaemia.
- High titres of ANCA.
- Treated with GCs and/or cyclophosphamide.

Tuberculosis

TB may present as a tuberculoma which may compromise hypothalamic or pituitary function. DI is common. Most patients have signs of TB elsewhere, but not invariably so. Transsphenoidal biopsy is therefore sometimes required. An alternative strategy is antituberculous treatment, with empirical GC treatment.

Further reading

Allen CE, et al. (2018). Langerhans-cell histiocytosis. N Engl J Med **379**, 856–68.

Freda PU, Post KD (1999). Differential diagnosis of sellar masses. Endocrinol Metab Clin North Am **28**, 81.

Makras P, Kaltsas G (2015). Langerhans cell histiocytosis and pituitary function. Endocrine **48**, 728–9.

Sagna Y, et al. (2019). Endocrine manifestations in a cohort of 63 adulthood and childhood onset patients with Langerhans cell histiocytosis. Eur J Endocrinol **181**, 275–85.

Lymphocytic hypophysitis

Background

This is a rare inflammatory condition of the pituitary.

Epidemiology

Lymphocytic hypophysitis occurs more commonly in ♀ and usually presents during late pregnancy or in the 1st year thereafter.

Pathogenesis

Ill-understood—probably autoimmune; ~25% of cases of lymphocytic hypophysitis have been associated with other autoimmune conditions—Hashimoto's thyroiditis in the majority, but also pernicious anaemia.

There is a recent association with immune checkpoint inhibitors (see ➲ Immune checkpoint inhibitors, pp. 81–2) (e.g. ipilimumab 9–14%), and corticotrophin deficiency does not usually recover. Gonadotrophin and thyrotrophin deficiency may show recovery in the long term.

Pathology

- Somatotroph and gonadotroph function are more likely to be preserved than corticotroph or thyrotroph function, unlike the findings in hypopituitarism due to a pituitary tumour. The posterior pituitary is characteristically spared, so that DI is not part of the picture, but there are occasional reports of coexisting or isolated DI, presumably because of different antigens.
- Lymphocytic hypophysitis has occasionally involved the cavernous sinus and extraocular muscles.
- Light microscopy typically reveals a lymphoplasmacytic infiltrate, occasionally forming lymphoid follicles, with variable destruction of the parenchyma and fibrosis.

Clinical features

- Mass effects, leading to headache and visual field defects.
- Often a temporal association with pregnancy.
- Hypopituitarism (ACTH and TSH deficiency, less commonly gonadotrophin deficiency and GHD).
- Posterior pituitary involvement and cavernous sinus involvement occur less commonly.

(See Box 2.26 for classification.)

Investigations

- Investigation of hypopituitarism is essential and may not be thought of because gonadotrophin secretion often remains intact, leaving the potentially life-threatening ACTH deficiency unsuspected.
- MRI shows an enhancing mass, with variable loss of hyperintense bright spot of the neurohypophysis, thickening of the pituitary stalk, and enlargement of the neurohypophysis. Suprasellar extension often appears tongue-like along the pituitary stalk. There may be central necrosis, but no calcification.
- Biopsy of the lesion is often required but may be avoided in the presence of typical features.

- The presence of antipituitary antibodies has been investigated by some groups and shown to be variably present. This is, however, a research tool and an unreliable marker.

Box 2.26 Classification of hypophysitis
- Lymphocytic hypophysitis.
- Xanthomatous—characterized by lipid-laden macrophages.
- Granulomatous: TB, sarcoidosis, syphilis.
- Plasmacytic/IgG4-related hypophysitis.
- Necrotizing hypophysitis.

Treatment
- Most often, no specific treatment is necessary. There is anecdotal evidence only of the effectiveness of immunosuppressive doses of GCs, e.g. prednisolone 60mg/day initially, then progressive reduction for 6 months. This has been reported to be associated with a reduction in mass and gradual recovery of pituitary function. However, relapse after discontinuing therapy is also reported.
- Spontaneous recovery may also occur.
- Surgery has also been used to improve visual field abnormalities.

Natural history
Variable—some progress rapidly to life-threatening hypopituitarism, while others spontaneously regress.

Relationship to other conditions
Lymphocytic hypophysitis remains an ill-understood condition but has been suggested to be the underlying cause of other conditions such as isolated ACTH deficiency and empty sella syndrome.

Further reading
Albarel F, et al. (2019). Management of endocrine disease. Immune check point inhibitors-induced hypophysitis. Eur J Endocrinol 181, R107–18.

Caturegli P, et al. (2005). Autoimmune hypophysitis. Endocr Rev 26, 599–614.

Faje AT, et al. (2014). Ipilimumab-induced hypophysitis: a detailed longitudinal analysis in a large co-hort of patients with metastatic melanoma. J Clin Endocrinol Metab 99, 4078–85.

Honegger J, et al. (2015). Treatment of Primary Hypophysitis in Germany. J Clin Endocrinol Metab 100, 3460–9.

Joshi MN, et al. (2018). Mechanisms in endocrinology. Hypophysitis: diagnosis and treatment. Eur J Endocrinol 179, R151–63.

Surgical treatment of pituitary tumours

Transsphenoidal surgery

❶ *Endoscopic approaches are controversial*

This is currently the favoured technique for pituitary surgery and is 1st line for virtually every case. It is preferred to the previously used technique of craniotomy because there is minimal associated morbidity as a result of the fact that the cranial fossa is not opened and there are therefore no immediate sequelae due to direct cerebral damage (particularly frontal lobe) and no long-term risk of epilepsy. There is reduced duration of hospital stay and improved cure rates, as there is better visualization of small tumours. Unfortunately, the technique may be inadequate to deal with very large tumours with extensive suprasellar extension. In these situations, craniotomy is required if adequate debulking is not possible following the transsphenoidal approach (TSA). (See Box 2.27 for indications for surgery; see Table 2.12 for complications.)

Preparation for transsphenoidal surgery

Pretreatment before surgery

- For patients with severe pharyngeal thickness and sleep apnoea, or high-output heart failure, medical therapy with long-acting SSAs preoperatively is suggested to reduce surgical risk from severe comorbidities.
- Pretreatment with *metyrapone* or *ketoconazole* to improve the condition of patients with Cushing's syndrome is often given for at least 6 weeks. This allows some improvement in healing and also improves the general state of the patient.
- Patients with macroprolactinomas will, in the majority of cases, have received treatment with dopamine agonists in any case, and surgery is usually indicated for resistance or intolerance. There is a risk of tumour fibrosis with long-term (>6 months) dopamine agonist therapy with bromocriptine.

Immediately preoperative

- Immediate preoperative treatment requires appropriate anterior pituitary hormone replacement—in particular, a decision as to whether perioperative GC treatment is required. The majority of microadenomas will not require perioperative hydrocortisone, but patients with Cushing's syndrome will require peri- and post-operative GC treatment. Patients with macroadenomas and an intact preoperative pituitary–adrenal axis do not usually require perioperative steroids, but those who are deficient or whose reserve has not been tested need to be given perioperative GCs. Preoperation TSH deficiency should be corrected with liothyronine (because of the potential for post-operative recovery), although others use levothyroxine, if necessary, with a plan to wean post-operatively in order to assess recovery. Ensure the patient is not taking aspirin.
- Prophylactic antibiotics are started in some centres the night before surgery to reduce the chances of meningitis.

Complications

(See also Box 2.28 and Table 2.12.)

- Patients should be informed about the possible complications of transsphenoidal surgery prior to consent. The commonest complications are DI, which may be transient or permanent (5% and 0.1%, respectively; often higher in Cushing's disease and prolactinoma), and the development of new anterior pituitary hormonal deficiencies (uncommon with microadenomas; ~10% of TSA for macroadenomas).
- Other complications include meningitis, CSF leak, visual deterioration, haemorrhage (rare), and transient hyponatraemia, usually 7–10 days post-operatively.
- Hyponatraemia may be ↓ by post-operative fluid restriction.

Box 2.27 Indications for pituitary surgery

- NFA.
- GH-secreting adenoma.
- ACTH-secreting tumour.
- Nelson's syndrome. (see Box 2.23).
- Prolactinoma—if patient is dopamine agonist-resistant or -intolerant.
- Recurrent pituitary tumour.
- Gonadotrophin-secreting tumour.
- TSH-secreting adenoma.
- Craniopharyngioma.
- Pituitary biopsy to define diagnosis, e.g. hypophysitis, pituitary metastases.
- Chordoma.
- Rathke's cleft cyst.
- Arachnoid cyst.

Box 2.28 Post-operative disorders of fluid balance

- Acute post-operative transient DI.
- Syndrome of inappropriate antidiuretic hormone (SIADH).
- Triphasic response: initial DI due to axon shock (hours to days), followed by antidiuretic phase due to uncontrolled release of ADH from damaged posterior pituitary (2–14 days), followed by DI due to depletion of ADH.
- Transient hyponatraemia (isolated 2nd phase) at 5–10 days post-operatively, usually mild and self-limiting.

Cerebral salt wasting

A rare, but important, complication of transsphenoidal surgery, more commonly seen after subarachnoid haemorrhage, is cerebral salt wasting (CSW) syndrome. This typically occurs at days 5–10 post-operatively and is associated with, often massive, urinary salt loss and hypovolaemia. It needs to be differentiated from SIADH which may also occur at this stage (often using CVP measurement to demonstrate hypovolaemia in CSW, compared with euvolaemia in SIADH). Management of CSW involves administration of saline, whereas fluid restriction is indicated for SIADH.

Table 2.12 Complications of transsphenoidal surgery

Complications of any surgical procedure	Anaesthetic-related
	Venous thrombosis and PE
Immediate	Haemorrhage
	Hypothalamic damage
	Meningitis
Permanent	Visual deterioration or loss
	Cranial nerve damage (e.g. oculomotor nerve palsies)
	Hypopituitarism
	DI
	SIADH
Transient	DI
	CSF rhinorrhoea
	Meningitis
	Visual deterioration
	Cerebral salt wasting

Further reading

Sterns RH (2008). Recurrent pituitary adenoma: role and timing of surgery. *J Am Soc Nephrol* **19**, 194–6.

Tampourlou M, et al. (2017). Outcome of nonfunctioning pituitary adenomas that regrow after primary treatment: a study from two large UK centers. *J Clin Endocrinol Metab* **102**, 1889–97.

Transfrontal craniotomy

Indications

- Pituitary tumours with major suprasellar and lateral invasion where transsphenoidal surgery is unlikely to remove a significant proportion of the tumour.
- Parasellar tumours, e.g. meningioma.

Complications

- In addition to the complications of transsphenoidal surgery, brain retraction can lead to cerebral oedema or haemorrhage.
- Manipulation of the optic chiasm may lead to visual deterioration.
- Vascular damage.
- Damage to the olfactory nerve.

Perioperative management

Similar to that for patients undergoing transsphenoidal surgery (see
Transsphenoidal surgery, p. 218).

Post-operative management

- Recovery is typically slower than after transsphenoidal surgery.
- Prophylactic anticonvulsants are administered for up to 1 year.
- The Driver and Vehicle Licensing Agency (DVLA) must be advised of surgery and relevant regulations to be followed.

Further reading

Laws ER, Thapar K (1999). Pituitary surgery. *Endocrinol Metab Clin North Am* **28**, 119.

Pituitary radiotherapy

Indications

(See Table 2.13.)

- Pituitary radiotherapy is an effective treatment used to reduce the likelihood of tumour regrowth following surgery, to further shrink a tumour, and to treat persistent hormone hypersecretion (usually after surgical resection or non-successful medical treatment).
- Pituitary radiotherapy is usually only administrable once in a lifetime.

Technique

(See Box 2.29 for focal forms of radiotherapy.)

- Conventional external beam 3-field radiotherapy is able to deliver a beam of ionizing irradiation accurately to the pituitary fossa.
- Accurate targeting requires head fixation in a moulded plastic shell to keep the head immobilized. The fields of irradiation are based on simulation using MRI or CT scanning, and the volume is usually the tumour margins plus 0.5cm in all planes. The preoperative tumour volume is used for planning, whereas post-drug (dopamine agonist) shrinkage films are used for prolactinomas. There are three portals: two temporal and one anterior.
- The standard dose is 4500cGy in 25 fractions over 35 days, but 5000cGy may be used for relatively 'radioresistant' tumours such as craniopharyngiomas.

Efficacy

Radiotherapy is effective in reducing the chance of pituitary tumour regrowth. Comparison of non-functioning tumour recurrence following surgery and radiotherapy with surgery alone shows that radiotherapy is effective in reducing the likelihood of regrowth (see Fig. 2.8).

Table 2.13 Indications for pituitary radiotherapy

Tumour	Aim of treatment
NFA	To shrink residual mass or reduce likelihood of regrowth
GH/PRL/ACTH-secreting tumour	To reduce persistent hormonal hypersecretion and shrink residual mass
Craniopharyngioma	To reduce likelihood of regrowth
Recurrent tumour	To shrink mass and reduce likelihood of regrowth

Box 2.29 Focal forms of radiotherapy

Stereotactic radiosurgery uses focused radiation to deliver a precise dose of radiation:

- Gamma knife 'radiosurgery'—ionizing radiation from a cobalt-60 source delivered by convergent collimated beams.
- Linear accelerator focal radiotherapy—photons focused on a stationary point from a moving gantry.
- Potential advantages are that a single high dose of irradiation is given which can be sharply focused on the tumour, with minimal surrounding tissue damage.
- Long-term data are required to demonstrate endocrine efficacy, but it may have a particular role in recurrent or persistent tumours which are well demarcated and surgically inaccessible, e.g. in the cavernous sinus.
- Potential limitations include proximity to the optic chiasm.

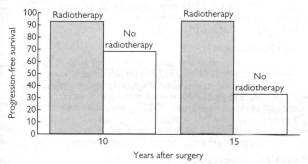

Fig. 2.8 Recurrence rates following radiotherapy.

Source: data from Gittoes NJL, Bates AS, Tse W, *et al.* (1998). Radiotherapy for non-functioning pituitary tumours. *Clin Endocrinol* 48, 331–7.

Complications of pituitary radiotherapy

Short term
- Nausea.
- Headache.
- Temporary hair loss at radiotherapy portals of entry.

Hypopituitarism

(See Fig. 2.9.)
- Anterior pituitary hormone deficiency occurs due to the effect of irradiation on the normal pituitary or hypothalamus, leading to reduced hypothalamic-releasing hormone secretion. The total dose of irradiation is one of the main determinants of the speed, incidence, and extent of hypopituitarism (see Table 2.14).
- The onset of hypopituitarism is gradual, and the order of development of deficiency is as for any other causes of developing hypopituitarism— namely, GH first, followed by gonadotrophin and ACTH, followed finally by TSH. Posterior pituitary deficiencies are very rare, but 2° temporary mild hyperprolactinaemia may be seen after about 2 years which gradually returns to normal.

Visual impairment

- The optic chiasm is particularly radioresistant but may undergo damage thought to be due to vascular damage to the blood supply. Visual deterioration typically occurs within 3 years of irradiation and is progressive.
- The literature suggests that the risk is greatest with high total and daily doses. A standard total dose of 4500cGy and a daily dose of 180cGy appear to pose very little, if any, risk to the chiasm.
- Our practice is to avoid administration of radiotherapy, where possible, when the chiasm is under pressure from residual tumour.

Radiation oncogenesis

- There is controversy as to whether pituitary irradiation leads to the development of 2nd tumours. There have been reports of sarcomas, gliomas, and meningiomas developing in the field of irradiation after 10–20 years. However, there are also reports of gliomas and meningiomas occurring in non-irradiated patients with pituitary adenomas. A retrospective review of a large series of patients given pituitary irradiation suggested a risk of a 2nd tumour of 1.9% by 20 years after irradiation, when compared to the normal population (but not patients with pituitary tumours).
- Subtle changes in neurocognition have also been suggested.

Further reading

Brada M, et al. (1992). Risk of second brain tumour after conservative surgery and radiotherapy for pituitary adenoma. *BMJ* **304**, 1343–6.

Jackson IMD, Noren G (1999). Role of gamma knife therapy in the management of pituitary tumours. *Endocrinol Metab Clin North Am* **28**, 133.

Loeffler JS, Shih HA (2011). Radiation therapy in the management of pituitary adenomas. *J Clin Endocrinol Metab* **96**, 1992–2003.

Minniti G, et al. (2016). Stereotactic radiotherapy and radiosurgery for non-functioning and secreting pituitary adenomas. *Rep Pract Oncol Radiother* **21**, 370–8.

Minniti G, et al. (2005). Risk of second brain tumor after conservative surgery and radiotherapy for pituitary adenoma: update after an additional 10 years. *J Clin Endocrinol Metab* **90**, 800–4.

Table 2.14 Development of new hypopituitarism at 10 years following pituitary radiotherapy

	No previous surgery (%)	Previous surgery (%)
Gonadotrophin deficiency	47	70
ACTH deficiency	30	54
Thyrotrophin deficiency	16	38

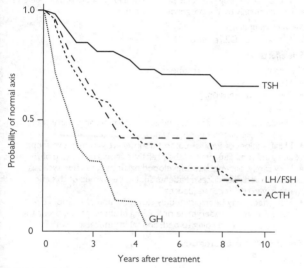

Fig. 2.9 Life-table analysis, indicating the probability of developing pituitary hormone deficiencies after conventional radiation therapy.

Reproduced with permission from Littley MD, Shalet SM, Beardwell CG, Ahmed, SR, et al. (1989). Q J Med 70:145–160 © Oxford University Press.

Drug treatment of pituitary tumours

Dopamine agonists

(See Box 2.30 for uses.)

Types

- *Bromocriptine*—the 1st ergot alkaloid to be used, short-acting, taken daily. Usually administered PO, although vaginal and IM formulations can be used and may reduce GI intolerance.
- *Quinagolide*—non-ergot, longer-acting, taken daily.
- *Cabergoline*—ergot derivative, long-acting, taken once or twice a week. This is the 1st drug of choice because of a lower incidence of side effects.
- *Less commonly used*—pergolide and lisuride.

Mechanism of action

- Activation of D2 receptors.

Side effects

Commonly at initiation of treatment

- Nausea.
- Postural hypotension.

Less common

- Headache, fatigue, nasal stuffiness, constipation, abdominal cramps, Raynaud-like phenomenon in hands.
- Manifestations of impulse control disorders (e.g. compulsive shopping and gambling). Patients and their relatives should be warned of this effect.
- Very rarely, patients have developed hallucinations and psychosis (usually at higher doses). Patients should be warned of this effect which can have serious consequences.
- Side effects may be minimized by slow initiation of therapy (e.g. 250 micrograms cabergoline or 1.25mg bromocriptine), taking the medication before going to bed, and taking the tablets with food.

Somatostatin analogues

(See Box 2.31 for uses.)

Mechanism of action

- Since the half-life of somatostatin is very short, longer-acting analogues were synthesized—octreotide and lanreotide. These have a half-life of 110min in the circulation and inhibit GH secretion 45× more actively than native somatostatin, with none of the rebound hypersecretion that occurs with somatostatin.
- SSAs act predominantly on somatostatin receptors 2 and 5. Unlike dopamine agonists, SSAs do not lead to dramatic tumour shrinkage, but some shrinkage is still seen in the majority of tumours.

Types

- Octreotide LAR® (10–30mg IM) administered every 4–6 weeks.
- Lanreotide Autogel® (60–120mg IM) administered every 28 days.
- SC octreotide (50–200 micrograms) administered usually three times daily.
- Pasireotide is a new SSA which has ↑ affinity for somatostatin receptor 5. It is licensed for use in Cushing's disease.

Box 2.30 Uses of dopamine agonists

Hyperprolactinaemia

(See ➲ Treatment of prolactinomas, pp. 164–7.)

- D2 receptor stimulation leads to inhibition of PRL secretion and reduction in cell size, leading to tumour shrinkage. The PRL level often falls before significant tumour shrinkage is seen.
- Problems may arise when patients are either intolerant of the medication or resistant. Cabergoline appears to be better tolerated than bromocriptine, and it is often worth trying an alternative in the case of intolerance, although true intolerance is probably a class effect. Dopamine agonist resistance macro- > microadenomas (10–25% patients) may be due to differences in receptor subtype (e.g. loss of D2 receptors) or possibly altered intracellular signalling.

GH-secreting tumours

- Although administration of levodopa to normal individuals leads to acute increase in GH due to hypothalamic dopamine and noradrenaline synthesis and inhibition of somatostatin secretion, >50% of patients with GH-secreting tumours given dopamine agonists have a fall in GH. Dopamine acts directly on somatotroph tumours to inhibit GH release.
- Patients with acromegaly often need larger doses of dopamine agonist than patients with prolactinomas, e.g. cabergoline 3mg/week. Tumour shrinkage is most likely if there is concomitant secretion of PRL from the tumour. Dopamine agonists are currently usually reserved for 2nd-line drug therapy in patients who are SSA-resistant or as a co-prescription with SSAs in patients with mixed GH- and PRL-secreting tumours.

Pregnancy

Bromocriptine is licensed for use in pregnancy, but cabergoline is not licensed in the UK, although it has not thus far been associated with any ↑ teratogenicity.

Box 2.31 Uses of somatostatin analogues

- Acromegaly.
- Carcinoid tumours.
- Pancreatic NETs.
- TSH-secreting pituitary tumours.

Side effects

- *Gallstones.* At least 20–30% of patients develop gallstones or sludge on octreotide (thought, by most, to antedate stone formation), but only 1%/year develop symptoms. The incidence is unknown on octreotide LAR® or lanreotide. Symptoms may occur particularly if SSA therapy is withdrawn (cholecystokinin active again).
- GI due to inhibition of motor activity and secretion, leading to nausea, abdominal cramps, and mild steatorrhoea. These usually settle with time.

- Injection site pain obviated by allowing the vial to warm to room temperature before injecting.
- Hair loss (<10%).

Growth hormone receptor antagonist

- Pegvisomant—treatment for acromegaly.

Mechanism of action

- Binds to GH receptor and induces internalization but blocks receptor signalling, leading to reduction in IGF-1 (but not GH) production.
- Studies suggest that it is the most potent available medical therapy. Normalization of IGF-1 in >90% of treated patients, if adequate dose, escape in 15.6%, and increase in tumour size in 9.4%.

Usage

- May be used with SSAs to decrease frequency of injections.

Problems

- High cost.
- Further data required on the effects on pituitary tumour growth.
- Occasional deterioration in liver biochemistry.
- IGF-1 used to monitor effectiveness of treatment.

Temozolomide

- An alkylating chemotherapeutic agent, effective in glioblastoma and NETs.
- It has been successfully used to treat pituitary carcinoma and invasive and aggressive pituitary adenomas.
- Response may be predicated by O-6-methylguanine DNA methyltransferase (MGMT) staining, which is lower in responders.

Further reading

McCormack AI, et al. (2011). Aggressive pituitary tumours: the role of temozolomide and the assessment of MGMT status. *Eur J Clin Invest* **41**, 1133–48.

Sandret L, et al. (2011). Place of cabergoline in acromegaly: a meta-analysis. *J Clin Endocrinol Metab* **96**, 1327–35.

Sherlock M, et al. (2011). Medical therapy in acromegaly. *Nat Rev Endocrinol* **7**, 291–300.

Trainer PJ, et al. (2000). Treatment of acromegaly with the growth hormone-receptor antagonist pegvisomant. *N Engl J Med* **342**, 1171–7.

Posterior pituitary

Physiology

The normal posterior pituitary is composed of neural tissue derived from ectodermal tissue of the diencephalon. Two hormones are synthesized, stored, and secreted from the neurohypophysis: arginine vasopressin (AVP) and oxytocin. The inferior hypophyseal arteries directly supply the posterior pituitary; venous drainage is into the cavernous sinus and internal jugular vein.

Pre-pro-vasopressin and secretion of AVP

AVP is a nonapeptide hormone, which is synthesized as a pre-prohormone in the supraoptic and paraventricular nuclei of the hypothalamus. It is then transported down the magnocellular neurones, via axonal transport to the posterior pituitary where it is stored in granules prior to release into the systemic circulation. Prior to secretion, the pre-prohormone is enzymatically cleaved into neurophysin and copeptin, which are biologically inert, and the active hormone AVP; the three distinct compounds are secreted in equimolar concentrations into the plasma.

Physiological release of AVP is solely determined by the ambient plasma osmolality. Osmoreceptors, situated in the subfornical organ (SFO) and organum vasculosum of the lamina terminalis (OVLT), in the anterior hypothalamus, are exposed to plasma via local fenestrations in the blood–brain barrier. Rising plasma osmolality triggers neural reflexes which lead to the release of AVP and the generation of the sensation of thirst, which leads to water intake. Lesions in the SFO and OVLT lead to impaired or absent thirst sensation, in addition to defective AVP secretion. Pathological falls in BP or blood volume are detected by baroreceptors, which can stimulate marked elevation in plasma AVP concentrations.

Vasopressin is transported to the kidneys where it binds to V2 receptors in the collecting ducts. Receptor binding activates the adenyl cyclase system and the generation of aquaporin 2 (AQ2) channels, which insert into the apical membrane, allowing reabsorption of water into the circulation, concentrating urine. When AVP is present in high concentration in the plasma, it binds to V1 receptors in vascular smooth muscle, acting as a powerful vasoconstrictor.

Measurement of plasma AVP by radioimmunoassay is technically difficult and only available in specialized labs. Although copeptin is biologically inert, it is easier and cheaper to measure, and recent studies have shown that it provides a good surrogate for measurement of AVP. The technical advantages of the copeptin assay dictate that it is likely to replace the measurement of AVP for diagnostic purposes.

Oxytocin

The main actions of oxytocin are relevant only in ♀ where it is involved in lactation and parturition. During childbirth, oxytocin binds to receptors in the uterus, predominantly the fundus, resulting in uterine contractions. Oxytocin also stimulates the production of prostaglandins. During lactation, oxytocin is released in a pulsatile pattern in response to suckling. It acts upon the myoepithelial cells in the breast tissue, which results in shortening and widening of the ducts, allowing milk to flow.

Diabetes insipidus

Definition

DI is the production of large volumes (>3L/24 hours) of dilute urine (urine osmolality <300mOsm/kg).

Classification

- Cranial DI is due to deficient AVP synthesis; 80% of AVP-secreting neurones must be lost to cause cranial DI.
- Nephrogenic DI results from renal resistance to circulating AVP.

Cranial

- Genetic, including DIDMOAD syndrome.
- Tumours, e.g. craniopharyngiomas, germinomas, metastases.
- Trauma, including head injury, surgery for pituitary adenomas.
- Inflammatory, e.g. hypophysitis, sarcoidosis, Langerhans cell histiocystosis, ANCA-associated vasculitis.
- Infections, e.g. meningitis, encephalitis, HIV disease.
- Vascular, e.g. subarachnoid haemorrhage, Sheehan's syndrome.
- Idiopathic—many idiopathic cases are autoimmune and associated with other autoimmune conditions.

Nephrogenic

- Genetic.
- Drugs, including lithium and demeclocycline.
- Metabolic, including hypercalcaemia, hypokalaemia, and hyperglycaemia.
- Chronic kidney disorder (CKD).
- Post-obstructive uropathy.

Primary polydipsia—'dipsogenic diabetes insipidus'

Clinical features

Adults present with polyuria, polydipsia, and thirst. Children with DI may present with failure to thrive, polydipsia, and enuresis.

The patient may have other features of underlying pathology, including headache, visual disturbance, or other endocrinopathy. Due to the role of cortisol in free water excretion, DI may only become apparent in hypopituitarism after replacement of GC.

Investigations

- Polyuria should be confirmed by asking the patient to measure a 24h urine output (normal <3L).
- Other causes of polyuria and polydipsia should be excluded. Absence of glycosuria excludes DM as a cause of polyuria. A corrected calcium and potassium should also be measured. Plasma sodium concentration is nearly always normal at diagnosis, as intact thirst preserves fluid intake. However, a low-normal plasma sodium concentration is suggestive of excess thirst. A baseline urine osmolality confirms dilute urine.
- A water deprivation test (see Box 2.32) can differentiate between DI and excess thirst; the addition of a desmopressin challenge helps differentiate between cranial and nephrogenic DI.

- The water deprivation test is time-consuming, unpleasant for the patient, and difficult to supervise; it is non-diagnostic in 30% of patients. Diagnostic accuracy is enhanced by adding the measurement of thirst using a visual analogue scale. Measurement of copeptin also increases diagnostic accuracy.

  (Interpretation of results is shown in Table 2.15.)
- Hypertonic saline—stimulated copeptin measurements have greater diagnostic accuracy than the water deprivation test (73% vs 95%) (see Box 2.33).
- Arginine-stimulated copeptin measurements may also be used.

Box 2.32 Water deprivation test
- Ensure normal thyroid and adrenal function prior to test.
- The patient should avoid cigarettes, alcohol, and caffeine for 24h prior to the test.
- The patient should fast overnight but can drink water until the beginning of the test.
- A starting weight should be obtained and 97% of this should be calculated.
- Weight should be monitored every hour, and the test stopped if >3% is lost.
- The patient should be observed closely throughout the test.
- Baseline plasma and urine osmolalities are performed, along with plasma sodium. The patient is then deprived of fluids for 8h.
- Samples are obtained for plasma osmolality and plasma sodium, and urine osmolality at 0, 2, 4, 6, and 8h. Hourly urine volumes should be noted. Measurement of copeptin, where available, is helpful.
- Thirst response to fluid deprivation should be assessed throughout the test using a visual analogue scale.
- At the end of water deprivation, desmopressin 2 micrograms IM is administered, and urine volume and osmolality are measured hourly for 4h.
- Free access to fluids is allowed in the period after desmopressin administration and the volume consumed should be measured.
- Interpretation of results is shown in Table 2.15.

Table 2.15 Interpretation of water deprivation test

Diagnosis	Urine osmolality (mOsm/kg) after fluid deprivation	Urine osmolality (mOsm/kg) after desmopressin
Normal	>750	>750
Cranial DI	<300	>750
1° polydipsia or partial DI	300–750	<750
Nephrogenic DI	<300	<300

Box 2.33 Stimulated copeptin measurements
- Discontinue diuretic and antidiuretic medication before test. No smoking/alcohol for 12h.
- Initial 250mL bolus of 3% saline, infusion continued at 0.15mL/kg/min.
- Blood samples for osmolality, sodium, urea, and glucose every 30min until 150mmol/L sodium is reached.
- Take copeptin measurement.
- Measure copeptin before and at peak sodium.

Interpretation
- Plasma copeptin <4.9pmol/L indicates complete or partial DI.
- >4.9pmol/L indicates 1° polydipsia or nephrogenic DI.

Further investigations
- MRI pituitary:
  - All patients with cranial DI should have an MRI pituitary if not contraindicated.
  - A normal MRI scan at presentation requires repeat imaging in 6–12 months to check for germinoma.
  - The commonest finding in cranial DI is an absent posterior pituitary bright spot.
  - A sellar mass in association with cranial DI excludes the diagnosis of pituitary adenoma; consider craniopharyngioma or granuloma.
- Serum ACE and CXR to check for sarcoid.
- IgG4.
- β-hCG and aFP to screen for germinoma—even if no mass on MRI—also in CSF.
- Vasculitis screen.
- If MRI shows no mass, check thyroid function, vitamin B12, and thyroid antibodies.

Pituitary stalk lesions
(See Box 2.34.)

Box 2.34 Pituitary stalk lesions
- 30% neoplastic, 20% inflammatory.
- 13% congenital, 39% unclear.
- 32% at least are anterior pituitary-deficient.
- Inflammatory—neurosarcoidosis, Langerhans cell histiocytosis, lymphocytic hypophysitis.
- Neoplastic—craniopharyngioma, metastatic cancer/lymphoma, germinoma, astrocytoma.

Treatment

If symptoms are mild and thirst is intact, patients may not require pharmacological management.

Cranial

- Desmopressin is the drug treatment of choice in cranial DI, given in 1–2 divided doses, according to severity of symptoms. Different formulations exist, e.g. oral, spray, according to preference.
- Desmopressin is a synthetic version of vasopressin which has been structurally altered to negate vasoconstrictor effects and increase the half-life.
- The aim of treatment is to improve QoL while avoiding treatment-induced hyponatraemia and associated complications.
- Dilutional hyponatraemia can be avoided by suggesting patient withholds desmopressin for a few hours 2–3 times per week, to allow mild polyuria to develop; this allows a washout of any excess water which has not been excreted.
- Regular follow-up is indicated to ensure symptom control, monitor for dilutional hyponatraemia, and screen for the appearance of germinoma and autoimmune disease in 'idiopathic DI'.

Nephrogenic

- Ensure adequate fluid intake and reduce salt intake.
- Correct underlying metabolic causes.
- Consider discontinuation of causative drugs, e.g. lithium.
- Thiazide diuretics, e.g. bendroflumethiazide or hydrochlorothiazide, can be used to reduce urine output and increase urine concentration.
- Amiloride can be used on its own or in addition to thiazide, particularly in lithium-induced nephrogenic DI.
- Prostaglandin synthetase inhibitors.

How do I manage adipsic DI?

Adipsic diabetes insipidus (ADI) is a rare clinical situation which occurs when damage to osmoreceptors in the anterior hypothalamus results in failure to respond to rising plasma sodium with appropriate fluid intake. It is associated with chronic hypernatraemia and is associated with significant morbidity and mortality. The commonest cause of adipsic DI is surgical clipping of aneurysms of the anterior communicating aneurysm, following subarachnoid haemorrhage. It has also been associated with extensive surgery for craniopharyngioma, TBI, neurosarcoidosis, and congenital causes.

Patients are susceptible to hypernatraemia, even when ambulant, but are particularly vulnerable during acute illness, particularly when vomiting occurs. Care must also be exercised when managing surgical patients with ADI, as hypernatraemia commonly occurs. In addition, acute hyponatraemia may develop, if the patients overdrinks.

Practical tips

* *Desmopressin*. A fixed prescription twice daily of desmopressin prevents excessive fluid loss from polyuria.
* *Fluid prescription*. Patients should be trained to drink a target volume per day. A target of 2L is usually sufficient or daily urine loss plus 500mL where urine measurement is possible.
* *Daily weights*. Fluctuations in body weight may indicate swings in hydration status, with dysnatraemia.
* *Regular monitoring of plasma sodium*. This group is prone to dysnatraemia and subsequent complications. They should therefore have frequent measurement of plasma electrolytes for continued monitoring.
* *Screening for hypothalamic complications*, particularly obstructive sleep apnoea and hypothalamic obesity.
* *Anticoagulation* during acute illness is helpful in preventing thrombotic complications of hypernatraemia.

Further reading

Catford S, et al. (2016). Pituitary stalk lesions: systematic review and clinical guidance. *Clin Endocrinol (Oxf)* **85**, 507–21.

Cuesta M, et al. (2017). Adipsic diabetes insipidus in adult patients. *Pituitary* **20**, 372–80.

Fenske W, et al. (2018). A copeptin-based approach in the diagnosis of diabetes insipidus. *N Engl J Med* 379, 428–39.

Garrahy A, et al. (2019). Diagnosis and management of central diabetes insipidus in adults. *Clin Endocrinol* **90**, 23–30.

Levy M, et al. (2019). Diabetes insipidus. *BMJ* **364**, i321.

Turcu AF, et al. (2013). Pituitary stalk lesions: the Mayo Clinic experience. *J Clin Endocrinol Metab* **98**, 1812–18.

Winzeler B, et al. (2019). Arginine-stimulated copeptin measurements in the differential diagnosis of diabetes insipidus: a prospective diagnostic study. *Lancet* **394**, 587–95. https://www.endocrinology.org/media/3627/ec-7-g8.pdf.

Hyponatraemia

Incidence

- Hyponatraemia occurs in 15–30% of hospitalized patients and is commoner in the elderly.
- It is associated with ↑ duration of hospital admission and ↑ mortality.
- Ambulant patients with hyponatraemia have ↑ falls, fractures, and osteoporosis.
- Hyponatraemia has been associated with ↑ mortality in all clinical conditions in which it has been studied.

Clinical features

Mild hyponatraemia may have no symptoms but is associated with ↑ falls, more fractures after falls, and osteoporosis. Neurological symptoms are a feature of rapid falls in plasma sodium. Acute severe hyponatraemia, developing over <48h, results in cerebral oedema, and when the patient presents with altered consciousness, seizures, or coma, this represents a medical emergency, which requires urgent intervention to elevate plasma sodium concentration.

Chronic hyponatraemia (>48h) allows cerebral adaptation, with a net shift of organic osmolytes out of brain cells, which allows equilibrium with the serum osmolality and fewer neurological symptoms. The associated gait disturbances, falls, and fractures still justify therapeutic intervention.

Causes

A number of clinical algorithms are available. The one used in our unit is shown in Table 2.16.

Table 2.16 Clinical algorithm for causes of hyponatraemia

Fluid status	Urinary sodium <30mmol/L	Urinary sodium >30mmol/L
Hypovolaemic	Diarrhoea Vomiting	Diuretic use Addison's disease MC deficiency Salt wasting nephropathy CSW
Euvolaemic	1° polydipsia Acute water intoxication Malnutrition Hypothyroidism	Syndrome of inappropriate antidiuresis (SIAD) GC deficiency
Hypervolaemic	Heart failure Liver cirrhosis Nephrotic syndrome	CRF Heart failure plus diuretics

Essential investigations

- Paired urine and plasma osmolalities.
- Urinary sodium.
- Renal function.
- TFTs.
- 9 a.m. cortisol >300nmol/L usually enough to exclude cortisol deficiency. Synacthen® test if high diagnostic suspicion.
- Drugs associated with hyponatraemia (see Box 2.35).

Management

Definitive management dependent on underlying cause; hypovolaemia requires fluid replacement, whereas hypervolaemia needs diuretic. Treatment of SIAD is shown in ➔ Management of SIAD, p. 240.

Two major guidelines have recently been published, outlining acute and chronic management of hyponatraemia.

The need for urgent treatment with hypertonic saline is determined by the presence of neurological symptoms, and not the severity of hyponatraemia. The risk of inducing osmotic demyelination in asymptomatic patients, by rapidly reversing hyponatraemia, does not justify the use of hypertonic saline. However, in patients with acute neurological compromise 2° to hyponatraemia, regardless of duration, treatment with 3% hypertonic saline is indicated. Recent data suggest improved outcomes (particularly neurological) with bolus vs continuous infusion regimens at 6h. (See Box 2.36 for suggested protocol for hypertonic saline.)

Box 2.35 Drugs associated with hyponatraemia

Vasopressin release or action stimulated.
- Antidepressants:
  - SSRIs, MAOIs, tricyclics, venlafaxine.
- Anticonvulsants:
  - Carbamazepine, valproate, lamotrigine.
- Antipsychotics:
  - Phenothiazines, butyrophenones.
- Anticancer drugs:
  - Vinca alkaloids, platinum, melphalan, cyclophosphamide, methotrexate.
- Antidiabetic drugs:
  - Chlorpropamide, tolbutamide.
- Others:
  - Opiates, interferon, NSAIDs, clofibrate, amiodarone.
  - PPIs.

Box 2.36 How do I manage severe hyponatraemia and overcorrection if it occurs?

- Hyponatraemia with associated neurological compromise has a high mortality due to cerebral oedema.
- The aim of emergency treatment is to acutely raise plasma osmolality, to cause an osmotic shift of water from the brain to plasma, causing a reduction in intracranial pressure.
- Patients should be managed in a medical high dependency or intensive care unit.
- 100mL of 3% saline should be administered via wide-bore cannula over 15min.
- Repeat plasma sodium should be measured at 1h.
- Target plasma sodium in first 6h of 4–6mmol/L.
- The target plasma sodium rise in the first 24h should be 8mmol/L, and no more than 12mmol/L.
- Two further boluses of 100mL of 3% hypertonic saline if the target plasma sodium has not been reached and neurological features persist.
- Once neurological symptoms have improved, then no further boluses are advised; slow correction to a target of 8mmol/L over 24h can continue.
- Caution is required as overcorrection may occur, particularly with the 3rd bolus.
- Patients at risk of osmotic demyelination—alcoholics, malnourished, liver disease—should have a plasma sodium target rise of 6mmol/L over 24h.
- Closely monitor urine output. Sudden aquaresis can be an early indication of rapid elevation in plasma sodium and an urgent sample for plasma sodium should be checked.
- If the change in plasma sodium exceeds the target, it should be relowered to reduce the risk of developing osmotic demyelination. IV infusion of glucose or SC desmopressin.

Further reading

Adrogue JH, Madias NE (2019). Hypernatremia. *N Engl J Med* **342**, 1581–9.

Garrahy A, et al. (2019). Continuous versus bolus infusion of hypertonic saline in treatment of symptomatic hyponatraemia caused by SIAD. *J Clin Endocrinol Metab* **104**, 3595–602.

Smith DM, et al. (2000). Hyponatraemia. *Clin Endocrinol (Oxf)* **52**, 667–78.

Spasovski G, et al. (2014). Clinical practice guideline on diagnosis and treatment of hyponatraemia. *Eur J Endocrinol* **170**, G1–47.

Verbalis JG, et al. (2013). Diagnosis, evaluation and treatment of hyponatraemia: expert panel recommendations. *Am J Med* **126**, S1–42.

SIAD

Diagnostic criteria

(See Box 2.37.)

> **Box 2.37 SIAD diagnostic criteria**
> - Euvolaemia.
> - Hypo-osmolality with hyponatraemia.
> - Inappropriate urine concentration (>100mOsm/kg).
> - Elevated urinary sodium concentration (>30nmol/L) with normal dietary salt intake.
> - Normal renal, adrenal, and thyroid function.
> - No recent diuretic use.

Causes

(See Table 2.17.)

Table 2.17 Causes of SIAD

Malignancy	Drugs	Respiratory	Intracranial	Miscellaneous
Lung	SSRI	Pneumonia	Tumour	Guillain–Barré syndrome
Nasopharyngeal	Carbamazepine	TB	Subarachnoid haemorrhage	Acute intermittent porphyria
Pancreatic	Tricyclic antidepressant	Vasculitis	Meningitis	Multiple sclerosis
GI tract	Chemotherapy	Abscess	Encephalitis	HIV
Mesothelioma	Levetiracetam	+ve pressure ventilation	Vasculitis	Idiopathic
Lymphoma	Haloperidol		TBI	
Sarcoma	Phenothiazines		Subdural haemorrhage	

Management of SIAD

- Any causative medications should be discontinued if possible.
- The underlying cause should be treated where possible.
- Acute severe hyponatraemia should be managed as a medical emergency, as outlined in Box 2.36.
- Chronic hyponatraemia may require drug treatment, with an aim to improve plasma sodium levels and treat symptoms.
- Several drug treatments have been used for ongoing management, including demeclocycline, oral urea, and V2 receptor antagonists.

Fluid restriction

- Fluid restriction remains the 1st-line treatment in most patients with SIAD; however, the evidence base is weak.
- Many patients will fail to have an adequate response or will find it difficult to adhere to fluid restriction limits.
- Several factors predict the likelihood of failure to respond to fluid restriction, including a baseline urine osmolality >500mOsm/kg and a urine output <1.5L/24h, or a Furst equation ratio >1.

V2 receptor antagonists

- The vaptans are V2 receptor antagonists which competitively bind to the V2 receptor in the kidney, preventing AVP-mediated antidiuresis and causing partial nephrogenic DI.
- Tolvaptan is a selective V2 receptor antagonist and is available as a tablet for use in euvolaemic hyponatraemia.
- A starting dose of 7.5mg tolvaptan can be used, with a dose titration every 24–48h if there is an inadequate response.
- The patient should have free access to oral fluids.
- Plasma sodium is measured every 6–8h in the first 24h, to screen for overcorrection. Overcorrection may occur if fluid intake is restricted or if baseline plasma sodium is <120mmol/L.
- The commonest side effect is polyuria. Liver damage has been reported in patients treated with high doses for polycystic kidneys, so regular LFT monitoring is indicated in chronic treatment.

Demeclocycline

- Demeclocycline is a tetracycline antibiotic which has been used 2nd line to manage SIAD.
- It inhibits adenylyl cyclase activation which occurs after binding of vasopressin to the V2 receptor in the kidney, therefore producing reversible nephrogenic DI.
- The therapeutic effect is variable and often delayed after starting treatment.
- Significant side effects may occur, including renal impairment and photosensitive rashes.
- There is no evidence base.

Urea

- Urea elevates plasma sodium by increasing water excretion and decreasing urinary sodium excretion.
- Urea-containing preparations are poorly tolerated due to taste.
- There are currently no commercially produced versions available.
- Empagliflozin (sodium–glucose cotransporter 2 (SGLT2) inhibitor) may be useful by causing inhibition of sodium–glucose transport in the tubule.

Further reading

Spasovski G, et al. (2014). Clinical practice guideline on diagnosis and treatment of hyponatraemia. *Eur J Endocrinol* **170**, G1–47.

Verbalis JG, et al. (2013). Diagnosis, evaluation and treatment of hyponatraemia: expert panel recommendations. *Am J Med* **126**, S1–42.

Stalk abnormalities

- Pituitary stalk lesions are rare sellar/suprasellar lesions.
- The normal pituitary stalk measures <3mm and tapers down towards the gland. It is hyperintense after administration of contrast.
- Stalk abnormalities rarely present with symptoms of hormonal dysfunction, but DI is the commonest endocrine manifestation. Lesions may present with symptoms of mass effect or as an incidental finding on cranial imaging.
- Metastases to the hypothalamic–pituitary area are rare but are commonest in the stalk.
- Stalk abnormalities may be due to three main aetiologies: congenital, inflammatory, and neoplastic, as outlined in Table 2.18.

Causes
(See Table 2.18.)

Table 2.18 Causes of stalk lesions

Congenital	Inflammatory	Neoplastic
Ectopic posterior pituitary	IgG4-related hypophysitis	Craniopharyngioma
Pituitary hypoplasia	Lymphocytic hypophysitis	Germinoma
Hypophyseal duplication	Immunotherapy-associated hypophysitis	Metastases, e.g. breast, lung
Rathke's cleft cyst	Neurosarcoidosis	Lymphoma
Pars intermedia cyst	ANCA-associated vasculitis	Pituicytomas
Vascular malformation	Langerhans cell histiocytosis Erdheim–Chester disease TB	Tanycytoma

Eating disorders

- Disabling, deadly, and costly mental disorders considerably impairing physical health and psychosocial functions.
- Increasing in the last 50 years.
- Six main disorders, including anorexia nervosa, bulimia nervosa, and binge eating disorders.

Anorexia nervosa

Features

- Typical presentation is a ♀ aged <25 with weight loss, amenorrhoea, and behavioural changes, including disturbed cognitive and emotional functioning.
- There is a long-term risk of severe osteoporosis associated with >6 months of amenorrhoea. There is loss of bone mineral content and bone density, with little or no recovery after resolution of the amenorrhoea. Bone loss occurs at 2.5% per annum.

Endocrine abnormalities

- Deficiency of GnRH, low LH and FSH, normal PRL, and low oestrogen in ♀ or testosterone in ♂.
- Elevated circulating cortisol (usually non-suppressible with dexamethasone).
- Low-normal thyroxine, reduced T_3, and normal TSH.
- Elevated resting GH levels.
- In addition, it is common to find various metabolic abnormalities, such as reduced magnesium, zinc, phosphorus, and calcium levels, in addition to hyponatraemia, hypoglycaemia, and hypokalaemia.
- Weight gain leads to a reversion of the prepubertal LH secretory pattern to the adult-like secretion. Administration of GnRH in a pulsatile pattern leads to normalization of the pituitary–gonadal axis, demonstrating that the 1° abnormality is hypothalamic.

Management

- The long-term treatment of these patients involves treatment of the underlying condition and then management of osteoporosis, although many patients will refuse oestrogen replacement.
- Resumption of menstrual function is important for recovery of spine BMD. Weight gain is important for hip BMD recovery. Oral contraceptives do not help BMD recovery.
- Anorexia may be persistent (69% at 9 years, 37% at 22 years).

Bulimia

Features

- Typically occurs in ♀ who are slightly older than the group with anorexia nervosa. Weight may be normal, and patients often deny the abnormal eating behaviour. Patients gorge themselves, using artificial means of avoiding excessive weight gain (laxatives, diuretic abuse, vomiting). This may be a cause of 'occult' hypokalaemia.
- These patients may, or may not, have menstrual irregularity. If menstrual irregularity is present, this is often associated with inadequate oestrogen secretion and anovulation.

Further reading

Miller KK, *et al.* (2006). Determinants of skeletal loss and recovery in anorexia nervosa. *J Clin Endocrinol Metab* **91**, 2931–7.

Mitchell JE, Peterson CB (2020). Anorexia nervosa. *N Engl J Med* **382**, 1343–51.

Treasure J, *et al.* (2020). Eating disorders. *Lancet* **395**, 899–911.

Hypothalamus

Anatomy and physiology

- The hypothalamus coordinates various endocrine, autonomic, and behavioural functions.
- It lies adjacent to the 3rd ventricle and superior to the pituitary gland.
- It is divided into anterior and medial regions.
- Within these regions lie distinct nuclei responsible for coordination of homeostatic mechanisms.
- Complete damage to the entire hypothalamus is not compatible with life.
- Each nucleus receives hormonal and/or neural inputs.
- Axons project directly into the posterior pituitary from the hypothalamus.
- Control of the anterior pituitary occurs via secretion of hormones into the local blood supply via the median eminence.

Hypothalamic syndromes

- Patients with significant hypothalamic damage may present with a hypothalamic syndrome which includes both endocrine and non-endocrine symptoms.
- Causes of hypothalamic damage include tumours, trauma, vascular events, post-radiotherapy, infections, and inflammatory disorders.
- The clinical syndrome depends on the site and extent of damage to the hypothalamus.
- Symptoms include dysthermia, somnolence, obesity, and disturbance of thirst mechanism, as outlined in Box 2.38.

Box 2.38 Hypothalamic syndrome effects

- Thermoregulation:
  - Hypothermia.
  - Hyperthermia.
- Appetite:
  - Hyperphagia and obesity.
  - Anorexia.
- Thirst:
  - Adipsia.
  - Polydipsia.
- Sleep disturbance:
  - Obstructive sleep apnoea.
  - Narcolepsy.
  - Abnormal sleep–wake cycle.
- Hypopituitarism, including DI.
- Hypothalamic seizures.

Pineal gland

- The pineal gland is situated adjacent to the 3rd ventricle.
- The main hormone synthesized and secreted from it is melatonin.
- Melatonin synthesis and release occur in a circadian fashion, with inhibition occurring 2° to polarization of photoreceptors in the retina.
- The role of melatonin in regulation of the reproductive axis is not fully understood in humans.

Pineal region tumours

- These are rare tumours, accounting for <1% of CNS tumours in adults and 3–8% in children.
- ♂ are more predominantly affected.
- They occur at any age; however, they peak in the 1st and 2nd decades.
- The commonest subtypes are germ cell tumours (50–75%), followed by pineal parenchymal tumours (14–27%).

Clinical features

- Symptoms of mass effect, including headache, nausea, and vomiting.
- Visual disturbance, including ocular palsies.
- DI.
- Precocious puberty.
- Abnormal growth.
- 2° amenorrhoea.
- Ataxia.
- Paraesthesiae.

Investigations

- MRI brain and spinal cord.
- Blood tumour markers (hCG, aFP, carcinoembryonic antigen (CEA)).
- Lumbar puncture for CSF analysis, including hCG, aFP, and cytology.
- Pituitary function assessment.

Treatment

- Management depends upon the histological tumour type.
- Surgical resection or debulking.
- Radiotherapy either to lesion only or to entire craniospinal region.
- Chemotherapy.

Further reading

Al-Hussaini M, et al. (2009). Pineal gland tumours: experience from the SEER database. *J Neuro Oncol* **94**, 351–8.

Adrenal

Jeremy Tomlinson

Anatomy

The normal adrenal glands weigh 4–5g. The cortex represents 90% of the normal gland and surrounds the medulla. The arterial blood supply arises from the renal arteries, aorta, and inferior phrenic artery. Venous drainage occurs via the central vein into the inferior vena cava (IVC) on the right and into the left renal vein on the left (see Figs. 3.1 and 3.2).

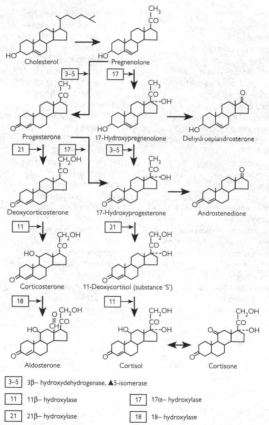

Fig. 3.1 Pathways and enzymes involved in the synthesis of GCs, MCs, and adrenal androgens from a cholesterol precursor.

Reproduced from Besser M and Thorner GM (1994). *Clinical Endocrinology* 2nd edn. Mosby. With permission from Elsevier.

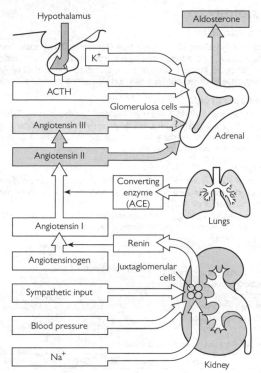

Fig. 3.2 Physiological mechanisms governing the production and secretion of aldosterone.

Reproduced from Besser M and Thorner GM (1994). *Clinical Endocrinology* 2nd edn. Mosby. With permission from Elsevier.

Physiology

Glucocorticoids

GC (cortisol 10–20mg/day) production (see Table 3.1) occurs from the zona fasciculata, and adrenal androgens arise from the zona reticularis (inner layer of the cortex). Both of these are under the control of ACTH, which regulates both steroid synthesis and also adrenocortical growth.

Mineralocorticoids

MC (aldosterone 100–150 micrograms/day) synthesis (see Table 3.1) occurs in the zona glomerulosa, predominantly under the control of the renin–angiotensin system (outer layer of the cortex) (see Fig. 3.2), although ACTH also contributes to its regulation.

Androgens

The adrenal gland (zona reticularis and zona fasciculata) also produces sex steroids in the form of DHEA and androstenedione. The synthetic pathway is under the control of ACTH.

Urinary steroid profiling provides quantitative information on the biosynthetic and catabolic pathways. Profiling can be useful in:

- MC hypertension.
- PCOS.
- CAH.
- Steroid-producing tumours.
- Precocious puberty/virilization.
- Hirsutism.
- Cushing's syndrome.
- Androgen resistance.

Table 3.1 Adrenal cortex steroid production

Adrenal cortex	Cortisol	Aldosterone	DHEA	DHEAS
Production rate/24h	10mg	100 micrograms	10mg	25mg
Half-life	80min	20min	20min	9h
Control	ACTH	Renin	ACTH	ACTH

Further reading

Storbeck KF, et al. (2019). Steroid metabolome analysis in disorders of adrenal steroid biosynthesis and metabolism. *Endocr Rev* **40**, 1605–25.

Taylor NF (2006). Urinary steroid profiling. *Method Mol Biol* **324**, 159–75.

Imaging

CT scanning

CT is the most widely used modality for imaging the adrenal glands. It is able to detect masses >5mm in diameter. It can be useful in differentiating between different adrenal pathologies, in particular by identifying benign adrenal tumours with high fat content (adrenocortical adenoma, adrenomyelolipoma), as indicated by precontrast tumour density <10HU (Hounsfield units) (see Fig. 3.3).

Magnetic resonance imaging

MRI can also reliably detect adrenal masses >5–10mm in diameter and, in some circumstances, provides additional information to CT, in particular by determining signal loss in opposed-phase, T_2-weighted sequences. Rapid signal loss is indicative of a benign tumour, whereas malignant tumours, and also PCCs, show a delay or lack in signal loss.

Ultrasound imaging

US detects masses >20mm in diameter, but normal adrenal glands are not usually visible, except in children. Body habitus and bowel gas can provide technical difficulties.

Normal adrenal

The normal adrenal cortex is assessed by measuring limb thickness and is considered enlarged at >5mm, approximately the thickness of the diaphragmatic crus nearby.

Radionucleotide imaging

- *123I-MIBG* is a guanethidine analogue, concentrated in some PCCs, paragangliomas, carcinoid tumours, and neuroblastomas, and is useful diagnostically. A different isotope 131I-MIBG may be used therapeutically, e.g. in malignant PCCs, when the diagnostic imaging shows MIGB uptake.
- *75Se 6β-selenomethyl-19-norcholesterol*. This isotope is concentrated in functioning steroid-synthesizing tissue and has, in the past, been used to image the adrenal cortex. However, high-resolution CT and MRI have largely replaced it in localizing functional adrenal adenomas.
- *123Iodo-metomidate* is an isotope that is derived from etomidate, which is a known 11β-hydroxylase (CYP11B1) inhibitor. Metomidate binds CYP11B1, which is specifically expressed in the adrenal gland, and thus iodo-metomidate single-photon emission computed tomography (SPECT) can identify adrenocortical tissue.
- *11C-metomidate* is another isotope of metomidate with a very short half-life (20min and therefore requires an on-site cyclotron for generation) but, when combined with PET-CT, has been used to aid lateralization in patients with 1° aldosteronism.

Positron emission tomography

PET can be useful in localizing tumours and metastases. Radiopharmaceuticals for specific endocrine tumours are being developed, e.g. 11C-metahydroxyephedrine for PCC—combined with CT (PET-CT), it may offer particular value in localizing occult neuroendocrine tumours. 11C-metomidate PET-CT has recently been shown to be of value for lateralization of aldosterone-producing adrenal masses.

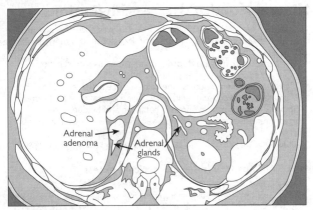

Fig. 3.3 Typical appearance of adrenal adenoma on CT scan.

Venous sampling

Adrenal vein sampling (AVS) (see ➲ Adrenal vein sampling, pp. 264–5) can be useful to lateralize an adenoma or to differentiate an adenoma from bilateral hyperplasia. It is technically difficult—particularly, catheterizing the right adrenal vein because of its drainage into the IVC. There is no widespread agreement on the exact protocol, e.g. consecutive or concurrent adrenal vein catherization, with and without concurrent or preceding ACTH stimulation. Usually, samples are drawn from the vena cava, superior and inferior to the renal veins, and separately from both adrenal veins, with subsequent determination of plasma aldosterone and serum cortisol levels (correct localization of the catheter in the adrenal vein is only confirmed when the adrenal:peripheral vein cortisol ratio is >5:1 with ACTH stimulation and >2:1 without). AVS is of particular value in lateralizing small aldosterone-producing adenomas that cannot be easily visualized on CT or MRI.

Further reading

Boland GW (2011). Adrenal imaging: from Addison to algorithms. *Radiol Clin North Am* **49**, 511–28.
Guest P (2011). Imaging of the adrenal gland. In: Wass JAH, Stewart PM (eds.). *Oxford Textbook of Endocrinology*. Oxford University Press, Oxford; pp. 763–73.
Hahner S, Sundin A (2011). Metomidate-based imaging of adrenal masses. *Horm Cancer* **2**, 348–53.
Monticone S, et al. (2015). Adrenal vein sampling in primary aldosteronism: towards a standardised protocol. *Lancet Diabetes Endocrinol* **3**, 296–303.
Pacak K, et al. (2004). Functional imaging of endocrine tumors: role of positron emission tomography. *Endocr Rev* **25**, 568–80.
Powlson AS, et al. (2015). Nuclear imaging in the diagnosis of primary aldosteronism. *Curr Opin Endocrinol Diabetes Obes* **22**, 150–6.
Wolley M (2020). Controversies and advances in adrenal venous sampling in the diagnostic workup of primary aldosteronism. *Best Pract Res Clin Endocrinol Metab* **34**, 101400.

Mineralocorticoid excess: definitions

The majority of cases of MC excess are due to excess aldosterone production, which may be 1° or 2°, and are typically associated with hypertension and hypokalaemia.

- *1° hyperaldosteronism* is a disorder of autonomous aldosterone hypersecretion with suppressed renin levels.
- *2° hyperaldosteronism* occurs when aldosterone hypersecretion occurs 2° to elevated circulating renin levels. This is typical of heart failure, cirrhosis, or nephrotic syndrome, but it can also be due to renal artery stenosis and, occasionally, a very rare renin-producing tumour (reninoma).
- Other MCs may occasionally be the cause of this syndrome (see Box 3.1).

Box 3.1 Causes of mineralocorticoid excess

Primary hyperaldosteronism
- Conn's syndrome (aldosterone-producing adrenal adenoma) 35%.
- Bilateral adrenal hyperplasia 60%.
- Glucocorticoid-remediable aldosteronism (GRA) <1%.
- Aldosterone-producing adrenal carcinoma <1%.

Secondary hyperaldosteronism
- Renal artery stenosis.
- Renal hypoperfusion.
- Cirrhosis.
- CCF.
- Nephrotic syndrome.
- Renin-secreting tumour.

Other mineralocorticoid excess syndromes
- Apparent MC excess (see ➔ Excess other mineralocorticoids, pp. 268–9).
- Liquorice ingestion (see ➔ Liquorice ingestion, p. 269) (inhibits 11β-hydroxysteroid dehydrogenase type 2 (11β-HSD2)): ↓ aldosterone, ↓ renin, ↓ K⁻ found in sweets, chewing tobacco, cough mixtures, herbal medicines.
- Deoxycorticosterone and corticosterone (see ➔ Deoxycorticosterone excess, p. 269).
- Ectopic ACTH secretion (see ➔ Ectopic ACTH syndrome, p. 269).
- CAH (see ➔ Congenital adrenal hyperplasia in adults, pp. 354–5).
- Exogenous MCs, e.g. carbenoxolone.

'Pseudoaldosteronism' due to abnormal renal tubular transport
- Bartter's syndrome (see ➔ Bartter's syndrome, pp. 282–3).
- Gitelman's syndrome (see ➔ Gitelman's syndrome, p. 284).
- Liddle's syndrome (see ➔ Liddle's syndrome, p. 280).

Primary aldosteronism

Epidemiology

Primary hyperaldosteronism is present in around 10% of hypertensive patients and an estimated 4–6% of hypertensive patients in 1° care. It is the most prevalent form of 2° hypertension and may be associated with more significant complications when compared to patients with matched essential hypertension. The commonest cause is bilateral adrenal hyperplasia (see Table 3.2).

Pathophysiology

Aldosterone causes renal sodium retention and potassium loss. This results in expansion of body sodium content, leading to suppression of renal renin synthesis. The direct action of aldosterone on the distal nephron causes sodium retention and loss of hydrogen and potassium ions, resulting in hypokalaemic alkalosis. However, serum potassium may not be significantly reduced and may be normal in up to 50% of cases.

Aldosterone has pathophysiological effects on a range of other tissues, causing cardiac fibrosis, vascular endothelial dysfunction, and nephrosclerosis.

Clinical features

- Moderately severe hypertension, which is often resistant to conventional therapy. There may be disproportionate left ventricular hypertrophy (LVH).
- Hypokalaemia is usually asymptomatic. Occasionally, patients may present with tetany, myopathy, polyuria, and nocturia (hypokalaemic nephrogenic DI) due to severe hypokalaemia.
- Observational studies highlight an association between 1° hyperaldosteronism and the risk for heart disease, atrial fibrillation and stroke, kidney disease, and metabolic syndrome. There may be an association with osteoporosis, although the mechanisms underpinning this are not clear.

Table 3.2 Causes of primary hyperaldosteronism

Condition	Relative frequency	Age	Pathology
Aldosteronoma (Conn's adenoma)	35%	3rd to 6th decade	Benign, adenoma, <2.5cm diameter, yellow because of high cholesterol content
Idiopathic hyperaldosteronism (bilateral adrenal hyperplasia)	60%	Older than Conn's, ♂ > ♀	Macronodular or micronodular hyperplasia
Adrenal carcinoma	Rare	5th to 7th decade (occasionally young)	Tumour >4cm in diameter— often larger, may be evidence of local invasion
GC-suppressible hyperaldosteronism	Rare	Childhood	Chimeric crossover between CYP11B1 and CYP11B2 genes results in an ACTH-responsive aldosterone synthase

Conn's syndrome—aldosterone-producing adenoma

Very high levels of the enzyme aldosterone synthase are expressed in tumour tissue. Recently, inactivating mutations in the potassium channel KCJN5 have been identified as the cause of disease in ~40% of aldosterone-producing adrenal adenomas. Very rarely, Conn's adenomas may be part of the MEN1 syndrome.

Mutations in other genes have now been implicated in the pathogenesis of aldosterone-producing adrenal adenomas, including *ATP1A1*, *ATP2B3*, *CTNNB1*, *CACNA1D*, *CACNA1H*, and *ARMC5*. Familial 1° hyperaldosteronism can now be classified as FH-I, II, III, and IV, depending on the gene mutation (see Table 3.3).

Genetic screening should be considered in individuals aged <20 years or in those with a family history of 1° aldosteronism or cerebrovascular accident (CVA) aged <40 years.

Table 3.3 Mutations associated with aldosterone-producing adenomas

	Genetic mutation	Mechanism of aldosterone excess
Familial hyperaldosteronism type I	Chimeric *CYP11B1* and *CYP11B2*	Also known as glucocorticoid-remediable aldosteronism (GRA) (see ➔ Glucocorticoid-remediable aldosteronism (FH-I), p. 259). Aldosterone excess driven by ACTH as a result of the formation of a chimeric *CYP11B1* and *CYP11B2* gene
Familial hyperaldosteronism type II	*CLCN2*	Mutations cause a gain of function, ↑ chloride permeability, depolarization, and calcium influx with *CYP11B2* upregulation
Familial hyperaldosteronism type III	*KCNJ5*	Altered sodium permeability of the mutant sodium channel, causing cellular depolarization and excess aldosterone secretion
Familial hyperaldosteronism type IV	*CACNA1H*	Impaired calcium channel inactivation, leading to excess aldosterone secretion

Further reading

Perez-Rivas LG, et al. (2019). Inherited forms of primary hyperaldosteronism: new genes, new phenotypes and proposition of a new classification. *Exp Clin Endocrinol Diabetes* **127**, 93–9.

Bilateral adrenal hyperplasia (bilateral idiopathic hyperaldosteronism)

This is the commonest form of 1° hyperaldosteronism in adults. Hyperplasia is more commonly bilateral than unilateral and may be associated with micronodular or macronodular hyperplasia. Note, however, that CT-demonstrable nodules have a prevalence of 2% in the general population (and rising with age), including hypertensive patients without excess aldosterone production. The pathophysiology is not known, although aldosterone secretion is very sensitive to circulating angiotensin II. The pathophysiology of bilateral adrenal hyperplasia is not understood, and it is possible that it represents an extreme end of the spectrum of low renin essential hypertension.

Glucocorticoid-remediable aldosteronism (FH-I)

This is a rare autosomal dominantly inherited condition due to the presence of a chimeric gene (8q22) containing the 5′ sequence, which determines regulation of the 11β-hydroxylase gene (*CYP11B1*) coding for the enzyme catalysing the last step in cortisol synthesis, and the 3′ sequence from the aldosterone synthase gene (*CYP11B2*) coding for the enzyme catalysing the last step in aldosterone synthesis. This results in the expression of aldosterone synthase in the zona fasciculata, as well as in the zona glomerulosa, and aldosterone secretion comes under ACTH control. GCs are the treatment of choice and lead to suppression of ACTH and of aldosterone production.
• Early hypertension and family history.
• Hybrid steroids (18OHcortisol and 18oxocortisol) elevated.

Aldosterone-producing carcinoma

Rare and usually associated with excessive secretion of other corticosteroids (cortisol, androgen, oestrogen). Hypokalaemia may be profound, and aldosterone levels very high. A tumour larger than 2.5cm associated with aldosterone excess has to be treated as suspicious.

Screening

Indications

- Patients resistant to conventional antihypertensive medication (i.e. not controlled) (BP >140/100mmHg on three agents).
- Hypertension (BP >150/100mmHg) associated with hypokalaemia (potassium <3.7mmol/L, irrespective of thiazide use). NB. ↓ potassium only present in 40%.
- Hypertension developing before age of 40 years.
- Adrenal incidentaloma.
- First-degree relative of patient with 1° aldosteronism and hypertension.
- Hypertension and family history of early-onset hypertension or stroke at young age.
- Hypertension and sleep apnoea.

Method

- Give oral supplements of potassium to control hypokalaemia; screening and confirmation should be carried out in the normokalaemic situation.
- There is no need to stop all concomitant antihypertensive medication for the 1st screening by paired plasma aldosterone and plasma renin measurements; the only medication that must be stopped are MC receptor antagonists (spironolactone, eplerenone) that must be stopped 4 weeks prior to diagnostic tests.
- *Measure aldosterone:renin ratio.*
- A high ratio is suggestive of 1° hyperaldosteronism (aldosterone (pmol/L)/plasma renin activity (PRA) (ng/mL/h) >750 or aldosterone (ng/dL)/PRA (ng/mL/h) >30–50). Note that newer assays that measure renin mass (rather than activity) will require the development of different cut-offs.
- Test results should be interpreted, having the effects of antihypertensive drugs in mind (see Table 3.4); β-blockers can cause false +ves, while ACE/AT1R blockers can cause false −ves in borderline cases. In doubt, the test can be repeated off these drugs for 2 weeks; BP can be controlled using doxazosin or calcium antagonists. False −ve results can also occur in patients with CRF due to upregulated plasma renin.

Confirmation of diagnosis

When there is spontaneous hypokalaemia, plasma renin below detection levels, and aldosterone concentrations >550pmol/L, there may be no need for confirmatory testing.

Confirmation of autonomous aldosterone production is made by demonstrating failure to suppress aldosterone in face of sodium/volume loading. This can be achieved by a number of mechanisms after optimizing test conditions as described.

- Test of choice—*saline infusion test*:
  - Contraindications: severe uncontrolled hypertension; cardiac arrhythmia, severe hyperprolactinaemia, severe chronic heart failure.
  - Administer 2L of normal saline over 4h.
  - Measure plasma aldosterone at 0, 2, 3, and 4h.
  - Aldosterone fails to suppress to <140pmol/L (140–280 equivocal) in 80–90% of 1° aldosteronism.
  - Most used test; caution in patients with fluid overload and/or evidence of heart failure.

- *Fludrocortisone suppression test:*
  - Give fludrocortisone 100 micrograms 6-hourly for 4 days.
  - Measure plasma aldosterone basally and on last day.
  - Aldosterone fails to suppress in 1° aldosteronism.
  - Caveat: difficult to execute in hypokalaemic, hypertensive patients.
- *Captopril challenge test:*
  - Give captopril 50mg PO after sitting for 1h.
  - Blood samples before, and at 1 and 2h (seated) for aldosterone.
  - Position = post-test aldosterone <30% of pretest values.

Table 3.4 Interpreting test results of aldosterone:renin ratios

Antihypertensive	Effect on renin	Effect on aldosterone	Net effect on ARR
β-blockers	↓	↑	↑
α1-blockers	↑	↑	↑
α2-sympathomimetics	↑	↑	↑
ACE inhibitors	↑	↓	↓
AT1R blockers	↑	↓	↓
Calcium antagonists	↑	↑	↑
Diuretics	(↑)	(↑)	↑/(↓)

- *Dietary sodium loading test:*
  - Patients are given instructions to take a diet with a high sodium content (sufficient to raise the sodium intake to 200mmol/day) for 3 days. If necessary, this can be achieved by adding supplemental sodium chloride tablets.
  - It is important to ensure that potassium is maintained as normal during this period, and potassium supplementation may also be required.
  - Failure to suppress aldosterone in 1° aldosteronism.
  - Caveat: cumbersome to execute, limited diagnostic value in populations with a high background sodium intake.
- Other tests, such as the captopril suppression test, are described but are of lesser value in this circumstance, lacking appropriate sensitivity or specificity in the diagnosis of 1° aldosteronism.
- A number of tests have been described that are said to differentiate between the various subtypes of 1° aldosteronism (solitary Conn's adenoma; bilateral adrenal hyperplasia; GRA). However, none of these are sufficiently specific to influence management decisions, and more specific investigations (imaging and AVS) are necessary if there is doubt. Additional tests, such as postural response of aldosterone and measurement of urinary 18-hydroxycortisol, have been largely superseded because of this. Diagnosis of GRA is best made using

a specific genetic test, rather than on the ability of dexamethasone (0.5mg 6-hourly for 3 days) to suppress aldosterone; the diagnosis is confirmed by genetic analysis (chimeric crossover between *CYP11B1* (11β-hydroxylase) and *CYP11B2* (aldosterone synthase) promoter regions that brings *CYP11B2* under the regulatory control of ACTH).

Further reading

Funder JW, *et al.* (2016). The management of primary aldosteronism: case detection, diagnosis, and treatment: an Endocrine Society clinical practice guideline. *J Clin Endocrinol Metab* **101**, 1889–916.

Localization and confirmation of differential diagnosis

CT/MRI scan

CT and MRI scanning are of value in identifying adrenal nodules >5mm in diameter. It should be noted, however, that the frequency of adrenal incidentalomas rises with age and for this reason, it is prudent to consider AVS if in doubt.

- In bilateral adrenal hyperplasia, both glands can appear enlarged or normal in size.
- Macronodular hyperplasia may result in identifiable nodules on imaging.
- A mass >4cm in size is suspicious of carcinoma but is unusual in Conn's syndrome.
- NB. In essential hypertension, adrenal nodules are described.

Adrenal vein sampling

Indicated in patients with bilateral adrenal changes and in older patients (age >50) with 1° aldosteronism who have an apparent solitary adenoma on scanning, as the incidence of adrenal nodules rises with age (3–4% at 40 years, 70–80% at 70 years). The procedure should only be undertaken in patients in whom surgery is feasible and desired.

Catheterization of the adrenal veins may not be necessary if there is a unilateral adrenal mass (>10mm and normal contralateral adrenal), in a young patient (aged <35years), with hypokalaemia at presentation and high aldosterone levels.

Aldosterone measurements from both adrenal veins allow a gradient between the two sides to be identified in the case of unilateral disease. It is the gold standard for differentiation between uni- and bilateral aldosterone production, but cannulating the right adrenal vein is technically difficult as it drains directly into the IVC. Cortisol measurements must also be taken concomitantly with aldosterone to confirm successful positioning within the adrenal veins. The adrenal:peripheral vein cortisol ratio is usually >5:1 with ACTH stimulation, and >2:1 without.

AVS should be carried out in specialist centres only; centres with <20 procedures per year have been shown to have poor success rates for bilateral catheterization of the adrenal vein (8–10%), thus producing mostly non-informative results, whereas experienced centres achieve around 70–80%.

Cortisol-corrected aldosterone ratios are used to determine lateralization. Using ACTH stimulation, a ratio of cortisol-corrected aldosterone ratio from high side to low side of >4:1 is indicative of unilateral aldosterone excess. A ratio of <3:1 is suggestive of bilateral aldosterone hypersecretion. Ratios between 3:1 and 4:1 can suggest either unilateral or bilateral disease. The AVS results must be cautiously interpreted in conjunction with the clinical setting; repeat AVS may be considered. Contralateral suppression of aldosterone secretion may be helpful. Without ACTH stimulation, a cortisol-corrected aldosterone lateralization ratio (high to low side) of >2:1 is likely to be consistent with unilateral disease.

Radiolabelled scanning

The iodocholesterol test has low sensitivity/specificity and offers no advantage over high-resolution CT or MRI with, where necessary, AVS. Recent data with ^{11}C-metomidate scanning are promising but warrant further confirmation prior to widespread use.

Treatment

Surgery

- Laparoscopic adrenalectomy is the treatment of choice for aldosterone-secreting adenomas and is associated with lower morbidity than open adrenalectomy.
- Surgery is not indicated in patients with idiopathic hyperaldosteronism, as even bilateral adrenalectomy may not cure the hypertension.
- Presurgical spironolactone treatment may be used to correct potassium stores before surgery.
- The BP response to treatment with spironolactone (50–400mg/day) before surgery can be used to predict the response to surgery of patients with adenomas.
- Hypertension is cured in about 70%.
- If it persists (more likely in those with long-standing hypertension and ↑ age), it is more amenable to medical treatment.
- Overall, 50% become normotensive within 1 month, and 70% within 1 year.
- Post-Conn's syndrome, adrenalectomy, a Synacthen® test should be performed to ensure non-suppressed contralateral adrenal function in case of co-secretion of cortisol from mineralocorticoid secreting adenoma in removed adrenal gland (27%).
- Adrenal carcinoma. Open surgery and post-operative adrenolytic therapy with *mitotane* is usually required, but the prognosis is usually poor (see ➋ Treatment of adrenal Cushing's syndrome, pp. 274–7).

Medical treatment

Medical therapy remains an option for patients with bilateral disease and those with a solitary adrenal adenoma who are unlikely to be cured by surgery, who are unfit for operation, or who express a preference for medical management.

- The MC receptor antagonist *spironolactone* (50–400mg/day; od administration) has been used successfully for many years to treat the hypertension and hypokalaemia associated with bilateral adrenal hyperplasia and idiopathic hyperaldosteronism.
- There may be a delay in response of hypertension of 4–8 weeks. However, combination with other antihypertensive agents (ACE inhibitors (ACEIs) and calcium channel blockers) is usually required.
- Spironolactone also interacts with the androgen and progesterone receptor, which contributes to its side effect. Side effects are common—particularly, gynaecomastia and impotence in ♂, menstrual irregularities in ♀, and GI effects.
- *Eplerenone* (50–200mg/day; bd administration due to shorter half-life and occasionally requiring tds administration) is an MC receptor antagonist without antiandrogen effects and hence greater selectivity and fewer side effects than spironolactone.
- Alternative drugs include the potassium-sparing diuretics *amiloride* and *triamterene*. Amiloride may need to be given in high doses (up to 40mg/day) in 1° aldosteronism, and monitoring of serum potassium is essential. Calcium channel antagonists may also be helpful.
- GRA can be treated with low-dose *dexamethasone* (0.25–0.5mg on going to bed). If needed, spironolactone and/or amiloride can be added.

Further reading

Funder JW (2020). Primary aldosteronism: where are we now? Where to from here? Horm Metab Res 52, 459–66.

Funder JW, et al. (2016). The management of primary aldosteronism: case detection, diagnosis, and treatment: an Endocrine Society clinical practice guideline. J Clin Endocrinol Metab **101**, 1889–916.

Heinrich DA, et al. (2019). Safety of medical adjustment and confirmatory testing in the diagnostic work-up of primary aldosteronism. Eur J Endocrinol **181**, 421–8.

Heinrich DA, et al. (2019). Adrenal insufficiency after unilateral adrenalectomy in primary aldosteronism: long-term outcome and clinical impact. J Clin Endocrinol Metab **104**, 5658–64.

Lechner B, et al (2019). Therapy of endocrine disease: medical treatment of primary aldosteronism. Eur J Endocrinol **181**, R147–53.

Morera J, Reznik Y (2019). Management of endocrine disease: the role of confirmatory tests in the diagnosis of primary aldosteronism. Eur J Endocrinol **180**, R45–58.

Mulatero P (2002). Drug effects on aldosterone/plasma renin activity ratio in primary aldosteronism. Hypertension **40**, 897–902.

O'Shea PM, et al. (2019). 11C-Metomidate PET/CT is a useful adjunct for lateralization of primary aldosteronism in routine clinical practice. Clin Endocrinol (Oxf) **90**, 670–9.

Seidel E, et al. (2019). Genetic causes of primary aldosteronism. Exp Mol Med **51**, 1–12.

Vaidya A, et al. (2018). Expanding spectrum of primary aldosteronism: implications for diagnosis, pathogenesis and treatment. Endocr Rev **39**, 1057–88.

Vilela LAP, Almeida MQ (2017). Diagnosis and management of primary aldosteronism. Arch Endocrinol Metab **61**, 305–12.

Williams TA, Reincke M (2018). Diagnosis and management of primary aldosteronism: the Endocrine Society guideline 2016 revisited. Eur J Endocrinol **179**, R19–29.

Williams TA, et al. (2017). Outcomes after adrenalectomy for unilateral primary aldosteronism: an international consensus on outcome measures and analysis of remission rates in an international cohort. Lancet Diabetes Endocrinol **5**, 689–99.

Young WF (2007). Primary aldosteronism—renaissance of a syndrome. Clin Endocrinol **66**, 607–18.

Excess other mineralocorticoids

Epidemiology

Occasionally, the clinical syndrome of hyperaldosteronism is not associated with excess aldosterone. This can be due either to an increase in an alternative MC or to an increased MC effect of cortisol.

These conditions are rare.

Apparent mineralocorticoid excess (AME)

- The MC receptor has an equal affinity for cortisol and aldosterone, but there is a 100-fold excess of circulating cortisol over aldosterone.
- The MC receptor is usually protected from the effects of stimulation by cortisol by the enzyme 11β-HSD2, which inactivates cortisol to cortisone.
- In AME, there is a deficiency of 11β-HSD2. This can be either caused by inactivating mutations in the corresponding gene encoded on chromosome 16q22 or due to exogenous intake of substances that inhibit 11β-HSD2 such as liquorice.
- Congenital absence (AR) of the enzyme or inhibition of its activity allows cortisol to stimulate the receptor and leads to severe, life-threatening hypertension.

Type 1 is seen predominantly in children, presenting with failure to thrive, thirst, polyuria, and severe hypertension, which can lead to brain haemorrhage in childhood or adolescence. The urinary cortisol over cortisone metabolites ratio (tetrahydrocortisol + allo-tetrahydrocortisol/tetrahydrocortisone) is raised to ten times normal.

Type 2 is a milder form that may be a cause of hypertension in adolescence/early adulthood.

However, multiple mutations have been found in the *11β-HSD2* gene for both types, and some authors believe there is a spectrum of disease—mild forms may present with salt-sensitive hypertension.

Biochemistry

- Suppression of renin and aldosterone.
- Hypokalaemic alkalosis.
- Urinary free cortisol/cortisone ratio ↑.
- Ratio of urinary tetrahydrocortisol and allo-tetrahydrocortisol to tetrahydrocortisone is raised (>10×) in type 1, but normal in type 2.
- Confirm with genetic testing (*11β-HSD2* gene).

Treatment

- *Dexamethasone* leads to suppression of ACTH secretion, reduced cortisol concentrations, and lowered BP in 60%. It has a much lower affinity for the MC receptor.
- Other antihypertensive agents are often required.
- One patient with hypertensive renal failure was cured with a renal transplant.

Liquorice ingestion
- Liquorice contains glycyrrhetinic acid which is used as a sweetener.
- It inhibits the action of 11β-HSD2, which allows circulating cortisol to get ↑ access to the MC receptor, causing hypertension.
- Liquorice can be found in sweets, chewing tobacco, cough mixtures, and some herbal medicines.

Ectopic ACTH syndrome
(See ➲ Cushing's syndrome due to ectopic ACTH secretion, pp. 752–3.)

In the syndrome of ectopic ACTH and in very severe Cushing's cases, the 11β-HSD2 protection is overcome because of high cortisol secretion rates, which saturate the enzyme, leading to impaired conversion of cortisol to cortisone. Therefore, cortisol has greater access to the MC receptor in the kidney, which results in hypokalaemia and hypertension.

Deoxycorticosterone excess
Two forms of CAH (see ➲ Congenital adrenal hyperplasia in adults, pp. 354–5) are associated with excess production of deoxycorticosterone (DOC), as they result in inhibition of enzymes downstream of DOC and thus lead to its accumulation. DOC acts as an agonist at the MC receptor, resulting in hypertension with suppression of renin.
- 17α-hydroxylase (CYP17A1) deficiency.
- 11β-hydroxylase (CYP11B1) deficiency.

GC replacement to inhibit ACTH is an effective treatment for these conditions.

Adrenal tumours, in particular adrenocortical carcinomas, rarely secrete excessive amounts of DOC. This may be concomitant with excessive aldosterone production, but occasionally, it may occur in an isolated fashion.

Adrenal Cushing's syndrome

Definition and epidemiology

- Cushing's syndrome results from chronic excess cortisol and is described in Chapter 2 (see ⮕ Definition of Cushing's disease, p. 178).
- The causes may be classified as ACTH-dependent and ACTH-independent. This section describes ACTH-independent Cushing's syndrome, which is due to adrenal tumours (benign and malignant), and is responsible for 10–15% cases of Cushing's syndrome.
- Adrenal tumours causing Cushing's syndrome are commoner in ♀. The peak incidence is in the 4th and 5th decades.
- Causes and relative frequencies of adrenal Cushing's syndrome in adults:
  - Adrenal adenoma 10%.
  - Adrenal carcinoma 2%. (NB. 50–60% of adrenocortical carcinomas (ACCs) associated with hormone excess).
  - Bilateral micronodular adrenal hyperplasia <1%.
  - Bilateral macronodular hyperplasia <1%.

Pathophysiology

(See Table 3.5.)

- Benign adrenocortical adenomas (ACAs) are usually encapsulated and <4cm in diameter. They are usually associated with pure GC excess.
- ACCs are usually >6cm in diameter, although they may be smaller and are not infrequently associated with local invasion and metastases at the time of diagnosis. Adrenal carcinomas are characteristically associated with excess secretion of several hormones; most frequently found is the combination of cortisol and androgen (precursors); occasionally, they may be associated with MC or oestrogen secretion.
- Bilateral adrenal hyperplasia may be micronodular (<1cm diameter) or macronodular (>1cm), but increasingly mixed cases of combined micro- and macronodular hyperplasia are observed.
- ACTH-dependent Cushing's results in bilateral adrenal hyperplasia; thus, one has to firmly differentiate between ACTH-dependent and independent causes of Cushing's before assuming bilateral adrenal hyperplasia as the 1° cause of disease.
- The majority of cases of ACTH-independent bilateral macronodular adrenal hyperplasia (AIMAH) do not have an identifiable cause.
- Abnormal expression of receptors that would not normally be expressed in the adrenal has been described as the cause of disease, including gastric inhibitory peptide (GIP), vasopressin, β-adrenoceptor, hCG/LH, and serotonin receptors.
- Several 'food-dependent' Cushing's syndrome cases have been described due to ectopic GIP receptor expression.
- Carney complex (see ⮕ Carney complex, pp. 666–8) is an AD condition characterized by a variable penetrance of atrial myxomas, spotty skin pigmentation (hyperlentiginosis), peripheral nerve tumours, and endocrine disorders, including Sertoli cell tumours and Cushing's syndrome due to PPNAD, which can be micro- or macronodular in appearance. PPNAD, in the context of Carney complex, has been shown to be caused by mutations in the *PRKAR1A* gene that encodes a regulatory subunit of protein kinase A (PKA), which is a key regulator of the adrenal ACTH response.

- McCune–Albright syndrome (see ⮕ McCune–Albright syndrome, pp. 654–5) can be associated with polyostotic fibrous dysplasia, unilateral café-au-lait spots, precocious puberty, and ACTH-independent Cushing's with bilateral macronodular adrenal hyperplasia, caused by activating mutations in the *GNAS-1* gene that encodes the Gs α protein, which is a key component of the transmembrane signal transduction cascade of the ACTH receptor. *GNAS-1* mutations have also been found in bilateral macronodular adrenal hyperplasia without other features of McCune–Albright's.
- Recent work has described phosphodiesterase (PDE) 11A and 8B mutations in patients with bilateral micronodular adrenal hyperplasia and ACTH-independent Cushing's.

Clinical features

- The clinical features of ACTH-independent Cushing's syndrome are as described in ⮕ Clinical features of Cushing's disease, p. 179.
- It is important to note that in patients with adrenal carcinoma, there may also be features related to excessive androgen production in ♀ and also a relatively more rapid time course of development of the syndrome.

Investigations

- Once the presence of Cushing's syndrome is confirmed (⮕ Clinical features of Cushing's disease, p. 179), subsequent investigation of the cause depends on whether ACTH is suppressed (ACTH-independent) or measurable/elevated (ACTH-dependent).
- Patients with ACTH-independent Cushing's syndrome do not suppress cortisol to <50% basal on high-dose dexamethasone testing and fail to show a rise in cortisol and ACTH following administration of CRH. (The latter test is often important when patients have borderline/low ACTH to differentiate pituitary-dependent disease from adrenal.)
- ACTH-independent causes are adrenal in origin, and the mainstay of further investigation is adrenal imaging by CT, which allows excellent visualization of the adrenal glands and their anatomy.
- Urinary steroid profiling can be helpful in identifying lesions that are more likely to be ACCs.

Table 3.5 Genetic causes of adrenal Cushing's syndrome

Adrenal lesion	Gene mutation	Clinical presentation
Cortisol secreting benign adrenal ademona	PRKACA somatic gain-of-function mutation	Sporadic adrenal Cushing's, no associated features
	CTNNB1 somatic loss-of-function mutation	Sporadic adrenal Cushing's, no associated features
	MEN1 loss-of-function mutation	MEN1
	APC loss-of-function mutation	Part of familial adenomatous polyposis and Gardner's syndrome
1° multinodular adrenal hyperplasia	Germline and somatic loss-of-function mutations in ARMC5	Sporadic adrenal Cushing's, no associated features
	Somatic mutation in MC2R	Sporadic adrenal Cushing's, no associated features
	Somatic GIPR amplification	Sporadic adrenal Cushing's, no associated features
	Germline PRKACA amplification	Sporadic adrenal Cushing's, no associated features
PPNAD	Germline loss-of-function mutation in PRKAR1A, uncharacterized defect in 2p16, germline PDE11A loss-of-function mutation	Sporadic adrenal Cushing's, no associated features
	Germline loss-of-function mutation in PRKAR1A, uncharacterized defect in 2p16, PRKACB amplification	Carney complex
Isolated micronodular adrenal disease	Germline PDE8B loss-of-function mutations	Sporadic adrenal Cushing's, no associated features
	Germline PDE11A loss-of-function mutations	Sporadic adrenal Cushing's, no associated features
	Germline PRKACA amplifications	Sporadic adrenal Cushing's, no associated features
1° bimorphic adrenocortical disease	Mosaic GNAS gain-of-function mutation	Part of McCune-Albright's syndrome

Treatment of adrenal Cushing's syndrome

(See ⊃ Treatment of Cushing's disease, pp. 186–8.)

Adrenal adenoma

- Unilateral adrenalectomy (normally laparoscopic) is curative.
- Post-operative temporary AI ensues because of long-term suppression of ACTH and the contralateral adrenal gland requiring GC replacement for up to 2 years.
- Steroid cover is therefore required.

Adrenal carcinoma

- Estimated incidence 0.7–2/million/year; peak age 40–60 years; ♀ > ♂.
- For staging classification, see Lughezzani et al. (2010) in ⊃ Further reading, p. 277.
- Treatment of ACCs should be carried out in a specialist centre by an MDT expert team (surgeons, oncologists, radiologists, pathologists, and endocrinologists with extensive expertise in treating ACCs). This improves survival.
- The 1° approach is surgical only by an experienced surgeon (>20 adrenalectomies per year), aiming at complete removal of the 1° tumour en bloc, including peritumoural fat without capsule violation. In cases of stage III disease with invasion of adjacent organs or venous thrombosis, a radical surgical approach with en bloc resection and removal of tumour thrombus, if necessary, in collaboration with vascular and cardiothoracic surgeons, is beneficial. Single metastases can also be approached surgically (lung, liver) or by RFA (liver). Surgical debulking can be helpful, even in metastatic disease, in cases of florid and difficult-to-control Cushing's, but needs to be carefully weighed against the resulting delay in initiating chemotherapy.
- Disease-free and total survival is defined by tumour stage and the presence or absence of capsule violation or invasion. Histopathology is notoriously difficult, as it insufficiently differentiates between benign and malignant tumours. It should be undertaken by an expert histopathologist and assessment includes using the Weiss score and the Ki67 index (see Table 3.6).
- The Ki67 index is the most predictive marker for recurrence of disease.
- Adjuvant therapy (see below) should be considered in those individuals with Ki67 >10% and those with advanced disease. However, even after successful and apparently complete removal of the 1° tumour, patients with Ki67 of 1%, indicative of benign disease, can later present with recurrence/metastasis. The majority of recurrences occur within 2–3 years of removal of the 1° tumour.
- Where complete surgical resection is not possible, radiotherapy, RFA, or chemoembolization may be considered.
- Continuing management includes:
  - Follow-up; regular cross-sectional imaging of chest, abdomen, and pelvis: 3-monthly for 2 years, then every 3–6 months for a further 3 years if completely resected.
  - Surveillance, depending on prognostic factors if advanced.
  - Regular hormone secretion assessment.

Table 3.6 Components of Weiss score (scores ≥3 are suggestive of malignancy)

Histological characteristics	Score
High nuclear grade	1
Mitotic rate >5/50 high-power field	1
Atypical mitotic figures	1
Clear cells comprising <25% of the tumour	1
Diffuse architecture (greater than one-third of the tumour)	1
Necrosis	1
Invasion of venous structures	1
Invasion of sinusoidal structures	1
Invasion of capsule of tumour	1
Total	**9**

- Adjuvant therapy:
  - Post-operative adjuvant treatment with the adrenolytic agent *mitotane* (*ortho-para* DDD) has been shown to prolong survival in high-risk patients, including those with no macroscopic residual tumour, but perceived as high risk due to stage III or Ki67 >10%.
  - It should be given for 2 years. Mitotane treatment should be monitored by experienced physicians; it is invariably associated with the development of GC deficiency, requiring permanent GC replacement. Due to induction of the major drug-metabolizing enzyme CYP3A4 by mitotane, a significant amount of hydrocortisone is immediately inactivated. Thus, patients on mitotane treatment require GC replacement with an ↑ dose, e.g. hydrocortisone 20–20–10mg. There are other important drug interactions with mitotane caused by induction of CYP3A4 (e.g. statins, benzodiazepines, opioid analgesics, oestrogen, and macrolide antibiotics). Monitoring of drug levels is mandatory to ensure that concentrations within the therapeutic range (14–20 micrograms/mL) are achieved in a timely fashion. Plasma mitotane level monitoring also limits unwanted side effects, including neurotoxic effects ('trouble talking, trouble walking') that usually occur when plasma levels increase above 20–25 micrograms/mL but resolve within days to weeks after transiently stopping mitotane treatment. Other possible side effects include diarrhoea, fatigue, allergic skin rashes, and moderate elevation of liver transaminases.
- Other drugs may be required to control cortisol hypersecretion (e.g. metyrapone, ketoconazole, and, in extreme cases, non-anaesthetic doses of etomidate).
- Metastatic disease/high risk of recurrence.
- Mitotane also represents the 1st-line treatment in metastatic adrenal cancer.

- In patients with metastatic disease occurring on mitotane treatment or in patients with rapidly progressive disease, cytotoxic chemotherapy should be initiated. The 1st choice is the so-called Berruti regimen ((EDP-M: cisplatin, etoposide, doxorubicin, and continued mitotane treatment). Newer treatment options, such as PI3 kinase inhibitors and IGF receptor antagonists, are currently under investigation.
- Adjuvant radiotherapy is not routinely used but may be considered by some.

Associated hereditary syndromes

- Li-Fraumeni.
- Lynch syndrome.
- MEN1.
- Familial adenomatous polyposis.

Bilateral adrenal hyperplasia

- Bilateral adrenalectomy is curative. Lifelong GC and MC treatment is required. In some cases of bilateral macronodular adrenal hyperplasia, there is a dominant, larger adrenal nodule on one side, and it has been described that unilateral adrenalectomy can lead to resolution of Cushing's for a number of years, but ultimately removal of the remaining adrenal may be necessary if Cushing's reoccurs due to further nodules developing.
- Medical treatment may be possible for some of the rare cases with aberrant receptors, e.g. octreotide for GIP-dependent disease.

Prognosis

- Adrenal adenomas, which are successfully treated with surgery, have a good prognosis and recurrence is unlikely. The prognosis depends on the long-term effects of excess cortisol before treatment—in particular, atherosclerosis and osteoporosis.
- The prognosis for adrenal carcinoma is very poor despite surgery.
- Prognosis of ACC: 3–4 years median survival.
  - 60–80% if confined to adrenal.
  - 30–50% if locally invasive.
  - 0–20% if metastatic.

Autonomous cortisol secretion (subclinical Cushing's syndrome)

- Describes a subset of 5–10% of patients with an adrenal incidentaloma with evidence of autonomous GC production, which, however, is insufficient to produce clinically overt Cushing's syndrome.
- A proportion with small adenomas may spontaneously normalize GC secretion.
- UFC measurement may be within the normal range, but there is failure to sufficiently suppress with low-dose (1mg) dexamethasone (9 a.m. cortisol levels 51–138nmol/L). ACTH may be low or suppressed.
- An associated risk of DM, osteoporosis, and hypertension has been reported and patients should be screened for these comorbidities. There is emerging evidence for ↑ cardiovascular mortality.
- Current data are insufficient to indicate the superiority of a surgical or non-surgical approach to management. Surgery may be considered on a case-by-case basis.
- An annual reassessment for cortisol excess and comorbidities should be performed, with treatment as indicated, aiming to reduce the risk of metabolic complications and fracture.
- Hypoadrenalism post-adrenalectomy has been reported due to suppression of the contralateral adrenal gland. Perioperative steroid cover is therefore required with re-evaluation post-operatively.

Further reading

Bancos I, et al. (2020). Urine steroid metabolomics for the differential diagnosis of adrenal incidentalomas in the EURINE-ACT study: a prospective test validation study; ENSAT EURINE-ACT Investigators. *Lancet Diabetes Endocrinol* **8**, 773–81.

Di Dalmazi G, et al. (2014). Cardiovascular events and mortality in patients with adrenal incidentalomas that are either non-secreting or associated with intermediate phenotype or sub-clinical Cushing's syndrome: a 15-year retrospective study. *Lancet Diabetes Endocrinol* **2**, 396–405.

Elhassan YS, et al. (2019). Natural history of adrenal incidentalomas with and without mild autonomous cortisol excess: a systematic review and meta-analysis. *Ann Intern Med* **171**, 107–16.

Fassnacht M, et al. (2012). Combination chemotherapy in advanced adrenocortical carcinoma. *N Engl J Med* **366**, 2189–97.

Fassnacht M, et al. (2016). Management of adrenal incidentalomas: European Society of Endocrinology clinical practice guideline in collaboration with the European Network for the Study of Adrenal Tumors. *Eur J Endocrinol* **175**, G1–34.

Fassnacht M, et al. (2018). European Society of Endocrinology Clinical Practice Guidelines on the management of adrenocortical carcinoma in adults, in collaboration with the European Network for the Study of Adrenal Tumors. *Eur J Endocrinol* **179**, G1–46.

Kroiss M (2011). Drug interactions with mitotane by induction of CYP3A4 metabolism in the clinical management of adrenocortical carcinoma. *Clin Endocrinol (Oxf)* **75**, 585–91.

Lacroix A, et al. (2001). Ectopic and abnormal hormone receptors in adrenal Cushing's syndrome. *Endocr Rev* **22**, 75–110.

Lughezzani G, et al. (2010). The European Network for the Study of Adrenal Tumors staging system is prognostically superior to the international union against cancer-staging system: a North American validation. *Eur J Cancer* **46**, 713–19.

Terzolo M, et al. (2007). Adjuvant mitotane treatment for adrenocortical carcinoma. *N Engl J Med* **356**, 2372–80.

Tritos N (2020). Adrenally directed medical therapies for Cushing syndrome. *J Clin Endocrinol Metab* **106**, 16–25.

Adrenal surgery

Adrenalectomy

Open adrenalectomy may still be necessary for large and complex pathology. However, laparoscopic adrenalectomy (first performed in 1992) has become the procedure of choice for removal of most adrenal tumours. Retrospective comparisons with open approaches suggest reduced hospital stay and analgesic requirements and lower post-operative morbidity. This may be improved even further by the recently introduced retroperitoneoscopic approach. However, there are few long-term outcome data on this technique. It is most useful in the management of small (<6cm) benign adenomas. Laparoscopic bilateral adrenalectomy, although technically demanding, offers a useful approach to patients with macronodular hyperplasia and in selected patients with ACTH-dependent Cushing's syndrome where alternative therapeutic options are not appropriate.

Myelolipoma
* Most discovered incidentally.
* <6cm unlikely to causes mass effect.
* Consider adrenalectomy with larger tumours, haematoma, or tumour growth.

Preoperative preparation of patients
* Cushing's: metyrapone or ketoconazole (see ➔ Medical treatment, pp. 187–8).
* PCC: α- and β-blockade (see ➔ Management, pp. 326–8).

Perioperative management
(See Box 3.2.)

Box 3.2 Perioperative management of patients undergoing adrenalectomy

Adrenal cortical tumours (benign and malignant)/bilateral adrenalectomy for Cushing's syndrome.

- Perioperative GC cover is required in all patients who fail to adequately suppress serum cortisol in the overnight 1mg dexamethasone suppression test. If in doubt, replace, as even 'silent' adenomas may be associated with subclinical excess cortisol, and hence suppression of the contralateral adrenal gland.
- Hydrocortisone is given as for pituitary surgery—100mg IM with the premedication and then continued every 6h for 24–48h, until the patient can take oral medication and is eating and drinking.
- This is changed to PO hydrocortisone at double replacement dose—20mg on waking, 10mg at lunchtime, and 10mg at 5 p.m.—and MC replacement commenced if bilateral adrenalectomy has been performed (100 micrograms of fludrocortisone daily). Electrolytes and BP guide adequacy of treatment. Normal replacement hydrocortisone (e.g. 10, 5, 5mg) can be commenced when the patient is recovered and may be omitted altogether if the patient did not have preoperative evidence of Cushing's syndrome/suppression of the contralateral gland/bilateral adrenalectomy. MC replacement is only required in patients who have had bilateral adrenalectomy.
- An SST (off hydrocortisone for at least 24h) is performed after at least 2 weeks to demonstrate adequate function of the contralateral adrenal. However, in patients with ACTH-independent Cushing's syndrome, it may take up to 2 years for full recovery of the contralateral adrenal gland, and thus the 1st assessment by SST should be done only after 3–6 months.
- The exception is patients undergoing adrenalectomy for MC-secreting tumours. These patients do not usually require perioperative GC replacement, but preoperative amiloride or spironolactone allows recovery of potassium stores and control of hypertension prior to surgery.

Further reading

Husebye E, et al. (2021). Adrenal insufficiency. *Lancet* **397**, 613.

Mihai R (2019). Open adrenalectomy. *Gland Surg* **8**(Suppl 1), S28–35.

Raffaelli M, et al. (2019). Laparoscopic adrenalectomy. *Gland Surg* **8**(Suppl 1), S41–52.

Renal tubular abnormalities

Background

Bartter's syndrome and Gitelman's syndrome are both associated with hypokalaemic alkalosis and the activation of the renin–angiotensin system, but without hypertension. In contrast, BP tends to be low in these conditions. Liddle's syndrome is associated with hypokalaemic alkalosis and hypertension, but with low renin and aldosterone levels.

Liddle's syndrome

A rare AD condition with variable penetrance that is caused by mutations in the gene encoding for the epithelial sodium channel (ENaC), usually by mutations in the gene encoding the β or γ subunit of ENaC, which is highly selective and located in the distal nephron. This leads to constitutive activation of sodium transport, independent of circulating MCs; consequently, 2° activation of sodium/potassium exchange occurs.

Features

- Hypokalaemia and hypertension.

Investigation

- Hypokalaemic alkalosis.
- Suppressed renin and aldosterone levels.

(See Table 3.4.)

Treatment

Hypertension responds to amiloride (doses up to 40mg/day), but not to spironolactone, because amiloride acts on the sodium channel directly, whereas spironolactone acts on the MC receptor.

Bartter's syndrome

Causes

Most commonly loss of function of the bumetanide-sensitive sodium–potassium–chloride (Na–K–2Cl) co-transporter in the thick ascending limb of the loop of Henle. Mutations in several genes have been reported to account for the phenotype and genetic classification (see Table 3.7).

Table 3.7 Genetic classification of Bartter's syndrome

Type	Inheritance	Genetic mutation	Comments
1	AR	SLC12A1	Na–K–2Cl co-transporter (NKCC2)
2	AR	KCNJ1	Rectified potassium channel (ROMK)
3	AR	CLCNKB	Chloride channel (ClC-Kb)
4a	AR	BSND	Barttin protein (accessory subunit for CLCNKA and B)
4b	AR	CLCNKA CLCNKB	Chloride channels (ClC-Ka, ClC-Kb)
5	AD	CASR	Calcium-sensing receptor

These encode regulatory ion channels (NKCC2, ROMK, CLCNKB). Inactivation of the co-transporter leads to salt wasting, activation of the renin–angiotensin system, and ↑ aldosterone which leads to ↑ sodium reabsorption at the distal nephron and causes hypokalaemic alkalosis. Reabsorption of calcium also occurs in the thick ascending loop, and thus inactivation leads to hypercalciuria. The lack of associated hypertension is thought to be due to ↑ prostaglandin production from the renal medullary interstitial tissue in response to hypokalaemia.

- Rare (~1/million) AR hypokalaemic metabolic alkalosis associated with salt wasting and normal or reduced BP.
- Usually presents at an early age (<5 years).
- Rare transient antenatal Bartter's syndrome can occur.

Features

- Intravascular volume depletion due to salt wasting.
- Seizures.
- Tetany.
- Muscle weakness.

There is also an antenatal variant which is a life-threatening disorder of renal tubular hypokalaemic alkalosis and hypercalciuria.

Investigations

- Hypokalaemic alkalosis.
- ↑ PRA and aldosterone.
- Hypercalciuria.
- Genetic testing

Treatment

- Potassium replacement—although often poorly tolerated in high doses.
- Potassium-sparing diuretics, e.g. amiloride, spironolactone, or eplerenone, may be helpful. However, they are usually inadequate in correcting hypokalaemia. Prostaglandin synthase inhibitors (non-steroidal anti-inflammatory drugs (NSAIDs)), e.g. indometacin 2–5mg/kg per day or ibuprofen, may be required.
- Sodium replacement may be required.

NB. Some conditions mimic Bartter's syndrome, e.g. aminoglycosides, bulimia.

Gitelman's syndrome

- Rare; 1/40,000.

Causes

- An inherited renal tubular disorder where loss of function in the thiazide-sensitive sodium–chloride (Na–Cl) transporter of the distal convoluted tubule (DCT) leads to renal salt wasting, hypovolaemia, and metabolic alkalosis.
- AR; due to mutations in the *SCL12A3* gene encoding the Na–Cl co-transporter.
- Hypovolaemia leads to activation of the renin–angiotensin system and ↑ aldosterone levels (2° hyperaldosteronism).
- Hypokalaemic alkalosis, in conjunction with hypocalciuria (? hypovolaemia and altered tubular handling) and hypomagnesaemia (due to downregulation of a magnesium-permeable channel in the DCT).
- Presents at older ages without overt hypovolaemia (essentially, a less severe phenotype of Bartter's syndrome).

NB. Some heterozygous carriers experience similar features.

Clinical features

Usually presents in late childhood/early adulthood.
- Salt craving.
- Muscle weakness (occasional tetany).
- Fatigue.
- Palpitations (prolonged corrected QT interval (QTc)).
- Joint pain.
- Hypertension can occur later (? 2° to hyperreninaemia).

Differential diagnosis

- Includes diuretic/laxative abuse.

Investigations

- Hypokalaemic alkalosis, in association with ↑ renin and aldosterone.
- Hypomagnesaemia (not in all).
- Hypocalciuria.
- ECG.
- Genetic testing.

Treatment

- Potassium and magnesium replacement (aim for potassium >3 and magnesium >0.6mmol/L).
- Potassium-rich foods include fresh fruit and vegetables—oranges, banana, kale spinach, and mushrooms—salmon, and coconut water.
- Magnesium-rich foods include cashew nuts, almond, and pumpkin seeds, and avocados, mackerel, and dark chocolate.
- Potassium-sparing diuretics may be required.
- Monitoring.
- Specialist review: 1–2 per year.
- Complications include ↑ risk of type 2 diabetes mellitus (T2DM) (mechanism unclear), proteinuria, and chronic renal disease.

(See Table 3.8.)

Table 3.8 Summary of features of renal tubular abnormalities

Syndrome[*]	BP	Renin	Aldosterone	Urinary calcium	Other
Bartter's	N	↑	↑	↑	
Gitelman's	N	↑	↑	↓	↓ magnesium
Liddle's	↑	↓	↓	N	

[*] All three conditions have hypokalaemic alkalosis.

N, normal.

Unexplained hypokalaemia

▶ Tricky issue

In some instances, despite extensive investigations (see algorithm approach below) to determine the aetiology of hypokalaemia, no specific cause can be identified. In these circumstances, it is appropriate to try and normalize potassium levels. This may include the use of potassium supplements and potassium-sparing diuretics. All should be used with careful monitoring of electrolyte levels.

Transcellular shifts

- Insulin.
- β-agonists.
- Refeeding syndrome.
- Alkalaemia.
- Rapid haemoptysis.
- Hypothermia.
- Thyrotoxic/familial periodic paralysis.
- ↓ intake (rare).
- ↑ loss

GI loss

- Diarrhoea.
- Laxatives.
- Vomiting.

Renal loss

- Normotension:
  - Diuretic therapy.
  - Bartter's syndrome.
  - Gitelman's syndrome.
  - Magnesium depletion.
- Hypertension:
  - High renin, high aldosterone: renal artery stenosis.
  - Low renin, high aldosterone: hyperaldosteronism.
  - Low renin, low aldosterone: Liddle's syndrome, AME, liquorice consumption.

Further reading

Fulchiero R, Seo-Mayer P (2019). Bartter syndrome and Gitelman syndrome. *Pediatr Clin North Am* **66**, 121–34.

Furuhashi M, et al. (2005). Liddle's syndrome caused by a novel mutation in the proline-rich PY motif of the epithelial sodium channel B-subunit. *J Clin Endocrinol Metab* **90**, 340–4.

Graziani G, et al. (2010). Gitelman syndrome: pathophysiological and clinical aspects. *QJM* **103**, 741–8.

Mrad FCC, et al. (2020). Bartter's syndrome: clinical findings, genetic causes and therapeutic approach. *World J Pediatr* **17**, 31–9.

Urwin S, et al. (2020). The challenges of diagnosis and management of Gitelman syndrome. *Clin Endocrinol* **92**, 3–10.

Mineralocorticoid deficiency

Epidemiology

Rare, apart from the hyporeninaemic hypoaldosteronism associated with DM.

Causes

Congenital
- 1° AI due to:
  - *CAH*—certain types, most commonly 21-hydroxylase deficiency, are associated with MC deficiency (see ➲ Congenital adrenal hyperplasia in adults, pp. 354–5).
  - *Congenital lipoid adrenal hyperplasia (CLAH)* caused by mutations in the genes encoding steroidogenic acute regulatory protein (StAR), responsible for rapid import of cholesterol into the mitochondrion, and the side chain cleavage protein (CYP11A1), responsible for the conversion of cholesterol to pregnenolone, i.e. the 1st step of steroidogenesis.
  - *Adrenal hypoplasia congenita (AHC)* caused by mutations in the genes encoding the transcription factors SF-1 (*NR5A1*) and DAX-1 (*NR0B1*) that play a crucial role in adrenal development.
  - *Adrenoleukodystrophy* affecting 1/20,000 ♂; very long-chain fatty acids (VLCFAs) cannot be oxidized in peroxisomes and accumulate in tissues and the circulation. CNS symptoms may be absent initially, in particular, in the milder form adrenomyeloneuropathy (AMN), but progressive demyelination can lead to hypertonic tetraparesis, dementia, epilepsy, coma, or death (in particular, in the early childhood-onset variant adrenoleukodystrophy).
- Rare *inherited disorders* of aldosterone biosynthesis.
- *Pseudohypoaldosteronism*—inherited resistance to the action of aldosterone (see ➲ Mineralocorticoid resistance, p. 769). AD and AR forms are described. Usually presents in infancy. Treated with sodium chloride.

Acquired
- All forms of non-congenital 1° AI (see ➲ Addison's disease, pp. 292–3). In 2° AI, the adrenals are anatomically intact, and thus regulation of MC secretion by the renin–angiotensin–aldosterone (RAA) system is intact.
- *Drugs*—heparin (heparin for >5 days may cause severe hyperkalaemia due to a toxic effect on the zona glomerulosa); ciclosporin.
- *Hyporeninaemic hypoaldosteronism*—interference with the renin–angiotensin system leads to MC deficiency and hyperkalaemic acidosis (type IV renal tubular acidosis), e.g. diabetic nephropathy. Treatment is fludrocortisone and potassium restriction. ACEIs may produce a similar biochemical picture, but here the PRA will be elevated, as there is no angiotensin II feedback on renin.

Treatment

- Fludrocortisone.

Adrenal insufficiency

Definition

AI is defined by the lack of cortisol, i.e. GC deficiency, and may be due to destruction of the adrenal cortex (1°, Addison's disease, and CAH; see ➔ Addison's disease, pp. 292–3) or due to disordered pituitary and hypothalamic function (2°).

Epidemiology

- Permanent AI is found in 5 in 10,000 population.
- The most frequent cause is hypothalamic–pituitary damage, which is the cause of AI in 60% of affected patients.
- The remaining 40% of cases are due to 1° failure of the adrenal to synthesize cortisol, with almost equal prevalence of Addison's disease (mostly of autoimmune origin, prevalence 0.9–1.4 in 10,000) and CAH (prevalence 0.7–1.0 in 10,000).
- AI due to suppression of pituitary–hypothalamic function by exogenously administered, supraphysiological GC doses for treatment of, for example, chronic obstructive pulmonary disease (COPD) or rheumatoid arthritis is much commoner (50–200 in 10,000 population). This is sometimes termed tertiary AI. Adrenal function can recover in some, but not all, patients following tapering and cessation of exogenous GC administration. This is likely to depend on cumulative previous exposure (dose and time) to GC treatment.

Causes of secondary adrenal insufficiency

Lesions of the hypothalamus and/or pituitary gland

- Tumours—pituitary tumour, metastases, craniopharyngioma.
- Infection—TB.
- Inflammation—sarcoidosis, histiocytosis X, haemochromatosis, lymphocytic hypophysitis.
- Iatrogenic—surgery, radiotherapy.
- Other—isolated ACTH deficiency, trauma.

Suppression of the hypothalamo–pituitary–adrenal axis
(See Box 3.3.)

Box 3.3 Adrenal suppression

- Inhaled steroids (20.5% fail SST)—beclometasone, fluticasone.
- Topical steroids—beclometasone, budesonide.
- Intranasal—beclometasone, fluticasone.
- GC administration.
- Chronic opiate administration.
- Cushing's disease (after pituitary tumour removal).

Features of secondary adrenal insufficiency

As 1° (see ➲ Adrenal insufficiency, pp. 288–90), except:
- Absence of pigmentation—skin is pale.
- Absence of MC deficiency.
- Associated features of underlying cause, e.g. visual field defects if pituitary tumour.
- Other endocrine deficiencies may manifest due to pituitary failure (see ➲ Hypopituitarism, pp. 138–9).
- Acute onset may occur due to pituitary apoplexy.

Isolated ACTH deficiency

- Rare.
- Pathogenesis unclear—may be autoimmune (associated with other autoimmune conditions and antipituitary antibodies described in some patients); can be associated with autoimmune hypothyroidism.
- Absent ACTH response to CRH.
- Often presents with unexplained hyponatraemia.
- *POMC* mutations and POMC processing abnormalities (e.g. proconvertase PC1).
- Some patients undergo spontaneous recovery; others progress to further pituitary deficiency. Thus, follow-up is essential.

Pathophysiology

Primary
- Adrenal gland destruction or dysfunction occurs due to a disease process which usually involves all three zones of the adrenal cortex, resulting in inadequate GC, MC, and adrenal androgen precursor secretion. The manifestations of insufficiency do not usually appear until at least 90% of the gland has been destroyed and are usually gradual in onset, with partial AI leading to an impaired cortisol response to stress and the features of complete insufficiency occurring later. Acute AI may occur in the context of acute septicaemia (e.g. meningococcal or haemorrhage). There is usually combined GC and MC deficiency.
- MC deficiency leads to reduced sodium retention and hyponatraemia and hypotension with ↓ intravascular volume, in addition to hyperkalaemia due to ↓ renal potassium and hydrogen ion excretion.
- Androgen deficiency presents in ♀ with reduced axillary and pubic hair and reduced libido. (Testicular production of androgens is more important in ♂.)
- Lack of cortisol −ve feedback increases CRH and ACTH secretion. Stimulation of skin melanocortin 1 receptors (MC1Rs) usually (80%) leads to pigmentation of the skin and other mucous membranes.

Secondary
- Inadequate ACTH results in deficient cortisol production (and ↓ androgens in ♀).
- There is no pigmentation because ACTH and POMC secretion is reduced. MC secretion remains normal, as its 1° regulator is the RAA system in kidneys and adrenal glands which are intact. However, hyponatraemia may be present due to mild SIADH arising from cortisol deficiency.
- The onset is usually gradual, with partial ACTH deficiency resulting in reduced response to stress. Prolonged ACTH deficiency leads to atrophy of the zona fasciculata and reduced ability to respond acutely to ACTH.
- Lack of stimulation of skin MC1Rs due to ACTH deficiency results in pale skin appearance.

Investigations

For pituitary/hypothalamic disease, see ➜ Investigations of hypopituitarism, p. 142. For long-term endogenous or exogenous GCs, see ➜ Autoimmune adrenalitis, pp. 294–5.

Addison's disease

Causes of primary adrenal insufficiency

- Autoimmune—commonest cause in the developed world (~70% of cases).
- Autoimmune polyglandular deficiency—type 1 or 2 (see ⊃ Autoimmune polyglandular syndrome (APS) type 1, p. 296).
- *Malignancy:*
  - Metastatic (lung, breast, kidney—adrenal metastases found in ~50% of patients, but symptomatic AI much less common and only observed with bilateral metastases).
  - Lymphoma (1° adrenal lymphoma, AI only if bilateral).
- Infiltration:
  - Amyloid.
  - Sarcoidosis.
  - Haemochromatosis.
- Infection:
  - TB (the medulla more frequently destroyed than the cortex).
  - Fungal, e.g. histoplasmosis, cryptococcosis.
  - Opportunistic infections in, for example, acquired immune deficiency syndrome (AIDS)—cytomegalovirus (CMV), *Mycobacterium intracellulare*, *Cryptococcus* (up to 5% of patients with AIDS develop 1° AI in the late stages).
- Vascular haemorrhage:
  - Anticoagulants.
  - Waterhouse–Friderichsen syndrome in meningococcal septicaemia.
- *Infarction*—e.g. 2° to thrombosis in antiphospholipid syndrome.
- *Adrenoleukodystrophy:*
  - Inherited disorder caused by mutations in the X-linked *ALD* gene that encodes the peroxisomal transporter protein ABCD1.
  - Diagnosed by measuring VLCFAs.
  - Presents in childhood and adolescence.
  - Progresses in 50% to quadriparesis and dementia, in association with adrenal failure (= cerebral ALS); milder-variant AMN (adrenomyelopathy) causes spinal neurology only, and AI may precede manifestations of neurological symptoms; in 10–20%, AI is the sole manifestation of disease.
- CAH see ⊃ Congenital adrenal hyperplasia in adults, pp. 354–5).
- Adrenal hypoplasia congenita—very rare familial failure of adrenal cortical development due to mutations/deletions in *NR0B1* (DAX-1), *NR5A1* (SF-1), *CDKN1C* (IMAGe syndrome), *POLE1* (IMAGe-like syndrome), *SAMD9* (MIRAGE syndrome), and *WNT4* (SERKAL syndrome).
- CLAH—very rare familial failure of adrenal steroidogenesis due to mutations in the genes encoding StAR (responsible for mitochondrial import of cholesterol) or the side chain cleavage enzyme CYP11A1 (responsible for conversion of cholesterol to pregnenolone, i.e. the 1st step of steroidogenesis).

- Familial glucocorticoid deficiency (FGD) due to mutations in genes encoding proteins involved in the regulation of ACTH action, e.g. the ACTH receptor MC2R or the MC2R accessory protein MRAP that transfers MC2R to the adrenal cell membrane to facilitate ACTH binding (see ➲ ACTH resistance and familial glucocorticoid deficiency, p. 298). Other genes with mutations leading to FGD include *MCM4* (minichromosome maintenance-deficient 4), *TXNRD2* (thioredoxin reductase), and *NNT* (nicotinamide nucleotide transhydrogenase).
- Triple A syndrome (*Achalasia*, *Addisonianism*, *Alacrimia*) (Allgrove syndrome):
  - Addison's due to ACTH resistance.
  - AR.
  - May get autonomic dysfunction, hypoglycaemia, and mental retardation.
  - Caused by mutations in the *AAAS* gene (12g13).
- Iatrogenic:
  - Bilateral adrenalectomy.
  - Drugs: ketoconazole, fluconazole, trilostane, abiraterone, etomidate, aminoglutethimide (inhibits cortisol synthesis), phenytoin, rifampicin (increases cortisol metabolism), mitotane (adrenolytic and increases cortisol metabolism).
  - Immunotherapy (CTLA4 and PD-1 inhibitors).

Autoimmune adrenalitis

- Mediated by humoral and cell-mediated immune mechanisms. Autoimmune insufficiency associated with polyglandular autoimmune syndrome is commoner in ♀ (70%).
- Adrenal cortex antibodies are present in the majority of patients at diagnosis, and although titres decline and eventually disappear, they are still found in ~70% of patients 10 years later. Up to 20% of patients/year with +ve adrenal antibodies develop AI. Antibodies to 21-hydroxylase are commonly found, although the exact nature of other antibodies that block the effect of ACTH, for example, are yet to be elucidated.
- Antiadrenal antibodies are found in <2% of patients with other autoimmune endocrine disease (Hashimoto's thyroiditis, DM, autoimmune hypothyroidism, hypoparathyroidism, pernicious anaemia). In addition, antibodies to other endocrine glands are commonly found in patients with autoimmune AI (thyroid microsomal in 50%, gastric parietal cell, parathyroid, and ovary and testis). However, the presence of antibodies does not predict subsequent manifestation of organ-specific autoimmunity.
- Polyglandular autoimmune conditions (see ➜ Autoimmune polyglandular syndrome (APS) type 1, p. 298; ➜ APS type 2, p. 297). The presence of 17-hydroxylase antibodies, in association with 21-hydroxylase antibodies, is a good marker of patients at risk of developing premature ovarian failure (POF) in association with 1° adrenal failure.
- Patients with T1DM and AITD only rarely develop autoimmune AI; ~60% of patients with Addison's disease have other autoimmune or endocrine disorders.

Clinical features

Chronic
- Anorexia and weight loss (>90%).
- Tiredness.
- Weakness—generalized, no particular muscle groups.
- Pigmentation—generalized, but commonest in skin areas exposed to friction or pressure (elbows and knees, and under bras and belts), mucosae, and scars acquired after onset of AI. Look at palmar creases in Caucasians.
- Dizziness and postural hypotension.
- GI symptoms—nausea and vomiting, abdominal pain, diarrhoea.
- Arthralgia and myalgia.
- Symptomatic hypoglycaemia—rare in adults.
- ↓ axillary and pubic hair and reduced libido in ♀.
- Pyrexia of unknown origin—rarely.
- Impaired QoL.

Associated conditions

- Vitiligo.
- Features of other autoimmune endocrinopathies.

Laboratory investigations
- Hyponatraemia.
- Hyperkalaemia.
- Elevated urea.
- Anaemia (normocytic normochromic).
- Elevated ESR.
- Eosinophilia.
- Mild hypercalcaemia—↓ absorption, ↓ renal absorption of calcium.

Autoimmune polyglandular syndrome (APS) type 1

- Also known as autoimmune polyendocrinopathy, candidiasis, and ectodermal dystrophy (APECED).
- AR with childhood onset.
- Chronic mucocutaneous candidiasis.
- Hypoparathyroidism (90%), 1° AI (60%).
- 1° gonadal failure (41%)—usually after Addison's diagnosis.
- 1° hypothyroidism.
- Rarely hypopituitarism, DI, T1DM.
- Associated chronic active hepatitis (20%), malabsorption (15%), alopecia (40%), pernicious anaemia, and vitiligo.
- Mutations in the *AIRE* (autoimmune regulator) gene located on chromosome 21p22.3.

Clinical pearls: screening for autoimmune conditions

Who?

The diagnosis should be considered where two out of three of the following have been diagnosed: chronic mucocutaneous candidiasis, hypoparathyroidism, and AI.

How?

Clinical assessment, combined with biochemical and endocrine screening to include thyroid, adrenal, pituitary, and gonadal function, glycated haemoglobin (HbA1c), liver chemistry, calcium and bone profile, and FBC.

Frequency?

Assessment on an annual basis unless there are symptoms during the intervening period, in which case appropriate investigations should be performed.

APS type 2

- Polygenic inheritance, association with HLADR3, CTL4, PTPN22, and CD25 regions, with mixed penetrance.
- Adult onset.
- AI (100%).
- 1° AITD (70%), mostly hypothyroidism, but also hyperthyroidism.
- T1DM (5–20%)—often before Addison's diagnosis.
- 1° gonadal failure in affected women (5–20%).
- Rarely DI (<0.1%).
- Associated vitiligo, myasthenia gravis, alopecia, pernicious anaemia, and immune thrombocytopenic purpura.

Eponymous syndromes

- Schmidt's syndrome:
  - Addison's disease, *and*
  - Autoimmune hypothyroidism.
- Carpenter syndrome:
  - Addison's disease, *and*
  - Autoimmune hypothyroidism, *and/or*
  - T1DM.

Management of APS

- Hormone replacement should be instigated as needed.
- Antibody screening can be helpful in predicting the development of further endocrinopathies (antibodies against TPO, glutamic acid decarboxylase-65, NALP5, and 21-hydroxylase).
- Patients should undergo a clinical assessment and examination, at least on an annual basis, to include biochemical screening for endocrinopathies.
- Patients with APS type 1 should be vaccinated against *Pneumococcus*, *Meningococcus*, and *Haemophilus influenzae* type b.

Further reading

Buonocore F, Achermann JC (2020). Primary adrenal insufficiency: new genetic causes and their long-term consequences. *Clin Endocrinol (Oxf)* **92**, 11–20.

Guo CJ, et al. (2018). The immunobiology and clinical features of type 1 autoimmune polyglandular syndrome (APS-1). *Autoimmun Rev* **17**, 78–85.

Hannon AM, et al. (2018). Clinical features and autoimmune associations in patients presenting with idiopathic isolated ACTH deficiency. *Clin Endocrinol* **88**, 491–7.

Husebye ES, et al. (2018). Autoimmune polyendocrine syndromes. *N Engl J Med.* **378**, 1132–41.

Siniscalchi C, et al. (2018). The Schmidt syndrome. *Acta Biomed* **88**, 499–501.

ACTH resistance and familial glucocorticoid deficiency

Causes

- Loss of function due to mutations in genes encoding key elements of ACTH signalling, including:
  - MC2R (ACTH receptor), FGD type 1.
  - MRAP (ACTH receptor accessory protein), FGD type 2.
- Usually diagnosed in the neonatal period or in early childhood.
- Presents with hypoglycaemic seizures, hyperpigmentation, recurrent infections, failure to thrive, collapse, and coma.
- Absent adrenarche is common.
- Tall stature and ↑ bone age (MC2R mutations).

Investigations

- Low cortisol with very high ACTH.
- Renin and aldosterone usually normal.
- Genetic testing provides a definitive diagnosis

Treatment

- Appropriate GC replacement.
- Achieving normalization of ACTH levels can be challenging.

Further reading

Flück CE (2017). Mechanisms in endocrinology: update on pathogenesis of primary adrenal insufficiency: beyond steroid enzyme deficiency and autoimmune adrenal destruction. *Eur J Endocrinol* **177**, R99–111.

Investigation of primary adrenal insufficiency

Electrolytes

• Hyponatraemia is present in 90%, and hyperkalaemia in 65%.
• Elevated urea.

Serum cortisol and ACTH

• Undetectable serum cortisol is diagnostic of AI, but basal cortisol is often in the normal range. Cortisol >550nmol/L precludes the diagnosis. At times of acute stress, an inappropriately low cortisol level is very suggestive of the diagnosis.
• A morning cortisol level >350nmol/L (depending on the assay) is highly likely to be associated with a pass on the SST and may avoid the need for further testing.
• Simultaneous 9 a.m. cortisol and ACTH will show elevated ACTH for the level of cortisol. This is a very sensitive means of detecting Addison's disease but performs poorly in less clear-cut cases.

NB. Drugs causing ↑ CBG (e.g. oestrogens) will result in higher total cortisol concentration measurements.

Response to ACTH

Short Synacthen® test

This test can be done at any time of the day.
• Following basal cortisol measurement, 250 micrograms of Synacthen® is administered IM, and serum cortisol checked at 30 and/or 60min.
• Serum cortisol should rise to a peak of 550nmol/L (note that this cut-off may depend on local assay conditions).
• Failure to respond appropriately suggests adrenal failure.
• A long Synacthen® test may be required to confirm 2° adrenal failure if ACTH is equivocal.
• Recent onset of 2° adrenal failure (up to 4 weeks) may produce a normal response to SST.

Long Synacthen® test

• Following a basal cortisol level, depot Synacthen® 1mg IM is administered, and serum cortisol measured at 30, 60, and 120min, and at 4, 8, 12, and 24h. A normal response is elevation in serum cortisol to >1000nmol/L.
• Differentiation of 2° from 1° adrenal failure can be made more reliably following 3 days of ACTH 1mg IM. This is because the test relies on the ability of the atrophic adrenal glands to respond to ACTH in 2° adrenocortical failure, whereas in 1° adrenal failure, the diseased gland is already maximally stimulated by elevated endogenous levels of ACTH and therefore is unable to respond to further stimulation.
• Serum cortisol responses within the first 60min are superimposable with the SST.
• There is a progressive rise in cortisol secretion in 2° AI, but little or no response on 1° AI.

Increased plasma renin activity (assessment of mineralocorticoid sufficiency)

This is one of the earliest abnormalities in developing 1° AI.

Thyroid function tests

Reduced thyroid hormone levels and elevated TSH may be due to a direct effect of GC deficiency (cortisol inhibits TRH) or due to associated auto-immune hypothyroidism; TSH is usually <10U/L in the former, and above 10 in the latter. Re-evaluation is therefore required after AI has been appropriately replaced for a few weeks. Initiation of thyroxine replacement prior to GC replacement can trigger an adrenal crisis, as thyroxine will speed up the inactivation of residual cortisol.

Establishing the cause of adrenal insufficiency

- *Adrenal autoantibodies* (detect antibodies to the adrenal cortex and, more recently, specific antibodies to 21-hydroxylase, side chain cleavage enzyme, and 17-hydroxylase). 21-hydroxylase antibodies are the major component of adrenal cortex antibodies and are present in 80% of recent-onset autoimmune adrenalitis. Adrenal cortex antibodies are not detectable in non-autoimmune 1° adrenal failure.
- *Imaging:*
  - Adrenal enlargement, with or without calcification, may be seen on CT of the abdomen, suggesting TB, infiltration, or metastatic disease. The adrenals are small and atrophic in chronic autoimmune adrenalitis.
  - Percutaneous CT-guided adrenal biopsy is occasionally required.
- *Specific tests*—e.g. serological or microbiological investigations directed at particular infections, VLCFAs (adrenoleukodystrophy) in ♂ and ♀ with antibody −ve isolated 1° AI.

Acute adrenal insufficiency (risk higher in primary disease)

Clinical features
- Shock.
- Hypotension (often not responding to measures such as inotropic support).
- Abdominal pain (may present as 'acute abdomen').
- Unexplained fever.
- Often precipitated by major stress such as severe bacterial infection, major surgery, and unabsorbed GC medication due to vomiting.
- Occasionally occurs due to bilateral adrenal infarction.

Investigations
- As for chronic.
- In the acute situation, if the diagnosis is suspected, an inappropriately low cortisol level (i.e. <600nmol/L) is often sufficient to make the diagnosis.

(See Box 3.4 for emergency management.)

Box 3.4 Emergency management of acute adrenal insufficiency

- This is a life-threatening emergency and should be treated if there is strong clinical suspicion, rather than waiting for confirmatory test results.
- Blood should be taken for urgent analysis of electrolytes and glucose, in addition to cortisol and ACTH.

Fluids

Large volumes of 0.9% saline may be required to reverse volume depletion and sodium deficiency. Several litres may be required in the first 24–48h, but caution should be exercised where there has been chronic hyponatraemia; in this circumstance, rapid correction of the deficit exposes the patient to risk of central pontine myelinolysis. If plasma sodium is <120mmol/L at presentation, aim to correct by no more than 10mmol/L in the first 24h.

Hydrocortisone

- A bolus dose of 100mg hydrocortisone is administered IV. Hydrocortisone 50mg IM (or IV) is then continued 6-hourly for 24–48h or until the patient can take oral therapy. A continuous infusion of hydrocortisone 200mg over 24h can also be considered as an alternative to 6-hourly injections. Double replacement dose hydrocortisone (20, 10, and 10mg PO) can then be instituted until well.
- Specific MC replacement is not required, as the high-dose GC has sufficient MC effects (40mg hydrocortisone equivalent to 100 micrograms fludrocortisone). Once the daily dose of GC is reduced to <50mg after a couple of days and the patient is taking food and fluids by mouth, fludrocortisone 100 micrograms/day can be commenced.

Glucose supplementation

Occasionally required because of risk of hypoglycaemia (low glycogen stores in the liver as a result of GC deficiency).

Investigate and treat precipitant

- This is often infection.

Monitoring treatment

- Electrolytes, glucose, and urea.

Treatment of primary adrenal insufficiency

Maintenance therapy

Glucocorticoid replacement

- Hydrocortisone is the treatment of choice for replacement therapy, as it is reliably and predictably absorbed and allows biochemical monitoring of levels.
- It is administered tds (or occasionally bd), e.g. 10mg immediately on waking, 5mg at midday, and 5mg at 4–5 p.m., or 15mg on waking and 5mg at midday.
- Longer-acting GC preparations can be advantageous in patients with co-incident T1DM, e.g. 3mg prednisolone on waking and 1mg at 5 p.m. They appear to be safe and well tolerated and potentially provide a more physiological replacement regimen.

Mineralocorticoid replacement

- Fludrocortisone (9-fluorohydrocortisone) is given at a dose of 100–150 micrograms daily; occasionally, lower (50 micrograms) or higher (200–250 micrograms) doses may be required. Aim to avoid significant postural fall in BP (>10mmHg).
- Plasma renin should be within the upper third of the normal reference range.
- Hydrocortisone 40mg has the equivalent MC effect of 100 micrograms fludrocortisone.
- Increase fludrocortisone if ambient temperature around 30, and consider adding slow sodium.

DHEA replacement

- DHEA synthesis is also deficient in hypoadrenalism, resulting in reduced production of adrenal androgen precursors and thus invariably androgen deficiency in affected women.
- DHEA replacement (25–50mg/day) may improve mood and well-being, as well as libido, in women with AI.
- DHEA is not available as a UK-licensed preparation but is available (on the Internet) from the USA as a dietary supplement.

Monitoring of therapy

Clinical

- For signs of GC excess, e.g. ↑ weight.
- BP (including postural change).
- Hypertension and oedema suggest excessive MC replacement, whereas postural hypotension and salt craving suggest insufficient treatment.

Biochemical

- Serum electrolytes.
- Plasma renin (elevated if insufficient fludrocortisone replacement).
- Cortisol day curves can be used to assess adequacy.

Intercurrent illness

- Mortality is ↑ in patients with adrenal failure, particularly associated with adrenal crisis; thus, patient education and rapid recognition are essential. Mortality data from the European Adrenal Insufficiency Registry (EU-AIR) (n = 2034 patients) reported mortality was 2–3× that in the general population.
- Cortisol requirements increase during severe illness or surgery.
- In patients with suspected or proven COVID-19 infection, high doses of GC supplementation (equivalent to hydrocortisone 20mg four times daily (qds)) are required (⅍ https://www.endocrinology.org/clinical-practice/clinical-guidance/adrenal-crisis/covid-19-adrenal-crisis-information/).
- For moderate elective procedures or investigations, e.g. endoscopy or angiography, patients should receive a single dose of 100mg hydrocortisone before the procedure.
- For major surgery, patients should receive 100mg IV or IM hydrocortisone with the premedication and receive:
  - 50mg IM (or IV) hydrocortisone 6-hourly (for 1–2 days until recovered), or
  - 200mg per 24h IV infusion hydrocortisone in 5% glucose before reverting rapidly to a maintenance dose.
- To cover severe illness, e.g. pneumonia, patients should receive 50mg IM (or IV) hydrocortisone 6-hourly until resolution of the illness.

  (See Box 3.5 for pregnancy.)

Drug interactions

Rifampicin
- Increases the clearance of cortisol.
- Double the usual dose of hydrocortisone.

Mitotane
- Increases CBG and induces CYP3A4, resulting in rapid inactivation of hydrocortisone.
- Double the usual dose of hydrocortisone, e.g. 20–10–10mg.
- Topiramate—also induces CYP3A4 and accelerates clearance of GCs.

Education of the patient

- Patient education is the key to successful management. Patients must be taught never to miss a dose. They should be encouraged to wear a MedicAlert/SOS bracelet or necklace and always to carry a steroid card (see Fig. 3.4). Sick day rules are shown in Fig. 3.5.
- Every patient should know how to double the dose of GCs during febrile illness and to get medical attention if unable to take the tablets because of vomiting. They should have a vial of 100mg hydrocortisone, with a syringe, diluent, and needle for times when parenteral treatment may be required (see Box 3.6).
- Prognosis in patients with Addison's disease—there is ↑ morbidity and mortality; this may relate to chronic over-replacement with GCs and under-replacement during times of crisis.

Box 3.5 Pregnancy

(See also ➲ The pituitary in pregnancy, p. 482.)
- During normal pregnancy:
  - CBG gradually increases.
  - Free cortisol increases in the 3rd trimester.
  - Progesterone increases, exerting an anti-MC effect.
  - Renin levels increase.
- In Addison's disease, therefore:
  - Initially continue the usual GC and MC replacement.
  - Increase hydrocortisone by 25–50% in the 3rd trimester.
  - Adjust MCs to BP and serum potassium (not renin).
- Severe hyperemesis gravidarum during the 1st trimester may require temporary parenteral therapy, and patients should be warned about this to avoid precipitation of a crisis.
- During labour and for 24–48h:
  - Hydrocortisone 100mg (IM or IV) at onset of active labour.
  - Parenteral GC therapy is then administered (50mg IM every 6h), or
  - Hydrocortisone 200mg IV in 5% glucose per 24h.
  - Fluid replacement with IV 0.9% saline may be required.

Box 3.6 Emergency pack contents for Addison's patients

- 100mg vial hydrocortisone.
- Water for injection.
- 2mL syringe.
- One green needle.
- One blue needle.
- Cotton wool.
- Plaster.

NB. Check the expiry date of hydrocortisone.

Steroid Emergency Card (Adult)

IMPORTANT MEDICAL INFORMATION FOR HEALTHCARE STAFF

THIS PATIENT IS PHYSICALLY DEPENDENT ON DAILY STEROID THERAPY as a critical medicine, to be given/taken as prescribed and never omitted or discontinued; missed doses, illness or surgery can result in adrenal crisis which requires emergency treatment.

Patients not on daily steroid therapy may also require emergency treatment, see reverse of card for links to further information.

Name...

Date of Birth .... NHS Number ....

Why steroid prescribed ....

Emergency Contact ....

If calling **999/111** describe symptoms (vomiting, diarrhoea etc) **AND** emphasise this is a likely Addison's/adrenal emergency or crisis

Emergency treatment of adrenal crisis

1) **EITHER** 100mg Hydrocortisone per i.v. or i.m. injection **followed by** 24 hr continuous i.v. infusion of 200mg Hydrocortisone in Glucose 5%

    OR 50mg Hydrocortisone i.v. or i.m. qds (100mg if severely obese)

2) Rapid rehydration with Sodium Chloride 0.9%

3) Liaise with endocrinology team

 Scan here for further information or search
https://www.endocrinology.org/adrenal-crisis

Fig. 3.4 NHS steroid card.

Reproduced from National Patient Safety Alert on Steroid Emergency Card to support early recognition and treatment of adrenal crisis in adults, under the Open Government License V3.0.

Sick Day Rule 1

Moderate intercurrent illness:
Fever, infection requiring antibiotics, surgical procedure under local anaesthesia
Double usual daily glucocorticoid dose

Sick Day Rule 2

Severe intercurrent illness, persistent vomiting (e.g. GI viral illnesses), during preparation for colonoscopy or in case of acute trauma or surgery

Hydrocortisone 100 mg intravenously at onset, followed by initiation of a continuous infusion of hydrocortisone 200 mg.24 h⁻¹
Or hydrocortisone 100 mg intramuscularly followed by 50 mg every 6 hours* i.m. or i.v.

Patient Education

Teach the patient and partner/parents how to self-administer and inject hydrocortisone. Provide them with a Hydrocortisone Emergency Injection kit (100 mg hydrocortisone sodium succinate for injection)

Addison's Disease Self Help Group (https://www.addisonsdisease.org.uk)
The Pituitary Foundations' websites (https://www.pituitary.org.uk).
Youtube video (Adrenal Crisis: when to give an emergency injection https://www.youtube.com/watch?time_continue=12&v=NpIEMIschTg).

Fig. 3.5 Sick day rules.

Reproduced from Simpson H et al (2020) "Guidance for the prevention and emergency management of adult patients with adrenal insuf-ficiency" *Clinical Medicine Journal* 20(4):371–378 with permission from Royal College of Physicians.

Further reading

Bancos I, et al. (2015). Diagnosis and management of adrenal insufficiency. *Lancet Diabetes Endocrinol* **3**, 216–26.

Hahner S (2018). Acute adrenal crisis and mortality in adrenal insufficiency: still a concern in 2018! Ann Endocrinol (Paris) 79, 164–6.

Husebye ES, et al. (2018). Autoimmune polyendocrine syndromes. *N Engl J Med* **378**, 1132–41.

Johannsson G, et al. (2015). Adrenal insufficiency: review of clinical outcomes with current glucocorticoid replacement therapy. *Clin Endocrinol (Oxf)* **82**, 2–11.

Lebbe M, Arlt W (2013). What is the best diagnostic and therapeutic management strategy for an Addison patient during pregnancy? Clin Endocrinol (Oxf) 78, 497–502.

Mitchell AL, Pearce SH (2012). Autoimmune Addison disease: pathophysiology and genetic complexity. *Nat Rev Endocrinol* **8**, 306–16.

Nilsson AG, et al. (2014). Prospective evaluation of long-term safety of dual-release hydrocortisone replacement administered once daily in patients with adrenal insufficiency. *Eur J Endocrinol* **171**, 369–77.

Prete A, et al. (2020). Prevention of adrenal crisis: cortisol responses to major stress compared to stress dose hydrocortisone delivery. *J Clin Endocrinol Metab* **105**, 2262–74.

Rushworth RL, et al. (2019). Adrenal crisis. *N Engl J Med* **381**, 852–61.

Sbardella E, et al. (2017). Baseline morning cortisol level as a predictor of pituitary-adrenal reserve: a comparison across three assays. *Clin Endocrinol (Oxf)* **86**, 177–84.

Simpson H, et al. (2020). Guidance for the prevention and emergency management of adult patients with adrenal insufficiency. *Clin Med* **20**, 371–8.

Wass JAH, Arlt W (2012). How to avoid precipitating an acute adrenal crisis. *BMJ* **345**, 6333.

Woodcock T, et al. (2020). Guidelines for the management of glucocorticoids during the perioperative period for patients with adrenal insufficiency: Anaesthesia 75, 654–63.

Woods CP, et al. (2015). Adrenal suppression in patients taking inhaled glucocorticoids is highly prevalent and management can be guided by morning cortisol. *Eur J Endocrinol* **173**, 633–42.

Long-term glucocorticoid administration

Both exogenous GC administration and endogenous excess GCs (Cushing's syndrome) lead to a −ve feedback effect on the hypothalamo–pituitary–adrenal axis (HPA), leading to suppression of both CRH and ACTH secretion and atrophy of the zona fasciculata and zona reticularis of the adrenal cortex. This can occur via all routes of exogenous steroid administration, including oral, inhaled, intra-articular, and topical.

Population studies suggest 20% of patients on inhaled GCs, and 15% of those on topical/nasal GCs, will fail an SST.

The HPA axis is sensitive to exogenous GC excess. However, the RAA axis continues to function when the GC excess ceases, while the HPA axis will suffer from lasting suppression. The time of recovery is likely to be dependent on the duration and dose of the preceding period of exposure to exogenous GC excess. (See Box 3.7 for steroid equivalents.)

Short-term steroids

- Any patient who has received GC treatment for <2 weeks is unlikely to have clinically significant adrenal suppression, and if the medical condition allows it, GC treatment can be stopped acutely. If patients are exposed to major stress within a week of stopping steroids, consideration should be given to providing acute GC cover.
- Patients who have received >2 weeks of GC treatment should be weaned.
- Exceptions to this are patients who have other possible reasons for adrenocortical insufficiency, who have received >40mg prednisolone (or equivalent), where a short course has been prescribed within 1 year of cessation of long-term therapy, or with evening doses (↑ HPA axis suppression).

Long-term steroids and weaning

- When patients are receiving supraphysiological doses (>5mg prednisolone or equivalent) of GC, dose reduction depends on the activity of the underlying disease requiring GC treatment. If GCs are still required for treatment of the underlying condition, then weaning with a view to GC discontinuation should not be undertaken.
- If the disease has resolved, the GC dose can be reduced to 5mg prednisolone. The speed of weaning should be considered on a case-by-case basis. Rapid weaning can result in symptoms of AI. Doses of prednisolone >10mg can often be reduced by 2.5–5mg/week. Doses of prednisolone <10mg can be weaned by 1–2mg per week.
- Once the patient is established on 5mg prednisolone, consider switching to hydrocortisone (15mg in the morning, 5mg at lunchtime, 5mg in early evening), as this has a shorter half-life and will therefore lead to less prolonged suppression of ACTH.
- A further daily hydrocortisone reduction (10mg in the morning, 5mg at lunchtime, 5mg in early evening) should be considered after 1–2 weeks, and an SST should then be performed. Once an SST demonstrates a normal response, hydrocortisone replacement can be stopped. Supplemental steroids during intercurrent illness are not required.

Cushing's syndrome

Patients with Cushing's syndrome on metyrapone or with recently treated disease, whatever the cause, may also have HPA axis suppression and may therefore need steroid replacement at times of stress.

Box 3.7 Steroid equivalents

- 1mg hydrocortisone.
- 1.5mg cortisone acetate.
- 0.2mg prednisolone.
- 0.0375mg dexamethasone.

4mg prednisolone ≡ 20mg hydrocortisone ≡ 0.75mg dexamethasone.

Further reading

Bensing S, et al. (2008). Increased death risk and altered cancer incidence pattern in patients with isolated or combined autoimmune primary adrenocortical insufficiency. Clin Endocrinol **69**, 697–704.

Crowley RK, et al. (2014). Central hypoadrenalism. J Clin Endocrinol Metab **99**, 4027–36.

Pofi R, et al. (2018). The short Synacthen (corticotropin) test can be used to predict recovery of hypothalamo-pituitary-adrenal axis function. J Clin Endocrinol Metab **105**, 3050–9.

Skov J, et al. (2019). Sex-specific risk of cardiovascular disease in autoimmune Addison disease—a population-based cohort study. J Endocrinol Metab **104**, 2031–40.

Woods CP, et al. (2015). Adrenal suppression in patients taking inhaled glucocorticoids is highly prevalent and management can be guided by morning cortisol. Eur J Endocrinol **173**, 633–42.

Adrenal incidentalomas

Definition and epidemiology

- An adrenal incidentaloma is an adrenal mass that is discovered incidentally upon imaging (e.g. CT chest or abdomen) carried out for reasons other than a suspected adrenal pathology.
- The incidental detection of an adrenal mass is becoming commoner, as increasing numbers of imaging procedures are performed and with technological improvements in imaging (~85% are benign and non-functioning).
- Autopsy studies suggest prevalence of adrenal masses of 1–6% in the general population.
- Imaging studies suggest that adrenal masses are present in 2–3% in the general population. Incidence increases with ageing, and 8–10% of 70-year olds harbour an adrenal mass, compared with <1% aged <20 years—thus an ↑ risk of significance in younger patients.

Importance

It is important to determine whether the incidentally discovered adrenal mass is:

- Malignant.
- Functioning and associated with excess hormonal secretion.

Differential diagnosis of an incidentally detected adrenal nodule (median % incidence and range)

- Non-functioning adrenal adenoma: 75% (71–84%).
- Cortisol-secreting adrenal adenoma causing Cushing's syndrome or autonomous cortisol secretion (subclinical Cushing's syndrome): 12% (1–29%).
- MC-secreting adrenal adenoma: 2.5% (1.6–3.3%).
- CAH.
- ACC: 8% (1.2–11%).
- Metastasis (most prevalent in breast, lung, kidney): 5% (0–18%).
- PCC: 7% (1.5–14%).
- Adrenal cysts: 5% (4–22%).
- Adrenal myelolipoma: 8% (7–15%).
- Haematoma.
- Ganglioneuroma: 4% (0–8%).

Special circumstances

- Bilateral adrenal masses: assess each adrenal lesion individually.
- Urgent assessment required if aged <40 years as higher incidence of malignancy.
- History of extra-adrenal malignancy: check plasma/urinary metanephrines to exclude PCC; FDG-PET is useful to assess the nature of adrenal lesion; biopsy only if indeterminate and having excluded hormonal secretion and PCC.

Investigations

- Clinical assessment for symptoms and signs of excess hormone secretion and signs of extra-adrenal carcinoma.
- UFC and overnight dexamethasone (1mg) suppression test.
- Plasma free metanephrines (most sensitive and specific screening test; alternatively, urinary metanephrine—however, more cumbersome and less specific) (see ➔ Plasma metanephrine measurement, p. 318).
- Aldosterone/renin ratio and serum potassium.
- *Imaging*:
  - A homogeneous mass with a low attenuation value prior to contrast administration (<10HU) on CT scan is likely to be a benign adenoma (low density = high fat content = benign), whereas a mass with high density (>20HU) has to be considered suspicious (differential diagnosis PCC/ACC/metastasis, but also lipid-poor adenoma). Current guidelines (2016) recommend no further imaging if <4cm, homogeneous, <10HU adrenal incidentalomas.
  - If indeterminate on CT, an MDT review may recommend interval repeat at 6 months of alternative imaging.
  - MRI scanning with chemical shift may be helpful.
  - 18F-FDG PET-CT scanning can also be considered to further delineate benign from malignant.
- Additional tests if adrenal carcinoma suspected:
  - 24h urinary excretion of corticosteroid metabolites.
  - DHEAS, 17α-OH progesterone, progesterone.
  - 17α oestradiol (in ♂ only).
  - Androstenedione, testosterone.
- Adrenal biopsy is not recommended unless all the following criteria are met:
  - The lesion is hormonally inactive.
  - The lesion has not been conclusively characterized as benign by imaging.
  - Management would be altered by knowledge of the histology.

Management

- Up to 20% of patients may develop hormonal excess during follow-up.
- Cortisol is the commonest excess hormone.
- Surgery if there is/are:
  - Evidence of a syndrome of hormonal excess attributable to the tumour.
  - Biochemical evidence of PCC.
  - Mass diameter >4cm (↑ likelihood of malignancy according to imaging or biochemistry—co-secretion of several corticosteroids indicative of malignancy—and definitely if >6cm in diameter).
  - Imaging features suggestive of malignancy (e.g. lack of clearly circumscribed margin, vascular invasion).
  - It should be noted that post-operative adrenal suppression may occur if, preoperatively, there is biochemical evidence of GC excess, and therefore, glucocorticoids may be necessary post-operatively.

- Non-surgical management:
  - As most adrenal incidentalomas are detected upon contrast CT, a follow-up investigation without contrast to determine precontrast tumour density is preferable; for larger nodules (>3cm), this might be combined with CT washout studies (<40% 15min after contrast indicative of malignancy).
  - In patients with a lesion <4cm and benign appearance on imaging (precontrast CT density <10HU) and no hormonal hypersecretion, further imaging is not required.
  - Repeat biochemical screening (if normal at presentation) should only be performed if there are new signs or symptoms or worsening comorbidities.
  - In patients with tumours >4cm not undergoing surgery, and those with tumours <4cm with indeterminate characteristics on imaging, a repeat non-contrast CT or MRI scan should be performed at 6 months. Surgical resection should be considered if there is a >20% increase in size (in addition to an absolute increase of >5mm). Changes smaller than this should prompt additional imaging in a further 6 months.

Further reading

Ebbehoj A, et al. (2020). Epidemiology of adrenal tumours in Olmsted County, Minnesota, USA: a population-based cohort study. *Lancet Diabetes Endocrinol* **8**, 894–902.

Fassnacht M, et al. (2016). Management of adrenal incidentalomas: European Society of Endocrinology clinical practice guideline in collaboration with the European Network for the Study of Adrenal Tumors. *Eur J Endocrinol* **175**, G1–34.

Mansmann G, et al. (2004). The clinically inapparent adrenal mass: update in diagnosis and management. *Endocr Rev* **25**, 309–40.

Sherlock M, et al. (2020). Adrenal incidentaloma. *Endocr Rev* **41**, 775–820.

Turner HE, et al. (1998). Pituitary, adrenal and thyroid incidentalomas. *Endocr Rel Cancer* **5**, 131–50.

Young WF Jr (2007). Clinical practice. The incidentally discovered adrenal mass. *N Engl J Med* **356**, 601–10.

Phaeochromocytomas and paragangliomas

Definition

- *PCCs and paragangliomas (PGLs) are collectively known as PPGL, and are chromaffin tumours arising from the adrenal medulla (PCC) or extra-adrenal sympathetic/parasympathetic (PPGL) which secrete catecholamines and are rare causes of hypertension.*
- *Sympathetic paraganglia occur as follows.* In prevertebral, paravertebral, thoracoabdominal, and pelvis area and close to the reproductive organs, prostate, bladder, liver, and organ of Zuckerkandl (at the bifurcation of the aorta). Tumours arising from this sympathetic tissue are termed extra-adrenal functional paraganglioma (eFPGL).
- *Parasympathetic paraganglia* are located close to major arteries and nerves, e.g. carotid body, glomus jugulare, vagal, tympanic, pulmonary, and aorta. Tumours arising from the parasympathetic nervous system are referred to as head and neck paraganglioma (HNPGL), and only a minority of those show endocrine activity (~25%).

Incidence

Rare tumours, accounting for <0.1% of causes of hypertension. However, it is a very important diagnosis due to:
- The development of potentially fatal hypertensive crises.
- The reversibility of all its manifestations after surgical removal of the tumour.
- The lack of long-term efficacy of medical treatment.
- The appreciable incidence of malignancy.
- The implications of the identification of an underlying genetic cause (>30% of cases, e.g. *RET* mutations and co-incident medullary carcinoma, *VHL* mutations and co-incident angiomas, or *SDHB* mutations and their potential for recurrent and malignant tumours) (see also ⊃ Chapter 13).

Epidemiology

- Equal sex distribution, and most commonly present in the 3rd and 4th decades. Up to 50% may be diagnosed postmortem.
- Tumours may be bilateral, particularly where part of an inherited syndrome (see Table 3.9).
- Thirty to 40% of PPGLs are genetic.
- Multiple tumours, extra-adrenal location, or evidence of malignancy are indicators of a high likelihood of an underlying genetic cause. (See Box 3.8 for who should be screened.)

Pathophysiology

Sporadic tumours are usually unilateral and <10cm in diameter. Tumours associated with familial syndromes are more likely to be bilateral and associated with pre-existing medullary hyperplasia.

Table 3.9 Genetically caused syndromes associated with phaeochromocytomas

Familial phaeochromocytomas	Isolated AD trait
MEN2A and 2B (see ⊃ MEN type 2, pp. 684–5)	Mutation in *RET* proto-oncogene (chromosome 10)
	1° hyperparathyroidism and MTC associated with PCC (adrenal phaeochromocytoma (aPCA))
	MEN2B also associated with marfanoid phenotype and mucosal neuromas (tongue) (see ⊃ MEN type 2, pp. 684–5)
von Hippel–Lindau (VHL) syndrome (⊃ von Hippel–Lindau disease, pp. 662–4)	Mutation of *VHL* tumour suppressor gene (chromosome 3)
	Renal cell carcinoma, cerebellar haemangioblastoma, retinal angioma, renal and pancreatic cysts
	PCCs (aPCA/eFPGL) in 25%
NF (see ⊃ Neurofibromatosis, pp. 658–60)	AD condition caused by mutations of *NF1* gene on chromosome 17
	PCCs (aPCA/eFPGL) in 1.0% and mostly late presentation (>30 years)
Succinate dehydrogenase (*SDH*) mutations	*SDHA*: rare AD cause of aPCA, eFPGL, and HNPGL
	SDHB: AD cause of aPCA, eFPGL, HNPGL, and renal cell carcinoma. High frequency of malignancy and extra-adrenal tumours
	SDHC: AD cause of HNPGL (rarely, also of aPCA and eFPGL)
	SDHD: AD cause of HNPGL, aPCA, and eFPGL (disease manifestation only in individuals with paternal inheritance of mutation)
SDHAF2 (succinate dehydrogenase complex assembly factor 2)	Rare AD cause of PCC and paraganglioma (aPCA, eFPGL, HNPGL)
TMEM127 (transmembrane encoding gene (chromosome 2q11))	AD cause of aPCA, eFPGL, and HNPGL
Prolyl hydroxylase domain gene mutations	*PHD1*: AD cause of paraganglioma (eFPGL) and polycythaemia
	PHD2/EGLN1: AD cause of paraganglioma (eFPGL) and polycythaemia
HIF2A (hypoxia-inducible factor 2 alpha gene)	AD cause of aPCA and eFPGL associated with polycythaemia, retinopathy, and duodenal somatostatinomas
MAX (*MYC*-associated factor X, a tumour suppressor susceptibility gene)	AD cause of aPCA, higher incidence of bilateral and malignant tumours (as in SDHD parent-of-origin effect: disease manifestation only in individuals with paternal transmission of mutation)

Familial phaeochromocytomas	Isolated AD trait
MDH2 (malate dehydrogenase 2 gene)	Small numbers of cases described (eFPGL)
FH (fumarate hydratase)	Rare cause of aPCA and eFPGL. Associated with cutaneous and uterine leiomyomas and renal cell carcinoma
KIF1B (kinesin family member 1B gene)	Very small numbers of cases described (aPCA)

Box 3.8 Who should be screened for the presence of a phaeochromocytoma?

- Patients with a family history of gene mutations causing PCC/paraganglioma.
- Patients with paroxysmal symptoms.
- Young patients with hypertension (onset age <30 years).
- Patients with resistant hypertension (>140/90mmHg on three agents).
- Patients developing hypertensive crisis during general anaesthesia/surgery.
- Patients with unexplained heart failure.
- Patients with an adrenal incidentaloma.

Malignancy

- ~15–20% are malignant, and these are characterized by local invasion or distant metastasis, rather than capsular invasion.
- Differentiating between benign and malignant tumours is difficult and mainly based on the presence of metastases, although chromosomal ploidy may be useful.
- Paragangliomas are more likely to be malignant and to recur.
- Typical sites for metastases are the retroperitoneum, lymph nodes, bone, liver, and mediastinum.

Secretory products

- Catecholamine secretion is usually adrenaline or noradrenaline and may be constant or episodic.
- Phenylethanolamine-*N*-methyltransferase (PNMT) is necessary for methylation of noradrenaline to adrenaline and is cortisol-dependent.
- Paragangliomas (exception—organ of Zuckerkandl) secrete noradrenaline only, as they lack PNMT.
- Small adrenal tumours tend to produce more adrenaline, whereas larger adrenal tumours produce more noradrenaline, as a proportion of their blood supply is direct, rather than corticomedullary, and therefore lower in cortisol concentrations.
- Pure dopamine secretion is rare and may be associated with hypotension. These tumours are more likely to be malignant.

- Other non-catecholamine secretory products may also be produced, including vasoactive intestinal polypeptide (VIP), neuropeptide Y, ACTH (associated with Cushing's syndrome), parathyroid hormone (PTH), and parathyroid hormone-related peptide (PTHrP).

Clinical features

- Sustained or episodic *hypertension* often resistant to conventional therapy (BUT: more and more PCCs are found incidentally following CT imaging, thus may not show any clinical signs and symptoms).
- The presence of palpitation, headaches, or sweating in a patient with hypertension should raise the diagnostic query of PCC.
- *General:*
  - Sweating and heat intolerance >80%.
  - Pallor or flushing.
  - Feeling of apprehension.
  - Pyrexia.
- *Neurological*—headache (throbbing or constant) (65%), paraesthesiae, visual disturbance, seizures.
- *Cardiovascular*—palpitations (65%), chest pain, dyspnoea, postural hypotension.
- *GI*—abdominal pain, constipation, nausea.
- *Skin*—livedo reticularis.
- *Endocrine*—paroxysmal thyroid swelling (noradrenaline-secreting).

Complications

- *Cardiovascular*—left ventricular failure, dilated cardiomyopathy (reversible), dysrhythmias.
- *Respiratory*—pulmonary oedema.
- *Metabolic*—carbohydrate intolerance, hypercalcaemia.
- *Neurological*—cerebrovascular, hypertensive encephalopathy.

Factors precipitating a crisis

- Straining.
- Exercise.
- Pressure on abdomen—tumour palpation, bending over.
- Surgery.
- Drugs:
  - Anaesthetics.
  - Unopposed β-blockade.
  - IV contrast agents.
  - Opiates.
  - Tricyclic antidepressants (TCAs).
  - Phenothiazines.
  - Metoclopramide.
  - Glucagon.

Investigations of phaeochromocytomas and paragangliomas

Demonstrate catecholamine hypersecretion

A 24h urine collection is the standard test for screening for a PCC. In a patient with suggestive symptoms, this is usually sufficient to confirm or exclude the diagnosis. False −ves are commoner when patients are asymptomatic and early in the disease. Particular care is needed in familial cases and incidentalomas, and in those in whom a general anaesthetic has precipitated a hypertensive episode. Metanephrines (either urine or plasma) offer more specific diagnostic tools than measurement of unmetabolized catecholamines and provide the best biochemical tests for diagnosing PCC (see Table 3.11 for sensitivity and specificity of tests).

24h urine collection for catecholamines/metanephrines

(See Tables 3.10 and 3.11.)

- Urine is collected into bottles containing acid (warn patient).
- Because of the episodic nature of catecholamine secretion, at least 2× 24h collections should be performed. It is useful to perform a collection while the patient is having symptoms if episodic secretion is suspected.
- Urinary metanephrines are of similar sensitivity, but of superior specificity, to urinary catecholamines. The sensitivity of urinary vanillylmandelic acid (VMA) is less than that of free catecholamines or metadrenalines and also influenced by dietary intake and should not be used.

NB. TCAs and labetalol interfere with adrenaline measurements and should be stopped for 4 days.

- For marginal elevation, urine collections should be repeated, avoiding nuts (walnuts), fruit (bananas and pineapple), potatoes, and beans.

Plasma metanephrine measurement

- Plasma metanephrines are the most sensitive test for detection of catecholamine excess and have only slightly lower specificity than urinary metanephrines (see Table 3.10).
- If plasma metanephrines are borderline, urinary metanephrines may be used for confirmation.
- Routine measurement requires controlled conditions—supine and cannulated for 30min; however, false +ves are rare; thus, screening can be carried out in the sitting position without 30min rest, and only borderline +ve cases require repeat after 30min supine rest.
- Plasma catecholamines are elevated by renal failure, caffeine, nicotine, exercise, and some drugs.
- Catecholamine levels in asymptomatic individuals investigated for an adrenal incidentaloma or due to a familial condition are often diagnosed at an earlier stage and may therefore have lower catecholamines.
- Plasma and urinary methoxytyramine levels are indicators of malignancy and can show isolated increases in patients with 'biochemically −ve' malignant PCC.

Table 3.10 Substances interfering with urinary catecholamine levels

↑ catecholamines	↓ catecholamines	Variable effect
α-blockers	MAOIs	Levodopa
β-blockers, e.g. phenoxybenzamine	Clonidine	TCAs
Levodopa	Guanethidine and other adrenergic neurone blockers	Phenothiazines
Drugs containing catecholamines, e.g. decongestants		Calcium channel inhibitors
Metoclopramide		ACEIs
Domperidone		Bromocriptine
Hydralazine		
Diazoxide		
Glyceryl trinitrate (GTN)		
Sodium nitroprusside		
Nicotine		
Theophylline		
Caffeine		
Amphetamine		

Table 3.11 Sensitivity and specificity of tests

Test	Sensitivity (%)	Specificity (%)
Plasma metanephrines	97	92
Urinary metanephrines	85	95
Urinary catecholamines	88	78
Urinary VMA	65	88
Clonidine suppression test	97	
MRI	98	70
CT	93	70
MIBG	80	95

Clonidine suppression tests
(See Box 3.9.)
  This test may be used to differentiate patients who have borderline cat-echolamine levels but may offer little advantage over the screening tests already described.
• *Clonidine 300 micrograms PO*—failure of suppression of plasma catecholamines into the normal range at 120 and 180min is suggestive of a tumour.

Provocative tests
These are not used routinely, as they do not enhance diagnostic accuracy and are potentially dangerous.

Localization of tumour

Imaging
• These are large tumours, in contrast to Conn's syndrome, and not easily missed with good-quality imaging to the bifurcation of the aorta; ~98% will be detected in the abdomen.
• <2% are in the chest, and 0.02% are in the head.
• Adrenal imaging (CT) with non-ionic contrast should be performed initially, then body imaging (ideally MRI) if tumour not localized in the adrenal.
• *MRI*. Bright hyperintense image on T_2.

Functional imaging
(See Table 3.12.)
• This aids localization, as well as characterization. The most useful 1st-line investigation is FDG-PET.

Positron emission tomography
• Several different tracers.
• ^{18}F-FDG and the noradrenaline analogue ^{11}C-metahydroxyephedrine (mHED) have both been used as radionucleotides.
• ^{18}F-fluorodopa (catecholamine precursor) is useful for head and neck paragangliomas.
• ^{68}Ga-labelled SSAs are also promising.

^{123}I-MIBG scan
(See Box 3.10.)
• *MIBG* is a chromaffin-seeking analogue. Imaging using MIBG is +ve in 60–80% of PCCs and may locate tumours not visualized on MRI, e.g. multiple and extra-adrenal tumours and also metastases of the 1° tumour.
• Specificity is nearly 100%.
• Performed preoperatively to exclude multiple tumours.
• NB. Phenoxybenzamine may lead to false −ve MIBG imaging, so these scans should be performed before commencing this drug where possible.

Further reading

Taïeb D, *et al.* (2014). Current approaches and recent developments in the management of head and neck paragangliomas. *Endocr Rev* **35**, 795–819.

Table 3.12 Sensitivity and specificity of imaging modalities for phaeochromocytoma

Imaging modality	1° (non-metastatic)		Head/neck PGL (%)	Metastatic (%)	SDHB metastatic (%)	Non-SDHB metastatic (%)	Bone metastases (%)
	Sensitivity (%)	Specificity (%)					
FDG-PET	77–88	90	67–76	74–82	83–100	49–67.3	76–93
FDOPA PET	67–93	100	92–100	45	20	75–93	–
FDA-PET	78–88	90	40–46	76	79–82	76–78	79–100
⁶⁸Ga-DOTATATE PET	73–100	86–100	100	92–100	98	97–100	100
MIBG	67–87	82–100	31–33	50–93	44–57	59–66	61–76
Octreoscan	28.5	75	64	68–89	59–81	–	–
CT/MRI	95–100	40–90	42–80	74	78	71–82	65–96

FDA, ^{18}F-fluorodopamine; FDG, ^{18}F-fluorodeoxyglucose; FDOPA, ^{18}F-fluorodopa; MIBG, metaiodobenzylguanidine; PGL, paraganglioma.

Reproduced from Turner H, Eastell R, and Grossman A (2018) *Endocrinology: Oxford Desk Reference* Oxford: Oxford University Press, with permission from Oxford University Press.

Box 3.9 Test procedures

Clonidine suppression test
- Patient supine and cannulated for 30min.
- Clonidine 300 micrograms PO.
- Plasma catecholamines measured at time 0, 120, and 180min.
- Failure to suppress into the normal range is suggestive of a tumour.
- False +ve rate of 1.5% in patients with essential hypertension.

Box 3.10 Drugs interfering with MIBG uptake in phaeochromocytoma[*]

- Opioids.
- Cocaine.
- Tramadol.
- TCAs:
  - Amitriptyline, imipramine.
- Sympathomimetics:
  - Phenylpropanolamine, pseudoephedrine, amphetamine, dopamine, salbutamol.
- Antihypertensives/cardiovascular agents:
  - Labetalol, metoprolol, amiodarone, reserpine, guanethidine, calcium channel blockers—nifedipine and amlodipine, ACEIs—captopril and enalapril.

[*] Should be discontinued 7–14 days prior to scan.

Screening for associated conditions

Up to 24% of patients with apparently sporadic PCCs may have a familial disorder, and high-risk patients should therefore be screened for the presence of associated conditions, even if asymptomatic.

Genetic testing

All patients with a PCC or paraganglioma should be considered for genetic testing to identify possible germline mutations. Genetic testing in non-syndromic PCC has shown a hereditary predisposition in 24%, of which 45% had germline mutations in *VHL*, 20% had mutations in *RET*, 18% had mutations in *SDHD*, and 17% had mutations in *SDHB*.
- Specific associated features may offer a guide as to the likely underlying genetic aetiology (see Table 3.9).
- Appropriate counselling before and after the test should be available.

MEN2

(See ➲ MEN type 2, pp. 684–5.)
- Serum calcium.
- Serum calcitonin (PCCs precede MTC in 10%).

VHL

(See ➲ von Hippel-Lindau disease, pp. 662–4.)
- Ophthalmoscopy—retinal angiomas are usually the 1st manifestation.
- MRI—posterior fossa and spinal cord.
- US of kidneys—if not adequately imaged on MRI of adrenals.

NF1

(See ➲ Neurofibromatosis, pp. 658–9.)
- Clinical examination for café-au-lait spots and cutaneous neuromas.

Succinate dehydrogenase (subunits A, B, C, D)

- The SDH enzyme consists of four subunits (A, B, C, and D). SDHC and SDHD anchor the two other components which form the catalytic core to the inner mitochondrial membrane. The enzyme is a component of Krebs' cycle and also regulates the downregulation of the transcription factor HIF1α.
- The D subunit gene is located on chromosome 11q21–23, and the B subunit on chromosome 1p35–6.
- Mutations in SDHB, SDHC, and SDHD may cause aPCA, eFPGL, and HNPGL.
- Mutations in SDHD have been associated with familial carotid body tumours.
- Germline SDHA mutations are associated with juvenile encephalopathy.
- SDH mutations show maternal imprinting, so that only carriers who inherit the mutation paternally are at risk of developing a tumour.
- Rates of penetrance and malignancy vary—SDHB mutation may be associated with a more malignant phenotype.

Other susceptibility genes
- *MAX* encodes transcription factor.
- *TMEM127* (linked to the mTOR (mammalian target of rapamycin) pathway).

Surveillance in presymptomatic carriers with familial phaeochromocytoma and paraganglioma syndromes

First-degree relatives of patients with familial PCC and paraganglioma syndromes should be offered genetic testing. In presymptomatic individuals, where mutations have been identified, the following investigations should be considered.
- Surveillance should start at least 5 years before the age of the youngest presentation within the family (usually between the age of 5 and 16 years).
- Clinical examination should be performed annually.
- Biochemical screening with plasma metanephrines should be performed annually.
- MRI (abdomen, neck, thorax) should be performed initially and then repeated every 2–3 years.
- Surveillance should continue at least until the age of 75 years and then reassessed on a case-by-case basis.
- For patients with asymptomatic mutations in *SDHD*, *SDHAF2*, and *MAX*, screening should only be undertaken if the mutation was paternally inherited (as imprinted).

Management

Medical

- It is essential that any patient is fully prepared with α- and β-blockade before receiving IV contrast or undergoing a procedure such as venous sampling or surgery.
- α-blockade must be commenced before β-blockade to avoid precipitating a hypertensive crisis due to unopposed α-adrenergic stimulation.
- *α-blockade*—commence phenoxybenzamine as soon as the diagnosis is made. Start at 10mg bd by mouth, and increase up to 20mg qds (doxazosin is an accepted alternative).
- *β-blockade*—use a β-blocker, such as propranolol 20–80mg 8-hourly by mouth, 48–72h after starting phenoxybenzamine and with evidence of adequate α-blockade (generally noted by a postural fall in BP).
- Calcium channel blockers can be useful if severe side effects with α- and β-blockade, inadequate BP control, to void severe hypotension with α-blockade.
- Treatment may need to be commenced in hospital. Monitor BP, pulse, and haematocrit. The goal is a BP of 130/80mmHg or less sitting and 100mmHg systolic standing, and pulse 60–70bpm sitting and 70–80bpm standing. Reversal of α-mediated vasoconstriction may lead to haemodilution (check Hb preoperatively).
- To ensure complete blockade before surgery, IV *phenoxybenzamine* (1mg/kg over 4h in 100mL of 5% glucose) can be administered 3 days before surgery. There is less experience with competitive α-adrenergic blockade such as prazosin.

  (See Table 3.13 for contraindicated drugs.)

Surgical

(Also considered in ⊃ Phaeochromocytoma, p. 326.)

- Surgical resection is curative in the majority of patients, leading to normotension in at least 75%.
- Mortality from elective surgery is <2%. It is essential that the anaesthetic and surgical teams have expertise of management of PCCs perioperatively.
- Surgery may be laparoscopic if the tumour is small and apparently benign. Careful perioperative anaesthetic management is essential, as tumour handling may lead to major changes in BP and also occasionally cardiac arrhythmias. *Phentolamine, nitroprusside,* or *IV nicardipine* are useful to treat perioperative hypertension, and *esmolol* or *propranolol* for perioperative arrhythmias. Hypotension (e.g. after tumour devascularization) usually responds to volume replacement but occasionally requires inotropic support.
- Risk factors for haemodynamic instability during surgery include a high noradrenaline concentration, a large tumour size, a postural drop after β-blockade, and a mean arterial pressure >100mmHg.

Table 3.13 Contraindicated drugs in phaeochromocytomas

Drug	Examples
β-blockers	Propranolol
D2 receptor antagonists	Metoclopramide Sulpiride Chlorpromazine
TCAs	Imipramine Amitriptyline Paroxetine Fluoxetine
MAOIs	
Sympathomimetics	Ephedrine Salbutamol Cocaine
Chemotherapeutic agents	
Opioid analgesics	
Neuromuscular-blocking agents	Tubocurarine Suxamethonium
Peptide and corticosteroid hormones	Glucagon ACTH Dexamethasone

Follow-up

- Cure is assessed by 24h urinary free catecholamine or plasma metanephrine measurements. However, catecholamines may remain elevated for up to 10 days following surgery. Follow-up assessments should therefore be performed until 2–6 weeks post-operatively. Thereafter, in the absence of symptoms, they should be measured annually (but as a matter of urgency with new clinical signs or symptoms).
- Cardiac involvement infrequent and this may persist after resection of the tumour.
- Imaging investigations should be performed 3 months post-operatively.
- Lifelong follow-up is essential to detect recurrence of a benign tumour or metastasis from a malignant tumour, as it is impossible to exclude malignancy on a histological specimen.
- Chromogranin A is also a useful marker (falsely elevated with proton pump therapy, steroids, liver and renal failure, essential hypertension, atrophic gastritis, prostatic carcinoma, and thyrotoxicosis).

Malignancy

- Malignant tumours require long-term α- and β-blockade. The TKI α-*methylparatyrosine* may help control symptoms.
- High-dose ^{131}I-MIBG can be used to treat metastatic disease. (Ensure patient avoids drugs blocking MIBG uptake (see Box 3.9) and are adequately blocked for catecholamie release.)
- RFA can be useful for hepatic/bone metastases (pretreatment blockade is essential).
- Radiolabelled SSAs have been evaluated.
- Chemotherapy, using *cyclophosphamide*, *vincristine*, and *dacarbazine* (CVD) has been associated with symptomatic improvement.
- Radiotherapy can be useful palliation in patients with bony metastases.
- Novel treatment options for malignant PCC are urgently needed, and current studies investigating VEGF inhibitors, e.g. sunitinib, and mTOR inhibitors have been investigated, depending on the mutation involved.

Prognosis

- Hypertension may persist in 25% of patients who have undergone successful tumour removal.
- The 5-year survival for 'benign' tumours is 96%, and the recurrence rate is <10%.
- The 5-year survival for malignant tumours is 44%.
- *SHB* gene mutations in patients are associated with shorter survival.

Further reading

Ayala-Ramirez M, et al. (2012). Treatment with sunitinib for patients with progressive metastatic pheochromocytomas and sympathetic paragangliomas. *J Clin Endocrinol Metab* **97**, 4040–50.

Eisenhofer G, et al. (2011). Measurements of plasma methoxytyramine, normetanephrine and metanephrine as discriminators of different hereditary forms of phaeochromocytoma. *Clin Chem* **57**, 411–20.

Erickson D, et al. (2001). Benign paragangliomas: clinical presentation and treatment outcomes in 236 patients. *J Clin Endocrinol Metab* **86**, 5210–16.

Ferreira VM, et al. (2016). Pheochromocytoma Is characterized by catecholamine-mediated myocarditis, focal and diffuse myocardial fibrosis, and myocardial dysfunction. *J Am Coll Cardiol* **67**, 2364–74.

Ilias I, et al. (2003). Superiority of 6-[18F]-fluorodopamine positron emission tomography versus [131I]-metaiodobenzylguanidine scintigraphy in the localization of metastatic pheochromocytoma. *J Clin Endocrinol Metab* **88**, 4083–7.

Lenders JW, et al. (2014). Pheochromocytoma and paraganglioma: an Endocrine Society clinical practice guideline. *J Clin Endocrinol Metab* **99**, 1915–42.

Murth A, et al. (2019). Genetic testing and surveillance guidelines in hereditarypheochromocytoma and paraganglioma. *J Intern Med* **285**, 187–204.

Nedmann HPH, et al. (2019). Pheochromocytoma and paraganglioma. *N Engl J Med* **381**, 552–65.

NGS in PPGL (NGSnPPGL) Study Group; Toledo RA, et al. (2017). Consensus Statement on next-generation-sequencing-based diagnostic testing of hereditary phaeochromocytomas and paragangliomas. *Nat Rev Endocrinol* **13**, 233–47.

Ploulin PF, et al. (2016). European Society of Endocrinology Clinical Practice Guideline for long-term follow-up of patients operated on for a phaeochromocytoma or a paraganglioma. *Eur J Endocrinol* **174**, G1–10.

Rimoldi SF, et al. (2014). Secondary arterial hypertension: when, who, and how to screen? *Eur Heart J* **35**, 1245–54.

Shah MH, et al. (2018). NCCN Guidelines Insights. Neuroendocrine and adrenal tumors. *J Natl Compr Cancer Netw* **16**, 693–702.

Chapter 4

Reproductive endocrinology

Waljit Dhillo, Melanie Davies, Channa Jayasena, and Leighton Seal

Reproductive physiology

Anatomy

- Normal adult ♂ testicular volume 15–30mL.
- Normal adult ♀ mean ovarian volume peaks at age 20 years to 7.7mL (reference range 4.8–12mL).
- Two gonadotrophins LH and FSH address two gonadal cell types, with feedback from sex steroids and inhibin.
- Three important cells of the gonad:
  - *Interstitial cells.* ♂ Leydig cells, ♀ theca cells—which are found in between the seminiferous tubules and follicles, respectively. Produce testosterone under LH drive.
  - *Cells supporting gametogenesis.* ♂ Sertoli cells, ♀ granulosa cells— secrete various hormones, including inhibin and anti-Müllerian hormone (AMH) under FSH drive. Inhibin inhibits FSH secretion from the pituitary gland, and AMH is responsible for suppressing ♀ sex organ development during sexual differentiation *in utero*. In adult ♀, AMH is produced in proportion to the number of antral follicles of 2–9mm in diameter and is therefore a marker of ovarian reserve. AMH peaks in a ♀ in her early twenties and falls from the age of 30 years onwards to undetectable levels at menopause.
  - *Germ cells.* ♂ continue to make new germ cells throughout adult life in the basal membrane of tubules. ♀ cease to make new germ cells after birth and are therefore born with all of the 'eggs' that they will ever make.
- Functional units:
  - ♂ *seminiferous tubules.* Make up 90% of testicular volume. Spermatogenesis occurs here in the presence of high intratesticular concentrations of testosterone. Made up of germ cells and Sertoli cells through which spermatogonia mature to be released into the lumen of the tubule.
  - ♀ *Graafian follicle.* Follicles develop from primordial, through to 1°, 2°, and antral to Graafian follicles. Primordial follicles are recruited in batches, with selection of a dominant follicle with a single central oocyte surrounded by granulosa cells which convert theca-derived testosterone to oestradiol. Follicles which do not proceed to ovulation become atretic.

Regulation of gonadal function

(See Fig. 4.1 for normal menstrual cycle.)

Hypothalamus

- *GnRH* is secreted by the hypothalamus in a pulsatile manner in response to stimuli from the cerebral cortex and limbic system via various neurotransmitters, e.g. leptin, kisspeptin, endorphins, catecholamines, and dopamine.
- GnRH release initially occurs during sleep in early puberty and then throughout the day in adulthood. It stimulates the secretion of *LH* and *FSH* by the pituitary gland. The pattern of GnRH secretion is crucial for normal gonadotrophin secretion. Faster pulse frequencies favour LH secretion, whereas slower frequencies favour FSH secretion.
- GnRH must be given in a pulsatile manner in order to stimulate the reproductive axis, whereas continuous administration leads to downregulation. Thus, long-acting GnRH analogues (e.g. goserelin, triptorelin, leuprorelin) can be used to suppress sex steroid levels, e.g. in the treatment of prostate cancer and endometriosis.

Pituitary

- LH drives interstitial cell synthesis and secretion of testosterone in both sexes and triggers ovulation in ♀. −ve feedback by sex steroids.
- FSH in ♂ drives Sertoli cell-mediated sperm maturation and production of seminiferous tubule fluid, as well as a number of substances thought to be important for spermatogenesis. FSH in ♀ drives granulosa cell-mediated aromatization of androgens to oestradiol. −ve feedback mainly by inhibin.

Gonads

- Testosterone and small amounts of androstenedione, DHEA, and dihydrotestosterone (DHT) are produced by *Leydig cells*. ♂ testosterone has a circadian rhythm, with maximum secretion at around 8 a.m. and minimum at around 9 p.m. ♀ testosterone production peaks at ovulation.
- Oestradiol production in ♂ mainly from peripheral conversion from androgens. In ♀, oestradiol rises with follicle maturation under FSH drive of granulosa cells. Oestradiol is also made by the placenta, adrenal, and corpus luteum.
- Progesterone is secreted from the corpus luteum, which is derived from luteinized granulosa cells in the remnants of the follicle following ovulation. Peak production occurs at the mid-luteal phase (day 21 of a 28-day cycle). It is also secreted from the placenta.

Regulation of gametogenesis

- Both FSH and LH are required for gametogenesis.
- LH ensures high intragonadal concentrations of testosterone (exogenous testosterone cannot substitute).
- FSH, through its action on Sertoli ♂ and granulosa ♀ cells, is vital for sperm and follicle growth, respectively.

- ♂. The whole process of spermatogenesis takes ~74 days, followed by another 12–21 days for sperm transport through the epididymis. This means that events which may affect spermatogenesis may not be apparent for up to 3 months, and successful induction of spermatogenesis treatment may take up to 2 years.
- ♀. From primordial follicle to 1° follicle, it takes about 180 days (a continuous process) and another 60 days to form a preantral follicle. An antral follicle may then proceed to become a dominant follicle under FSH drive over 2–3 weeks and ovulate following the mid-cycle LH surge.

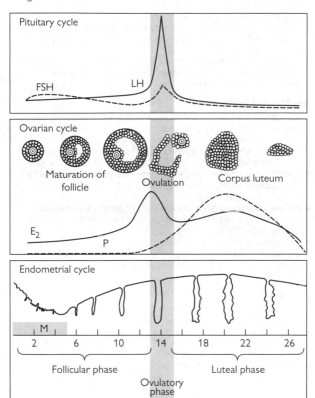

Fig. 4.1 The normal menstrual cycle.

Reproductive physiology

Sex steroid transport

- Testosterone daily production rate in ♂ is 5–15mg; 2–4% of total testosterone circulates as free biologically active hormone.
  - The rest is bound to proteins, particularly albumin (~38%) and SHBG (~60%).
  - Testosterone is bound to albumin with lower affinity than to SHBG, such that albumin-bound testosterone also can be regarded as 'bioavailable'.
  - Several equations are used to estimate free testosterone; free androgen index ((total testosterone/SHBG) × 100) is of limited value in men, and web-based calculators of free testosterone taking into account SHBG and albumin, e.g. Vermeulen equation, have better validation.
- Androstenedione is only about 6% SHBG-bound.
- Oestradiol daily production rate in ♀ is 40–400 micrograms; 2–3% of free oestradiol is biologically active; the rest is bound to SHBG.

Sex steroid metabolism

- Testosterone is converted in target tissues to the more potent androgen DHT in the presence of the enzyme 5α-reductase. There are multiple 5α-reductase isoenzymes; type 2 is the isoenzyme responsible for DHT synthesis in the genitalia, genital skin, and hair follicles. It is therefore essential for normal ♂ virilization and sexual development.
- Testosterone may alternatively be converted into oestradiol through the action of the aromatase enzyme, found in greatest quantities in the testes and adipose tissue.
- Many effects previously attributed to testosterone are now known to be mediated by oestrogen—especially closure of epiphyses and maintenance of bone density.
- Testosterone and its metabolites are inactivated in the liver and excreted in the urine.
- Oestradiol is conjugated in the liver to sulphates and glucuronates and then extracted in the urine.

Androgen action

- Both testosterone and DHT exert their activity by binding to androgen receptors, DHT more avidly than testosterone.
- ♂ sexual differentiation during embryogenesis.
- Development and maintenance of ♂ 2° sex characteristics after puberty.
- Normal ♂ sexual function and behaviour.
- Spermatogenesis.

Oestrogen action

- Oestradiol binds to α (reproductive tissues) and β (bone, brain, heart, etc.) receptors.
- Development of ♀ 2° sex characteristics.
- Increase in fat stores.
- Increase in vaginal wall and uterine thickening.
- Regulation of gonadotrophin secretion.

Progesterone action

- Involved in ovulation, implantation, and pregnancy.
- Regulation of uterine function during the menstrual cycle, controlling cyclical changes in proliferation and decidualization.
- Smooth muscle relaxation.
- CNS effects, including mood modulation.

Further reading

De Ronde W, et al. (2003). The importance of oestrogens in males. Clin Endocrinol **58**, 529–42.
Vermeulen A, et al. (1999). Critical evaluation of simple methods for the estimation of free testosterone in serum. J Clin Endocrinol Metab **84**, 3666–72.

Hirsutism

Definition

Hirsutism is excessive terminal hair that appears in a ♂ pattern in ♀ as a result of ↑ androgen production or ↑ skin sensitivity to androgens. (See Table 4.1 for causes; see Box 4.1 for signs of virilization.)

Physiology of hair growth

- Before puberty, the body is covered by fine, unpigmented hairs called vellus hairs.
- During adolescence, androgens convert vellus hairs into coarse, pigmented terminal hairs in androgen-dependent areas.
  - The extent of terminal hair growth depends on the concentration and duration of androgen exposure, as well as on the sensitivity of the individual hair follicle.
  - Idiopathic hirsutism refers to those with normal investigations and presumably greater-than-average androgen receptor sensitivity.
- The reason different body regions respond differently to the same androgen concentration is unknown but may be related to the number of androgen receptors in the hair follicle. Genetic factors play an important role in the individual susceptibility to circulating androgens, as evidenced by racial differences in hair growth.

Androgen production in women

In ♀, testosterone is secreted primarily by the ovaries and adrenal glands, although a significant amount is produced by the peripheral conversion of androstenedione and DHEA. Ovarian androgen production is regulated by LH, whereas adrenal production is ACTH-dependent. The predominant androgens produced by the ovaries are testosterone and androstenedione, and the adrenal glands are the main source of DHEA. Circulating testosterone is mainly bound to SHBG, and it is the free testosterone which is biologically active. Testosterone is converted to DHT in the skin by the enzyme 5α-reductase. Androstenedione and DHEA are not significantly protein-bound (see Fig. 4.2).

Table 4.1 Causes of hirsutism

Ovarian	PCOS	95%
	Androgen-secreting tumours	<1%
Adrenal	CAH	1%
	Cushing's syndrome	<1%
	Androgen-secreting tumours	<1%
	Acromegaly	<1%
	Severe insulin resistance	<1%
Idiopathic	Normal US and endocrine profile	3%
Drugs	For example, ciclosporin, danazol, diazoxide	

Box 4.1 Signs of virilization
- Frontal balding.
- Deepening of voice.
- ↑ muscle size.
- Clitoromegaly.

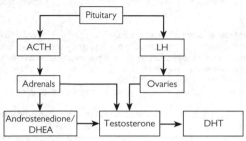

Fig. 4.2 Regulation of androgen production in ♀.

Evaluation of hirsutism

(See Box 4.2 for androgen-independent hair growth.)

Androgen-dependent hirsutism

Normally develops following puberty. Hairs are coarse and pigmented and typically grow in ♂ pattern. It is often accompanied by other evidence of androgen excess such as acne, oily skin and hair, and ♂ pattern alopecia.

History

- *Age and rate of onset of hirsutism.* Slowly progressive hirsutism following puberty suggests a benign cause, whereas rapidly progressive hirsutism of recent onset requires further immediate investigation to rule out an androgen-secreting neoplasm.
- *Menstrual history.* ? oligomenorrhoea
- Presence of other evidence of *hyperandrogenism*, e.g. acne or bitemporal hair recession.
- *Drug history.* Some progestins used in oral contraceptive preparations may be androgenic (e.g. norethisterone) (see Box 4.2).
- Treatments are often based on subjective appearance, so be cautious if there is a great disparity between subjective and objective assessment. Consider psychological background.

Physical examination

- Distinguish between *androgen-dependent* and *androgen-independent* hair growth (hypertrichosis).
- Assess the *extent* and *severity* of hirsutism. The Ferriman–Gallwey score is a tool that assesses the degree of hair growth in 11 regions of the body (see Fig. 4.3). Total scores >4–6, depending on ethnicity, define hirsutism.
- *Virilization* should be looked for only in suspected cases of severe hyperandrogenism (see Box 4.1).
- *Acanthosis nigricans* is indicative of insulin resistance which can be associated with PCOS.
- *Rare causes* of hyperandrogenism, such as Cushing's syndrome and acromegaly, should be ruled out.

Laboratory investigation

Serum testosterone should be measured in all ♀ presenting with hirsutism. If this is <5nmol/L, then the risk of a sinister cause for her hirsutism is low. Further investigations and management of the individual disorders will be discussed in the following chapters.

Imaging

Pelvic US may be useful to diagnose PCOS (see ➲ Investigations of PCOS, pp. 344–5). Idiopathic hirsutism refers to those with normal ovarian morphology, but this distinction is not clear-cut, as the level of detection of polycystic ovary morphology on US is operator-dependent.

Management

Management is largely either pharmacological or direct hair removal. For the majority of women who are not seeking fertility, oral contraceptives are front-line treatment. Lower oestrogen-dose, low-risk progestin oral contraceptives are recommended in women with a higher risk of VTE (e.g. obese or over 39 years old).

Box 4.2 Androgen-independent hair growth

Excess vellus hairs over face and trunk, including forehead. It does not respond to antiandrogen treatment.

Causes of androgen-independent hair growth
- Drugs, e.g. phenytoin, ciclosporin, glucocorticoids.
- Anorexia nervosa.
- Hypothyroidism.
- Familial.

For direct hair removal, electrolysis is preferred over photoepilation for those with blonde or white hair.

❶ Potential complications of photoepilation may occur in women of colour. Women of Mediterranean or Middle Eastern background should be warned of potential paradoxical hair growth. Unintentional injury is more likely to occur with darker skin pigmentation.

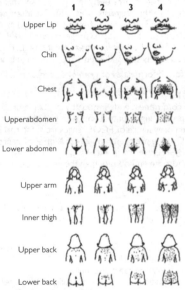

Fig. 4.3 The Ferriman–Gallwey score.

Reprinted from Rosenfield R.L (1986) "Pilosebaceous physiology in relation to hirsutism and acne" *Clin Endocrinology and Metabolism* 15(2):341–362, with permission from Elsevier.

Further reading

Barrionvevo P, et al. (2018). Treatment options for hirsutism: a systematic review and network meta-analysis. *J Clin Endocrinol Metab* **103**, 1258–64.

Koulori O, Conway G (2009). Management of hirsutism. *BMJ* **338**, 823–6.

Loriaux DL (2012). An approach to the patient with hirsutism. *J Clin Endocrinol Metab* **97**, 2957–68.

Martin KA, et al. (2018). Evaluation and treatment of hirsutism in premenopausal women: an Endocrine Society clinical guideline. *J Clin Endocrinol Metab* **103**, 1233–57.

Polycystic ovary syndrome

Definition

- A heterogeneous clinical syndrome characterized by hyperandrogenism, menstrual irregularity, and polycystic ovary morphology in which other causes of androgen excess have been excluded (see Boxes 4.3 and 4.4). It is supported by hyperinsulinaemia/glucose intolerance.
- The diagnosis is further supported by the presence of characteristic ovarian morphology on US in at least one ovary. Note the misnomer: the ovarian appearance refers to >12 follicles per ovary, i.e. polyfollicle syndrome by Rotterdam criteria, or more recently ≥20 follicles per ovary by the 2018 international guidelines.
- A distinction is made between polycystic ovary morphology on ultrasound (PCO) and PCOS—the syndrome, where PCO is also associated with other clinical features of PCOS such as hyperandrogenism or menstrual disturbance. Many causes of hyperandrogenism mimic features of PCOS, including PCO morphology (see Box 4.4 for other causes of hyperandrogenism that can be considered prior to the diagnosis of PCOS). The international PCOS guidelines recommend that CAH should be excluded in all patients with a measurement of 17-hydroxyprogesterone (17OHP) during the follicular phase. Investigations for rarer conditions such as Cushing's syndrome should only be conducted if there is a high index of suspicion.

(See Fig. 4.4 for abnormalities of hormone secretion in PCOS.)

Epidemiology

- PCOS is the commonest endocrinopathy in ♀ of reproductive age; >95% of ♀ presenting to outpatients with hirsutism have PCOS.
- The estimated prevalence of PCOS ranges from 5% to 13%. Polycystic ovaries on US alone are present in 20–25% of ♀ of reproductive age.
- First-degree ♂ relatives of ♀ with PCOS have ↑ prevalence of metabolic syndrome and obesity than the general population.

Pathogenesis

(See Fig. 4.4.)

The fundamental pathophysiological defect is unknown, but both genetic and environmental factors are thought to play a role.

Genetic

- Familial aggregation of PCOS in 50% of ♀. A family history of T2DM is also commoner in ♀ with PCOS.
- PCOS is probably a polygenic disorder.
- Implicated genes include those of the insulin pathway, testosterone biosynthesis enzymes, and obesity-related genes, including the *FTO* gene.

Hyperandrogenism
- The main source of hyperandrogenaemia is the ovaries, although there may also be adrenal androgen hypersecretion, particularly in lean women with PCOS.
- The biochemical basis of ovarian dysfunction is unclear. Studies suggest an abnormality of cytochrome P450c17 activity, but this is unlikely to be the 1° event, but rather an index of ↑ steroidogenesis by ovarian theca cells.
- There is also an increase in the frequency and amplitude of GnRH pulses, resulting in an increase in LH concentration (present in ~50% of ♀), although this may be blunted in obese ♀.

Box 4.3 2003 Joint European Society of Human Reproduction and Embryology and American Society of Reproductive Medicine Consensus on the diagnosis criteria for PCOS (Rotterdam criteria)

At least two out of three of the following:
- Oligo-/amenorrhoea.
- Hyperandrogenism (clinical or biochemical).
- Polycystic ovaries on US.
- Exclusion of other disorders:
  - CAH, hyperprolactinaemia, Cushing's if indicated.

Source: data from The Rotterdam ESHRE/ASRM-Sponsored PCOS Consensus Workshop Group (2004) 'Revised 2003 consensus on diagnostic criteria and long-term health risks related to polycystic ovary syndrome' *Fertility and Sterility* 81(1):19–25.

Box 4.4 Other causes of hyperandrogenism
- CAH.
- Acromegaly.
- Cushing's syndrome.
- Testosterone-secreting tumours (most commonly arrhenoblastoma)

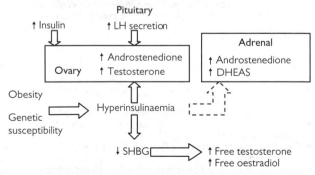

Fig. 4.4 Abnormalities of hormone secretion in PCOS.

Hyperinsulinaemia
- ~70% of ♀ with PCOS are insulin-resistant, depending on the definition. The defect in insulin sensitivity appears to be selective, mainly affecting the metabolic effects of insulin (effects on muscle and the liver), but sparing the ovaries where insulin acts as a co-gonadotrophin to amplify LH-mediated testosterone synthesis. Hyperinsulinaemia is exacerbated by obesity but can also be present in lean ♀ with PCOS.
- T2DM four times higher than age-matched controls and tends, on average, to occur 4 years younger than in unaffected ♀ population.
- There is also evidence in a number of ♀ with PCOS of insufficient β-cell response to a glucose challenge, which is known to be a precursor to T2DM.
- Insulin also inhibits SHBG synthesis by the liver, with a consequent rise in free androgen levels.

Features
- *Onset of symptoms*. Symptoms often begin around puberty, after weight gain, or after stopping the oral contraceptive pill (OCP) but can present at any time.
- *Oligo-/amenorrhoea* (70%). Due to anovulation. *Hirsutism* (66%):
  - 25% of ♀ also suffer from acne or ♂ pattern alopecia. Virilization is not a feature of PCOS.
  - There is often a family history of hirsutism or irregular periods.
  - Slower onset of hirsutism makes a distinction from adrenal or ovarian tumours which are rapidly progressive and more likely to be associated with virilization and higher testosterone concentrations.
  - <1% of hirsute ♀ have non-classic CAH (see ➔ Clinical presentation, p. 355), and this should be excluded, particularly in ♀ with significantly raised serum testosterone levels.
- *Obesity* (50%). Symptoms worsen with obesity, as it is accompanied by ↑ testosterone concentrations as a result of hyperinsulinaemia. Acanthosis nigricans may be found in 1–3% of insulin-resistant ♀ with PCOS.
- *Infertility* (30%). PCOS accounts for 75% of cases of anovulatory infertility. The risk of spontaneous miscarriage is also thought to be higher than in the general population, mainly because of obesity.
- *Depression/mood disturbance*.
- *Obstructive sleep apnoea*.

Rule out an androgen-secreting tumour
If there is:
- Evidence of virilization.
- Testosterone >5nmol/L (or >3nmol/L in post-menopausal ♀).
- Rapidly progressive hirsutism.
- *CT of adrenals or US of ovaries* will detect tumours >1cm.
- *Selective venous sampling* occasionally necessary to locate virilizing tumours undetected by imaging.
- *Ovarian suppression test* using GnRH analogues can establish ovarian origin of androgens.
- Adrenal tumours usually co-secrete cortisol as part of Cushing's syndrome.

Risks associated with PCOS

Type 2 diabetes mellitus

T2DM is 2–4 times commoner in ♀ with PCOS. IGT affects 10–30% of ♀ with PCOS, and gestational diabetes is also more prevalent. The prevalence of DM is ↑ in all ♀ with PCOS but is highest in the obese group. The most important risk factor is family history of T2DM.

Dyslipidaemia

Several studies have shown an ↑ risk of hypercholesterolaemia, hypertriglyceridaemia, and low high-density lipoprotein cholesterol (HDL-C) in ♀ with PCOS. However, epidemiological studies of ♀ with PCOS have yet to conclusively demonstrate ↑ mortality.

Endometrial hyperplasia and carcinoma

In anovulatory ♀, endometrial stimulation by unopposed oestrogen results in endometrial hyperplasia. Several studies have also shown that this results in a 2- to 4-fold excess risk of endometrial carcinoma in ♀ with PCOS. Thus, it is recommended to induce at least 3–4 withdrawal bleeds per year to reduce this risk in amenorrhoeic ♀.

Arterial disease

Meta-analyses suggest a 2-fold risk of arterial disease in ♀ with PCOS relative to ♀ without PCOS.

Pregnancy in women with PCOS

Adverse pregnancy outcome

1. ↑ miscarriage ×2–3.
2. ↑ risk gestational diabetes.
3. ↑ hypertension ×3–4.
4. ↑ lower-segment Caesarean section (LSCS) rate odds ratio (OR) 1.2.

Further reading

Khomami MB, et al. (2010). Polycystic ovary syndrome and adverse pregnancy outcomes: current state of knowledge, challenges and potential implications for practice. *Clin Endocrinol (Oxf)* **88**, 761–9.

Investigations of PCOS

The aims of investigations are mainly to exclude serious underlying disorders and to screen for complications, as the diagnosis is primarily clinical (see Box 4.3).

Confirmation of diagnosis

- Testosterone concentration:
  - Often normal in ♀ with PCOS, and serum androgen concentrations do not reflect the degree of hirsutism because of variable androgen receptor sensitivity.
- LH concentration:
  - The higher the LH level, the more likely the risk of anovulation and infertility.
  - Cannot be used to diagnose PCOS, as it is raised in only half of ♀.
- SHBG:
  - Low in 50% of ♀ with PCOS, owing to the hyperinsulinaemic state, with a consequent increase in circulating free androgens.
  - Useful indirect marker of insulin resistance, although can be low in obesity more generally.
- Free androgen index (FAI) = 100 × (total testosterone/SHBG).
- AMH made by preantral follicles and raised in PCOS. Can be a useful non-invasive alternative to US, but AMH does not yet form part of the diagnostic criteria, whereas PCO morphology does (poor sensitivity, but useful if elevated).
- Pelvic US of ovaries and endometrium:
  - US criteria for PCO defined as >20 follicles between 2 and 9mm in diameter or ovarian volume >10cm³. NB: if using transabdominal US, a volume of >10mL should be used, as follicle number is unreliable.
  - US is sensitive, but not specific (occurs in CAH and Cushing's). Usually transvaginal, but transabdominal possible in experienced hands. False −ve results common in non-specialist scans.
  - Measurement of endometrial thickness is of major importance in the diagnosis of endometrial hyperplasia in the presence of anovulation. Endometrial hyperplasia is diagnosed if the endometrial thickness is >10mm.
  - Transvaginal US will also identify 90% of ovarian virilizing tumours.
  - US should not be used for the diagnosis of PCOS if within 8 years of menarche due to high incidence of multifollicular ovaries around puberty.

Associated endocrinopathy

- *Serum PRL.* In the presence of infertility or oligo-/amenorrhoea.
  - Mild hyperprolactinaemia (<2000mU/L) is present in up to 30% of ♀ with PCOS.
- 17OHP level:
  - Used to exclude late-onset (non-classic) CAH.
  - Indicated in those with testosterone concentrations in excess of 5nmol/L or with evidence of virilization.

- May also perform a Synacthen® test if basal 17OHP does not exclude CAH, to look for an exaggerated rise in 17OHP in response to ACTH in the presence of non-classic 21-hydroxylase deficiency (see ➔ Clinical presentation, p. 355).
- If the patient is ovulating, then all 17OHP measurements should be performed during the follicular phase of the cycle to avoid false +ves due to pregnancy.
- DHEAS and androstenedione concentrations:
  - Both can be moderately raised in PCOS, although DHEAS is traditionally considered an adrenal androgen.
  - Adrenal androgen excess may be of particular relevance in lean ♀ with PCOS.
  - Do not need to be measured routinely in ♀ with PCOS, but indicated if serum testosterone >5nmol/L, in the presence of rapidly progressive hirsutism, or in the presence of virilization.
- Other:
  - Depending on clinical suspicion, e.g. UFC or overnight dexamethasone suppression test if Cushing's syndrome is suspected, or IGF-1 if acromegaly is suspected—but not routinely.

Screening for complications

- *Serum lipids and blood glucose.* All obese ♀ with PCOS should have an annual fasting glucose and fasting lipid profile. Consider OGTT in those with a family history of T2DM; studies have suggested fasting plasma glucose (FGP) is insufficient in predicting dysglycaemia.
- *OGTT if BMI ≥25kg/m², age >40 years, history of gestational diabetes mellitus (GDM) or family history of T2DM, or non-Caucasian ethnicity (NICE).*
- All ♀ with PCOS who fall pregnant should be screened for GDM.

Management of PCOS

The management of PCOS should be personalized to the patient's symptoms, i.e. hirsutism, oligo-/anovulation, and oligo-/amenorrhoea, taking into consideration the need for contraception. Patients and prescribers should be aware that some drugs are used off licence.

Weight loss

Studies have uniformly shown that weight reduction in obese ♀ with PCOS improves insulin sensitivity and significantly reduces hyperandrogenaemia. Obese ♀ are less likely to respond to antiandrogens and fertility treatment. With a loss of 5%, ♀ with PCOS show improvement in hirsutism, restoration of menstrual regularity, and fertility.

Metformin

(*Off-licence use—inform patient.*)

In obese and lean insulin-resistant ♀ with PCOS, metformin (1–2.5g daily) improves insulin sensitivity, with a corresponding reduction in serum androgens (by 11%) and LH concentrations and an increase in SHBG levels. Metformin may regulate menstruation by improving ovulatory function, but improved live birth rate is not established. Metformin does not seem to improve response rates to ovulation induction using clomifene citrate or gonadotrophins. Evidence suggests that metformin is no better than lifestyle at improving metabolic risk and progression to T2DM. Metformin is usually stopped at the diagnosis of pregnancy, as benefit in pregnancy is not proved outside of established GDM.

There have been few long-term studies looking at the effect of metformin on hirsutism, but it appears that its effects are modest at best, and most ♀ with significant hirsutism will require an antiandrogen.

♀ should be warned of its GI side effects. In order to minimize these, they should be started on a low dose (500mg od) which may be ↑ gradually to a therapeutic dose over a number of weeks. A modified-release preparation can be used if GI side effects are an issue.

Hirsutism

Pharmacological treatment of hirsutism (see Table 4.2) is directed at slowing the growth of new hair. It can be combined with mechanical methods of hair removal such as electrolysis and laser therapy. Therapy is most effective when started early. There is slow improvement over the first 6–12 months of treatment. Patients should be warned that facial hair is slow to respond, treatment is prolonged, and symptoms may recur after discontinuation of drugs. Adequate contraception is mandatory during pharmacological treatment of hirsutism because of possible teratogenicity.

Ovarian androgen suppression

Combined oral contraceptive pill (COCP)
- The oestrogen component increases SHBG levels and thus reduces free androgen concentrations; the progestogen component inhibits LH secretion, and thus ovarian androgen production.
- The effect of the COCP alone on hair growth is modest, so it may be combined with an antiandrogen.

Table 4.2 Pharmacological treatment of hirsutism

Ovarian androgen suppression	Combined OCP
Adrenal androgen suppression	Corticosteroids (rarely)
Androgen receptor antagonists	Spironolactone (off licence)
	Cyproterone acetate (CPA)
	Flutamide
Reductase inhibitor	Finasteride
Insulin sensitizers	Metformin (off licence)
Topical inhibitors of hair follicle growth	Eflornithine

- Co-cyprindiol (e.g. Dianette®, which contains CPA 2mg), or Yasmin®, which contains drospirenone, may have additional benefit because the progestogens are antiandrogenic. However, they may carry a greater risk of VTE and benefit of these brands over 3rd-generation COCP has not been established. So 1st-line treatment with brands such as Cilest®, Marvelon®, and Femodene® is appropriate if contraception is desired.

Androgen receptor blockers

These are most effective when combined with oral contraceptives. All are contraindicated in pregnancy. They act by competitively inhibiting the binding of testosterone and DHT to the androgen receptor.

Spironolactone
- Antiandrogen of choice, particularly in overweight ♀.
- *Dose.* 100–200mg a day.
- *Side effects.* Polymenorrhoea if not combined with the COCP. A fifth of ♀ complain of GI symptoms when on high doses of spironolactone. Potassium levels should be monitored (risk of hyperkalaemia), and other potassium-sparing drugs should be avoided.

Cyproterone acetate
- *Dose.* 25–100mg, days 1–10 of the pill cycle, in combination with the COCP.
- *Side effects.* Amenorrhoea if given alone for prolonged periods or in higher doses. *Progesterone side effects.* Hepatic toxicity rare, but monitoring of liver function 6-monthly is recommended.
- A *washout period* of 3–4 months is recommended prior to attempting conception.

Flutamide
- A potent antiandrogen.
- *Dose.* 125–250mg a day; 1mg/kg daily may be effective and associated with a lower frequency of hepatic adverse effects. Monitor LFTs pretreatment and monthly for first 4 months, then as indicated.
- *Side effects.* Dry skin, nausea in 10%. However, there is a 0.4% risk of hepatic toxicity, and it should therefore be used with extreme caution. Patients should be advised to avoid pregnancy.

5α-reductase inhibitors
Block the conversion of testosterone to the more potent androgen DHT.
- Finasteride:
  - *Dose.* 1–2.5mg a day. A weak antiandrogen.
  - *Side effects.* No significant adverse effects.
  - Can be used as monotherapy, or combined with other antiandrogens or COCP.
  - Adequate contraceptive measures are mandatory because of its teratogenicity. In addition, pregnancy should not be attempted until at least 3 months after drug cessation.

Eflornithine 11.5%
- Irreversibly blocks the enzyme ornithine decarboxylase which is involved in growth of hair follicles.
- It is administered as a topical cream on the face to reduce new hair growth. Studies have shown its efficacy in the management of mild facial hirsutism, following at least 8 weeks of treatment. Treatment should be discontinued if there is no benefit at 4 months. It is not a depilatory cream and so must be combined with mechanical methods of hair removal.
- *Side effects.* Skin irritation with burning or pruritus, acne, hypersensitivity.

Amenorrhoea
- A minimum of a withdrawal bleed every 3 months minimizes the risk of endometrial hyperplasia.
- *Treatment:*
  - COCP.
  - Cyclical progestogen: desogestrel (e.g. Cerazette®) is a progesterone-only contraceptive pill with minimal androgenic properties. Medroxyprogesterone acetate 5–10mg bd for 12 days of each calendar month. Norethisterone should be avoided, as it is more androgenic.
  - Metformin (up to 1g bd) which also improves lipoprotein pattern.

Infertility
Ovulation induction regimens are indicated. Obesity adversely affects fertility outcome, with poorer pregnancy rates and higher rates of miscarriage, so weight reduction should be strongly encouraged.

Letrozole
- Inhibits aromatase (reduces oestrogen production), leading to reduced −ve feedback and thus ↑ gonadotrophins.
- Improved live birth and pregnancy rates, compared to clomifene citrate, when used to cause ovulation.
- It has a short half-life and does not deplete oestradiol receptors throughout the body like clomifene citrate.
- Was not used for many years due to concerns about congenital malformations, now thought to be unfounded.
- Currently remains off-label, thus clomifene citrate currently still used as 1st-line agent.

Clomifene citrate
- A selective oestrogen receptor modulator (SERM). Inhibits oestrogen −ve feedback, ↑ FSH secretion, and thus stimulates ovarian follicular growth.
- *Dose.* 25–150mg a day from day 2 of menstrual cycle for 5 days.
- *Response rates.* 80% ovulation rate, 67% pregnancy rate.
- *Complications.* 8% twins, 0.1% higher-order multiple pregnancy. Risk of ovarian neoplasia following prolonged clomiphene treatment remains unclear, so limit treatment to a maximum of six cycles.

Metformin
- Use remains controversial but probably does not improve pregnancy rates in insulin-resistant, particularly overweight, ♀ with PCOS.
- Emerging reports of higher BMI/↑ rates of obesity in children exposed to metformin *in utero*, but generally thought to be safe in pregnancy. No reported teratogenic or neonatal complications.
- *Dose.* Start at 500mg od with largest meal to minimize GI side effects; to be ↑ gradually to 1g bd. If ovulation restored following 6 months of treatment, then continue for up to 1 year. If pregnancy does not occur, then consider other treatments.
- *Side effects.* Nausea, bloating, diarrhoea, vomiting.

Gonadotrophin preparations (human menopausal gonadotrophin (hMG) or FSH)
- Used in those unresponsive to clomifene citrate. Low-dose step-up regimens show better response rates and fewer complications by increasing the chance of achieving monofollicular growth, e.g. 75IU/day for 2 weeks, then increase by 37.5IU/day every 7 days, if required.
- 94% ovulation rate and 50% pregnancy rate.
- *Complications.* Hyperstimulation, multiple pregnancies.
- Close ultrasonic monitoring is essential.

Surgery
- Laparoscopic ovarian diathermy or laser drilling may restore ovulation in up to 90% of ♀, with cumulative pregnancy rates of 80% within 8 months of treatment. Particularly effective in slim ♀ with PCOS and high LH concentrations.
- Invasive and could adversely affect ovarian reserve.
- *Complications.* Surgical adhesions, although usually mild.

In vitro fertilization (IVF)
- In ♀ who fail to respond to ovulation induction.
- Approximately a third will have a live birth following each IVF cycle.

Acne

Treatment for acne should be started as early as possible to prevent scarring. All treatments take up to 12 weeks before significant improvement is seen. All treatments, apart from benzoyl peroxide, are contraindicated in pregnancy.

Mild-to-moderate acne
- *Topical benzoyl peroxide 5%.* Bactericidal properties. May be used in conjunction with oral antibiotic therapy to reduce the risk of developing resistance to antibiotics. *Side effects*: skin irritation and dryness. Add oral antibiotics if no improvement after 2 months of treatment.

Moderate-to-severe acne
- *Topical retinoids*, e.g. tretinoin, isotretinoin. Useful alone in mild acne or in conjunction with antibiotics in moderately severe acne. Continue as maintenance therapy to prevent further acne outbreaks. *Side effects*: irritation, photosensitivity. Apply high-factor sunscreen before sun exposure. Avoid in acne involving large areas of skin.
- *Oral antibiotics*, e.g. oxytetracycline 500mg bd, doxycycline 100mg od, or minocycline 100mg od. Tetracyclines should not be used during pregnancy. Response usually seen by 6 weeks, and full efficacy by 3 months. Continue antibiotics for 2 months after control is achieved. Prescription usually given for a course of 3–6 months. Continue topical retinoids and/or benzoyl peroxide to prevent further outbreaks.
- *COCP and antiandrogens.* As for hirsutism.

Severe acne
- *Isotretinoin.* Very effective in ♀ with severe acne or acne which has not responded to other oral or topical treatments. Used early, it can minimize scarring in inflammatory acne. However, it is highly toxic and can only be prescribed by a consultant dermatologist. Also consider referring ♀ who develop acne in their 30s or 40s and ♀ with psychological problems as a result of acne. Isotretinoin must not be used during pregnancy.

Further reading

Deng Y, et al. (2017). Steroid hormone profiling in obese and nonobese women with polycystic ovary syndrome. *Sci Rep*, **7**, 14156.

Diamanti-Kandarakis E, Dunaif A (2012). Insulin resistance and the polycystic ovary syndrome revisited: an update on mechanisms and implications. *Endocr Rev* **33**, 981–1030.

Dunaif A (1997). Insulin resistance and polycystic ovary syndrome: mechanism and implications for pathogenesis. *Endocr Rev* **18**, 774–800.

Ehrmann DA (2005). Polycystic ovary syndrome. *N Engl J Med* **352**, 1223–36.

Ehrmann DA, Rychlik D (2003). Pharmacological treatment of polycystic ovary syndrome. *Semin Reprod Med* **21**, 277–83.

Hoeger KM, et al. (2021). Update on PCOS: consequences, challenges, and guiding treatment. *J Clin Endocrinol Metab* **106**, e1071–83.

Ledger WL, Clark T (2003). Long-term consequences of polycystic ovary syndrome. Guideline no. 33. Royal College of Obstetricians and Gynaecologists, London.

Legros RS, et al.; Endocrine Society (2013). Diagnosis and treatment of polycystic ovary syndrome: an Endocrine Society clinical practice guideline. *J Clin Endocrinol Metab* **98**, 4565–92.

Lord JM, et al. (2003). Insulin sensitizing drugs for polycystic ovary syndrome. *Cochrane Database Syst Rev* **3**, CD003053.

Neithardt AB, Barnes RB (2003). The diagnosis and management of hirsutism. *Semin Reprod Med* **21**, 285–93.

Nestler JE (2008). Metformin for the treatment of the polycystic ovary syndrome. *N Engl J Med* **358**, 47–54.

Palomba S (2009). Evidence-based and potential benefits of metformin in the polycystic ovary syndrome: a comprehensive review. *Endocr Rev* **30**, 1–50.

Paradisi R (2010). Retrospective observational study on the effects and tolerability of flutamide in a large population of patients with various kinds of hirsutism over a 15-year period. *Eur J Endocrinol* **163**, 139–4.

Pierpoint T, et al. (1998). Mortality of women with polycystic ovary syndrome at long term follow up. J Clin Epidemiol **51**, 581–6.

Randeva HS, et al. (2012). Cardiometabolic aspects of the polycystic ovary syndrome. Endocr Rev **33**, 812–41.

Teede H, et al (2018). Recommendations from the international evidence-based guideline for the assessment and management of polycystic ovary syndrome. Clin Endocrinol **89**, 251–68.

The Rotterdam ESHRE/ASRM-sponsored PCOS Consensus Workshop Group (2004). Revised 2003 Consensus on diagnostic criteria and long-term health risks related to polycystic ovary syndrome. Hum Reprod **19**, 41–7.

Tsilchorozidou T, et al. (2004). The pathophysiology of polycystic ovary syndrome. Clin Endocrinol (Oxf) **60**, 1–17.

Post-menopausal hirsutism

Causes

- Hyperthecosis (commonest cause).
- Virilizing tumour:
  - Adrenal.
  - Ovarian.
- Drugs (as for hirsutism; see ➔ Hirsutism, p. 336).
- Cushing's.

GnRH suppression test can help differentiate, as suppresses ovarian testosterone production in hyperthecosis. Venous sampling may be required, as tumours may be very small and difficult to visualize on standard imaging.

Treatment

Of cause

- Finasteride/spironolactone.
- Offer oophorectomy.
- GnRH analogues.

Further reading

Alpañés M, et al. (2012). Management of postmenopausal virilization. *J Clin Endocrinol Metab* **97**, 2581 8.

Congenital adrenal hyperplasia in adults

Definition

CAH is a group of inherited disorders characterized by deficiency of an enzyme necessary for cortisol biosynthesis. This can lead to an increase of precursors and diversion to other steroid pathways such as androgen or MC production.

- >90% of cases are due to 21α-hydroxylase deficiency.
- Clinical presentation depends on severity of mutation. Wide clinical spectrum, from presentation in neonatal period with salt wasting and virilization to non-classic CAH in adulthood.
- Complete enzyme deficiency will present in infancy due to MC/ corticosteroid deficiency with a salt wasting crisis (classic) and ambiguous genitalia in ♀ (see ⭢ Chapter 7).
- Partial enzyme deficiency may present in later life with hyperandrogenism or premature puberty (non-classic).
- AR.

Epidemiology

- Carrier frequency of classic CAH 1:50–1:100 in Caucasians.
- Carrier frequency of non-classic CAH 19% in Ashkenazi Jews, 13.5% in Hispanics, 6% in Italians, and 3% in other Caucasians.

Pathogenesis

Genetics

- *CYP21* encodes the 21α-hydroxylase enzyme, located on the short arm of chromosome 6 (chromosome 6p21.3). In close proximity is the *CYP21* pseudogene, with 90% homology but no functional activity.
- 21α-hydroxylase deficiency results from gene mutations, partial gene deletions, or gene conversions in which sequences from the pseudogene are transferred to the active gene, rendering it inactive. There is a correlation between the severity of the molecular defect and the clinical severity of the disorder. Non-classic CAH is usually due to a point mutation (single base change); missense mutations result in simple virilizing disease, whereas a gene conversion or partial deletion usually results in presentation in infancy, with salt wasting or severe virilization.
- Other rare genetic causes are listed in Table 4.3.

Biochemistry

(See Fig. 4.5.)

- 21α-hydroxylase deficiency results in aldosterone and cortisol deficiency. Loss of −ve feedback from cortisol results in ACTH hypersecretion, and this causes adrenocortical hyperplasia and accumulation of steroid precursors 'above' the enzyme deficiency, including progesterone and 17OHP. These are then shunted into androgen synthesis pathways, resulting in testosterone and androstenedione excess.
- 11β-hydroxylase is the next commonest enzyme deficiency, but in addition to causing hyperandrogenism, it can lead to accumulation of 11-deoxycorticosterone which acts on the MC receptor to cause hypertension and hypokalaemia.

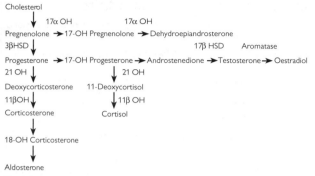

Fig. 4.5 Adrenal steroid biosynthesis pathway.

Clinical presentation

Classic CAH

- Most patients are diagnosed in infancy, and their clinical presentation is discussed elsewhere (see ⊃ Congenital adrenal hyperplasia, p. 493).
- *Problems persisting into adulthood.* Sexual dysfunction and subfertility in ♀, particularly in salt wasters. Reconstructive genital surgery is required in the majority of ♀ who were virilized at birth to create a suitable vaginal introitus. With improvement of medical care, normal pregnancy rates (90%) can be achieved.
- In ♂, high levels of adrenal androgens suppress gonadotrophins, and thus testicular function. ↑ ACTH results in the development of testicular adrenal rest tissues (TARTs). These are always benign but may be misdiagnosed as testicular tumours. TARTs can be destructive, leading to testicular failure. Spermatogenesis is often low if CAH is poorly controlled.
- There is a significant risk of adrenal crises over lifetime.
- There is an impaired QoL.
- Emerging evidence to suggest ↑ cardiovascular risk and ↑ mortality.

Non-classic CAH

- Due to partial deficiency of 21α-hydroxylase. GC and aldosterone production is normal, but there is overproduction of 17OHP, and thus androgens.
- Presents with hirsutism (60%), acne (33%), and oligomenorrhoea (54%), often around the onset of puberty. Only 13% of ♀ present with subfertility.
- Polycystic ovaries on US are common, and adrenal incidentalomas or hyperplasia are seen in 40%.
- Asymptomatic in ♂. The effect of non-classic CAH on ♂ fertility is unknown.

Investigations of CAH in adults

Because of diurnal variation in adrenal hormonal secretion, all investigations should be performed at 9 a.m.

Diagnosis of non-classic CAH—17OHP measurement

Timing of measurement

- Screen in the follicular phase of the menstrual cycle. 17OHP is produced by the adrenals and the corpus luteum, so false +ve results may occur if measured in the luteal phase of the cycle.

Interpretation of result

If having menstrual cycles, measure in the follicular phase.

- <6nmol/L—normal.
- >30nmol/L—CAH and proceed to additional tests.
- 6–30nmol/L—proceed to ACTH stimulation test. A 5th will have non-classic CAH.

ACTH stimulation test

- Measure 17OHP 60min after ACTH (250 micrograms) administration, and cortisol at 30min.
- An exaggerated rise in 17OHP is seen in non-classic CAH (60min 17OHP 30–300nmol/L).
- Patients with classic CAH typically have 60min 17OHP levels >300nmol/L.
- 17OHP level <30nmol/L post-ACTH excludes the diagnosis.
- Levels of 30–45nmol/L may suggest heterozygosity or non-classic CAH.
- Cortisol response to ACTH stimulation measured at 30min is usually mildly low or normal in non-classic CAH and low in classic CAH.

Other investigations

24h urine steroid metabolite profile

- Provides a gold standard test for all forms of CAH and is able to distinguish between differing genetic causes.
- A normal urinary steroid profile excludes a diagnosis of CAH and therefore should be considered in all cases and especially where there is clinical uncertainty or discordant results.

Androgens

- In poorly controlled classic CAH in ♀, testosterone and androstenedione levels may be in the adult ♂ range. Dehydroepiandrosterone sulphate levels are usually only mildly, and not consistently, elevated in CAH.
- Circulating testosterone, and particularly androstenedione, is elevated in non-classic CAH, but there is a large overlap with levels seen in PCOS, so serum androgen concentrations cannot be used to distinguish between the disorders.

Renin

- PRA elevated due to aldosterone deficiency.
- A proportion of ♀ with non-classic CAH may also have mildly elevated renin concentrations.

ACTH
- Greatly elevated in poorly controlled classic CAH.
- Usually normal levels in non-classic CAH.

  (See Table 4.3 for a list of enzyme deficiencies in CAH.)

Genetic testing
- Provides the definitive diagnosis where specific mutations are identified.
- Should be offered to all patients (and to their partners if pregnancy is being planned).
- Allows putative correlations between genotype and phenotype to be made.

Table 4.3 Enzyme deficiencies in CAH

Enzyme deficiency	Incidence (per births)	Clinical features
Classic 21α-hydroxylase (CYP21A2)	1:10,000– 1:15,000	Salt wasting, ambiguous genitalia in ♀, precocious pubarche in ♂
Non-classic 21α-hydroxylase (partial deficiency) (CYP21A2)	1:27–1:1000	Hirsutism, oligomenorrhoea in pubertal ♀, asymptomatic in ♂
11β-hydroxylase (CYP11B1)	1:100,000	Ambiguous genitalia, virilization, hypertension
3β-hydroxysteroid dehydrogenase type 2 (HSD3B2)	Rare	Mild virilization, salt wasting in severe cases
P450 oxidoreductase (POR)	Rare	Ambiguous genitalia, skeletal malformation (Antley–Bixler syndrome). Possible maternal virilization in pregnancy. No postnatal virilization
17α-hydroxylase (CYP17A1)	Rare	Delayed puberty in ♀, pseudohermaphroditism in ♂, hypertension, hypokalaemia
StAR, lipoid CAH	Rare	Classic and non-classic forms with degrees of genital ambiguity and AI, including salt wasting
Cholesterol side chain cleavage (CYP11A1)	Rare	Classic and non-classic forms with degrees of genital ambiguity and AI, including salt wasting

Management of CAH in adults

- Transition clinic—this is helpful for adolescent patients, and a joint clinic with a paediatrician, an adult endocrinologist, a reproductive specialist, and a urologist is helpful.

The aims of treatment of CAH in adulthood under specialist care are:
- To maintain normal energy levels and weight, and avoid adrenal crises.
- To minimize hyperandrogenism and restore regular menses and fertility in ♀.
- To avoid GC under- or over-replacement.
- To treat stress with adequate extra GC.
- To suppress ACTH-driven adrenal androgen secretion.

Classic CAH

- Hydrocortisone (tds) should be considered as the 1st-line treatment, although longer-acting GCs can be used.
- *Prednisolone.* Total dose 5–7.5mg/day, given in two divided doses, which is no longer a reverse circadian pattern.
- Occasional patients who are not controlled on prednisolone may be treated with nocturnal dexamethasone instead (0.25–0.5mg nocte). Occasionally, additional progesterone to induce withdrawal bleeds.
- The optimum dose is the minimum dose required to normalize serum androgens. Dose titration should be achieved using androstenedione, rather than 17OHP, to guide management (data from CHASE study).
- As with other forms of AI, GC doses should be doubled during illness. This is discussed in detail elsewhere (see ➲ Intercurrent illness, pp. 304–7).
- All patients (children and adults) with classic salt wasting CAH require MC replacement. Fludrocortisone 50–200 micrograms/day is given as a single daily dose. Fludrocortisone dose should be titrated according to clinical symptoms, electrolytes, postural BP, and renin measurements.
- Addition of androgen receptor antagonists/OCP may be required for hyperandrogenic symptoms. Spironolactone is relatively contraindicated in CAH due to potential for salt wasting.
- Bilateral adrenalectomy reduces the risk of virilization in ♀ and allows for ↓ GC doses; however, it also carries surgical risk and is not recommended for patients discordant with steroid treatment. Furthermore, due to the potential for ovarian, retroperitoneal, or TART, adrenalectomy may not effectively control hyperandrogenaemia. Thus, it is occasionally considered in those with unsatisfactory outcome with conventional medical management, but it is not routinely recommended.
- Periodic testicular US is useful in ♂ with CAH to monitor for TARTs.
- *Pregnancy.* Patient and partners require prior *CYP21* mutation analysis at the earliest opportunity to enable genetic counselling. If partner is a carrier, 50% risk of affected child (1 in 63 is a carrier of the 21OH gene).
- *Bone health should be monitored.*

Non-classic CAH

- Treatment should only be considered in symptomatic individuals or in the context of pregnancy.
- *Oligo-/amenorrhoea.* Prednisolone 2.5–5mg/day may be used but is often reserved to normalize ovulatory function. If asymptomatic, avoid use of GC. If previously treated, give option of discontinuing therapy when adult height achieved.
- *Stress dosing.* Recommended for major trauma, surgery, and childbirth only if suboptimal cortisol response to SST.
- *Hirsutism and acne.* May alternatively, and more effectively, be treated as for PCOS (see ➜ Management of PCOS, pp. 346–51). Spironolactone should be avoided because of the potential risk of salt wasting, and thus hyper-reninaemia.
- If plasma renin level is elevated, then fludrocortisone, given in a dose sufficient to normalize renin concentrations, may improve adrenal hyperandrogenism.
- ♂ may not require treatment. The occasional ♂ may need GCs to treat subfertility, although excess GC may suppress gonadotrophins.
- In adult patients with adequate adrenal cortisol reserve, consideration should be given to withdrawing GC therapy if symptoms have improved.

Management of pregnancy in CAH

- *Maternal classic CAH.* Genotyping of the partner may be used as 1st line. Alternatively, screen patient/partner using basal ± ACTH-stimulated 17OHP levels (see ➜ Investigations of CAH in adults, pp. 356–7), and if levels are elevated, proceed to genotyping. If heterozygote, then preimplantation genetic diagnosis during IVF treatment or prenatal treatment of fetus may be considered.
- Physiological prednisolone or hydrocortisone rarely needs adjusting in pregnancy (↑ by 20–25% during the 3rd trimester). Fludrocortisone doses do not normally need to be adjusted. Routine biochemical markers cannot be used in pregnancy, so treat symptomatically. Dexamethasone crosses the placenta, so should not be used unless aiming to suppress fetal adrenal function (see ➜ Treatment (commenced before 7 weeks' gestation), p. 360).
- Adjust fludrocortisone against BP, but alteration during pregnancy is not normally required.
- Placental aromatase protects the fetus from maternal androgens; >200 pregnancies reported to mothers with CAH—no case of fetal virilization recorded, so monitoring testosterone not required.
- >75% Caesarean section rate because of masculinized pelvis and surgical scarring following vaginoplasty.
- ↑ risk of GDM.
- Routine GC boost at onset of active labour.

Prenatal treatment of pregnancies at risk of CAH

Aim of prenatal treatment is to prevent virilization of an affected ♀ fetus.

- Only to be considered if previous child from same partner with CAH or known mutations in both parents. Mutations must be identified well before trying to conceive (this cannot be done on the run).
- NOT for mothers with CAH, unless partner is a known carrier of a severe mutation.
- Only to be considered by experienced unit. Current guidelines consider this still in the realms of research, as long-term outcome of dexamethasone exposure to unaffected fetuses is unknown.

Treatment (commenced before 7 weeks' gestation)

- Dexamethasone (20 micrograms/kg maternal body weight), in three divided doses a day, crosses the placenta and reduces fetal adrenal hyperandrogenism. If possible/., aim to collect circulating DNA at 5/40, and if ♀ fetus, commence dexamethasone from 7/40.
- Discontinue if ♂ fetus.

Outcome

- 50–75% of affected ♀ do not require reconstructive surgery.

Monitoring of treatment

Annual follow-up is usually adequate in adults.

- *Clinical assessment.* Measure BP and weight. Look for evidence of hyperandrogenism and GC excess. Amenorrhoea in ♀ usually suggests inadequate therapy but may have to be accepted, as often cannot be achieved without excessive doses of GC. Try progesterone for withdrawal bleed. Consider the use of intermittent progesterone-induced withdrawal bleeds.
- Androstenedione levels can be used to titrate GC dose (aiming for mid- to upper-normal range).
- Suppressed levels of 17OHP, testosterone, and renin are an indication of overtreatment. Normalizing will often result in complications from supraphysiological doses of GCs. Therefore, use androstenedione as a guide, but do not aim for suppression in order to avoid adverse effects of overtreatment, as well as clinical features.
- Modestly raised or high normal levels of 17OHP, testosterone, and renin are optimal. ACTH monitoring is not useful.
- Consider bone density which may be reduced by supraphysiological steroid doses.
- Testicular function requires special attention. Low LH is a sign of raised adrenal androgens. Raised FSH may follow adrenal rests as a sign of testicular failure. US testis every 2 years. Consider sperm count/ storage if adrenal rests are present.
- US ovaries not useful routinely, as PCO morphology is common.
- In men, testicular adrenal rest tumours may develop (up to 94%). Consider 5-year adrenal imaging. Their detection may prevent infertility later. Consider semen cryopreservation. US screening of the scrotum is suggested every 2 years.

Prognosis

Emerging evidence suggests that patients with CAH may have ↑ cardiovascular and metabolic risk and this may translate to reduced life expectancy. Improvement in medical and surgical care has also improved QoL for most sufferers. However, there are additional unresolved issues:

- *Height.* Despite optimal treatment in childhood, patients with CAH are, on average, significantly shorter than their predicted genetic height. Studies suggest that this may be due to overtreatment with GCs during infancy.
- *Fertility.* Mainly a problem in ♂ with poorly controlled classic CAH and adrenal rests.
- *Adrenal incidentalomas.* Benign adrenal adenomas have been reported in up to 50% of patients with classic CAH. ♂ with CAH may develop gonadal adrenocortical rests.
- *Psychosexual issues.* Gender dysphoria common in ♀. A significant number of ♀ with classic CAH, despite adequacy of vaginal reconstruction, are not sexually active.

Further reading

Arlt W, et al. (2010). Health status of adults with congenital adrenal hyperplasia: a cohort study of 203 patients. *J Clin Endocrinol Metab* **95**, 5110–21.

Aycan Z, et al. (2013). Prevalence and long-term follow-up outcomes of testicular adrenal rest tumours in children and adolescent males with congenital adrenal hyperplasia. *Clin Endocrinol (Oxf)* **78**, 667–72.

El-Maouche D, et al. (2017). Congenital adrenal hyperplasia. *Lancet* **390**, 2194–210.

Engels M, et al. (2019). Testicular adrenal rest tumors: current insights on prevalence, characteristics, origin, and treatment. *Endocr Rev* **40**, 973–87.

Falhammar H, et al. (2014). Increased mortality in patients with congenital adrenal hyperplasia due to 21-hydroxylase deficiency. *J Clin Endocrinol Metab* **99**, E2715–21.

Jenkins-Jones S, et al. (2018). Poor compliance and increased mortality, depression and healthcare costs in patients with congenital adrenal hyperplasia. *Eur J Endocrinol* **178**, 309–20.

Joint LWPES/ESPE CAH Working Group (2002). Consensus statement on 21-hydroxylase deficiency from the Lawson Wilkins Paediatric Endocrine Society and the European Society for Paediatric Endocrinology. *J Clin Endocrinol Metab* **87**, 4048–53.

Merke DP (2008). Approach to the adult with congenital adrenal hyperplasia due to 21-hydroxylase deficiency. *J Clin Endocrinol Metab* **93**, 653–60.

Merke DP, Auchus RJ (2020). Congenital adrenal hyperplasia due to 21-hydroxylase deficiency. *N Engl J Med* **383**, 1248–61.

Miller WL (2018). Mechanisms in endocrinology: Rare defects in adrenal steroidogenesis. *Eur J Endocrinol* **179**, R125–41.

New MI (2006). Extensive clinical experience: nonclassical 21-hydroxylase deficiency. *J Clin Endocrinol Metab* **91**, 205–14.

New MI, et al. (2001). Prenatal diagnosis for congenital adrenal hyperplasia in 532 pregnancies. *J Clin Endocrinol Metab* **86**, 5651–757.

Ogilvie CM, et al. (2006). Congenital adrenal hyperplasia in adults: a review of medical, surgical and psychological issues. *Clin Endocrinol (Oxf)* **64**, 2–11.

Premawaradhana LDKE, et al. (1997). Longer term outcome in females with congenital adrenal hyperplasia: the Cardiff experience. *Clin Endocrinol (Oxf)* **46**, 327–32.

Speiser PW, White PC (2003). Congenital adrenal hyperplasia. *N Engl J Med* **349**, 776–88.

Speiser PW, et al. (2018). Congenital adrenal hyperplasia due to steroid 21-hydroxylase deficiency: an Endocrine Society clinical practice guideline. *J Clin Endocrinol Metab* **103**, 4043–88.

Tamhane S, et al. (2018). Cardiovascular and metabolic outcomes in congenital adrenal hyperplasia: a systematic review and meta-analysis. *J Clin Endocrinol Metab* **103**, 4097–103.

Androgen-secreting tumours

Definition

Rare tumours of the ovary or adrenal gland which may be benign or malignant, which cause virilization in ♀ through androgen production (differential diagnosis in post-menopausal woman ovarian hyperthecosis).

Epidemiology and pathology

Androgen-secreting ovarian tumours

- 75% develop before the age of 40 years.
- Account for 0.4% of all ovarian tumours; 20% are malignant.
- Tumours are 5–25cm in size. The larger they are, the more likely they are to be malignant. They are rarely bilateral.
- Two major types:
  - Sex cord stromal cell tumours: often contain testicular cell types.
  - Adrenal-like tumours: often contain adrenocortical or Leydig cells.
- Other tumours, e.g. gonadoblastomas and teratomas, may also, on occasion, present with virilization.

Androgen-secreting adrenal tumours

- 50% develop before the age of 50 years.
- Larger tumours, particularly >4cm, are more likely to be malignant.
- Usually with concomitant cortisol secretion as a variant of Cushing's syndrome.
- 45% of ACCs present with Cushing's syndrome, 25% with both Cushing's and hyperandrogenism, and 10% with hyperandrogenism alone (↑ chance of ACC rather than adrenal adenoma).

Clinical features

- *Onset of symptoms.* Usually recent onset of rapidly progressive symptoms.
- *Hyperandrogenism:*
  - Hirsutism of varying degree, often severe; ♂ pattern balding and acne are common.
  - Usually oligo-/amenorrhoea.
  - Infertility may be a presenting feature.
- *Virilization.* (see Box 4.1) Indicates severe hyperandrogenism, is associated with clitoromegaly, and is present in 98% of ♀ with androgen-producing tumours. Not usually a feature of PCOS.
- *Other:*
  - Abdominal pain.
  - Palpable abdominal mass.
  - Ascites.
  - Symptoms and signs of Cushing's syndrome present in many of ♀ with adrenal tumours.

Investigations

- A total testosterone level >5nmol/L should prompt further evaluation for a testosterone-secreting ovarian or testicular tumour, or ovarian hyperthecosis (see ➲ Causes, p. 352).
- Start with ovarian US, and consider adrenal imaging if US −ve or high DHEA. Occasional venous sampling of gonadal vein for androgens. >50% suppression testosterone suggests ovarian in origin.

- 90% of DHEA/DHEAS are produced in the adrenal glands. They are weak androgens, but small amounts are converted to androstenedione and then testosterone. The concentrations of DHEAS are 100–1000 times higher than those of DHEA. DHEAS levels do not strongly identify an adrenal malignant cause of hyperandrogenism, although values >18.9 micromol/L require further evaluation.

(See Fig. 4.6.)

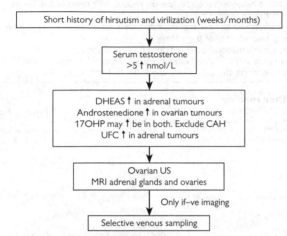

Fig. 4.6 Investigation of androgen-secreting tumours.

Management

Surgery
- Adrenalectomy or ovarian cystectomy/oophorectomy.
- Curative in benign lesions.

Adjunctive therapy
- Malignant ovarian and adrenal androgen-secreting tumours are usually resistant to chemotherapy and radiotherapy. Spironolactone/CPA if benign.

Prognosis

Benign tumours
- Prognosis excellent.
- Hirsutism improves post-operatively, but clitoromegaly, ♂ pattern balding, and deep voice may persist.

Malignant tumours
- *Adrenal tumours.* 20% 5-year survival. Most have metastatic disease at the time of surgery.
- *Ovarian tumours.* 30% disease-free survival and 40% overall survival at 5 years.

Athletics

- The 2018 International Association of Athletics Federation (IAAF) released guidelines state that people with disorders of sexual differentiation competing in women's events must reduce their testosterone to <5nmol/L for a continuous period of at least 6 months (e.g. by use of hormonal contraceptives) if running 400m to 1 mile races.
- If this is exceeded, the athlete must reduce their testosterone levels or compete in different classes.
- It is important to note that this ruling does *not* question either the sex or gender identity of the athlete.
- In non-international competitions of any sort, the athlete may compete in the ♀ class without restrictions, and for international competitions, this only affects the 400m to 1 mile categories.

Further reading

Hamilton-Fairley D, Franks S (1997). Androgen-secreting tumours. In: Sheaves R, Jenkins PJ, Wass JAH (eds.) *Clinical Endocrine Oncology*. Blackwell Science, Oxford; pp. 323–9.
Rothman MS, Wierman ME (2011). How should postmenopausal androgen excess be evaluated? Clin Endocrinol (Oxf) 75, 160–4.

Menstrual function disorder—assessment and investigation

Definitions

- *Oligomenorrhoea* is defined as reduction in the frequency of menses to <9 periods a year.
- 1° *amenorrhoea* is failure of menarche by the age of 16 years. Prevalence ~0.3%.
- 2° *amenorrhoea* refers to cessation of menses for >3 months in ♀ with previous regular menstrual cycles or <3 periods per year. Prevalence ~3%.

(See Table 4.4 for WHO categorization.)

Aetiology

Although the list of causes is long (see Box 4.5 for causes), the majority of cases of 2° amenorrhoea can be accounted for by four conditions:
- PCOS.
- Hypothalamic amenorrhoea (HA).
- Hyperprolactinaemia.
- Ovarian failure.

Table 4.4 WHO categorization of hypogonadism

WHO group	LH and FSH	Clinical
I	↓	HH/HA
II	→	PCOS
III	↑	Premature ovarian insufficiency (POI)

Box 4.5 Causes of amenorrhoea

Physiological
- Pregnancy and lactation.
- Post-menopause.

Iatrogenic
- Depot medroxyprogesterone acetate.
- Levonorgestrel-releasing intrauterine device.
- Progesterone-only pill (POP).

Pathological—primary
- Chromosomal abnormalities—50%:
  - Turner syndrome.
  - Other X chromosomal disorders.
  - *FGFR1* mutation.
- 2° hypogonadism—25%:
  - Kallmann syndrome.
  - Pituitary disease.
  - HA.
- Genitourinary malformations—15%:
  - Imperforate hymen.
  - Absence of uterus, cervix, or vagina, e.g. *Rokitansky syndrome*, *androgen insensitivity syndrome*.
- Other—10%:
  - CAH.
  - PCOS.

  Most causes of 2° amenorrhoea can also cause 1° amenorrhoea.

Pathological—secondary
- Ovarian—70%:
  - PCOS.
  - POF.
- Hypothalamic—15%:
  - HH.
  - HA.
  - Weight loss/excess exercise.
  - Infiltrative lesions of the hypothalamus.
  - Drugs, e.g. opiates.
- Pituitary—5%:
  - Hyperprolactinaemia.
  - Hypopituitarism.
- Uterine—5%:
  - Intrauterine adhesions—*Asherman's syndrome*.
- Other endocrine disorders—5%:
  - Thyroid dysfunction.
  - Hyperandrogenism—Cushing's syndrome, CAH, tumour.

Menstrual function disorder—clinical evaluation

PCOS is the only common endocrine cause of amenorrhoea with normal oestrogenization—all other causes are oestrogen-deficient. ♀ with PCOS therefore are at risk of endometrial hyperplasia, and all others are at risk of osteoporosis.

History

- Oestrogen deficiency, e.g. hot flushes, reduced libido, dyspareunia.
- Hypothalamic dysregulation, e.g. exercise and nutritional history, body weight changes, emotional stress, recent or chronic physical illness.
- In 1° amenorrhoea—history of breast development, history of cyclical pain, age of menarche of mother and sisters.
- In 2° amenorrhoea—duration and regularity of previous menses, family history of early menopause or familial autoimmune disorders, or galactosaemia.
- Anosmia may indicate Kallmann syndrome.
- Hirsutism or acne.
- Galactorrhoea.
- History suggestive of pituitary, thyroid, or adrenal dysfunction.
- Drug history—e.g. causes of hyperprolactinaemia (see ➡ Box 2.13, p. 161), chemotherapy, hormonal contraception, recreational drug use.
- Obstetric and surgical history.

Physical examination

- Height, weight, BMI.
- Features of Turner syndrome or other dysmorphic features.
- 2° sex characteristics.
- Galactorrhoea.
- Evidence of hyperandrogenism or virilization.
- Evidence of thyroid dysfunction.
- Anosmia, visual field defects.

Amenorrhoea with normal gonadotrophins—WHO group II

In routine practice, a common differential diagnosis is between mild version of PCOS and HA. The distinction between these conditions may require repeated testing, as a single snapshot may not discriminate and both conditions may coexist. PCOS is more often oestrogen-replete, and thus clomifene citrate (an antioestrogen) or letrozole (aromatase inhibitor) are good options to induce ovulation for fertility. HA is oestrogen-deficient and will therefore be less likely to respond to clomifene citrate. HRT for bone protection, or ovulation induction with pulsatile GnRH (1st-line if available) or gonadotrophins, e.g. hMG if desiring conception. (For comparison, see Table 4.5.)

Table 4.5 Comparison of two common causes of amenorrhoea with normal gonadotrophins

	PCOS	HA
Exercise intensity	Any	High, contributing to available energy deficit
Androgen excess	Common	Rare
BMI usually	Any, ↑ prevalence with ↑ BMI	<21
LH	↔ or ↑ pulsatility	↓ (associated with FSH-predominant secretion)
Polycystic ovaries	90%	20%
Risk of endometrial hyperplasia	↔ or ↑ (oestradiol usually preserved)	↔ (low oestradiol state)

Menstrual function disorder—investigations

(See Fig. 4.7.)
- Is it 1° or 2° ovarian dysfunction?
  - FSH, LH, TFTs, oestradiol, PRL.
- US:
  - Ovarian and uterine morphology—exclude anatomical abnormalities, PCOS, and Turner syndrome.
  - Note that PCO morphology is present in 20% of all ♀; thus, most ♀ do not have the additional features of hyperandrogenism or oligo-/amenorrhoea to constitute the syndrome (PCOS) (see ➔ Polycystic ovary syndrome, pp. 340–3).
  - Endometrial thickness—to assess oestrogen status (<14mm premenopausal and <5mm post-menopausal, although depends on stage of menstrual cycle).
- Other tests, depending on clinical suspicion:
  - Induce withdrawal bleed with progesterone (e.g. 10mg medroxyprogesterone acetate bd for 7 days). If a bleed occurs, then there is adequate oestrogen priming and endometrial development. This test has poor specificity and sensitivity and has been abandoned in favour of US in many centres.
  - Serum testosterone in the presence of hyperandrogenism.
  - Karyotype in ovarian failure or disorder of sex development (DSD) suspected (absent uterus).
  - MRI of the pituitary fossa if FSH low or in the presence of hyperprolactinaemia.
  - Bone density if long-term oestrogen deficiency.

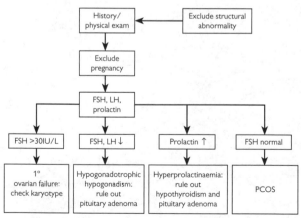

Fig. 4.7 Investigation of amenorrhoea.

Management of amenorrhoea

- Treat underlying disorder, e.g.:
  - Dopamine agonists for prolactinomas.
  - Pituitary surgery for pituitary tumours.
  - Eating disorder clinic in anorexia nervosa.
- Treat oestrogen deficiency—oestrogen/progestogen preparations.
- Treat infertility (see ⊃ Infertility, pp. 444–6).
- In PCOS with endometrial hyperplasia—progesterone withdrawal bleed, and consider hysteroscopy in resistant cases. Aim to induce a minimum of 3–4 withdrawal bleeds per year for endometrial health.

(See Box 4.6 for progesterone sensitivity.)

> **Box 4.6 Progesterone sensitivity**
> - Skin condition occurs regularly premenstrually—settling with onset of menses.
> - Dermatoses includes eczema, pompholyx, urticaria, and erythema multiforme.
> - Autoantibodies present (+ve challenge test).

Functional hypothalamic amenorrhoea (FHA)

- Chronic anovulation associated with excess exercise, weight loss, or stress, often in combination in the absence of other identified causes.
- Investigation indicated if >45-day cycle length and/or >3 months of amenorrhoea.

Evaluation

History
- Diet.
- Eating disorder.
- Exercise—amount/intensity/frequency.
- Stress and psychology, e.g. perfection, exams, performance.
- Drugs/complementary therapy/substances.
- Mood and sleep.
- Periods/OCP usage, etc.
- Features of organic causes, e.g. galactorrhoea, headaches, hirsutism, acne, family history, autoimmune disease, systemic disease.

Endocrine investigations
- TFTs, PRL, LH/FSH/oestradiol (E2), testosterone ± DHEAS, 17OHP.
- Exclude pregnancy.
- Pelvic US.
- Consider MRI pituitary and dual-energy absorptiometry (DXA).

Treatment
- Correction of energy balance.
- Reassurance; may take 1 year or more of normal weight and exercise to recover regular menses.
- Psychological support, e.g. CBT.
- Consider short-term oestrogen with progesterone.
- Avoid ovulation induction unless BMI normal.

Further reading

Baird DT (1997). Amenorrhoea. *Lancet* **350**, 275–9.

Beswick SJ, et al. (2002). A recurrent rash treated by oophorectomy. *QJM* **95**, 636–7.

Coutifaris C, et al. (2018). Case 29-2018: a 31-year-old woman with infertility. *N Engl J Med* **379**, 1162–72 [complete androgen insensitivity syndrome].

Gordon C, et al. (2017). Functional hypothalamic amenorrhea: an Endocrine Society clinical practice guideline. *J Clin Endocrinol Metab* **102**, 1413–39.

Hickey M, Balen A (2003). Menstrual disorders in adolescence: investigation and management. *Hum Reprod Update* **9**, 493–504.

Premature ovarian insufficiency

Definition

Premature ovarian insufficiency (POI) is a clinical syndrome defined by loss of ovarian activity in ♀ aged <40 years. It is characterized by amenorrhoea or oligomenorrhoea, oestrogen deficiency, and elevated gonadotrophins.

Epidemiology

- Prevalence is 1% of ♀ <40 years and 0.1% of ♀ <30 years.
- Accounts for 10% of all cases of 2° amenorrhoea.
- ~80% have no identifiable cause.

Causes of POI

- Chromosomal abnormalities (10% overall, 20% in 1° amenorrhoea):
  - Turner syndrome (see ➲ Turner syndrome in adulthood, p. 382).
  - Other X chromosomal abnormalities, e.g balanced translocation.
- Gene mutations:
  - Fragile X (*FMR1*) premutations.
  - Galactosaemia.
  - Rare single gene defects that are not yet part of routine testing (e.g. *NOBOX, FSHR, FOXL2, BMP15*).
- Familial, without identifiable genetic cause.
- Autoimmune disease (<20%).
- Iatrogenic (increasing %):
  - Chemotherapy.
  - Pelvic radiotherapy.
  - Pelvic surgery.
- Other:
  - Enzyme deficiencies, e.g. 17-hydroxylase deficiency.
  - Infections, e.g. mumps.
  - ? environmental toxins.
- Unknown (the majority of cases).

Pathogenesis

POI is the result of accelerated depletion of ovarian germ cells. POI is usually progressive and permanent, although a remitting or fluctuating course is possible. The term 'resistant ovary syndrome' is no longer used for this mild form of POI that gradually progresses to amenorrhoea. Conversely, 'ovarian dysgenesis' refers to the severe form with early onset and 1° amenorrhoea.

Clinical presentation

- *Menstrual disturbance*: Oligomenorrhoea or amenorrhoea (may be 1° or 2°).
- *Symptoms of oestrogen deficiency*:
  - 75% of ♀ with 2° amenorrhoea due to POI report hot flushes, night sweats, mood changes, fatigue, or dyspareunia; symptoms may precede the onset of menstrual disturbance.
  - POI may have a fluctuating course, with intermittent symptoms.
  - Symptoms do not occur in 1° amenorrhoea.

- *Relevant history:*
  - Previous chemotherapy, pelvic radiotherapy, or pelvic surgery.
  - Family history in 20% of patients.
  - Autoimmune disorders: screen for symptoms/signs (see Box 4.7).
- Ovarian function can resume, albeit transiently, usually within a year of diagnosis in idiopathic POI. Spontaneous pregnancies have been recorded in 5% of ♀ with POI.

Box 4.7 Autoimmune diseases and POI

- Autoimmunity underlies up to 20% of cases of POI.
- In 10–40% of these ♀, a second autoimmune disorder is present:
  - Autoimmune thyroid disease 25%.
  - Addison's disease 10%.
  - T1DM 2%.
  - Myasthenia gravis 2%.
  - B12 deficiency.
  - SLE is also more common.
- Autoimmune endocrinopathies:
  - 60% of ♀ with APS type 1 (see ➜ Autoimmune polyglandular syndrome (APS) type 1, p. 296).
  - 25% of ♀ with APS type 2 (see ➜ APS type 2, p. 297).
- Steroid cell antibodies are +ve in 60–100% of patients with Addison's disease in combination with POI. The presence of +ve steroid cell antibodies in ♀ with Addison's disease confers a 40% risk of ultimately developing POI. Other ovarian antibodies have little predictive value.

Investigation of POI

Diagnosis

Diagnosis is based on menstrual history with biochemical confirmation.

- Diagnosis is confirmed by serum FSH >30mIU/L on at least two occasions at least a month apart.
- LH also elevated but to lesser extent than FSH.
- Serum oestradiol levels are usually low.
- Anti-Müllerian hormone (AMH) is not recommended for diagnosis of POI.
- Pelvic ultrasound is not required for diagnosis; it may show ovarian activity, which is associated with spontaneous pregnancy.
- Ovarian biopsy is not used, as it has no diagnostic value.

Tests of causation

- Karyotype: ♀ with Y chromosomal material are at risk of gonadoblastoma and should be referred for bilateral gonadectomy.
- Fragile X premutation screening: Identification of carrier status is important for family members.
- Autoimmunity screening: Test for antibodies to thyroid, adrenal, parietal cell, and intrinsic factor. Ovarian antibodies are rarely +ve as the test has poor sensitivity. ♀ with +ve adrenal antibodies require further testing for Addison's disease (see ➜ Addison's disease, pp. 292–3).

Further assessment
- TSH, free T4; prevalence of thyroid dysfunction in POI is ~20%.
- Vitamin B12.
- Bone mineral densitometry; risk of osteopenia/osteoporosis.

Consequences of POI
- Infertility: This may be the most distressing aspect of POI. Spontaneous pregnancy has been reported in 5%, so all women must be informed that pregnancy is possible, even though conventional fertility treatments are not effective (often a difficult paradox to describe).
- Osteoporosis, increasing the risk of fragility fracture.
- Cardiovascular disease: POI is an independent risk factor for ischaemic heart disease.
- Cognitive and neurological sequelae (increased risk of parkinsonism, dementia) have been identified in ♀ with surgical menopause.
- Mortality is slightly increased, due to cardiovascular and osteoporotic complications, reducing life expectancy by ~2 years in untreated POI.

Management of POI

Sex hormone replacement therapy (HRT)

For a full review of HRT, see ➲ Menopause, p. 384.

- Exogenous oestrogen is required to alleviate symptoms and prevent the long-term complications of oestrogen deficiency.
- Exogenous progestogen is required for 12–14 days a month to prevent endometrial hyperplasia (unless prior hysterectomy).
- Standard doses of HRT may be sub-physiological for young ♀.
- When initiating HRT, take into account duration of amenorrhoea; if oestrogen deficient for >12 months, start on lower dose to prevent side effects, titrate up to full dose by 6 months.
- Doses used in HRT are not contraceptive and do not suppress spontaneous ovarian follicular activity. Women who do not wish to conceive may use combined oral contraception (COC) instead of HRT; oestrogen-deficiency symptoms can recur in pill-free week.
- Low-dose androgen replacement therapy may improve fatigue and poor libido persisting despite adequate oestrogen replacement.
- HRT should be continued at least until the age of 50 years, the mean age of natural menopause.

Fertility

- 5% spontaneous fertility rate in ♀ with POI
- Egg donation is the only effective fertility treatment. Birth rate >30% per cycle. Hormone therapy is required for endometrial preparation and early pregnancy support. Outcomes are poor in ♀ with uterine damage after pelvic radiotherapy.
- Other treatments have not been shown to be effective:
  - Ovulation induction therapy.
  - Glucocorticoid therapy in autoimmune POI.
  - FSH suppression.
- Fertility preservation can be offered to ♀ at high risk of POI (e.g. before chemo/radiotherapy, Turner syndrome mosaicism with retained ovarian function (see ➲ Turner syndrome in adulthood, p. 382), but is not possible after onset of POI.

Psychology

- The psychological impact of POI is significant, affecting self-esteem and relationships. Supportive counselling should be offered.
- Reactive depression is common at diagnosis and may return at critical times, such as pregnancy in a close friend.

Monitoring treatment

Assess adequacy of treatment by symptom control and bone mineral densitometry (baseline measurement, repeated after 3-5 years). Suboptimal bone mass may be due to a combination of factors, including delay in initiating HRT, poor compliance with HRT, and oestrogen 'underdosing'.

Turner syndrome in adulthood

Commonest X-chromosome abnormality, affecting 1:2500 live ♀ births. Result of complete or partial absence of an X chromosome.

Clinical features

Short stature and gonadal dysgenesis; 80% of affected ♀ have 1° amenorrhoea.

Characteristic phenotype

Webbed neck, micrognathia, low-set ears, high arched palate, widely spaced nipples, cubitus valgus.

Other associated conditions

- Aortic coarctation, bicuspid aortic valve, and other left-sided congenital heart defects.
- Congenital renal anomalies, horseshoe kidney.
- Lymphoedema.
- ENT conditions, hearing loss.
- Hypothyroidism, coeliac disease, inflammatory bowel disease.
- Osteoporosis, skeletal abnormalities.

Diagnosis

Made on karyotype (see Table 4.6). Features are milder in ♀ with mosaic karyotype.

Table 4.6 Correlation of karyotype with phenotype

Karyotype	Phenotype
45, X (50%)	Most severe phenotype
	High incidence of cardiac and renal abnormalities
46, Xi(Xq) (20%)	↑ prevalence of thyroiditis, inflammatory bowel disease, and deafness
45,X/46, XX (10%)	Least severe phenotype
	Fewer comorbidities
	Spontaneous puberty and menses in up to 40%
46, Xr(X) (10%)	Spontaneous menses in 33%
	Congenital anomalies uncommon
	Cognitive dysfunction in those with a small ring chromosome
45, X/46, XY (6%)	Risk of gonadoblastoma (recommend gonadectomy)
Other (4%)	

Management in adults

- Sex hormone replacement therapy.
- Treat associated conditions.

Follow-up

- Annual health surveillance: BMI, BP, TFT, LFT, lipids, blood glucose.
- 3- to 5-yearly: echocardiogram, bone densitometry, and audiometry.
- 5-yearly: thyroid and coeliac autoantibodies, GTT.

Further reading

European Society of Human Reproduction and Embryology, POI guideline development group (2015). Management of women with premature ovarian insufficiency. ℛ https://www.eshre.eu/Guidelines-and-Legal/Guidelines/Management-of-premature-ovarian-insufficiency

Davies MC, Cartwright B (2012). What is the best management strategy for a 20-year-old woman with premature ovarian failure? *Clin Endocrinol (Oxf)* **77**, 182–6.

Nelson LM (2009). Clinical practice. Primary ovarian insufficiency. *N Engl J Med* **360**, 606–14.

Webber L, et al. (2017). HRT for women with premature ovarian insufficiency: a comprehensive review. *Human Reproduction Open* **2017**, 2 hox007.

Gravholt CH, et al. (2017). Clinical practice guidelines for the care of girls and women with Turner syndrome: proceedings from the 2016 Cincinnati International Turner Syndrome meeting. *Eur J Endocrinol* **177**, G1-G70.

Cameron-Pimblett A, et al. (2017). The Turner syndrome life course project: karyotype-phenotype analyses across the lifespan. *Clin Endocrinol (Oxf)* **87**, 532–8. ℛ https://www.daisynetwork.org (patient support organization)

Menopause

Definition

- The *menopause* is the permanent cessation of menstruation as a result of ovarian failure and is a retrospective diagnosis made after 12 months of amenorrhoea. The average age at menopause is 51 years in developed countries (range 45–55 years).
- The *perimenopause* encompasses the menopause transition and the 1st year following the last menstrual period.

Physiology

- Ovaries have a finite number of germ cells, with maximal numbers at 20 weeks of intrauterine life. Thereafter, there is a gradual reduction in the number of follicles, speeding up in the late reproductive years, until the store of oocytes is depleted at the time of the menopause.
- There are familial and environmental influences; smokers reach menopause ~2 years earlier.
- The mechanisms regulating the rate of attrition of follicles are not clear. AMH and inhibin B are ovarian glycoproteins, produced by follicles, as they develop from preantral to antral stages, which may participate in ovarian paracrine regulation.

(See Table 4.7 for hormonal changes.)

Diagnosis

- Menopause is a clinical diagnosis in ♀ aged >45 years.
- Routine biochemistry (FSH, oestradiol measurement) is not necessary for confirmation.
- AMH measurement adds nothing in routine practice.

Long-term consequences

- *Osteoporosis.* During the late perimenopause and early postmenopause there is an accelerated loss of bone mineral, rendering post-menopausal ♀ more susceptible to osteoporotic fractures.
- *IHD.* Post-menopausal ♀ are 2–3 times more likely to develop IHD than premenopausal ♀, even after age adjustments. The menopause is associated with an increase in risk factors for atherosclerosis, including less favourable lipid profile, ↓ insulin sensitivity, and ↑ thrombotic tendency.
- *Dementia.* ♀ are more likely to develop Alzheimer's disease than ♂. It is suggested that oestrogen deficiency may play a role in the development of dementia.

Table 4.7 Hormonal changes during the menopausal transition

	Premenopause (from age 36 years)	Early perimenopause	Advanced perimenopause	Menopause
Menstrual cycle	Regular, ovulatory	Irregular, often short cycles, increasingly anovulatory	Oligo-menorrhoea	Amenorr-hoea
FSH	Rising but within normal range	Intermittently raised, especially in follicular phase	Persistently ↑	↑↑
AMH	Declining	Low/undetectable	Low/undetectable	Un-detectable
E2	Normal	Fluctuating, may be high normal	Normal/low	Low

Clinical presentation of menopause

Menstrual disturbances

Cycles gradually become increasingly variable in length from about 4 years prior to the menopause. Shortening of the cycle may be an early warning. Oligomenorrhoea often precedes permanent amenorrhoea. In 10% of ♀, menses cease abruptly, with no preceding transitional period.

Vasomotor symptoms (~75%)

Hot flushes and night sweats are the cardinal symptoms of oestrogen deficiency. Although the exact mechanism is uncertain, it appears to involve the central nervous system and autonomic thermoregulatory pathway. Symptoms are experienced by 75% of women in Western countries, 25% of these being severely affected. There are marked differences in the % of women reporting symptoms across countries and ethnic backgrounds. Vasomotor symptoms improve with time and eventually resolve, but the median duration is 7 years.

Sexual dysfunction (~40%)

This has both physical and psychosexual components. Vaginal dryness resulting from urogenital atrophy may result in dyspareunia. Additionally, falling androgen and oestrogen levels may reduce sexual arousal and libido.

Urinary symptoms (~50%)

Atrophy of urethral and bladder mucosa after the menopause and ↓ sensitivity of α-adrenergic receptors of the bladder neck in the perimenopausal period. This may result in urinary frequency and incontinence.

Mood changes (25–50%)

Anxiety, low mood, and irritability are common problems at the time of menopause. ♀ with a history of affective disorders are at ↑ risk of mood disturbances in the perimenopausal period. Cognitive changes with forgetfulness and difficulty in concentration are often reported and may be partly attributed to fatigue due to night waking.

Musculoskeletal symptoms

Joint and muscle aches are commonly reported by women in menopause.

Evaluation of menopause if HRT is being considered

History

- Perimenopausal symptoms and their severity.
- Bleeding pattern.
- Assess risk factors for:
  - cardiovascular disease,
  - osteoporosis,
  - breast cancer,
  - thromboembolic disease.
- Medical history e.g. active liver disease.
- Family history, e.g. VTE.

See Box 4.8 for contraindications to HRT.

Examination

- BP, BMI.
- Breast examination if symptomatic.
- Consider pelvic examination for dyspareunia.

Investigations

- Menopause is a clinical diagnosis in women >45 years.
- *FSH* is not usually required, nor helpful, as levels fluctuate markedly in the perimenopausal period and may not correlate with symptoms.
- *Breast screening (mammography)* should be offered as per national screening programme guidelines; it may be indicated prior to starting ERT only in high-risk ♀.
- *Cervical screening (cervical smear)* should be offered as per national screening programme guidelines.
- *Pelvic ultrasound, hysteroscopy,* and *endometrial biopsy* may be required in ♀ with abnormal uterine bleeding, for whom gynaecological review is essential before initiating HRT.

Box 4.8 Summary of contraindications to HRT

Absolute
- Undiagnosed vaginal bleeding
- Pregnancy
- Recent VTE or arterial thromboembolic event
- Endometrial cancer
- Breast cancer

Significant—seek advice
- Past/family history of VTE
- Active liver disease
- Ischaemic heart disease
- Cerebrovascular disease
- Hypertriglyceridaemia
- Previous endometrial cancer
- Previous breast cancer

Contraception in the perimenopause

- Be aware that raised FSH in the perimenopause may not necessarily indicate infertility. Contraception, if desired, should continue until amenorrhoeic for 1 year in women aged >50 years and 2 years in women aged 40–50 years.
- Diagnosis of menopause can be difficult in women using hormonal contraception, which may cause altered bleeding patterns. Combined hormonal contraception suppresses gonadotrophins. FSH measurement may be used to diagnose menopause in amenorrhoeic women using progestogen-only contraception.

Alternatives to HRT in treatment of symptoms of menopause

Lifestyle measures

Alcohol and caffeine can provoke vasomotor symptoms, and reduction or avoidance is usually beneficial. Physically active women tend to suffer less from menopausal symptoms, and exercise improves psychological health and quality of life in symptomatic women.

Vaginal lubricants and moisturisers

'Moisturisers' can be more effective than the water-based vaginal lubricants used during intercourse, as they may contain hydrocolloids, adhering to the vaginal walls and retaining moisture for longer.

Plant-based (herbal) remedies

See Table 4.8.

Cognitive behavioural therapy (CBT)

CBT can be used to alleviate low mood or anxiety that arises as a result of menopause and to manage vasomotor symptoms.

SNRIs and SSRIs

These have been confirmed to reduce vasomotor symptoms, although less effectively than HRT. They act at lower doses than required for depression. The SNRI venlafaxine has been the most studied and the SSRIs escitalopram/citalopram and paroxetine are similarly effective. These agents are not recommended as first-line therapy ahead of HRT but are useful in women with contraindications to HRT, e.g. breast cancer (although some SSRIs interact with tamoxifen).

Gabapentin

Gabapentin has also been shown to reduce the frequency and severity of hot flushes. Side effects include dizziness, somnolence, and weight gain.

Clonidine

Clonidine is less effective, reducing the occurrence of flushes by 20%, and is often associated with disabling side-effects, such as dizziness, drowsiness, and dry mouth.

Treatment for osteoporosis

The SERM raloxifene can be used for prevention and treatment of osteoporosis; however, it may exacerbate vasomotor symptoms. Bisphosphonates, e.g. alendronic acid and risedronate, are non-hormonal therapies for osteoporosis. See also ➔ Treatment of osteoporosis, p. 552–3.

Table 4.8 Plant-based treatments for symptoms of menopause

Remedy	Efficacy and safety
Phytoestrogens: plant-derived substances with slight oestrogen-like activity. They include isoflavones, found in soy beans, chickpeas, and red clover, and lignans, found in cereals and seeds	Epidemiological studies suggest women with diets high in isoflavones have ↓ rates of menopausal symptoms, osteoporosis, and cardiovascular disease. Data from clinical trials are inconclusive. The effect on vasomotor symptoms is modest at best. Soy protein may have a favourable effect on plasma lipid concentrations and thus cardiovascular risk. However, the daily dose required is unclear. Data regarding effects on bone and breast cancer risk are inconclusive. Phytoestrogen supplements cannot be recommended for disease prevention in peri- and post-menopausal ♀
Chinese herbal remedies	Uncertain efficacy, and not recommended because of potential for toxicity; drug interactions have been reported
St John's wort	Shown to be effective in treating mild to moderate depression in peri- and post-menopausal women, but not proven to be effective for vasomotor symptoms. Numerous drug interactions require caution in use
Other herbal products: these include black cohosh, ginseng, sage, evening primrose oil, *Agnus castus*, *Ginkgo biloba*	None of these have sufficient supportive evidence to recommend use

Hormone replacement therapy

HRT is established as the most effective therapy for menopausal symptoms. The aim of treatment for perimenopausal ♀ is to alleviate symptoms and optimize QoL. The majority of women with mild symptoms will not require HRT. For ♀ with a contraindication to HRT or who are intolerant of it, offer non-hormonal therapies (see ➔ Alternatives to HRT in treatment of symptoms of menopause, p. 390.).

Benefits of HRT

Hot flushes

Respond very well to oestrogen therapy in a dose-dependent manner. Start with a low dose, and increase gradually, as required, to control symptoms. Higher doses may be required in younger ♀ or in those whose symptoms develop abruptly post-oophorectomy.

Vulval and vaginal atrophy

HRT improves vaginal dryness and dyspareunia. Vaginal oestrogen therapy should be offered before systemic HRT. With modern preparations systemic absorption is minimal, allowing long-term use without risk of endometrial hyperplasia or systemic adverse effects.

Urinary symptoms

HRT may improve stress and urge incontinence as well as urinary frequency and predilection to cystitis. Vaginal oestrogen therapy should be offered before systemic HRT.

Osteoporosis

HRT has been shown to increase BMD in the lumbar spine by 3–5% and at the femoral neck by about 2% by inhibiting bone resorption. The influential Women's Health Initiative (WHI) trial (see Box 4.9) confirmed that HRT ↓ the risk of both hip and vertebral fractures by 30%. HRT is not primarily used for bone protection, however.

Colorectal cancer

The WHI showed a 20% ↓ in the incidence of colon cancer in HRT users. However, HRT should not be prescribed to prevent colorectal cancer.

Common side effects of HRT and troubleshooting

- *Breast tenderness* usually subsides within 3–6 months of use. If troublesome, reduce oestrogen dose, then build up slowly.
- *Mood changes* are usually associated with progestogen therapy; manage by changing the type of progestogen or route of administration.
- *Irregular vaginal bleeding* may be a problem in ♀ on a continuous combined preparation. This should only be prescribed for women who have had no spontaneous bleeds for a year. Usually settles within 3–6 months. Prolonged bleeding must be investigated (see Box 4.10).
- *No withdrawal bleeds* on cyclical therapy usually indicates poor compliance or inadequate dosage

Risks of HRT

Breast cancer

There is an ↑ risk of breast cancer in HRT users which is related to the duration of use. Estimates of risk have been contentious, and higher in observational than in randomized studies. For women starting HRT aged 50

Box 4.9 Summary of WHI hormone therapy trials

- *Trial design.* Randomized controlled trial of the effects of HRT on healthy asymptomatic post-menopausal ♀. Mean follow-up on combined HRT 5.6 years, oestrogen alone 7.2 years. Extended follow-up to 13 years.
- *Participants.* >27,000 women aged 50–79 (mean age 63 years). 70% were overweight or obese, and 50% were current or past smokers.
- Outcomes. Trial stopped early because of ↑ risk of breast cancer, heart disease, stroke and VTE with combined HRT, ↑ stroke with oestrogen-alone.

(See also Table 4.9.)

- *Controversies:*
  - whether results can be extrapolated to younger HRT users. For women <60 results were largely reassuring, and if taking oestrogen alone, findings were of benefit
  - whether different HRT preparations or routes of administration have the same benefit/risk profile.
    WHI used oral-conjugated oestrogens and medroxyprogesterone acetate, but newer HRT is now used, e.g. biosimilar hormones and transdermal HRT.

Reference: ℔ https://www.whi.org

Box 4.10 Investigation for irregular uterine bleeding

- *Sequential cyclical HRT.* Check compliance, as missed tablets can cause breakthrough bleeding. Refer if recurrent bleeding (≥3 cycles) or ↑ in the duration / intensity of bleeding.
- *Continuous combined HRT.* Refer if bleeding continues after 3-6 months of use, or earlier if bleeding is heavy or prolonged, or if bleeding starts after a spell of amenorrhoea.
- *Endometrial assessment.* Pelvic ultrasound (transvaginal) is essential in ♀ with irregular uterine bleeding. Endometrial thickness of <5mm excludes disease in 96–99% of cases, a sensitivity similar to that of endometrial biopsy. However, specificity is poor, so if the endometrium is >5mm (as it will be in 50% of post-menopausal ♀ on HRT), endometrial biopsy will be required to rule out carcinoma.

and taking it for 5 years (the typical scenario), the background rate of breast cancer is 13 cases/1000 women, and an additional 8 cases would occur on HRT. (See Table 4.9.) The risk increases with prolonged use, and falls after discontinuing HRT.

The risk is low in ♀ on oestradiol alone (an additional 3 cases/1000 women at 5 years). Sequential HRT is associated with less risk than continuous combined HRT. These findings suggest that progestogens are implicated in pathogenesis. Mortality has not been shown to be ↑ in ♀ developing breast cancer on HRT.

Women at high risk of breast cancer

♀ with familial risk of breast cancer may use HRT for severe vasomotor symptoms, after discussion, as there is little evidence that the risk is ↑ further; dose and duration should be minimized. Women undergoing risk-reducing bilateral oophorectomy prior to menopause may require HRT.

Past history of breast cancer

Avoid HRT in ♀ with a past history of breast cancer. Individual circumstances may be considered (e.g. length of disease-free follow-up, hormone sensitivity of tumour).

Venous thromboembolism

Oral HRT is associated with ≤3-fold ↑ risk of VTE, resulting in an extra 2 cases/10,000 woman-years. The risk is highest in the first year of HRT usage. Transdermal E2 at standard doses has not been shown to ↑ risk of VTE in healthy women. Transdermal therapy is therefore preferred for women at increased risk, including BMI >30kg/m².

Personal or family history of VTE

Women with a personal history of VTE or relevant family history need individualized advice. HRT is contraindicated in thrombophilic states. Even with -ve thrombophilia screen, risk is slightly ↑ and if HRT is prescribed it should be transdermal. A very small number of women will use HRT whilst on long-term anticoagulation.

Cerebrovascular disease

Oral HRT has been shown to i the risk of ischaemic stroke ≤1.5-fold, but events are rare in menopausal women as baseline risk is strongly age-dependent. HRT should not be used in ♀ with a history of cerebrovascular disease or atrial fibrillation, unless they are anticoagulated.

Endometrial cancer

Unopposed oestrogen causes dose-dependent ↑ in the risk of endometrial hyperplasia and cancer incidence doubles after 5 years of use, so it is not prescribed unless women have had a hysterectomy. The addition of progestogen given sequentially for ≥10 days/cycle reduces this risk, and eliminates it when given continuously.

Women with cured stage I endometrial tumours may safely take HRT.

Ovarian cancer

Long-term use of HRT may be associated with slight ↑ risk of ovarian cancer (1 case/1000 women with 10 years of use).

Gallstones

The risk of gallstones is ↑ 2-fold in HRT users.

Migraine

Migraines may increase in severity and frequency with oestrogen. Providing there are no focal neurological signs associated with the migraine, a trial of HRT is worthwhile. Transdermal therapy minimizes the risk.

Endometriosis and uterine fibroids

Growth of uterine fibroids is unlikely on HRT.

Recurrence of endometriosis on HRT is uncommon, but a bleed-free regimen is chosen to minimize the risk.

Liver disease

In ♀ with impaired liver function, use transdermal therapy to avoid hepatic metabolism, and monitor LFTs. Do not use HRT in the presence of active liver disease or liver failure.

Areas of uncertainty with HRT

Cardiovascular disease)

The effect of HRT on CVD has been controversial. Data from numerous observational studies suggest that HRT may reduce the risk of developing CVD by up to 50%. However, randomized placebo-controlled trials, e.g. the Heart and Oestrogen-Progestin Replacement Study (HERS), failed to show that HRT protects against IHD, and indeed in the WHI trial more events were recorded on HRT.

Current interpretation is that HRT does not increase cardiovascular risk if started aged <60. Oestrogen alone may even be beneficial. However, HRT should not be prescribed to prevent cardiovascular disease. HRT may be used cautiously in individual patients with cardiovascular risk factors if these are appropriately managed.

Cognitive function

In the immediate post-menopause, HRT may improve certain aspects of cognitive function. There is good evidence that HRT does not prevent cognitive decline in older postmenopausal women and indeed may have a negative effect.

Table 4.9 Risks and benefits of HRT

	Risks over 5 years		Total risks up to age 69	
	Cases per 1000 women with no HRT use	Extra cases per 1000 women using HRT	Cases per 1000 women with no HRT use	Extra cases per 1000 women after using HRT for 5 years
Breast cancer risks associated with HRT of various types				
All combined HRT	13	+8	63	+17
Sequential HRT	13	+7	63	+14
Continuous combined HRT	13	+10	63	+20
Oestrogen alone	13	+3	63	+5
Other risks associated with combined oestrogen and progestogen				
Endometrial cancer	2	—	10	—
Ovarian cancer	2	+<1	10	+<1
VTE	5	+7	26	+7
Stroke	4	+1	26	+1
CHD	14	—	88	—
Fracture of femur	1.5	—	12	—

Source: Data from Medicines and Healthcare Products Regulatory Agency. ♫ https://www.cas.mhra.gov.uk

HRT regimens

How do I... choose the right HRT for my patient?

HRT regimens may seem complex, but the principles are straightforward. Use the lowest effective dose of oestrogen for the shortest duration (typically 3-5 years) to relieve symptoms. Higher doses may be required by younger women and after surgical menopause, but can then be reduced gradually.

Progestogen must be added to protect the endometrium, except in women who have had a hysterectomy. See Fig. 4.8.

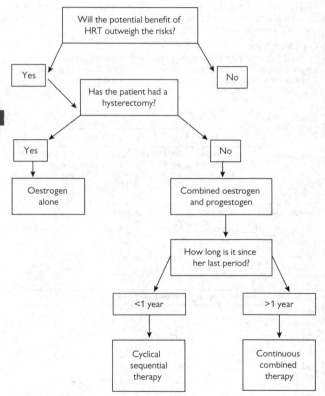

Fig. 4.8 How do I... choose the right HRT.

Route of oestrogen administration

- *Oral route* is the most popular. First-pass hepatic metabolism results in ↑ thrombotic risk. May be associated with nausea and may exacerbate liver disease.
- *Transdermal patches* avoid first-pass effect and are thus ideal in ♀ with liver disease or hypertriglyceridaemia, and in women with ↑ risk of VTE. Skin reactions are uncommon; rotate patch sites to avoid this.
- *Gels* have the advantages of patches, but skin irritation is less common.
- *Implants* are not commonly used. If side effects develop, implants are difficult to remove. They may release oestradiol for a prolonged period, and progestagen must be continued until oestrogen levels are undetectable.
- *Topical oestrogen.* Vaginal administration of very low-dose oestradiol as a tablet, cream, or ring, is used specifically to treat symptoms of urogenital atrophy. In these doses it does not cause systemic effects.

Types of oestrogen and progestogen

- All modern HRT preparations contain oestradiol.
- There is a range of synthetic progestogen preparations, from dydrogesterone (the least androgenic) through medroxyprogesterone acetate and levonorgestrel to norethisterone (the most androgenic).
- Micronized progesterone is physiological.
- The levonorgestrel intrauterine system is increasingly popular as the progestogen component of HRT, giving endometrial protection for at least 4 years and achieving amenorrhoea in most women.

Sequential cyclical regimen

Progestogen is given for a minimum of 10 days a month, in a cyclical regimen to produce monthly withdrawal bleed. (See Fig. 4.8.)

Continuous combined regimen

Progestogen is given daily, in a lower dose, to avoid endometrial build-up. Although breakthrough bleeding may occur in the early months, 90% of ♀ have amenorrhoea by 1 year. (See Fig. 4.8.)

Tibolone

A synthetic steroid with mixed oestrogenic, progestogenic, and weak androgenic activities. An alternative form of continuous HRT, with little stimulation of the endometrium. It alleviates vasomotor symptoms, may improve mood and libido, and is protective against osteoporosis. Risks of VTE and breast cancer similar to oestrogen; <10% of ♀ may experience vaginal bleeding on tibolone.

Stopping HRT

- In 75% of ♀, vasomotor symptoms settle within 5 years. Consider stopping HRT after 5 years of treatment.
- The dose of HRT should be gradually reduced over weeks, as sudden withdrawal of oestrogen may precipitate the return of vasomotor symptoms.

Androgen replacement therapy

- Androgens are thought to play a role in maintaining bone density and muscle strength, sexual function, and cognitive function in ♀. The major androgens in premenopausal ♀ are androstenedione and testosterone, which is produced by both the ovaries and adrenal glands roughly equally, and >90% bound to SHBG and albumin. The amount of testosterone produced pre-menopause is actually greater than oestrogen. Effects are both direct and through peripheral conversion to oestrogen.
- Total and free serum androstenedione and testosterone levels fall by up to 50% after the menopause.
- *Indications for androgen replacement therapy.* Poor well-being and libido despite adequate ERT in ♀ with ovarian failure.
- *Administration.* No licensed preparation available in UK for ♀; transdermal preparations for ♂ may be used off-label in appropriate doses (e.g. one sachet of 50mg for daily use by ♂ should last 10 days for ♀). Systemic HRT should be prescribed before a trial of testosterone. Avoid in active liver disease, polycythaemia, history of hormone-sensitive breast cancer. Allow 3-6 months to assess response.
- *Monitoring.* Serum testosterone; consider LFT, lipid profile.
- *Side effects and risks.* Hirsutism, acne. Virilization can occur with excessive dose. Adverse changes to lipid profile commonly occur, but effect on cardiovascular risk is unknown. Long-term effects of androgen therapy on the endometrium and breast are unknown.

Other hormonal therapies

- Progestagens can be used; megestrol acetate reduces hot flushes by up to 70%, but use is limited by side effects, e.g. weight gain.
- Dehydroepiandrosterone (DHEA) used vaginally for atrophic symptoms appears effective; there is not sufficient evidence for systemic use for bone mass, libido, and flushes.

Further reading

Avis NE, *et al.* (2015). Duration of menopausal vasomotor symptoms over the menopausal transition. *JAMA Intern Med* **175**(4), 531-9.

Collaborative group on hormonal factors in breast cancer (2019). Type and timing of menopausal hormone therapy and breast cancer risk: individual participant meta-analysis of the worldwide epidemiological evidence. *Lancet* **394** ,1159-68.

Davis SR, *et al.* (2008). Testosterone for low libido in postmenopausal women not taking estrogen. *N Engl J Med* **359**, 2005–17.

NICE (2015, updated 2019). Menopause: diagnosis and management. [NG23].

Rees MCP, Panay N (2010). Alternatives to HRT for the management of symptoms of the menopause. *RCOG Scientific Impact paper no.6.*

Rymer J, *et al.* (2003). Making decisions about hormone replacement therapy. *BMJ* **326**, 322–6.

Santoro N, *et al.* (2017). Menstrual cycle hormone changes in women traversing menopause: study of women's health across the nation. *J Clin Endocrinol Metab* **102**(7), 2218–29.

Somboonporn W, *et al.* (2005). Testosterone for peri and postmenopausal women. *Cochrane Database Syst. Rev* **4**, CD 004509. doi:10.1002/14651858.CD004509.pub2

Writing Group for Women's Health Initiative Investigators (2002). Risks and benefits of estrogen plus progestin in healthy postmenopausal women: principal results from the Women's Health Initiative randomized controlled trial. *JAMA* **288**, 321–33.

Hormonal contraception

Hormonal contraception: overview

- Hormonal contraception is the most widely used type of contraception in Europe and North America. It is also commonly prescribed for non-contraceptive benefits (e.g. control of hirsutism).
- Health professionals giving advice on contraception need knowledge of the full range of alternative methods (i.e. intrauterine contraception, barrier methods, and ♂ and ♀ sterilization).
- Acceptability of the contraceptive method determines its use.
- Non-contraceptive use still requires full discussion of risks and side effects, and contraceptive efficacy.

Formulations

- Combined hormonal contraception:
  - pills
  - patch
  - ring.
- Progestogen-only contraception:
  - pills
  - depot injection
  - implant
  - intrauterine system.
- Emergency contraception.

Combined hormonal contraception

Overview

- Very effective contraception, with method failure rate of <1%, although with typical use at least 5 pregnancies/100 users occur in the first year.
- Acts by preventing ovulation by suppressing gonadotrophins through HPO axis; progestogen also acts on cervical mucus and tubal motility

Route of administration

- Oral:combined oral contraceptive pill, 'The Pill' (COC).
- Transdermal (patch changed weekly).
- Vaginal ring (worn continuously for 21 days).

Data on the COC is generally extrapolated to other versions of combined hormonal contraception (CHC).

Regimen

- All types of CHC are usually taken cyclically in a 21/7 regimen, 3 weeks of medication followed by a 1-week break during which withdrawal bleeding occurs.
- Tailored regimens reduce the frequency or length of the hormone-free interval with extended or continuous administration of CHC. A common example is 'tri-cycling', 9 weeks of CHC followed by 1 week's break.
- Most COC are monophasic (fixed dose). Multiphasic COC (varying doses through the cycle) carry no particular advantage and cannot be used in extended regimens.

Types of oestrogen/progestogen

Oestrogens

- Ethinylestradiol (EE) is standard. COC, as estradiol, is available in three strengths: 20, 30, and 35 micrograms EE. The lowest dose may reduce side effects but provides less menstrual control, so 30micrograms is commonly prescribed.
- 17β-oestradiol (as estradiol) is now available in COC and may have a better safety profile than EE, but data are limited as yet.

Progestogens

- First generation: norethisterone (NET).
- Second generation: levonorgestrel (LNG).
- First-line COCs contain NET or LNG as they have the lowest risk of thrombosis, but more androgenic side effects. (EE 30micrograms + LNG 150micrograms is the most commonly prescribed COC).
- Third generation: *desogestrel, gestodene,* and *norgestimate* are less androgenic but may carry ↑ risk of thromboembolism.
- Fourth generation: *drospirenone*. Anti-androgenic and anti-mineralocorticoid properties; used in the treatment of acne and hirsutism in PCOS.
- Unclassified: *cyproterone acetate*. Anti-androgenic, marketed in combination with EE 35micrograms for the treatment of acne and hirsutism rather than as COC. Higher VTE risk.

Non-contraceptive benefits

Acne and hirsutism
- All COCs reduce free testosterone concentration by suppressing ovarian production of androgens and by ↑ hepatic SHBG production. Use COCs containing anti-androgenic progestogens.

PCOS
- COC can be used to manage acne, hirsutism, and menstrual irregularity. Be aware of ↑ VTE risk in obese women.

Menstrual disorders
- COC improves menorrhagia by ↓ menstrual flow and also ↓ dysmenorrhoea and improves premenstrual symptoms. Offer tailored regimens to ↓ frequency of bleeds. Continuous regimens can reduce the risk of recurrent endometriosis after surgery.

POI
- COC improves vasomotor symptoms and prevents bone mineral loss, offer to ♀ with POI who require contraception.

Cancer
- The risks of ovarian, endometrial, and colon cancer are all reduced by COC use. With long-term use ≥10 years, ovarian and endometrial cancer incidence is halved. Risk reduction persists long after discontinuation of COC.

Table 4.10 CHC contraindications

Absolute	Relative
History of heart disease, ischaemic or valvular	Migraine without focal aura
Pulmonary hypertension	Hypertension
History of arterial or venous thrombosis	Sickle cell disease
History of cerebrovascular disease	Inflammatory bowel disease Gallstones
High risk of thrombosis, known thrombophilia, e.g. factor V Leiden, antiphospholipid antibodies	Family history of thrombosis Obesity
Liver disease	Hyperlipidaemia
Migraine if severe or with focal aura	Diabetes mellitus
Breast or genital tract cancer	Family history of breast cancer
Pregnancy	Smoking
Two or more relative contraindications	Age >35 years
	Otosclerosis

CHC side effects

- Breakthrough bleeding (more likely with 20micrograms COC; check compliance).
- Low mood, reduced libido.
- Nausea.
- Fluid retention and weight gain.
- Breast tenderness and enlargement.
- Headache.
- Chloasma.

CHC risks

Venous thromboembolism

- VTE risk in ♀ on the COC is ↑ 3- to 3.5-fold, compared to background risk of 2/10,000 non-pregnant ♀ per year.
- Risk of VTE is highest in the 1st year of use.
- VTE risk ↑ with age and obesity. COC is not advisable if BMI >35kg/m².
- VTE risk is affected by EE dose and progestogen type; it is lower with 1st- and 2nd generation progestogens, ~ 6/10,000, than with anti-androgenic progestogens, 9-12/10,000.
- Transdermal/vaginal CHC appear to carry the same VTE risk.

Arterial thrombosis

- Current COC users have slightly ↑ risk of myocardial infarction and ischaemic stroke, but absolute risk is very small.
- Avoid CHC in women with multiple risk factors (see Table 4.10). There is a 10-fold excess risk of IHD in ♀ smokers aged >35 years on COC.
- Risk of arterial thrombosis relates to EE dose.
- Migraine with aura is a risk factor for ischaemic stroke and CHC should be avoided.
- Risk of haemorrhagic stroke does not seem to be ↑ by COC.

Hypertension

- May be provoked by COC and, if already present, may be more resistant to treatment.

Hepatic disease

- Raised hepatic enzymes may be seen in ♀ on COC. The incidence of benign hepatic tumours is also ↑.

Gallstones

- The risk of developing gallstones is slightly ↑ by COC (RR = 1.2).

Breast cancer

- COC usage is associated with a slightly ↑ risk of breast cancer (RR = 1.2 compared to never-users), which may be related to duration of use.
- The RR of developing breast cancer returns to normal 10 years after discontinuing COC.

Cervical cancer

- The use of COC for >5 years appears to be associated with an excess risk of cervical cancer (RR = 1.9).
- The risk reduces over time after discontinuing COC use.

Practical prescribing issues

Age and BMI

- ♀ with no risk factors for arterial or venous thrombosis may continue to use COC until the age of 50 years.
- Those with risk factors, particularly smokers, should avoid COC after the age of 35 years.
- Because obesity affects risk of VTE, MI and ischaemic stroke, for ♀ with BMI >35kg/m² the risks of COC generally outweigh the benefits.

Breakthrough bleeding

Causes include:

- Genital tract disease.
- Missed pill.
- Gastroenteritis.
- Drug interactions, e.g. hepatic enzyme inducers.

Breakthrough bleeding is to be expected with continuous use; extended regimens advise a 4- to 7-day break if bleeding occurs.

Antibiotics and COC use

- Broad-spectrum antibiotics interfere with intestinal flora, reducing bioavailability of the COC. Additional methods of contraception should be used.

Surgery and CHC use

- Stop CHC at least 4 weeks before major surgery and any surgery to the pelvis or legs. Advise on alternative contraception.
- Do not restart until fully mobile for at least 2 weeks.
- If emergency surgery, then stop CHC and give antithrombotic prophylaxis.

Progestogen-only contraception

Overview

- There are few medical restrictions on the use of progestogen-only contraception (POC), making it a suitable choice for most ♀ with contraindications to CHC.
- Efficacy of oral POC (POP) is less than CHC.
- The intrauterine system (IUS), implant and depot injection are forms of long-acting reversible contraception (LARC). These methods are very effective, with failure rate well below 1% per year, and are not user dependent. They are recommended where unintended pregnancy would carry serious health risks, e.g. ♀ with complex congenital heart disease.
- Intrauterine and injectable POC are suitable for women on enzyme-inducing drugs.

Route of administration and regimens

- Oral: progestogen-only pill (POP) taken daily at same time with no pill-free interval.
- Injectable: Depot injection administered IM or SC every 3 months.
- Implant: single flexible plastic rod inserted SC in the upper arm every 3 years.
- Intrauterine: IUS, T-shaped plastic intrauterine device replaced every 3-5 years.

Mode of action

- The POP makes cervical mucus viscid and thus hostile to sperm, and also impairs Fallopian tube function and implantation. POPs suppress ovulation to a variable extent.
- POPs have a short duration of action and a 2nd generation POP taken more than 3h late is considered 'missed'.
- Depot injection and implant inhibit ovulation as well as thickening cervical mucus.
- The IUS thickens cervical mucus, thins the uterine lining to prevent implantation, and partially suppresses ovulation.

Types of progestogen

- Oral: POPs contain either 2nd generation progestogens, levonorgestrel or norethisterone, or 3rd generation desogestrel. Although comparative data on efficacy are lacking, desogestrel suppresses ovulation in >90% of cycles compared to 50-60% with other POPs.
- Injectable: Depot medroxyprogesterone acetate.
- Implant: etonogestrel.
- Intrauterine: levonorgestrel.

Non-contraceptive benefits

- Reduction in menstrual bleeding and pain. Desogestrel is the most effective POP for menstrual control. IUS generally induces amenorrhoea at 6-12 months.
- The IUS is frequently used in treatment of menorrhagia, dysmenorrhea, endometrial hyperplasia, and endometriosis. The LNG-IUS can also be used as the progestogen component of HRT.

Side effects
- Breakthrough bleeding. An irregular bleeding pattern is common, and may lead to ♀ discontinuing POC (e.g. one-third have the implant removed early).
- Follicular cysts are common but transient.
- Fluid retention, breast tenderness, headache, nausea (all less common in POC users than in CHC users), acne, low mood.

Risks
- Breast cancer risk is slightly ↑ in users of injectable POC but has not been identified with POP use.
- IUS insertion can be complicated by perforation, infection, or expulsion.

Emergency contraception

Refers to contraception that a woman can use after unprotected sexual intercourse to prevent pregnancy. The most effective option is insertion of a copper intrauterine contraceptive device (IUCD). Two single-dose oral agents are available; ulipristal acetate is slightly more effective than levonorgestrel.

Oral agents

- These are not effective after ovulation has occurred and do not provide ongoing contraception.
- Their efficacy might be reduced by obesity and in women taking enzyme-inducing drugs.
- Side effects: headache, nausea—if vomiting occurs within 3h of administration, the dose should be repeated. Menstrual upset (period often delayed).
- If pregnancy does occur, there is no evidence of teratogenesis.

Levonorgestrel

- A progestogen, also used in COC and HRT.
- Requires a single dose of 1.5mg taken within 72h of intercourse, and certainly within 96h.
- Overall pregnancy rate 0.6-2.6%.
- Acts by inhibiting ovulation and must be taken before the LH surge occurs.

Ulipristal acetate

- A progesterone receptor modulator with a partial progesterone antagonist effect.
- Requires a single dose of 30mg taken as soon as possible after intercourse, and no later than after 120h.
- Overall pregnancy rate 1-2%.
- Appears to work by delaying ovulation, so that ejaculated sperm are no longer viable.
- Rare but serious cases of liver injury, including hepatic failure requiring liver transplantation, have been reported with continuous use of ulipristal acetate for uterine fibroids. There are no concerns about use for emergency contraception.

IUCD

- The copper IUCD is the most effective method of emergency contraception, and the only one to provide ongoing contraception.
- Effective if inserted up to 5 days after ovulation and up to 5 days after intercourse.
- Overall pregnancy rate <0.1%.
- Acts both to reduce likelihood of fertilization by effect of copper on gametes and also to prevent implantation by endometrial reaction to IUCD.
- Risks: pelvic infection, uterine perforation, and pain.

Further reading

The Faculty of Sexual and Reproductive Healthcare has comprehensive up-to-date guidelines on all forms of contraception, available freely online at ♒ https://www.fsrh.org.

The British National Formulary lists the multiple (frequently changing) preparations available for hormonal contraception at ♒ https://www.bnf.nice.org.uk

Faculty of Sexual and Reproductive Healthcare. (2016, amended 2019). UK medical eligibility criteria for contraceptive use. ♒https://www.fsrh.org/documents/ukmec-2016/

Faculty of Sexual and Reproductive Healthcare. (2017). Emergency contraception. ♒ https://www.fsrh.org/standards-and-guidance/fsrh-guidelines-and-statements/emergency-contraception/

Morch LS, et al. (2017). Contemporary hormonal contraception and the risk of breast cancer. N Engl J Med **377**, 2228-39.

Nash Z, et al. (2020). Tailored regimens for combined hormonal contraceptives. BMJ **368**, m200.10

Male hypogonadism

Definition

Failure of testes to produce adequate amounts of testosterone.

Epidemiology

- Klinefelter's syndrome (XXY) (see $\supset$ Klinefelter's syndrome, p. 418) is the commonest congenital cause and is thought to occur with an incidence of 2:1000 live births.
- Acquired hypogonadism is even commoner, affecting 1:200 ♂.
- Higher incidence (2%) in men >40 years due to 1% annual drop in testosterone levels.

Evaluation of male hypogonadism

Presentation

- Failure to progress through puberty.
- Sexual dysfunction.
- Infertility.
- Non-specific symptoms, e.g. lethargy, reduced libido, mood changes, weight gain.

The clinical presentation depends on:

- Age of onset (congenital vs acquired).
- Severity (complete vs partial).
- Duration (functional vs permanent).

Secondary hypogonadism

Definition

Hypogonadism as a result of hypothalamic or pituitary dysfunction.

Diagnosis

- Low 9 a.m. serum testosterone.
- Low normal or low LH and FSH.

Causes

(See Box 4.11.)

Congenital hypogonadotrophic hypogonadism (CHH: Kallmann syndrome)
A genetic disorder characterized by failure of episodic GnRH secretion ±
anosmia. Results from disordered migration of GnRH-producing neurones
into the hypothalamus.

Epidemiology
- Incidence of 1 in 10,000 ♂.
- ♂:♀ ratio = 4:1.

Diagnosis
- Anosmia in 75%.
- ↑ risk of cleft lip and palate, sensorineural deafness, cerebellar ataxia,
  and renal agenesis.
- Low testosterone, LH, and FSH levels.
- Rest of pituitary function normal.
- Normal MRI pituitary gland and hypothalamus; absent olfactory bulbs
  may be seen on MRI.
- Normalization of pituitary and gonadal function in response to
  physiological GnRH replacement.

Genetics
- Most commonly, a result of an isolated gene mutation with variable
  inheritance patterns.
- Several genes involved, including *KAL1*, *FGFR1*, *FGF8*, *PROK2*, *FDFR8*,
  ProkR2, and *ANOS1*.
- *KAL1* gene mutation, responsible for some cases of X-linked Kallmann
  syndrome, is located on Xp22.3. It has a more severe reproductive
  phenotype.
- Mutations of *FGFR1* (fibroblast growth factor receptor 1) gene, located
  on chromosome 8p11, are associated with the AD form of Kallmann
  syndrome. Affected ♂ have ↑ likelihood of undescended testes
  at birth.
- 12–15% incidence of delayed puberty in families of subjects with
  Kallmann syndrome, compared with 1% in general population.
- ♂ with AD form (*FGFR1* mutation)—50% transmitted to offspring who
  have ↑ likelihood of undescended testes at birth.

Management
- Androgen replacement therapy.
- When fertility is desired, testosterone is stopped and exogenous
  gonadotrophins are administered (see ➲ Management of male
  infertility, pp. 456–7).

Box 4.11 Causes of secondary hypogonadism
- CHH:
  - Normosmic.
  - Anosmic (Kallmann syndrome).
  - Other genetic causes, e.g. mutations of *GnRHR* or *GPR54* genes.
  - Fertile eunuch syndrome.
  - CAH (*DAX-1* gene mutation).
- Acquired:
  - Functional.
  - Obesity.
  - T1DM or T2DM.
  - Exercise, weight loss, or systemic illness.
  - Illicit drugs: anabolic steroids.
  - Drug treatment: opioids, SSRIs.
  - Hyperprolactinaemia.
  - Syndromic, e.g. Prader–Willi, Laurence–Moon–Biedl, CHARGE syndrome.
- Structural:
  - Tumours, e.g. pituitary adenoma, craniopharyngioma, germinoma.
  - Infiltrative disorders, e.g. sarcoidosis, haemochromatosis.
  - Head trauma.
  - Pituitary surgery or radiotherapy.

Normosmic CHH
- Indistinguishable from Kallmann syndrome, apart from the absence of anosmia. >90% of patients are ♂.
- Several causative genes identified (e.g. *KISS1*, *TAC3*, *GNRH1*), so no longer termed idiopathic HH (IHH).
- ♂ with acquired IHH may go through normal puberty and have normal testicular size, but present with infertility or poor libido and potency. May be temporary, with normalization of gonadal function after stopping GnRH or testosterone therapy.

Fertile eunuch syndrome
- Incomplete GnRH deficiency. Enough gonadotrophins to maintain normal spermatogenesis and testicular growth, but stimulate insufficient testosterone for adequate virilization.
- May not require gonadotrophin therapy for treatment.
- Rare X-linked or AR disease, caused by a mutation in the *DAX* gene which is located on the X chromosome.
- Presents with 1° adrenal failure in infancy.
- Hypothalamic hypogonadism is also present.

Structural
- Usually associated with other pituitary hormonal deficiencies.
- In children, craniopharyngiomas are the commonest cause. Cranial irradiation for leukaemia or brain tumours may also result in 2° hypogonadism.
- The commonest lesions in adulthood are prolactinomas.

Systemic illness
Severe illness of any kind may cause HH (see ⊃ Box 4.13).

Drugs
- Anabolic steroids and opioids may cause 2° hypogonadism.
- All drugs causing hyperprolactinaemia (see Box 2.13) will also cause hypogonadism.
- Immunotherapy rarely.

Prader–Willi syndrome
- A congenital syndrome, affecting 1:25,000 births, caused by loss of an imprinted gene on paternally derived chromosome 15q11–13.
- It should be suspected in infancy in the presence of characteristic facial features (almond eyes, downturned mouth, strabismus, thin upper lip), severe hypotonia, poor feeding, and developmental delay. The child then develops hyperphagia due to hypothalamic dysfunction, resulting in severe obesity. Other characteristic features include short stature, small hands and feet, HH, and learning disability.
- T2DM occurs in 15–40% of adults.

Laurence–Moon–Biedl syndrome
- Congenital syndrome characterized by severe obesity, gonadotrophin deficiency, retinal dystrophy, polydactyly, and learning disability.

Haemochromatosis
(See Box 4.12.)

> **Box 4.12 Haemochromatosis**
> *Complications*
> - Central and 1° hypogonadism.
> - DM.
> - Liver cirrhosis.
> - Addison's disease.
>
> Diagnosed by genotyping.

Relative energy deficiency in sport (RED-S)
Characteristics
Where an athlete has insufficient *energy* intake *relative* to the amount of training being undertaken.
- Weight loss.
- Reduced haemoglobin (Hb).
- ↑ SHBG.
- ↑ cortisol and abnormal TFTs (sick euthyroidism).
- Relatively rapid recovery.
- GH resistance.

Differential diagnosis
- Anabolic steroid administration (atrophic testes, reduced SHBG, ↑ Hb).

Further reading

Boehm U, *et al*. (2015). Expert consensus document: European Consensus Statement on congenital hypogonadotropic hypogonadism—pathogenesis, diagnosis and treatment. *Nat Rev Endocrinol* **11**, 547–64.

Wong HK, et al. (2019) Reversible male hypogonadotropic hypogonadism due to energy deficit. *Clin Endocrinol* **91**, 3–9

Hypogonadotrophic hypogonadism

Definition

Hypogonadism as a result of gonadotrophin deficiency.

Diagnosis

- Low LH, FSH, oestradiol, and testosterone.
- Rest of pituitary function normal.
- MRI: small pituitary gland, normal hypothalamus.
- Small gonads.
- Absent or delayed puberty, 1° amenorrhoea.
- Tall stature from delayed closure of epiphyses.
- Anosmia and absent olfactory bulbs on MRI in Kallmann syndrome.

Causes

(See Box 4.13.)

CHARGE syndrome

The association of coloboma, heart anomaly, choanal atresia, retardation, and genital and ear anomalies (may be deaf, mute, and/or blind). A proportion also has HH.

> **Box 4.13 Systemic illness resulting in hypogonadism**
> - Any acute illness (e.g. myocardial infarction (MI), sepsis, head injury).
> - Severe stress.
> - Haemochromatosis.
> - Endocrine disease (Cushing's syndrome, hyperprolactinaemia).
> - Liver cirrhosis.
> - CRF.
> - Chronic anaemia (thalassaemia major, sickle cell disease).
> - GI disease (coeliac disease, Crohn's disease).
> - AIDS.
> - Rheumatological disease (rheumatoid arthritis).
> - Respiratory disease (e.g. COPD, cystic fibrosis (CF)).
> - Cardiac disease (e.g. CCF).

X-linked adrenal hypoplasia congenita

Rare X-linked or AR disease, caused by a mutation in the *DAX* gene, which is located on the X chromosome.
- Presents with 1° adrenal failure in infancy.
- Hypothalamic hypogonadism is also present.

Management

- Androgen replacement therapy (see ➲ Androgen replacement therapy, pp. 426–7).
- ERT.
- When fertility is desired, testosterone is stopped and exogenous gonadotrophins are administered (see ➲ Management of female infertility, pp. 452–5).

Primary hypogonadism

Due to testicular failure with normal hypothalamus and pituitary function. (See Box 4.14 for clinical characteristics.)

Diagnosis

- Low 9 a.m. fasting serum testosterone.
- Elevated LH and FSH.

Causes

Genetic

Klinefelter's syndrome

The commonest congenital form of 1° hypogonadism identified to affect 1:2000 live births, but thought to be undiagnosed in many other men. Clinical manifestations will depend on the age of diagnosis. Patients with mosaicism tend to have less severe clinical features.

- Adolescence:
  - Small, firm testes (mean 5mL).
  - Gynaecomastia.
  - Tall stature (↑ leg length).
  - Other features of hypogonadism.
  - Psychological problems are common.
- Adulthood:
  - Reduced libido and erectile dysfunction.
  - Gynaecomastia (50%).
  - Reduced facial hair.
  - ↑ fat-to-lean mass or obesity.
  - Infertility.
- Risks:
  - T2DM.
  - Osteoporosis.
  - Thromboembolism.
  - Malignancies, e.g. extragonadal germ cell tumours.
- Diagnosis:
  - Karyotyping: 47,XXY in 80%; higher-grade chromosomal aneuploidies (e.g. 48,XXXY) or 46,XY/47,XXY mosaicism in the remainder.
  - Low testosterone, elevated FSH and LH.
  - Elevated SHBG and oestradiol.
  - Azoospermia.
- Management:
  - Lifelong androgen replacement.
  - May need surgical reduction of gynaecomastia.
  - Fertility: microdissection testicular sperm extraction (mTESE) retrieves sperm in a minority of cases. Sperm is used to fertilize eggs of partner using intracytoplasmic sperm injection (ICSI) (see ➔ Management of male infertility, pp. 456–7). However, still unclear what proportion of patients can be successfully treated.

Box 4.14 Testicular dysfunction—clinical characteristics of male hypogonadism

Testicular failure occurring before onset of puberty
- Testicular volume <5mL.
- Penis <5cm long.
- Lack of scrotal pigmentation and rugae.
- Gynaecomastia.
- High-pitched voice.
- Central fat distribution.
- Eunuchoidism:
  - Arm span 1cm greater than height.
  - Lower segment > upper segment.
- Delayed bone age.
- No ♂ escutcheon.
- ↓ body and facial hair.

Testicular failure occurring after puberty
- Testes soft, volume <15mL.
- Normal penile length.
- Normal skeletal proportions.
- Gynaecomastia.
- Normal ♂ hair distribution, but reduced amount.
- Pale skin, fine wrinkles.
- Central fat distribution.
- Osteoporosis.
- Anaemia (mild).

Other chromosomal disorders
- XX ♂:
  - Due to an X to Y translocation, with only a part of the Y present in one of the X chromosomes.
  - Incidence 1:10,000 births.
  - Similar clinical and biochemical features to Klinefelter's syndrome. In addition, short stature and hypospadias may be present.
- XX/XO (mixed gonadal dysgenesis):
  - Occasionally, phenotypically ♂ with hypospadias and intra-abdominal dysgenetic gonads.
  - Bilateral gonadectomy is essential because of the risk of neoplasia, followed by androgen replacement therapy.
- XYY syndrome:
  - Taller than average, but often have 1° gonadal failure with impaired spermatogenesis.
- Y chromosome microdeletions:
  - Causes oligo-/azoospermia. Testosterone levels are not usually affected. Normal clinical phenotype.
- Noonan's syndrome:
  - AD disorder, with an incidence of 1:1000 to 1:2500 live births.

- 46,XY karyotype and 2° external genitalia. However, several stigmata of Turner syndrome (dysmorphic facial features, short stature, webbed neck, ptosis, low-set ears, lymphoedema) and ↑ risk of cardiac anomalies (valvular pulmonary stenosis and hypertrophic cardiomyopathy). Most have cryptorchidism and 1° testicular failure. May have a bleeding diathesis.

Cryptorchidism

- 10% of ♂ neonates have undescended testes, but most of these will descend into the scrotum eventually, so that the incidence of post-pubertal cryptorchidism is <0.5%.
- 15% of cases have bilateral cryptorchidism.

Consequences

- 75% of ♂ with bilateral cryptorchidism are infertile.
- 10% risk of testicular malignancy; highest risk in those with intra-abdominal testes.
- Low testosterone and raised gonadotrophins in bilateral cryptorchidism.

Treatment

- *Orchidopexy.* Best performed before 18 months, certainly before age od 5 years, in order to reduce the risk of later infertility. But can risk causing epididymal obstruction and obstructive azoospermia.
- *Gonadectomy.* In patients with intra-abdominal testes, followed by androgen replacement.

Orchitis

- 25% of ♂ who develop mumps after puberty have associated orchitis, and 25–50% of these will develop 1° testicular failure.
- HIV infection may also be associated with orchitis.
- 1° testicular failure may occur as part of an autoimmune disease.

Chemotherapy and radiotherapy

- Cytotoxic drugs, particularly alkylating agents, are gonadotoxic. Infertility occurs in 50% of patients following chemotherapy for most malignancies, and a significant number of ♂ require androgen replacement therapy because of low testosterone levels.
- Germ cells are radiosensitive, so hypogonadism can occur as a result of scattered radiation during the treatment of Hodgkin's disease, for example.
- All men should be offered sperm cryopreservation prior to cancer therapy.

Other drugs

- Sulfasalazine, colchicines, and high-dose GCs may reversibly affect testicular function.
- Alcohol excess will also cause 1° testicular failure.

Chronic illness

- Any chronic illness may affect testicular function, in particular CRF, liver cirrhosis, and haemochromatosis.

Testicular trauma

Testicular torsion is another common cause of loss of a testis, and it may also affect the function of the remaining testis.

Clinical assessment of hypogonadism

History

- *Developmental history.* Congenital urinary tract abnormalities, e.g. hypospadias, late testicular descent, or cryptorchidism.
- *Delayed or incomplete puberty.*
- *Infections,* e.g. mumps, orchitis.
- *Abdominal/genital trauma.*
- *Testicular torsion.*
- *Anosmia.*
- *Drug history,* e.g. sulfasalazine, antihypertensives, chemotherapy, cimetidine, radiotherapy; alcohol, previous anabolic steroids, and recreational drugs also important.
- *General medical history.* Chronic illness, particularly respiratory, neurological, and cardiac.
- *Gynaecomastia.* Common (see ⊃ Gynaecomastia, pp. 430–1) during adolescence. Recent-onset gynaecomastia in adulthood—must rule out oestrogen-producing tumour.
- *Family history.* Young's syndrome (reduced fertility, bronchiectasis, and rhinosinusitis), CF, Kallmann syndrome.
- *Sexual history.* Erectile function, frequency of intercourse, sexual techniques. Absence of morning erections suggests an organic cause of erectile dysfunction.

Physical examination

- Body hair distribution.
- Muscle mass and fat distribution.
- Eunuchoidism.
- Gynaecomastia.
- Assess visual fields and sense of smell.
- Genital examination:
  - *Pubic hair.* Normal ♂ escutcheon.
  - *Phallus.* Normal >8cm length and >3cm width.
  - *Testes.* Size (using Prader orchidometer) and consistency (normal >15mL and firm).
  - Look for nodules or areas of tenderness.

Hormonal evaluation of testicular function

Serum testosterone

- Diurnal variation in circulating testosterone, peak levels occurring in early morning; 20% suppression following glucose ingestion.
- Measure serum testosterone between 8 and 10 a.m. when patient is fasted. If level is low, this should be repeated.

Sex hormone-binding globulin

- Only 2–4% of circulating testosterone is unbound; 50% is bound to SHBG, and the rest to albumin.
- Concentrations of SHBG should be taken into account when interpreting a serum testosterone result. SHBG levels may be affected by a variety of conditions (see Table 4.11).
- It is important to measure SBHG when testosterone values at 9 a.m. are under the normal range. The Vermeulen equation has 98% correlation to measured free testosterone (which is therefore never needed).

Gonadotrophins
Raised FSH and LH in 1° testicular failure and inappropriately low in pituitary or hypothalamic hypogonadism. Should always exclude hyperprolactinaemia in 2° hypogonadism.

Oestradiol
Results from the conversion of testosterone and androstenedione by aromatase. (See Box 4.15 for causes of elevated oestradiol.) Request serum oestradiol level if gynaecomastia is present or a testicular tumour is suspected.

Table 4.11 Factors affecting SHBG concentrations

Raised SHBG	Low SHBG
Androgen deficiency	Hyperinsulinaemia
GH deficiency	Obesity
Ageing	Acromegaly
Thyrotoxicosis	Androgen treatment
Oestrogens	Hypothyroidism
Liver cirrhosis	Cushing's syndrome/GC therapy, nephrotic syndrome

---

Box 4.15 Causes of raised oestrogens in ♂
- Neoplasia:
  - Testicular.
  - Adrenal.
  - Hepatoma.
- 1° testicular failure.
- Liver disease.
- Thyrotoxicosis.
- Obesity.
- Androgen resistance syndromes.
- Antiandrogen therapy.

Inhibin B and AMH
Gonadal glycoproteins secreted into the circulation. Useful markers of normal testicular functions; low if 1° testicular failure, and normal if pituitary/hypothalamic dysfunction. But testicular volume is an excellent surrogate if these tests are unavailable.

Other investigations
- Scrotal US (if concerned about tumour).
- Semen analysis (♂ with low sperm count may have reduced fertility; difficult to interpret in patients taking testosterone replacement therapy).
- >20 × 10⁶ million is normal. It is possible to conceive with a sperm count of 1–20 × 10⁶. It is unlikely to conceive with a count of 1 × 10⁶ million.
- Dynamic tests (hCG and clomifene stimulation tests) are of limited clinical value and are thus rarely performed routinely.

Further reading

Aksglaede L, Juul A (2013). Testicular function and fertility in men with Klinefelter syndrome: a review. *Eur J Endocrinol* **168**, R67–76.

Caronia LM, et al. (2013). Abrupt decrease in serum testosterone levels after an oral glucose load in men: implications for screening for hypogonadism. *Clin Endocrinol (Oxf)* **78**, 291–6.

Corona G, et al. (2017). Sperm recovery and ICSI outcomes in Klinefelter syndrome: a systematic review and meta-analysis. *Hum Reprod Update* **23**, 265–75.

Lanfranco F, et al. (2004). Klinefelter's syndrome. *Lancet* **364**, 273–83.

Miller JF (2012). Approach to the child with Prader–Willi syndrome. *J Clin Endocrinol Metab* **97**, 3837–44.

Petak SM, et al.; American Association of Clinical Endocrinologists (2002). American Association of Clinical Endocrinologists Medical Guidelines for clinical practice for the evaluation and treatment of hypogonadism in adult male patients—2002 Update. *Endocr Pract* **8**, 440–56.

Semple RK, Topaloglu AK (2010). The recent genetics of hypogonadotrophic hypogonadism—novel insights and new questions. *Clin Endocrinol (Oxf)* **72**, 427–35.

Androgen replacement therapy

Treatment aims

- To improve libido and sexual function.
- To improve mood and well-being.
- To improve muscle mass and strength. Testosterone has direct anabolic effects on skeletal muscle and has been shown to increase muscle mass and strength when given to hypogonadal men. Lean body mass is also ↑, with a reduction in fat mass.
- To prevent osteoporosis. Hypogonadism is a risk factor for osteoporosis. Testosterone inhibits bone resorption, thereby reducing bone turnover. Its administration to hypogonadal ♂ has been shown to improve BMD and reduce the risk of developing osteoporosis. Testogel in older men with low testosterone has been shown to lead to similar effects as bisphosphonates after 1 year.

Androgen replacement therapy does not restore fertility—indeed, it suppresses normal spermatogenesis. ♂ with 2° hypogonadism who desire fertility may be treated with gonadotrophins to initiate and maintain spermatogenesis (see ➜ Management of male infertility, pp. 456–7). Prior testosterone therapy will not affect fertility prospects but should be stopped before initiating gonadotrophin treatment. ♂ with 1° hypogonadism will not respond to gonadotrophin therapy and may require surgical sperm retrieval or donor insemination.

Indications for treatment

- In ♂ with established 1° or 2° hypogonadism of any cause.

  (See Table 4.12 for contraindications.)
- Treatment should be begun slowly in prolonged and/or severe hypogonadism (in case of priapism).

NB. Weight reduction is associated with a rise in testosterone.

Pretreatment evaluation

Clinical evaluation

History or symptoms of:
- Prostatic hypertrophy.
- Breast or prostate cancer.
- CVD.
- Sleep apnoea.

Examination

- Rectal examination of prostate.
- Examination for gynaecomastia.

Laboratory evaluation

- Prostate-specific antigen (PSA) (NB. PSA is often low in hypogonadal ♂, rising to normal age-matched levels with androgen replacement).
- Hb and haematocrit (Hct) are excellent long-term biomarkers of testosterone status. In older men, unexplained anaemia may be the presenting feature of hypogonadism.
- Cholesterol profile.

  (See Box 4.16 for monitoring.)

Table 4.12 Contraindications for androgen replacement therapy

Absolute	Relative
Prostate cancer*	Benign prostate hyperplasia
Breast cancer	Polycythaemia
	Sleep apnoea

* In patients with low recurrence risk, this is no longer an absolute contraindication. Check current guidance.

Box 4.16 Monitoring of therapy
- Three months after initiating therapy, and then 6- to 12-monthly:
  - Clinical evaluation—relief of symptoms of androgen deficiency and excluding side effects.
  - Serum testosterone (trough).
  - Rectal examination of the prostate (if >40 years).
  - PSA (if >40 years) (NB. Age-related reference range).
  - Hb and Hct (target <0.54).
  - Serum lipids.[1]

References
1. Al-Sharefi A, Quinton R (2018). Hiding in a plain sight: a high prevalence of androgen deficiency due to primary hypogonadism among acute medical inpatients with anaemia. *Clin Endocrinol (Oxf)* **89**, 527–9.

Further reading
Bhasin S, et al. (2018). Testosterone therapy in men with hypogonadism: an Endocrine Society clinical practice guideline. *J Clin Endocrinol Metab* **103**, 1715–44.

Shankara-Narayana N, et al. (2020). Rate and extent of recovery from reproductive and cardiac dysfunction due to androgen abuse in men. *J Clin Endocrinol Metab* **105**, 1827–39.

Risks and side effects of androgen replacement therapy

(See Table 4.13 for testosterone preparations.)

Prostatic disease

- It is now accepted that testosterone therapy does *not* cause prostate cancer but could accelerate the growth of an incidental tumour.
- Patients above 40 years of age need regular prostate surveillance.
- Testosterone replacement therapy may therefore induce symptoms of bladder outflow obstruction in ♂ with prostatic hypertrophy.
- There is a growing body of evidence supporting testosterone treatment for men with treated prostate cancer under urological follow-up.
- Men who cannot have testosterone replacement therapy owing to prostate cancer need bone protection.
  - Lifestyle modification: smoking cessation, avoiding excessive alcohol consumption, maintaining an active lifestyle.
  - Pharmacological interventions: calcium and vitamin D supplementation (see ➔ Treatment of osteoporosis, pp. 552–3).

Polycythaemia (Hct >0.54)

Testosterone stimulates erythropoiesis via hepcidin, which leads to ↑ iron uptake and erythropoiesis. Androgen replacement therapy may increase Hct levels, particularly in older ♂. It may be necessary to reduce the dose of testosterone in ♂ with clinically significant polycythaemia. Testosterone injections have a higher risk of polycythaemia than transdermal preparations. Thus, conversion to transdermal testosterone, as well as dose reduction, can be helpful.

Cardiovascular disease

This is a highly controversial topic. One RCT stopped early due to excess cardiovascular events in the testosterone group, but other studies suggest +ve effects on glycaemic control. The NIH Testosterone Trials observed a greater increase in coronary artery plaque volume in older men taking testosterone vs placebo. The US Food and Drug Administration requires doctors to warn patients about cardiovascular risks, but the European Medicines Agency (EMA) concludes that the evidence between testosterone therapy and cardiac disease is inconsistent.

Other

- Acne.
- Gynaecomastia is occasionally enhanced by testosterone therapy, particularly in peripubertal boys. This is the result of conversion of testosterone to oestrogens.
- Obstructive sleep apnoea may be exacerbated by testosterone therapy.
- Hepatotoxicity only with oral 1/α alkylated testosterones.
- Mood swings are uncommon.
- Exogenous androgen therapy in men.
- Suppressed testicular function may take 6–18 months to recover.
- Supplemented testicular function may take 6–18 months to recover.
- ↑ VTE risk, peaking in first 3 months.

Table 4.13 Testosterone preparations

Preparation	Dose	Advantages	Problems
IM testosterone esters	250mg every 2–3 weeks Monitor pre-dose serum testosterone (should be above the lower limit of normal)	2- to 3-weekly dosage Effective, cheap	Painful IM injection Contraindicated in bleeding disorders Wide variations in serum testosterone levels between injections which may be associated with symptoms
Testosterone undecanoate (e.g. 'Nebido'®)	1g 3-monthly (after loading dose)	Convenience of infrequent injections	Cough post-injection
Testosterone implants	100–600mg every 3–6 months Monitor pre-dose serum testosterone	Physiological testosterone levels achieved 3- to 6-monthly dosing	Minor surgical procedure Risk of infection and pellet extrusion (3–10%). Must remove pellet surgically if complications of androgen replacement therapy develop
Transdermal gel (1%, 2%)	5–10g (1%), 2–4g (2%) gel daily	Physiological testosterone levels achieved Convenience	Skin reactions (rare) Possible person-to-person transfer through direct skin contact
Oral, e.g. testosterone undecanoate and mesterolone (analogue of DHT)	40mg tds, 25mg tds	Oral preparations	Highly variable efficacy and bioavailability Rarely achieves therapeutic efficacy Multiple daily dosing
Buccal testosterone	30mg bd	Physiological testosterone levels achieved	Local discomfort, gingivitis, bitter taste Twice-daily dosing

Further reading

Basaria S, et al. (2010). Adverse events associated with testosterone administration. N Engl J Med **363**, 109–22.

Bhasin S, et al. (2018). Testosterone therapy in men with hypogonadism: an Endocrine Society clinical practice guideline. J Clin Endocrinol Metab **103**, 1715–44.

Budoff MJ, et al. (2017). Testosterone treatment and coronary artery plaque volume in older men with low testosterone. JAMA **317**, 708–16.

Handelsman DJ, Zajac JD (2004). Androgen deficiency and replacement therapy in men. Med J Aust **180**, 529–35.

Gynaecomastia

Definition

- Enlargement of the ♂ breast, as a result of hyperplasia of the glandular tissue, to a diameter of >2cm (see Fig. 4.9). Common; present in up to one-third of ♂ <30 years and in up to 50% of ♂ >45 years. Mostly benign; cancer only found in ~1% of ♂ breast enlargement.

(See Box 4.17 for causes.)
- Incidence increasing.

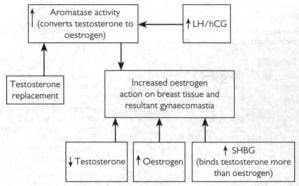

Fig. 4.9 Hormonal influences on gynaecomastia.

Box 4.17 Causes of gynaecomastia

(See Fig. 4.9 for hormonal influences.)

- Physiological:
  - Neonatal.
  - Puberty—about 50% of boys develop transient gynaecomastia.
  - Idiopathic—about 25% of all cases.
- Drugs (possible mechanisms: oestrogen-containing, androgen receptor blockers, inhibiting androgen production):
  - Oestrogens, antiandrogens, testosterone.
  - hCG therapy for spermatogenesis induction.
  - Spironolactone, ACEIs, calcium antagonists, digoxin.
  - Alkylating agents.
  - Alcohol, marijuana, heroin, methadone.
  - Cimetidine, PPI.
  - Ketoconazole, metronidazole, antituberculous agents, TCAs, dopamine antagonists, opiates, benzodiazepines.
  - Antiretroviral drugs.
  - Imatinib (chronic myeloid leukaemia).
  - Statins.
- Hypogonadism:
  - $1°$.
  - $2°$.
- Tumours:
  - Oestrogen- or androgen-producing testicular or adrenal tumours.
  - hCG-producing tumours, usually testicular, e.g. germinoma; occasionally ectopic, e.g. lung.
  - Aromatase-producing testicular or hepatic tumours.
- Endocrine:
  - Thyrotoxicosis.
  - Cushing's syndrome.
  - Acromegaly.
  - Androgen insensitivity syndromes.
- Systemic illness:
  - Liver cirrhosis.
  - CRF.
  - HIV infection.
  - Malnutrition.

Evaluation of gynaecomastia

History

- Duration and progression of gynaecomastia.
- Further investigation warranted if:
  - Rapidly enlarging gynaecomastia.
  - Recent-onset gynaecomastia in a lean post-pubertal ♂.
  - Painful gynaecomastia.
- Exclude underlying tumour, e.g. testicular cancer.
- Symptoms of hypogonadism. Reduced libido, erectile dysfunction.
- Symptoms of systemic disease, e.g. hepatic, renal, and endocrine disease.
- Drug history, including recreational drugs, e.g. alcohol, anabolic steroids.

Physical examination

- *Breasts:*
  - Pinch breast tissue between thumb and forefinger—distinguish from fat.
  - Measure glandular tissue diameter. Gynaecomastia if >2cm.
  - If >5cm, hard, or irregular, investigate further to exclude breast cancer.
  - Look for galactorrhoea.
- *Testicular palpation:*
  - Exclude tumour.
  - Assess testicular size—? atrophy.
- 2° *sex characteristics.*
- Look for evidence of *systemic disease*, e.g. chronic liver or renal disease, thyrotoxicosis, Cushing's syndrome, chronic cardiac or pulmonary disease.

Investigations

(See Fig. 4.10.)

Baseline investigations

- Serum testosterone.
- Serum oestradiol.
- LH and FSH.
- PRL.
- SHBG.
- hCG.
- LFTs.

Additional investigations

- If testicular tumour is suspected, e.g. raised oestradiol/hCG: testicular US.
- If adrenal tumour is suspected, e.g. markedly raised oestradiol: dehydroepiandrostenedione; abdominal CT or MRI scan.
- If breast malignancy is suspected: mammography; FNAC/tissue biopsy.
- If lung cancer is suspected, e.g. raised hCG: chest radiograph.
- Other investigations, depending on clinical suspicion, e.g. renal or thyroid function.

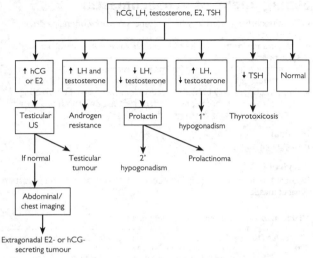

Fig. 4.10 Investigations of gynaecomastia.

Management of gynaecomastia

- Treat underlying disorder when present. Withdraw offending drugs where possible.
- Reassurance in the majority of idiopathic cases. Often resolves spontaneously.
- Treatment may be required for cosmetic reasons or to alleviate pain and tenderness.
- Drug treatment only partially effective. May be of benefit in treating gynaecomastia of recent onset. Risk of reduced BMD with prolonged use of drugs blocking oestrogen effects.

Medical

(See Table 4.14.)

Surgical

Reduction mammoplasty may be required in ♂ with severe and persistent gynaecomastia.

Table 4.14 Medical treatment of gynaecomastia

Tamoxifen (10–30mg/day)	Antioestrogenic effects. Particularly effective in reducing pain and swelling if used in gynaecomastia of recent onset. A 3-month trial before referral for surgery may be of benefit. Off-label use, ↑ risk of VTE
Clomifene (50–100mg/day)	Antioestrogenic. May be effective in reducing breast size in pubertal gynaecomastia
Danazol (300–600mg/day)	Non-aromatizable androgen. May also reduce breast size in adults. Its use is limited by side effects, particularly weight gain and acne. Only licensed medication for gynaecomastia
Testolactone (450mg/day)	Aromatase inhibitor. May be effective in reducing pubertal gynaecomastia. However, tamoxifen appears to be more effective and better tolerated
Anastrozole (1mg/day)	Another aromatase inhibitor. Clinical trials have failed to show a beneficial effect on gynaecomastia, compared with placebo

Further reading

Ali SN, et al. (2017). Which patients with gynaecomastia require more detailed investigation? Clin Endocrinol (Oxf) 88, 360–3.

Carlson HE (2011). Approach to the patient with gynecomastia. J Clin Endocrinol Metab 96, 15–21.

Khan HN, Blarney RW (2003). Endocrine treatment of physiological gynaecomastia. BMJ 327, 301–2.

Koch T, et al. (2020). Marked increase in incident gynecomastia: a 20-year national registry study, 1998–2017. J Clin Endocrinol Metab 105, 3134–40.

Testicular tumours

Epidemiology

- 6/100,000 ♂ per year.
- Incidence rising, particularly in North West Europe (see Table 4.15 for classification).

Risk factors

- Cryptorchidism.
- Gonadal dysgenesis.
- Infertility.

Classification

(See Table 4.15.)

Prognosis

Seminomas

- 95% cure for early disease; 80% cure for stages II/IV.
- ↑ incidence of 2nd tumours and leukaemias 20 years after therapy.

Non-seminoma germ cell tumours

- 90% cure in early disease, falling to 60% in metastatic disease.
- ↑ incidence of 2nd tumours and leukaemias 20 years after therapy.

Stromal tumours

- Excellent prognosis for benign tumours.
- Malignant tumours are aggressive and poorly responsive to treatment.

Table 4.15 Classification of testicular tumours

Tumours		Tumour markers
Germ cell tumours (95%)	Seminoma	None
	Non-seminoma	hCG, aFP, CEA Oestradiol
	Mixed	
Stromal tumours (2%)	Leydig cell	
	Sertoli cell	
Gonadoblastoma (2%)		
Other (1%)	Lymphoma	
	Carcinoid	

Further reading

Griffin JE, Wilson JD (1998). Disorders of the testes and male reproductive tract. In: Wilson JD, Foster DW, Kronenberg HM, Larson PR (eds.) *Williams Textbook of Endocrinology*, 9th edn. WB Saunders, Philadelphia, PA; pp. 819–76.

Erectile dysfunction

Definition

The consistent inability to achieve or maintain an erect penis sufficient for satisfactory sexual intercourse. Affects ~10% of ♂ and >50% of ♂ >70 years.

Physiology of male sexual function

- The erectile response is the result of the coordinated interaction of nerves, smooth muscle of the corpora cavernosa, pelvic muscles, and blood vessels.
- It is initiated by psychogenic stimuli from the brain or physical stimulation of the genitalia, which are modulated in the limbic system, transmitted down the spinal cord to the sympathetic and parasympathetic outflows of the penile tissue.
- Penile erectile tissue consists of paired corpora cavernosa on the dorsum of the penis and the corpus spongiosum. These are surrounded by fibrous tissue known as the tunica albuginea.
- In the flaccid state, the corporeal smooth muscle is contracted, minimizing corporeal blood flow and enhancing venous drainage.
- Activation of the erectile pathway results in penile smooth muscle relaxation and cavernosal arterial vasodilatation. As the corporeal sinuses fill with blood, the draining venules are compressed against the tunica albuginea, so venous outflow is impaired. This results in penile rigidity and an erection.
- Corporeal vasodilatation is mediated by parasympathetic neuronal activation, which induces nitric oxide release by the cavernosal nerves. This activates guanylyl cyclase, thereby increasing cyclic guanosine monophosphate (cGMP) and causing smooth muscle relaxation.
- Detumescence occurs after inactivation of cGMP by the enzyme PDE, resulting in smooth muscle contraction and vasoconstriction.
- Ejaculation is mediated by the sympathetic nervous system.

Pathophysiology

Erectile dysfunction may thus occur as a result of several mechanisms:
- Neurological damage.
- Arterial insufficiency.
- Venous incompetence.
- Androgen deficiency.
- Penile abnormalities.

Evaluation of erectile dysfunction

History

Sexual history
- Extent of the dysfunction, and its duration and progression.
- Presence of nocturnal or morning erections.
- Abrupt onset of erectile dysfunction which is intermittent is often psychogenic in origin.
- Progressive and persistent dysfunction indicates an organic cause.

Symptoms of hypogonadism
- Reduced libido, muscle strength, and sense of well-being.

Full medical history
- For example, DM, liver cirrhosis, and neurological, cardiovascular, or endocrine disease.
- Intermittent claudication suggests a vascular cause.
- A history of genitourinary trauma or surgery is also important.
- Recent change in bladder or bowel function may indicate a neurological cause.
- Psychological history.

Drug history
- Onset of impotence in relation to commencing a new medication.

Social history
- Stress.
- Relationship history.
- Smoking history.
- Recreational drugs, including alcohol.

Physical examination

- Evidence of 1° or 2° hypogonadism.
- Evidence of endocrine disorders:
  - Hyperprolactinaemia, thyroid dysfunction, hypopituitarism.
  - Other complications of DM, if present.
- Evidence of neurological disease:
  - Autonomic or peripheral neuropathy.
  - Spinal cord lesions.
- Evidence of systemic disease, e.g.:
  - Chronic liver disease.
  - Chronic cardiac disease.
  - Peripheral vascular disease.
- Genital examination:
  - Assess testicular size—? testicular failure
  - Penile abnormalities, e.g. Peyronie's disease.

  (See Box 4.18 for causes of erectile dysfunction.)

Investigation of erectile dysfunction

Baseline investigations
- Serum morning fasting testosterone.
- LFTs.
- PRL, LH, and FSH if serum testosterone low.
- Renal function.

Box 4.18 Causes of erectile dysfunction

- Psychological (20%):
  - Stress, anxiety.
  - Psychiatric illness.
- Drugs (25%):
  - Alcohol.
  - Antihypertensives, e.g. diuretics, β-blockers, methyldopa.
  - Cimetidine.
  - Marijuana, heroin, methadone.
  - Major tranquillizers.
  - TCAs, benzodiazepines.
  - Digoxin.
  - GCs, anabolic steroids.
  - Oestrogens, antiandrogens.
- Endocrine (20%):
  - Hypogonadism (1° or 2°).
  - Hyperprolactinaemia.
  - DM (30–50% of ♂ with DM >6 years).
  - Thyroid dysfunction.
- Neurological:
  - Spinal cord disorders.
  - Peripheral and autonomic neuropathies.
  - Multiple sclerosis.
- Vascular:
  - PVD.
  - Trauma.
  - DM.
  - Venous incompetence.
- Other:
  - Haemochromatosis.
  - Debilitating diseases.
  - Penile abnormalities, e.g. priapism, Peyronie's disease.
  - Prostatectomy.

- Fasting blood glucose.
- Serum lipids.
- TFTs.
- Serum ferritin (haemochromatosis).

Additional investigations

Rarely required. To assess vascular causes of impotence if corrective surgery is contemplated:

- *Intracavernosal injection* of a vasodilator, e.g. alprostadil E1 or papaverine. A sustained erection excludes significant vascular insufficiency.
- *Penile Doppler ultrasonography.* Cavernous arterial flow and venous insufficiency are assessed.

Management of erectile dysfunction

Treat underlying disorder or withdraw offending drugs where possible.

Androgens

This should be 1st-line therapy in ♂ with hypogonadism (see ➜ Androgen replacement therapy, pp. 426–7). Hyperprolactinaemia, when present, should be treated with dopamine agonists, and the underlying cause of hypogonadism treated.

Phosphodiesterase inhibitors

(See Table 4.16 and Box 4.19.)
- Act by enhancing cGMP activity in erectile tissue by blocking the enzyme PDE-5, thereby amplifying the vasodilatory action of nitric oxide, and thus the normal erectile response to sexual stimulation.
- Trials indicate 50–80% success rate.

Alprostadil

- Alprostadil results in smooth muscle relaxation and vasodilatation.
- It is administered intraurethrally and then absorbed into the erectile bodies.
- 60–66% success rate.
- *Side effects.* Local pain.

Intracavernous injection

- 70–100% success rate, highest in men with non-vasculogenic impotence.
- Alprostadil is a potent vasodilator. The dose should be titrated in 1-microgram increments until the desired effect is achieved in order to minimize side effects.
- Papaverine, a PDE inhibitor, induces cavernosal vasodilatation and penile rigidity but causes more side effects.
- *Side effects:*
  - Priapism in 1–5%. Patients must seek urgent medical advice if an erection lasts >4h.
  - Fibrosis in the injection site in up to 5% of patients. Minimize risk by alternating sides of the penis for injection and injecting a maximum of twice a week.
  - Infection at injection site is rare.
- *Contraindication.* Sickle cell disease.
- *Injection technique.* Avoid the midline, so as to avoid urethral and neurovascular damage. Clean the injection site; hold the penis under slight tension, and introduce the needle at 90°. Inject after the characteristic 'give' of piercing the fibrous capsule. Apply pressure to the injection site after removing the needle to prevent bruising.

Vacuum device

Results are good, with 90% of ♂ achieving a satisfactory erection. The flaccid penis is put into the device and air is withdrawn, creating a vacuum which then allows blood to flow into the penis. A constriction band is then placed on to the base of the penis, so that the erection is maintained. This should be removed within 30min.
- *Side effects.* Pain, haematoma.

Table 4.16 PDE-5 inhibitors

	Sildenafil	Vardenafil	Tadalafil
Dose (mg/day)	50–100	10–20	10–20
Recommended interval between drug administration and sexual activity	60min	30–60min	>30min
Half-life (h)	3–4	4–5	17
Adverse effects (%)			
Headaches	15–30	7–15	7–20
Facial flushing	10–25	10	1–5
Dyspepsia	2–15	0.5–6	1–15
Nasal congestion	1–10	3–7	4–6
Visual disturbance	1–10	0–2	0.1

Box 4.19 PDE-5 inhibitors—contraindications and cautions

Contraindications
- Recent MI/stroke.
- Unstable angina.
- Current nitrate use, including isosorbide mononitrate/GTN.
- Hypotension (<90/50mmHg).
- Severe heart failure.
- Severe hepatic impairment.
- Retinitis pigmentosa.
- Ketoconazole or HIV protease inhibitors.

Cautions (reduce dose)
- Hypertension.
- Heart disease.
- Peyronie's disease.
- Sickle cell anaemia.
- Renal or hepatic impairment.
- Elderly.
- Leukaemia.
- Multiple myeloma.
- Bleeding disorders, e.g. active peptic ulcer disease.

Avoid concomitant opiates, including dihydrocodeine—may get prolonged erections (opiates increase cGMP in nerve endings).

Penile prosthesis

- Usually tried either in ♂ reluctant to try other forms of therapy or when other treatments have failed. They may be semi-rigid or inflatable.
- *Complications*. Infection, mechanical failure.

Psychosexual counselling

Particularly for ♂ with psychogenic impotence and in ♂ who fail to improve with the above therapies.

Surgical

- Rarely indicated, as results are generally disappointing.
- Revascularization techniques may be available in specialist centres.
- Ligation of dorsal veins may restore erectile function temporarily in men with venous insufficiency, although rarely permanently.

Further reading

Beckman TJ, et al. (2006). Evaluation and medical management of erectile dysfunction. *Mayo Clin Proc* **81**, 385–90.

Cohan P, Korenman SG (2001). Erectile dysfunction. *J Clin Endocrinol Metab* **86**, 2391–4.

Fazio L, Brick G (2004). Erectile dysfunction: management update. *CMAJ* **170**, 1429–37.

Shamloul R, Ghanem H (2013). Erectile dysfunction. *Lancet* **381**, 153–65.

Infertility

Definition

- Subfertility, defined as failure of pregnancy after 1 year of unprotected regular (×2/week) sexual intercourse, affects ~15% of all couples.
- Couples who fail to conceive after 1 year of regular unprotected sexual intercourse should be investigated.
- If there is a known predisposing factor or the ♀ partner is aged >35 years, then investigation should be offered earlier.

Causes

(See Boxes 4.20 and 4.21, and Fig. 4.11.)
- ♀ factors (e.g. anovulation, tubal damage) 45%.
- ♂ factors (e.g. oligospermia) 30%.
- Unexplained subfertility ~25% (depending on intensity of investigation).
- Both ♀ and ♂ factors may coexist in ~40% of couples.

Box 4.20 Causes of female infertility

Anovulation
- PCOS (80% of anovulatory disorders).
- POI (5% of anovulatory disorders).
- HA (weight-/exercise-induced).
- HH.
- Hyperprolactinaemia.
- Structural hypothalamic/pituitary disease.
- Thyroid dysfunction.
- Drugs, e.g. anabolic steroids.
- Previous surgery, e.g. ovarian cystectomy.
- Systemic illness.

Tubal disorders
- Infective, e.g. *Chlamydia*.
- Endometriosis.
- Previous pelvic surgery.

Uterine abnormalities
- Congenital anomalies.
- Intrauterine adhesions.
- Cervical factors (e.g. surgery).
- Uterine (intracavitary) fibroids.

The ♀ age is a major determinant of fecundity; fertility declines markedly after the age of 35.

Obesity reduces fertility in both ♀ and ♂, and also affects pregnancy outcome.

Smoking is associated with subfertility and also affects pregnancy outcome.

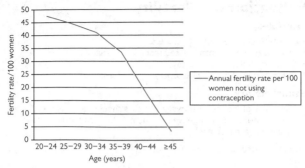

Fig. 4.11 The effect of maternal age on the average rate of pregnancy, calculated on the basis of studies in ten different populations that did not use contraceptives.

Reprinted from NICE (2013) 'Fertility problems – assessment and treatment' CG156 🕾 https://www.nice.org.uk/guidance/cg156. With permission from NICE.

Box 4.21 Causes of male infertility

Primary gonadal dysfunction/failure
- Idiopathic.
- Genetic, e.g. Klinefelter's syndrome, Y chromosome microdeletions, immotile cilia/Kartagener's syndrome, CF.
- Congenital cryptorchidism.
- Orchitis.
- Testicular torsion or trauma.
- Chemotherapy/testicular radiotherapy.
- Other toxins, e.g. alcohol, anabolic steroids.
- Drugs, e.g. spironolactone, corticosteroids, sulfasalazine.
- Systemic illness.
- Varicocele.

Secondary gonadal failure
- HH.
- Structural hypothalamic/pituitary disease.
- Hyperprolactinaemia.

Obstructive
- Congenital.
- Infective.
- Post-surgical.

Other
- Sperm autoimmunity.
- Erectile dysfunction.
- ♂ age has slight effect on fertility.
- Obesity reduces fertility in both ♀ and ♂.
- Smoking tobacco, vaping, and cannabis reduce semen quality.

Evaluation of infertility

Principles
- Investigate both ♀ and ♂ partners.
- Undertake pre-pregnancy assessment for ♀ partner.
- Offer psychological support.
- Refer to specialist multidisciplinary fertility clinic.

Sexual history
- Frequency of intercourse? Every 2–3 days should be encouraged.
- Use of lubricants? These have detrimental effect on semen quality.
- Psychosexual difficulties?

Female factors

History
- Age (see Fig. 4.11).

Menstrual history
- Length and regularity of menstrual cycle: cycle of 25–35 days indicates ovulation; oligo-/amenorrhoea suggests anovulation.
- Dysmenorrhoea? Menorrhagia? Severe menstrual symptoms are suggestive of endometriosis.
- Irregular bleeding?

Gynaecological and obstetric history
- Details of previous pregnancies. Ectopic pregnancy suggests tubal damage; complicated miscarriage/termination of pregnancy may cause intrauterine adhesions; Caesarean delivery may also cause adhesions.
- Pelvic inflammatory disease (PID)? Implies tubal damage (each episode of acute PID causes infertility in 10–15% of cases).
- Sexually transmitted disease? Predisposes to tubal damage.
- Previous pelvic surgery? Predisposes to pelvic adhesions.
- Dyspareunia? If deep pain, may be due to endometriosis.

Symptoms of endocrine disorders
- Hot flushes may be indicative of oestrogen deficiency.
- Spontaneous galactorrhoea may be due to hyperprolactinaemia.

Medical history
- DM, thyroid or pituitary dysfunction, and other systemic illnesses.

Lifestyle factors
- Excessive physical exercise (e.g. distance running) or weight loss >10% in 1 year, may cause hypothalamic amenorrhoea/hypogonadism.
- Smoking, alcohol, and recreational drugs can affect fertility.

Drug history
- Drugs that may cause hyperprolactinaemia (see Box 2.13).
- Chemotherapy/radiotherapy may cause ovarian failure.

Family history
- Suggestive of risk of POF, PCOS, and endometriosis.

Physical examination
- *BMI:* outside the range of 18.5–29kg/m² adversely affects fertility and pregnancy.
- *Hyperandrogenism?* Indicative of PCOS. Rarely, may detect virilization/DSD.
- *Galactorrhoea?* Suggests hyperprolactinaemia.
- *Pelvic examination:* fibroids, endometriosis.

Investigations
(See Fig. 4.12.)

Assess ovulatory function
- Home ovulation kit testing of urinary LH ± E2 is reliable in regular cycles; basal body temperature charts less reliable.
- Mid-luteal progesterone, timed 7 days before expected onset of menses. Values >30nmol/L consistent with ovulation.
- Consider ovulation tracking by serial US if uncertain.

Assess ovarian reserve
- Serum FSH, LH, and E2 on days 2–6 of the menstrual cycle (day 1 = 1st day of menses). FSH >10IU/L is indicative of reduced ovarian reserve. FSH >30IU/L indicates ovarian insufficiency.
- Antral follicle count (number of small follicles visible on pelvic US) assesses oocyte pool.
  - AMH measurement reflects the size of the oocyte pool and is useful in clinical practice, being stable throughout the menstrual cycle and relatively unaffected by hormonal contraception. It is an early marker of oocyte depletion.

Assess pelvic anatomy
- Pelvic US (transvaginal) for uterine and ovarian anatomy.

Assess tubal patency
- Hysterosalpingography (HSG) (uses X-ray) or hysterosalpingo contrast sonography (HyCoSy) (uses US).
- Laparoscopy and dye test remain the 'gold standard' for pelvic and tubal assessment.

Exclude infection
- Send vaginal discharge for bacteriology.
- Test for *Chlamydia trachomatis* by swab, urine, or serology.

Pre-pregnancy assessment
- Rubella immunity.
- Cervical cytology (follow national screening guidelines).
- Haemoglobinopathy screening.
- Virology screening for HIV, hepatitis B, and hepatitis C.
- Advice on smoking, alcohol, diet and exercise, folic acid, and vitamin D.

Further assessment if indicated
- In ♀ with irregular/absent menstrual cycles, measure TSH, FT₄, and serum PRL, as well as FSH, LH, and E2.
- In ♀ with clinical evidence of hyperandrogenism, measure serum testosterone, and consider SHBG and 17OHP.
- In ♀ with hyperprolactinaemia or otherwise unexplained HH, arrange pituitary MRI.

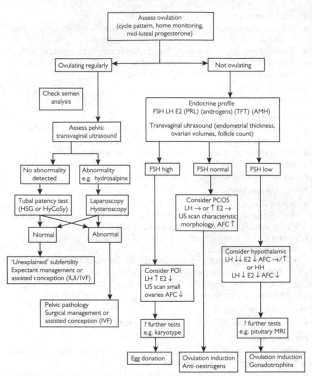

Fig. 4.12 Investigation and management of ♀ infertility.

Male factors

History
- *Testicular injury or surgery.*
- *Previous infection*, e.g. mumps orchitis, sexually transmitted disease, epididymitis.

Symptoms of androgen deficiency (may be asymptomatic)
- Reduced libido and potency.
- Reduced frequency of shaving.

Drug history
- Recreational drugs, excessive alcohol, and anabolic steroids may all contribute to hypogonadism.
- Drugs affecting spermatogenesis, e.g. sulfasalazine, methotrexate.
- Chemotherapy/radiotherapy may cause 1° testicular failure.

Medical history
- Bronchiectasis may be associated with epididymal obstruction (Young's syndrome) or severe asthenospermia (immotile cilia syndrome).

Physical examination
- BMI.
- 2° sexual characteristics:
  - Rarely may detect hypogonadism.
  - Eunuchoid habitus (see Box 4.14) suggestive of prepubertal hypogonadism.
  - Gynaecomastia may suggest hypogonadism.
- External genitalia:
  - Penile/urethral abnormalities, epididymal thickening.
- Testicular size measured using orchidometer:
  - Normal 15–25mL.
  - Reduced to <15mL in hypogonadism.
  - In Klinefelter's syndrome, testes are often <5mL.
  - In ♂ with azoospermia and normal testicular size, suspect genital tract obstruction, e.g. congenital absence of vas deferens.

Investigations
(See Fig. 4.13.)

Semen analysis
Essential in the diagnostic work-up of any infertile couple. Semen collection should be performed by masturbation after 3 days of sexual abstinence (see Table 4.17 for interpretation of results).
- If *normal*, then a ♂ cause is excluded.
- If *abnormal*, then repeat semen analysis 6–12 weeks later.
- If *azoospermia*, repeat and measure FSH, LH, and testosterone.
- If *asthenospermia*, i.e. immotile sperm, consider immunological infertility or infection (prostatic infection characterized by high semen viscosity and pH, and leucocytes in semen).

Further investigations
- Endocrine profile:
  - ↑ FSH and ↑ LH, with low testosterone in testicular failure.
  - ↑ FSH with normal LH and testosterone can occur in disordered spermatogenesis.
  - ↓ FSH, LH, and testosterone indicate 2° hypogonadism. Arrange MRI of the pituitary gland and hypothalamus.
- Infection screening in ♂ with leucocytospermia.
- Scrotal US may aid diagnosis of chronic epididymitis. Infertile ♂ are at ↑ risk of testicular tumours.
- Genetic tests: ♂ with 1° testicular failure may have abnormal karyotype or Y chromosome deletions. ♂ with Klinefelter's syndrome (47,XXY) may present with infertility.
- Sperm antibodies in semen should not be measured routinely, as specific treatment is rarely effective.
- Testicular biopsy is rarely diagnostic but may be used to retrieve sperm for assisted reproduction techniques.
- Sperm function tests are not performed routinely, as they are not sufficiently predictive of fertility outcome.

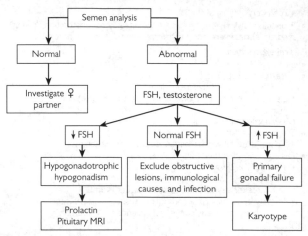

Fig. 4.13 Investigation of ♂ infertility.

Table 4.17 WHO criteria for normal semen analysis

Test	Normal values (based on 95th centile for fertile men)	Nomenclature for abnormal values
Volume	≥1.5mL	Aspermia (no ejaculate)
pH	≥7.2	
Total sperm number	≥39 × 10⁶/ejaculate	
Sperm concentration	≥15 × 10⁶/mL	Oligozoospermia
		Azoospermia (no sperm in ejaculate)
Motility	≥32% progressive motility	Asthenospermia
Morphology	≥4% normal forms	Teratospermia
Live sperm	≥58%	Necrospermia
Leucocytes	<1 × 10⁶/mL	Leucocytospermia

Source: data from World Health Organization, Department of Reproductive Health and Research (2010). WHO laboratory manual for the examination and processing of human semen. Fifth edition.

Further reading

Agarwal A, et al. (2021). Male infertility. Lancet **397**, 319–33.
Guzick DS, et al. (2001). Sperm morphology, motility, and concentration in fertile and infertile men. N Engl J Med **345**, 1388–93.

Management of female infertility

Anovulation

Hypogonadotrophic (WHO class I)

- Treat hyperprolactinaemia with dopamine agonists.
- Address functional (hypothalamic) amenorrhoea with lifestyle changes to gain weight/reduce exercise.
- Then may need ovulation induction (see ➋ Ovulation induction, p. 458).

Normogonadotrophic (WHO class II)

- Usually PCOS; 1st-line treatment is weight loss if obese.
- Ovulation induction (see ➋ Ovulation induction, p. 458).

Hypergonadotrophic (WHO class III)

- Ovarian stimulation has poor results if FSH >15IU/L.
- Spontaneous pregnancy is still possible in early POI.
- Egg donation is only effective treatment in established POI.

Tubal infertility

- IVF achieves better pregnancy rates than surgical tubal reconstruction, with a lower risk of ectopic pregnancy.
- Hydrosalpinges reduce IVF success rates. Laparoscopic salpingectomy should be offered prior to IVF.
- Surgical treatment of mild tubal disease may be offered, usually by laparoscopy for distal tubal damage, or hysteroscopic cannulation for proximal obstruction.
- Surgical reversal of sterilization is highly successful.

Endometriosis

- Medical therapies (e.g. progestogens, GnRH agonists) do not improve fertility.

Minimal/mild

- Laparoscopic destruction of superficial disease improves chance of pregnancy. Resection of ovarian endometriomas may improve ovarian folliculogenesis, and thus fertility, but can reduce ovarian reserve.
- Assisted reproductive techniques (ARTs) (see Table 4.18).

Moderate/severe

- Surgery may improve fertility. However, IVF offers the best chance of pregnancy.

Uterine factors

- Intracavity fibroids, polyps, and intrauterine septae can be resected hysteroscopically.
- Intrauterine adhesions can be divided hysteroscopically, but the endometrium may not regenerate fully.
- Intramural fibroids may also reduce fertility and, if large, may require myomectomy. Fibroid embolization is not recommended for ♀ wishing fertility because it affects uterine blood flow.

Table 4.18 Assisted reproductive techniques

Technique	Indications	Pregnancy rates	Notes
Intrauterine insemination (IUI) (usually offered 3–6 cycles)	Donor insemination Psychosexual infertility (Can be used, though not sufficient evidence of efficacy, for unexplained infertility) Mild oligospermia Mild endometriosis	<15% per cycle	Washed and prepared motile spermatozoa are injected into the uterine cavity through a catheter just before ovulation Superovulation improves success rates but is associated with an ↑ risk of multiple pregnancy
IVF	Most forms of infertility, unless severe ♂ factor (Donor sperm may be used)	30% birth rate per embryo transferred in women under the age of 35 years Success rates markedly reduced in women over 40 years of age The main risks of IVF are ovarian hyperstimulation and multiple pregnancy	After superovulation, ovarian follicles are aspirated under transvaginal US guidance. Eggs are fertilized with prepared sperm *in vitro*. Embryo transfer into the uterine cavity is performed after 3–6 days. Luteal support is required, using progesterone supplementation
ICSI	♂ infertility. ICSI allows IVF to be offered in severe oligospermia	Pregnancy rates equivalent to standard IVF There is a small risk of sex chromosome abnormalities (1%) in ♂ conceived following ICSI	Viable spermatozoa are injected directly into oocytes. Spermatozoa may be derived from an ejaculate or aspirated from the epididymis or testis in men with obstructive azoospermia
Egg donation	POI, maternal age-related infertility	Pregnancy rates are better than with standard IVF, and not affected by patient's age	Donated eggs are fertilized *in vitro* with partner's sperm. Hormonal support (oestrogen and progesterone) is required before and after embryo transfer

Risks of ART

Ovarian hyperstimulation syndrome (OHSS) is a condition specific to ovarian stimulation (see ➔ Gonadotrophins, p. 423). It is a potentially fatal syndrome of ovarian enlargement and ↑ vascular permeability, with accumulation of fluid in the peritoneal, pleural, and pericardial cavities.

- OHSS is more severe if pregnancy occurs due to endogenous hCG production. Avoid by freezing all embryos and using an agonist trigger, instead of hCG, in at-risk cycles.
- Mild OHSS occurs in up to 25% of stimulated cycles and results in abdominal bloating and nausea. It resolves with bed rest and fluid replacement.
- Severe OHSS, associated with hypotension, markedly enlarged ovaries, ascites, and pleural and pericardial effusions, occurs in <0.1%. ♀ need to be hospitalized and resuscitated, as there is mortality from disseminated intravascular coagulation and PE. Management should be led by an expert reproductive endocrinologist.
- Risk factors for OHSS are multiple follicles, young age, PCOS, and previous OHSS.
- *Multiple pregnancy* increases the risk of all pregnancy complications, particularly prematurity. The rate of multiple pregnancies in IVF has come down from 1:4 to 1:10 over the last 20 years, and elective single embryo transfer is advised in women aged <37.
- *Bleeding* into the pelvis after egg harvest is uncommon.
- *Pelvic infection* arising from the cervix or vagina during ART is uncommon.
- *VTE* risk is ↑ as high circulating oestrogen during stimulation (and early pregnancy) produces a hypercoagulable state.
- *Risk of malignancy.* Infertility is associated with an ↑ risk of ovarian cancer. Large studies on IVF populations are reassuring on the risk of breast cancer but confirm a slight ↑ risk of ovarian cancer. Endometrial hyperplasia and endometrial cancer risk is ↑ in anovulatory women with PCOS, especially if obese.

Management of male infertility

Hypogonadotrophic hypogonadism

- Gonadotrophins: hCG 1500–2000IU IM ×2/week. Most also require FSH/hMG 150IU SC ×3/week. Monitor serum testosterone and testicular size.
- Once testes are >8mL, semen analysis every 3–6 months. Takes at least 2 years to maximize spermatogenesis. Normalization of spermatogenesis in 80–90% of ♂.
- Once spermatogenesis is induced, it may be maintained by hCG alone.

Idiopathic semen abnormalities

- There is insufficient evidence for the use of antioestrogens, gonadotrophins, or androgens in idiopathic disorders of spermatogenesis.
- IVF using ICSI can overcome all degrees of oligospermia.
- Varicocele has controversial association with subfertility. There is insufficient evidence that surgery improves pregnancy rates.

Obstructive azoospermia

- Reversal of vasectomy will result in successful pregnancy in up to 50% of cases within 2 years.
- Microsurgery is possible for most other causes, with successful pregnancies in 25–35% of couples within 18 months of treatment. During surgery, sperm is often retrieved and stored for future IVF/ICSI.

Primary testicular failure

- In selected cases of azoospermia, mTESE may obtain sufficient spermatozoa for ICSI.
- Donor insemination.

Unexplained infertility

Definition

Subfertility despite sexual intercourse occurring at least twice weekly, normal semen analysis, proven ovulation, and patent tubes.

Prognosis

- This depends on duration of subfertility and the woman's age. If investigations are normal after 1 year trying to conceive, there is a 50% chance of pregnancy within the next year. However, if trying >3 years, pregnancy chances are low and ART should be considered. In ♀ >35 years of age, treatment should be expedited.

Treatment options

- Expectant management.
- Superovulation (using clomifene or low-dose gonadotrophins) with IUI may be offered to couples with a relatively short duration of subfertility and ♀ partner aged <37.
- IVF should be offered for prolonged unexplained subfertility and couples where ♀ partner aged ≥37.

Ovulation induction

Indications

Anovulation due to:
- PCOS.
- Hypopituitarism.
- HH.

Note that aim of treatment is unifollicular ovulation, in contrast to 'controlled ovarian hyperstimulation' for IVF.

Pretreatment assessment

- Exclude thyroid dysfunction and hyperprolactinaemia.
- Confirm normal semen analysis.
- Baseline pelvic US is essential to exclude ovarian/uterine abnormalities.
- Confirm tubal patency (see ➔ Investigations, p. 447) prior to gonadotrophin use and/or after failed clomifene use.
- Pre-pregnancy checks.
- Optimize lifestyle: smoking cessation, maintain normal BMI, exercise in moderation, and limit alcohol intake.

Oral agents

Antioestrogens

Mode of action

On hypothalamic–pituitary–ovarian (HPO) axis by lack of normal −ve feedback. ↑ pulse frequency of GnRH, which increases FSH and LH release, thereby stimulating ovarian folliculogenesis (may have antioestrogen effect on the endometrium, cervix, and vagina).

Indications

- Normogonadotrophic anovulation, PCOS.
- May also be used in unexplained infertility.
- Requires normal HPO axis, therefore ineffective in HH.

Types

- Clomifene citrate 50–100mg—SERM. Most widely used agent.
- Tamoxifen 20–40mg—very similar to clomifene.
- Letrozole 2.5–5mg—selective aromatase inhibitor. Recently recommended as 1st-line agent, with higher efficacy and lower multiple pregnancy rate than clomifene.

Administration

- May have to induce bleed by giving a progestagen for 10 days.
- Start on days 2–5 of menstrual cycle. Spontaneous ovulation should occur 5–10 days later.
- Must monitor with US 'follicle tracking' to confirm effectiveness and avoid multiple pregnancies.
- May ensure ovulation by administration of 10,000IU of hCG mid cycle when leading follicle is at least 20mm.
- Remain on optimum dose for ≥6 ovulations.

Efficacy
- 80–90% ovulate, with conception rates of 50–60% in first six ovulatory cycles.

Side effects
- Uncommon. With clomifene, hot flushes in 10%, pelvic pain in 5%, nausea in 2%, headache, mood changes, and visual disturbances in 1.5%.
- Multiple pregnancies in 7–10%.
- OHSS in <1%.
- Association with ovarian cancer (previously reported with use of clomifene) is uncertain, but treatment duration should be limited to 6–12 months.

Metformin
- May be used as a sole agent in women with PCOS with anovulatory infertility, and does not require US monitoring, but is less effective than antioestrogens.
- May be used in combination with clomifene to increase efficacy in women resistant to clomifene alone.
- Use may be limited by GI side effects.

Ovarian diathermy
- Laparoscopic ovarian diathermy, using electrocautery to drill 4–10 points on the surface of the ovaries, may be used in ♀ with PCOS who have failed to conceive on oral therapy.
- It is most effective in slim ♀ with amenorrhoeic PCOS and high LH, in whom it can achieve an ovulation rate of >80% and a pregnancy rate of >60% (comparable to gonadotrophin therapy without the risk of multiple pregnancies or OHSS).
- There is a small risk of pelvic adhesions and a theoretical risk of POF following ovarian diathermy.

Gonadotrophins
Indications
- HH (hypothalamic or pituitary origin) (requires hMG = FSH + LH).
- ♀ with PCOS who are resistant to 1st-line therapy (may use hMG or FSH).

Aim
- To induce monofollicular ovulation. Close monitoring with transvaginal US is essential.

Dose and administration
Several regimens available. Low-dose step-up approach widely used:
- Start on day 3 of (induced) menses at 50–75IU/day. Titrate the dose upwards, at no less than weekly intervals, according to follicle development.
- Administer hCG 5000–10,000IU to trigger ovulation when the dominant follicle >18mm in diameter.
- Ovulation is only triggered with <3 mature follicles >14mm in diameter. If ≥3 mature follicles, then abandon cycle and advise avoidance of intercourse.
- May use gonadotrophins for a total of six cycles. If unsuccessful, then consider IVF.

Efficacy
- 80–85% pregnancy rate after six cycles.

Adverse effects
- Multiple pregnancies 10–20%.
- *OHSS* (see ➔ Risks of ART, p. 454).

Use of gonadotrophins in ART
- *Superovulation* for IUI treatment aims to develop 2–3 mature follicles.
- *Controlled ovarian hyperstimulation* for IVF aims to develop multiple follicles. This requires strategies to prevent premature ovulation before eggs can be collected, either a GnRH agonist, usually started in the mid-luteal phase of the preceding cycle, or a GnRH antagonist started in the mid-follicular phase of stimulation.

Pulsatile GnRH
- *Indications.* Hypothalamic hypogonadism with normal pituitary function.
- *Dose and administration.* Pulsatile GnRH using an infusion pump, worn continuously, which delivers an SC dose of GnRH every 90min. Unfortunately, this is no longer marketed in the UK.
- *Efficacy.* Cumulative pregnancy rate of 70–90%. Avoids the risk of OHSS and multiple pregnancies associated with gonadotrophins.

Human Fertilisation and Embryology Act (UK)
The Human Fertilisation and Embryology Authority (HFEA) is a statutory body set up in 1991 to inspect, monitor, and license fertility centres offering IVF, ICSI, IUI, and treatments with donor gametes, and also to regulate all research involving human embryos. It is required to keep a register of all IVF treatment cycles and of all children born as a result of IVF or donor gametes. The HFEA also provides information to couples seeking fertility treatment or potential donors.

The HFEA is accountable to the Secretary of State for Health and advises government ministers, as required, particularly regarding new developments in fertility technology or research.

Fertility preservation

Fertility may be affected by chemotherapy, pelvic radiotherapy, or surgery. The outcome depends on gender, age, chemotherapeutic agents used (alkylating agents are highly gonadotoxic), and the cumulative dose of chemo-/radiotherapy.

Pathophysiology

- In ♂, the Leydig cells are relatively resistant, so endocrine function may be preserved, even in azoospermic ♂. Some recovery of spermatogenesis may occur over 1–2 years.
- In ♀, destruction of ovarian follicles causes oestrogen deficiency (POI) (see ➔ Premature ovarian insufficiency, pp. 376–8), as well as loss of fertility.

Indications for fertility preservation

- Cancer therapies (may be classified into low, medium, and high risk); use of cytotoxic drugs for benign disease, e.g. stem cell transplants for haemoglobinopathies; gender transition; surgery for recurrent ovarian cysts; elective ('social') egg freezing to avoid age-related infertility.

Sperm cryopreservation

- ♂ patients should be offered semen storage prior to commencing treatment. Semen is mixed with cryoprotectant, divided into aliquots, and stored in liquid nitrogen vapour. Thawed samples are used in ICSI. Only a minority (≤15%) of men use their stored samples.

Embryo cryopreservation

- Offered to ♀ with established partner. (NB. Consent to use embryos requires both partners.) Requires ovarian stimulation and egg harvest, usually with a 'random start' protocol of gonadotrophins with GnRH antagonist, taking 2–3 weeks. For oestrogen-sensitive conditions (breast cancer), an antioestrogen is given during stimulation. Well-established freezing techniques.

Egg cryopreservation

- Available to ♀ without a partner. Requires ovarian stimulation, as for embryo freezing. Utilizing the technique of vitrification, success rates using stored oocytes can now equate to fresh IVF.

Ovarian cryopreservation

- Possible for prepubertal patients or adult ♀ when there is insufficient time for egg collection, but not yet an established technique. Patients must be fit enough to undergo a surgical procedure. At laparoscopy, all or part of an ovary is removed and cortical strips (containing immature oocytes) are frozen. Subsequent reimplantation of tissue gives a high chance of restoring endocrine function, but this is transient. Pregnancy rates are uncertain (? 25%). *In vitro* maturation of follicles has not yet been achieved.

Ovarian suppression

- The use of GnRH analogues during chemotherapy for breast cancer has been shown in three recent RCTs to reduce the rate of subsequent amenorrhoea. Further data are needed on pregnancy rates.

Testicular tissue

- For prepubertal boys, there is no effective option for fertility preservation. Testicular tissue storage is experimental.

Further reading

Adoption UK. ℘ https://www.adoptionuk.org/

Daisy Network. [Offers patient support and information for women with POI]. ℘ https://www.daisynetwork.org/

Farhat R, et al. (2010). Outcome of gonadotropin therapy for male infertility due to hypogonadotrophic hypogonadism. Pituitary **13**, 105–10.

Fertility Network UK. [The UK's leading patient-focused fertility charity, providing free support, advice, and information for anyone affected by fertility issues]. ℘ https://fertilitynetworkuk.org/

Human Fertilisation and Embryology Authority (2019). Fertility treatment 2017: trends and figures. ℘ https://www.hfea.gov.uk/media/2894/fertility-treatment-2017-trends-and-figures-may-2019.pdf

Human Fertilisation and Embryology Authority (HFEA). [The government regulator responsible for fertility clinics and research; the HFEA website provides free impartial patient information on ART and also information on UK clinics]. ℘ https://www.hfea.gov.uk/

National Institute for Health and Care Excellence (2013, updated 2017). Fertility problems: assessment and treatment. ℘ https://www.nice.org.uk/guidance/cg156

Oktay K, et al. (2018). Fertility preservation in patients with cancer: ASCO clinical practice guideline update. J Clin Oncol **36**, 1994–2001.

Royal College of Obstetricians and Gynaecologists (2016). Management of ovarian hyperstimulation syndrome. Green-top guideline no. 5. ℘ https://www.rcog.org.uk/en/guidelines-research-services/guidelines/gtg5/

Teede HJ, et al.; International PCOS Network (2018). Recommendations from the international evidence-based guideline for the assessment and management of polycystic ovary syndrome. Clin Endocrinol (Oxf) **89**, 251–68.

Yasmin E, et al.; British Fertility Society Policy and Practice Committee (2013). Ovulation induction in WHO type 1 anovulation: guidelines for practice. Hum Fertil (Camb) **16**, 228–34.

Gender dysphoria in adults

Definition

Gender dysphoria is defined as a marked difference between the individual's expressed/experienced gender and the gender others would assign him or her, and it must continue for at least 6 months by the *Diagnostic and Statistical Manual of Mental Disorders*, 5th edition (DSM-5). In children, the desire to be of the other gender must be present and verbalized. As defined, this condition causes clinically significant distress or impairment in social, occupational, or other important areas of functioning. Importantly, this condition is no longer part of the mental health chapter in the DSM. The *International Classification Diseases 11* (ICD-11) will include the condition of gender incongruence of adult and adolescence where there is a marked incongruence between experience/expressed gender and assigned gender of at least 6 months duration accompanied by a desire to either be rid of the primary sex characteristics of your birth gender or acquire some or all of the secondary sex characteristics of your desired gender. Importantly distress is not part of the definition of gender incongruence.

Epidemiology

Estimated prevalence of 0.5–1.3% of birth-assigned ♂, and 0.4–1.2% of birth-assigned ♀, identify as a transgender person ♀.

Aetiology

- Unknown and controversial.
- Some evidence that it may have a neurobiological basis. There appear to be sex differences in the size and shape of certain nuclei in the hypothalamus. Transgender women (a person who is birth-assigned ♂ who has transitioned to ♀) have been found to have ♀ differentiation of one of these nuclei, whereas transgender men (a person who is birth-assigned ♀ who has transitioned to ♂) have been found to have a ♂ pattern of differentiation.
- This does not explain the phenomenon of non-binary people (a person who does not identify as either ♂ or ♀), and psychosocial models of gender development are also important in considering the aetiology of gender non-conformity.

Management

Standards of care

- Multidisciplinary approach among psychiatrists, psychologists, endocrinologists, and surgeons. The patient should be counselled about the treatment options, risks, and implications, and realistic expectations should be discussed.
- Endocrine disorders should be excluded prior to the use of gender hormone therapy, i.e. ensure normal physical development, gonadotrophins, SHBG, PRL, testosterone, and oestradiol. Karyotype is only indicated if there is clinical evidence of a possible intersex state.
- Psychosocial assessment and follow-up are essential before definitive therapy. The gender dysphoria should be shown to have been persistently present for at least 6 months.

- The aim of treatment programme is to help the individual consolidate their gender identity and social role, and this is usually accompanied by an improvement in psychological function. Hormone therapy is an adjunct to induce the 2° sex characteristics of the desired gender to make the physical expression of the person's gender more congruent with their internal sense of gender. This should continue for at least 1 year before surgery.
- Psychological follow-up and expert counselling should be available, if required, throughout the programme, including after surgery.
- In adolescents, puberty can be reversibly halted by GnRH analogue therapy to prevent irreversible changes in the wrong gender until a permanent diagnosis is made.

(See Table 4.19.)

Table 4.19 Monitoring of therapy

- Every 3 months for 1st year.
- Hormonal therapy is lifelong, indefinitely, then every 6 months for 2 years, then annually.
- Therefore, patients should be followed up.

♂ to ♀	♀ to ♂
• BP, BMI	• BP, BMI
• LFTs	• LFTs
• Serum lipids and glucose	• Serum lipids
• Oestradiol, PRL, testosterone	• Testosterone
• Mammogram (>50 years)	• FBC (exclude polycythaemia)

Hormonal manipulation

See Table 4.20 for contraindications.

Table 4.20 Contraindications to hormone manipulation

Feminization	Masculinization
Prolactinoma	CVD
History of breast cancer	Active liver disease
Previous thromboembolism (if not anticoagulated)	Polycythaemia
Active liver disease	Breastfeeding
	Pregnancy
Relative contraindications	
IHD	IHD
Cerebrovascular disease	Cerebrovascular disease
Other contraindication to oestrogen therapy	Other contraindication to testosterone therapy

Transgender women
- Suppress ♂ 2° sex characteristics (GnRH analogue leuprorelin 11.25mg every 12 weeks or goserelin 10.8mg every 12 weeks) to prevent a testosterone flare that can occur; may use CPA 100mg od for first 2 weeks. In Europe, CPA 50–100mg od is used long term.
- Induce ♀ 2° sex characteristics:
  - Estradiol valerate or hemihydrate 2–8mg od.
  - Oestrogen patches 25–200 micrograms twice per week.
  - Oestrogen gel 0.5–4mg od.
- *Aims:*
  - Breast development—maximum after 2 years of treatment.
  - Development of ♀ fat distribution.
  - Reduced body hair and smoother skin. However, facial hair is often resistant to treatment.
  - Reduced muscle bulk and strength.
  - Reduction in testicular size.
  - Hormonal manipulation has little effect on voice.
- Adjust oestrogen dose, depending on plasma oestradiol levels.
- *Side effects* (particularly while on high-dose EE2 + CPA therapy):
  - Hyperprolactinaemia.
  - VTE.
  - Abnormal liver enzymes.
  - Depression.
  - ↑ in cardiovascular events

Transgender men
- Induce ♂ 2° sex characteristics, and suppress ♀ 2° sex characteristics: parenteral testosterone (see Table 4.21).
- *Aims:*
  - Cessation of menstrual bleeding.
  - Atrophy of uterus and breasts.
  - Increase muscle bulk and strength.
  - Deepening of voice (after 6–10 weeks).
  - Hirsutism.
  - ♂ body fat distribution.
  - Increase in libido.
- *Side effects:*
  - Acne (in 40%).
  - Weight gain.
  - Abnormal liver function.
  - Adverse lipid profile.
  - Polycythaemia

Gender reassignment surgery
- Performed at least 12 months after establishing the desired gender role.
- A 2nd psychiatric/psychological opinion should be sought prior to referral for surgery.

Feminizing genital surgery
- Bilateral orchidectomy and resection of the penis.
- Construction of a vagina and labia minora.
- Clitoroplasty.

Not available on the NHS
- Breast augmentation.
- Facial feminization surgery.

Table 4.21 Maintenance hormone regimens in the treatment of transsexualism

Feminization (post-surgery)	Masculinization (pre- and post-surgery)
Estradiol valerate or hemihydrate (PO) 2–8mg od	Testosterone 250mg IM every 2–4 weeks
Estradiol valerate (transdermal) 50–200 micrograms 2×/week	Testosterone gel 25–100mg
Estradiol gel 0.5–4mg od	Testosterone undecanoate 1000 mg every 9–15 weeks
Notes	
Over the age of 40, topical preparations are chosen to minimize cardiovascular risk	Testosterone gel has a lower risk of polycythaemia

Transgender men
- Bilateral mastectomy and ♂ chest reconstruction.
- Hysterectomy and salpingo-oophorectomy.
- Phalloplasty and testicular prostheses.
- Metoidioplasty.

Prognosis

- Significantly ↑ morbidity in transgender women (RR 2- to 20-fold from thromboembolism).
- Hyperprolactinaemia and elevation in liver enzymes are self-limiting in the majority of cases.
- The risk of osteoporosis is not thought to be ↑ in transgender people.
- There may be a slightly ↑ risk of breast cancer in transgender women.
- Cosmetic results from reconstructive surgery, particularly in transgender men, remain suboptimal.
- There is an ↑ risk of depressive illness and suicide in transgender individuals which is reduced with treatment.

Further reading

Barrett JD (2007). Transsexual and Other Disorders of Gender Identity: A Practical Guide to Management. Radcliffe, Abingdon.

Bouman WP, Arcelus J (2017). The Transgender Handbook: A Guide for Transgender People, their Families and Professionals. Nova Science Publishers, Hauppauge, NY.

Coleman E, et al. (2011). Standards of care for the health of transsexual, transgender, and gender-nonconforming people, version 7. *International Journal of Transgenderism*, **13**, 165–232.

Hembree WC, et al. (2017). Endocrine treatment of gender-dysphoric/gender-incongruent persons: an Endocrine Society clinical practice guideline. *Endocr Pract* **23**, 1437.

Richards C, et al. (2016). Non-binary or genderqueer genders. *Int Rev Psychiatry* **28**, 95–102.

Seal LJ (2016). A review of the physical and metabolic effects of cross-sex hormonal therapy in the treatment of gender dysphoria. *Ann Clin Biochem* **53**(Pt 1), 10–20.

Wylie K, et al. (2013). Good practice guidelines for the assessment and treatment of adults with gender dysphoria. ℛ https://www.rcpsych.ac.uk/docs/default-source/improving-care/better-mh-policy/college-reports/cr181-good-practice-guidelines-for-the-assessment-and-treatment-of-adults-with-gender-dysphoria.pdf?sfvrsn=84743f94_4

Endocrinology in pregnancy

Catherine Williamson and Rebecca Scott

The thyroid in pregnancy

(See ➔ Anatomy, pp. 2–3.)

The maternal thyroid

- Thyroid size: ↑ by 10–20% due to hCG stimulation; exacerbated by relative iodine deficiency.
- TBG: ↑ concentration due to ↓ hepatic clearance plus ↑ oestrogen-mediated synthesis.
- TSH: often ↓ initially due to thyroid stimulation by hCG; thereafter ↓ returns towards normal. Upper limit ~0.5IU/L lower than non-pregnant TSH. TSH does not cross the placenta. (See Fig. 5.1.)
- Total T_4 and T_3: ↑ in proportion to rise in TBG.
- FT_4 and FT_3: levels may increase in 1st trimester due to hCG stimulation but fall as TBG ↑. In 2nd and 3rd trimesters, levels may be below the limit of the non-pregnant reference range, in part as placental deiodinase degrades maternal thyroid hormone. Small quantities nevertheless do cross the placenta and are essential in early fetal neurological development.
- TRH: levels do not change in pregnancy. TRH does cross the placenta but does not affect the fetal thyroid axis.
- Iodine stores: ↓ due to ↑ renal clearance and transplacental transfer to fetus. The WHO recommends 200 micrograms of iodine/day supplementation in pregnancy. Iodine crosses the placenta, so excessive quantities can suppress the fetal thyroid, causing hypothyroidism and goitre.

The fetal thyroid

- TRH, TSH, and T_4 are first detectable at 8–10 weeks' gestation.
- The fetal hypothalamic–pituitary–thyroid axis is not functionally mature until 18–20 weeks' gestation, so the fetus is dependent on placental transfer of maternal T_4 to protect from hypothyroidism.

Clinical practice point

Reference ranges

- Local trimester-specific reference ranges for TFTs should be used in pregnancy; otherwise risk overdiagnosing subclinical and overt hypothyroidism.
- If local ranges not available, 4mU/L should be used as upper limit for TSH reference range, and remember FT_4 goes below the non-pregnant range in the 3rd trimester. (See Table 5.1 for examples of reference ranges.)

Clinical practice point

Screening for thyroid disease in pregnancy

- There is no evidence for routine thyroid function screening in pregnancy. Only check TFTs in women with known thyroid disease or if high suspicion of new-onset disease.

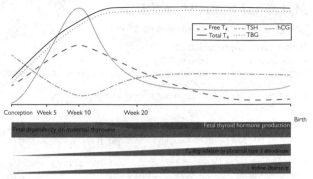

Fig. 5.1 Changes in thyroid physiology during pregnancy.

Reprinted from Korevaar T. et al. (2017) Thyroid disease in pregnancy: new insights in diagnosis and clinical management. *Nature Reviews Endocrinology* 13, 610–622, with permission from Springer.

Table 5.1 Examples of trimester-specific reference ranges for TSH (mIU/L) and FT$_4$ (pmol/L)

	Zhang et al.[1]		Xing et al.[2]		Cotzias et al.[3]	
	TSH	FT$_4$	TSH	FT$_4$	TSH	FT$_4$
T$_1$	0.02–3.78	13.93–26.49	0.07–3.96	9.16–18.12	0–5.5	1–16.5
T$_2$	0.47–3.89	12.33–19.33	0.27–4.53	8.67–16.21	0.5–3.5	29–15.5
T$_3$	0.55–4.91	11.38–19.21	0.48–5.4	7.8–13.90	0.5–4	8–14.5

References

1. Zhang D, *et al.* (2019). Trimester-specific reference ranges for thyroid hormones in pregnant women. *Medicine* **98**, e14245.
2. Xing J, *et al.* (2016). Trimester- and assay-specific thyroid reference intervals for pregnant women in China. *Int J Endocrinol* **2016**, 3754213.
3. Cotzias C, *et al.* (2008). A study to establish gestation-specific reference intervals for thyroid function tests in normal singleton pregnancy. *Eur J Obstet Gynecol Reprod Biol* **137**, 61–6.

Maternal hyperthyroidism

(See ➋ Thyrotoxicosis in pregnancy, pp. 50–4.)

Gestational thyrotoxicosis

- Due to thyroid stimulation by hCG.
- Typically associated with hyperemesis gravidarum (most women do not have symptoms of thyrotoxicosis).
- Hydatidiform moles can cause particularly severe gestational thyrotoxicosis.

Pathological thyrotoxicosis

- Usually due to exacerbation of known Graves' disease, toxic nodules, or goitre.
- New diagnosis of Graves' in pregnancy is unusual, occurring in ~0.05% of pregnancies. This is because untreated thyrotoxicosis is often associated with oligo-/amenorrhoea.
- Pre-existing Graves' may flare in the 1st trimester, typically improves in the 2nd and 3rd trimesters, and then flares again post-partum in response to maternal immune changes.

Maternal hyperthyroidism

- Incidence:
  - Gestational thyrotoxicosis: 1–3% pregnancies.
  - Pathological thyrotoxicosis: 0.2% of pregnancies.
- Maternal complications: arrhythmia, heart failure, pre-eclampsia, thyroid storm.
- Fetal complications: miscarriage, intrauterine death, adverse effect on neurological development, preterm birth, IUGR. TRAb can cross the placenta and cause fetal or neonatal thyrotoxicosis.

Management of hyperthyroidism in pregnancy

Gestational thyrotoxicosis

- This is usually transient. Can control symptoms with propranolol 40mg tds.

Pathological thyrotoxicosis

- Propranolol 40mg tds to control symptoms.
- ATDs are the treatment of choice but cross the placenta.
  - PTU: 0.9% risk of malformations. Congenital abnormalities are typically genitourinary. Maternal risk of liver failure.
  - Carbimazole: 1.7% risk of malformation. These include aplasia cutis, choanal and oesophageal atresia, and other intestinal abnormalities.
  - The risk remains 1.7% for those converted from carbimazole to PTU in the 1st trimester or 3 months pre-pregnancy.
  - The MHRA recommends women on carbimazole should be on effective contraception; however, women should be counselled it is safer to be treated with carbimazole in pregnancy than to have uncontrolled hyperthyroidism.
  - Do not use block-and-replace regimens.

- Monitor TFTs every trimester, every 4 weeks after a dose change, and 6 weeks post-partum.
- RAI: contraindicated in pregnancy, and pregnancy should be avoided for 6 months after RAI therapy.
- Thyroidectomy: rarely needed unless there is a significant reaction to ATDs (e.g. agranulocytosis) or drug resistance.
- Surgery should be planned in the 2nd trimester.

Clinical practice point
- Distinguishing pathological and gestational thyrotoxicosis can be difficult.
- Therefore, check TFTs in women with hyperemesis; look for signs of Graves', and check TPO/TRAbs to confirm pathological thyrotoxicosis.

Clinical practice point
- PTU is recommended in women trying to conceive, but aim to have women stable on PTU for at least 3 months prior to conception.
- If a woman conceives on carbimazole, she should continue on this throughout pregnancy.

Clinical practice point
- Breastfeeding and ATDs: carbimazole doses of up to 20mg daily should be given in divided doses to decrease fetal exposure. PTU is thought to be safe; it does enter breast milk, so small changes in infant TFTs have been reported, but there are no reported cases of infant liver damage from PTU.

Hyperemesis gravidarum

- Characterized by severe vomiting and weight loss.
- Typically begins in early pregnancy (6–9 weeks' gestation), and resolves by 20 weeks' gestation.
- Biochemical hyperthyroidism is seen in two-thirds of affected women, but T_3 is less commonly elevated. Women have no other evidence of thyroid disease.
- Mechanism: hCG has TSH-like effect, thus stimulating the thyroid gland and suppressing TSH secretion. Degree of thyroid stimulation correlates with severity of vomiting. Genetic studies implicate growth differentiating factor 15 (GDF15) and its receptor.
- Diagnosis: hyperemesis may be associated with hyponatraemia, hypokalaemia, low serum urea, raised Hct, ketonuria, and metabolic hypochloraemic alkalosis.
- Dehydration can increase the risk of thromboembolism. Treatment: antiemetics, fluids, and vitamin replacement. Steroids may be needed. Thromboprophylaxis when admitted. ATDs are not required and do not improve symptoms of hyperemesis.

Overt maternal hypothyroidism

- Definition: TSH >10mIU/L with FT$_4$ of any level OR TSH >4mIU/L with FT$_4$ below lower limit of trimester-specific reference range.
- Prevalence: 1–2% of pregnancies.
- Common causes:
  - Hashimoto's thyroiditis.
  - Previous radioiodine therapy.
  - Previous thyroidectomy.
  - Previous post-partum thyroiditis.
  - Hypopituitarism.
- Maternal complications: miscarriage, pre-eclampsia.
- Fetal complications: premature delivery, low birthweight, impaired neurological development.

Preconception counselling

- In women on levothyroxine, aim TSH in lower half of non-pregnant reference range.
- Once pregnancy confirmed, urgently check TFTs; if not possible, increase levothyroxine dose by 30% to ensure optimal early neurological development, and check TFTs as soon as possible.
- Aim for TSH in lower half of local reference ranges for outside of pregnancy.

During pregnancy

- Treat with levothyroxine—start at 100 micrograms daily if a new diagnosis.
- Armour thyroid and liothyronine are not recommended.
- Aim for TSH within local normal trimester-specific range (see Table 5.1).

Post-partum

- Return to pre-pregnancy doses of thyroxine, and check thyroid function in 4 weeks.

Subclinical maternal hypothyroidism

- Definition: TSH > upper limit of trimester-specific reference range, but <10IU/L, with FT$_4$ in the normal range.
- Maternal complications: may increase risk of miscarriage, preterm birth, hypertension, and eclampsia.
- Fetal complications: inconsistent evidence for effect on fetal birthweight. No evidence that it affects fetal cognitive development.
- Treatment: studies of thyroxine started at the end of the 1st trimester show no improvement in gestational age, pre-eclampsia, birthweight, neonatal complications, or childhood IQ. Studies with thyroxine started earlier in pregnancy are lacking. Do recommend treatment if TSH >4 or above the trimester-specific normal range, regardless of FT$_4$.
- Natural history: 2–5% per year progress to frank hypothyroidism.

Isolated hypothyroxinaemia

- Definition: TSH within the trimester-specific reference range, but FT_4 below the lower limit for that trimester.
- Risk factors: iodine deficiency and excess; raised BMI.
- Maternal complications: none known.
- Fetal complications: mild impairment in neurocognitive tests demonstrated in childhood.
- Treatment: there is no evidence that treatment with levothyroxine improves outcomes, so treatment is not recommended.

Euthyroid but TPO antibody positive

- Maternal risks: ↑ risk of miscarriage, developing overt hypothyroidism, and post-partum thyroiditis.
- Fetal complications: risk of preterm birth.
- Treatment: no robust evidence that treatment with levothyroxine improves pregnancy rates or outcomes; however, low-dose levothyroxine can be considered in women who are TPO +ve and euthyroid and have recurrent pregnancy loss.
- Do check TFTs in 3rd trimester and 3 months post-partum to look for evolving thyroid disease. Up to 20% develop frank hypothyroidism by the 3rd trimester.

Post-partum thyroid dysfunction

- Prevalence: 5–10% of women within 1 year of delivery or miscarriage; 3× commoner in women with T1DM; commoner in women who are TPOAb +ve.
- Aetiology: chronic autoimmune thyroiditis (see ➔ Other types of thyroiditis, pp. 80–3).
- Clinical presentation:
  - Hyperthyroidism (32%): develops within 4 months of delivery; typically presents as fatigue. Most spontaneously resolve in 2–3 months but can be followed by hypothyroidism, so check TFTs every 4–6 weeks. Rarely, propranolol used to control symptoms in thyrotoxic phase.
  - Hypothyroidism (43%): develops 4–6 months after delivery. Symptoms may be mild and non-specific. There may be an ↑ risk of post-partum depression. Treat with levothyroxine if TSH >10 or TSH 4–10 and symptomatic. However, need to recheck TFTs every 6–8 weeks and wean off thyroxine if appropriate.
  - Hyperthyroidism followed by hypothyroidism (25%): spontaneous recovery in 80% within 6–12 months of delivery.
- Prognosis:
  - Recurrence in future pregnancies in 25% of women.
  - Permanent hypothyroidism develops in up to 30% of women within 10 years.
  - If treatment is withdrawn, then annual TSH measurements are essential.

Clinical practice point

- Assess all women with possible post-partum depression for thyroid dysfunction.

Clinical practice point

- All women with post-partum thyroiditis should have annual TFTs, looking for hypothyroidism.

Clinical practice point

- Consider checking thyroid function in early pregnancy and post-partum in all those at ↑ risk of thyroid dysfunction, e.g. underlying DM, autoimmune disorders, previous treatment with alemtuzumab and checkpoint inhibitors.

Fetal thyroid disease due to maternal thyroid disorders

Fetal hyperthyroidism

- Women with Graves' disease treated with RAI or surgery may still have high antibody levels.
- All women with previous or current Graves' disease should have TRAbs measured in 1st trimester to identify at-risk pregnancies.
- Occurs after week 25 of gestation due to transplacental transfer of TRAbs that stimulate the fetal thyroid.
- Fetal complications: IUGR, fetal goitre, tachycardia, cardiac failure.
- Management: give the mother ATDs. Monitor fetal heart rate (aim <140bpm), growth, and goitre size.

Neonatal thyrotoxicosis

- Develops in 1% of infants born to thyrotoxic mothers, usually due to transplacental passage of stimulating TRAbs.
- Transient, usually subsides by 6 months.
- Symptoms develop from 2 days postnatally.
- Up to 30% mortality if untreated.
- Associated with high levels of maternal TRAbs in 2nd and 3rd trimesters.
- Treat with ATDs and β-blockers.

Fetal hypothyroidism

- Very rare occurrence following treatment of mother with high doses of ATDs (typically >30mg carbimazole, with maternal FT_4 suppression), particularly in the latter half of pregnancy.
- Fetal complications: fetal bradycardia, fetal goitre, abnormal skeletal and neurological development.
- Diagnosis: hypothyroidism can be confirmed with fetal cord blood from cordocentesis.
- Management: cases are monitored by the paediatric team and treated with levothyroxine if hypothyroidism is persistent.

Thyroid cancer in pregnancy

(See ➔ Thyroid cancer and pregnancy, p. 114.)

Further reading

Alexander EK, et al. (2017). 2017 guidelines for the American Thyroid Association for the diagnosis and management of thyroid disease during pregnancy and the postpartum. *Thyroid* **27**, 315–89.

Cotzias C, et al. (2008). A study to establish gestation-specific reference intervals for thyroid function tests in normal singleton pregnancy. *Eur J Obstet Gynecol Reprod Biol* **137**, 61–6.

Dhillon-Smith RK, et al. (2019). Levothyroxine in women with thyroid peroxidase antibodies before conception. *N Engl J Med* **380**, 1316–25.

Haddow JE, et al. (1999). Maternal thyroid deficiency during pregnancy and subsequent neuro-psychological development of the child. *N Engl J Med* **341**, 549–55.

Iijima S (2019). Current knowledge about the in utero and peripartum management of fetal goitre associated with maternal Graves' disease. *Eur J Obstet Gynecol Reprod Biol X* **3**, 100027.

Korevaar TIM, et al. (2017). Thyroid disease in pregnancy: new insights in diagnosis and clinical management. *Nat Rev Endocrinol* **13**, 610–22.

Lazarus JH, et al. (2012). Antenatal thyroid screening and childhood cognitive function. *N Engl J Med* **366**, 493–501.

Napier C, Pearce SHS (2015). Rethinking antithyroid drugs in pregnancy. *Clin Endocrinol (Oxf)* **82**, 475–7.

Royal College of Obstetricians and Gynaecologists (2016). *The management of nausea and vomiting of pregnancy and hyperemesis gravidarum*. Green-top guideline no. 69. ℅ https://www.rcog.org.uk/globalassets/documents/guidelines/green-top-guidelines/gtg69-hyperemesis.pdf

Seo GH, et al. (2018). Antithyroid drugs and congenital malformation: a nationwide Korean cohort study. *Ann Intern Med* **168**, 405–13.

Wiles K (2019). Management for women with subclinical hypothyroidism in pregnancy. *Drug Ther Bull* **57**, 22–6.

Xing J, et al. (2016). Trimester- and assay-specific thyroid reference intervals for pregnant women in China. *Int J Endocrinol* **2016**, 3754213.

Zhang D, et al. (2019). Trimester-specific reference ranges for thyroid hormones in pregnant women. *Medicine* **98**, e14245.

Calcium metabolism in pregnancy

- There are ↑ calcium requirements in pregnancy; 25–30g is transferred to the baby.
- The placenta and mammary glands produce PTHrP, causing ↑ intestinal absorption and renal resorption of calcium, plus ↑ bone resorption, maintaining serum calcium despite transfer to fetus and to baby through breast milk.

Primary hyperparathyroidism in pregnancy

Incidence

- Rare—8 cases in 100,000 in women of childbearing age. Maternal hypercalcaemia may improve due to fetal transfer of calcium.

Diagnosis

- Raised PTH in the presence of raised serum and urinary calcium.
- US to localize the adenoma; sestamibi/SPECT-CT not recommended.
- Women of childbearing age are younger than those typically with 1° hyperparathyroidism (PHPT), so perform genetic screen for MEN1 and 2, plus familial PHPT (see ⊃ Tumour surveillance in MEN type 1, p. 681).

Symptoms

- Recurrent miscarriage, severe headache, gestational hypertension, ureteric calculi, and hyperemesis—but often incidental biochemical finding.

Maternal complications

- Hyperemesis, nephrolithiasis, peptic ulcers, pancreatitis, hypertension, pre-eclampsia, recurrent miscarriage.

Fetal complications

- IUGR, preterm delivery, intrauterine and neonatal death due to neonatal hypocalcaemia (normally present at days 5–14 with poor feeding, tetany, and convulsions).

Management

- Refer for multidisciplinary management in a specialist centre as recommended by NICE guideline on management of PHPT in pregnancy.
- Aim to keep calcium <2.8mmol/L with PO or IV hydration.
- If this cannot be maintained, consider surgery in 2nd trimester.
- Ensure vitamin D replete.
- Cinacalcet has been used in some cases in 2nd and 3rd trimesters.
- Bisphosphonates should not be given, as they cross the placenta to affect fetal skeletal development.

Hypoparathyroidism

- Incidence and cause: very rare. Mostly subsequent to neck surgery.
- Maternal and fetal outcomes: very little evidence about conception or pregnancy outcomes, but may cause miscarriage, fetal hypocalcaemia, and neonatal rickets.
- Management: treat with calcium, calcitriol, and vitamin D supplements. Aim to keep calcium within the lower reference range, checking calcium levels every 3–4 weeks throughout pregnancy, as supplement requirements may increase or decrease in pregnancy. Avoid treatment with thiazide diuretics or synthetic PTH.

Pregnancy- and lactation-associated osteoporosis

- Pregnancy- and lactation-associated osteoporosis is rare.
- Typically presents as vertebral fractures in the 3rd trimester or post-partum—present with back pain.
- Underlying mechanism is not fully understood.
- Treat with bisphosphonates after pregnancy.

Further reading

DiMarco AN, et al. (2019). Seventeen cases of primary hyperparathyroidism in pregnancy: a call for management guidelines. *J Endocr Soc* **3**, 1009–21.

Hardcastle SA, et al. (2019). Pregnancy-associated osteoporosis: a UK series and literature review. *Osteoporos Int* **30**, 939–48.

Khan AA, et al. (2019). Hypoparathyroidism in pregnancy: review and evidence-based recommendations for management. *Eur J Endocrinol* **1800**, R37–44.

Leere JS, Vestergaard P (2019). Calcium metabolic disorders in pregnancy: primary hyperparathyroidism, pregnancy induced osteoporosis and vitamin D deficiency in pregnancy. *Endocrinol Metab Clin North Am* **48**, 643–55.

National Institute for Health and Care Excellence (2019). *Hyperparathyroidism (primary): diagnosis, assessment and initial management.* NICE guideline [NG132]. https://www.nice.org.uk/guidance/ng132

The pituitary in pregnancy

Normal anatomical changes during pregnancy

- *Size:* the anterior pituitary increases by up to 70% during pregnancy. Greatest enlargement is during the first 3 days post-partum. May take 1 year to shrink to near pre-pregnancy size in non-lactating women.
- *MRI:* enlarged anterior pituitary gland, but stalk is midline, so any deviation may suggest an adenoma. The posterior pituitary may not be seen in late pregnancy.
- *PRL:* marked lactotroph hyperplasia during pregnancy. Serum PRL increases dramatically and remains high in breastfeeding; it falls to pre-pregnancy levels ~2 weeks post-partum in the non-lactating woman.
- *Gonadotrophin axis:* −ve feedback from the high levels of oestrogen, progesterone, and PRL cause undetectable levels of LH and FSH during pregnancy. GnRH response is blunted. Marked reduction in size and number of gonadotrophs.
- *Thyroid axis:* TSH is suppressed in early pregnancy due to ↑ hCG levels but returns to normal during 2nd and 3rd trimesters. No change in size or shape of TSH-secreting cells. Total thyroid hormones increase in pregnancy, but free hormone levels often fall in later pregnancy due to ↑ TBG.
- *GH axis:* placental GH production causes reduced pituitary GH secretion, and blunted GH response to hypoglycaemia. IGF-1 levels are normal/high in pregnancy. No change in GH-secreting cells.
- *Cortisol axis:* corticotroph number is stable. CRH and ACTH are both produced by the placenta, so levels rise progressively through pregnancy. This, plus oestrogen-induced CBG, leads to progressive increases in maternal cortisol levels in pregnancy. Urinary cortisol levels also increase. Diurnal variation is generally preserved. There is incomplete suppression of cortisol, following dexamethasone suppression test, and an exaggerated response of cortisol to CRH stimulation in normal pregnancy. Placental 11β-hydroxysteroid dehydrogenase inactivates most GCs, protecting the fetus from hypercortisolism.
- *Posterior pituitary:* placental production of vasopressinase plus changes in the osmostat lower serum osmolality by about 10mOsm/kg, with serum sodium usually at the lower end of the normal range in pregnancy. Placental vasopressinase can unmask or worsen DI in pregnancy.

Prolactinoma in pregnancy

Pre-pregnancy

- Prolactinomas reduce fertility—probably responsible for 7–20% of ♀ infertility. Cabergoline restores fertility more effectively than bromocriptine.

In pregnancy

- Maternal risks: ↑ tumour size with potential for visual field defects, headaches, and DI.
- Risk of significant tumour enlargement:
  - Microadenoma <1%.
  - Macroadenoma 15–20%.
  - Macroadenoma treated with surgery and/or radiotherapy before pregnancy 4–7%.
- Fetal risk: none known.

Treatment in pregnancy

- In women with microadenomas, stop dopamine agonists once pregnant; assess visual fields to confrontation each trimester. There is 40–60% remission of prolactinoma after pregnancy.
- In women with macroadenomas, can often stop dopamine agonists and monitor visual fields each trimester; however, in women with invasive prolactinomas or prolactinomas abutting the chiasm, continuing dopamine agonists in pregnancy may be advised. In these women, if stable, can continue dopamine agonists until ~36 weeks' pregnancy, and then consider stopping to allow breastfeeding, with appropriate clinical monitoring.
- In women with visual field defects and/or new headache, arrange an urgent MRI scan and formal visual fields. In those with symptomatic growth of prolactinomas, cabergoline or bromocriptine is advised.
- In rare cases, transsphenoidal pituitary surgery in the 2nd trimester may be needed.
- MRI scan should be performed in the post-partum period to look for tumour growth, particularly in macroadenomas.

Dopamine agonists in pregnancy

Bromocriptine

- Well established to be safe in pregnancy, with no increase in congenital abnormalities or problems with psychological development.
- However, when bromocriptine was used to suppress lactation, there were ↑ numbers of strokes and ischaemic cardiac events. It is therefore no longer recommended for suppression of lactation and should be used with care in women with hypertensive disorders and pre-eclampsia in pregnancy.

Cabergoline
- Not licensed for use in pregnancy, but increasing evidence for safety in pregnancy, with no ↑ risk of fetal loss or congenital abnormalities, and is often better tolerated than bromocriptine.
- There is a risk of cardiac valve abnormalities in Parkinson's patients who take cabergoline at higher doses for sustained periods; this has *not* been replicated in the pregnant population, nor in the fetus. However, echocardiography is currently recommended prior to treatment and during treatment, with the frequency depending on the dose (see ➔ Box 2.15).
- In women with macroadenomas well managed on cabergoline, it is reasonable to continue treatment in pregnancy, but this indication is unlicensed.

Quinagolide
- Not recommended, as associated with ↑ risk of congenital abnormalities.

Breastfeeding and prolactinomas
- There are no contraindications to women with prolactinomas breastfeeding; however, those on dopamine agonists will be unable to breastfeed.

Further reading
Molitch M (2015). Endocrinology in pregnancy: management of the pregnant patient with a prolactinoma. *Eur J Endocrinol* **172**, R205–13.

Cushing's syndrome

- Pregnancy is rare in women with untreated Cushing's syndrome as they have oligo- or amenorrhoea.
- *Causes:* adrenal disease commoner than pituitary in pregnancy.
- *Maternal complications:* hypertension, GDM, pre-eclampsia, heart failure, wound infections, psychiatric disorders.
- *Fetal complications:* intrauterine death (23%), IUGR, neonatal hypocortisolism, and respiratory distress.
- *Clinical diagnosis:* can be difficult as many symptoms overlap those of pregnancy (weight gain, fatigue, emotional lability, striae, acne, hypertension, glucose intolerance). Purple striae, proximal myopathy, and hypokalaemia should increase clinical suspicion.
- *Biochemical diagnosis is difficult:* plasma and urinary cortisol both rise during pregnancy, with urinary cortisol being >3× upper limit of normal by term. There are no internationally agreed pregnancy-specific values for dynamic tests for Cushing's (low- or high-dose dexamethasone suppression tests), and many normal women fail to suppress cortisol production following a low-dose dexamethasone suppression test. Late-night cortisol levels can be helpful, as diurnal variation is preserved in pregnant women; elevated levels at midnight can suggest Cushing's syndrome.
- *Management:*
  - Treatment of comorbidities (hypertension, DM) is essential.
  - Surgery is the 1st-choice treatment and is safest in the 2nd trimester. Reduces perinatal mortality and maternal morbidity.
  - There is limited experience of drugs; metyrapone most commonly used, and doses <2g/day are generally well tolerated, although its use may be associated with pre-eclampsia and fetal hypoadrenalisim. Cabergoline can be used in pituitary-dependent Cushing's.
  - Vaginal delivery may be preferred to minimize the risk of poor wound healing.

Acromegaly

- Fertility may be reduced in acromegaly due to hyperprolactinaemia and 2° hypogonadism. Most reported cases conceive after treatment, though women have conceived with active acromegaly.
- In an acromegalic pregnancy, there is an increase in pituitary GH, as well as the normal rise in placental GH.
- *Maternal complications:* exacerbation of hypertension (45%), heart disease, hyperglycaemia (32%)—ensure the woman is screened for hypertension in pregnancy and GDM.
- *Diagnosis:* difficult due to secretion of placenta GH which is not distinguished from pituitary GH in many assays; also IGF-1 increases in normal pregnancy.
- *Management:*
  - Consider stopping medication and manage expectantly, unless the tumour bulk causes headache and/or visual disturbance.
  - Severe headache may be treated with bromocriptine or SC octreotide.
  - Visual fields should be checked every trimester, but tumour enlargement is relatively rare (<10%).
  - SSAs cross the placenta and may cause fetal growth restriction, so should be used with care.
  - Cabergoline or bromocriptine can be used, and octreotide has been used to stabilize a large, sight-threatening adenoma.
  - Surgery, ideally in the 2nd trimester, is possible if the tumour causes significant problems.
  - Treatment may be deferred until after delivery in the majority of patients.
  - SSAs cross in breast milk.

Further reading

Jallad RS, et al. (2018). Outcome of pregnancies in a large cohort of women with acromegaly. *Clin Endocrinol (Oxf)* **88**, 896–907.

Non-functioning pituitary adenomas

- These tumours are the 2nd commonest pituitary tumours but are rarely reported in pregnancy.
- *Maternal complications:* symptomatic tumour expansion occurs in up to 25%, presenting with headache and visual disturbance.
- *Fetal complications:* nil noted.
- *Management:* visual fields each trimester; bromocriptine can be used to reduce the size of lactotrophs if visual field defects occur.

Hypopituitarism in pregnancy

- *Causes:* pre-existing hypopituitarism due to pituitary surgery or pituitary radiotherapy, lymphocytic hypophysitis, Sheehan's syndrome.
- *Symptoms:*
  - Often associated with infertility that requires gonadotrophin stimulation/ovulation induction.
  - During pregnancy, look for signs of adrenal crisis (hypotension, weight loss, fatigue, hyponatraemia, collapse).
  - SST can be used in pregnancy with trimester-specific ranges (see ➔ Addison's disease in pregnancy, p. 492).
  - Post-partum, often presents as agalactia, fatigue, weight loss, and loss of axillary and pubic hair, as well as signs of hypoadrenalism (collapse, hyponatraemia, hypotension) and signs of hypothyroidism.
- *Management:*
  - *Hydrocortisone:* dose may need to be ↑ in the 3rd trimester, as the increase in CBG will reduce the bioavailability of hydrocortisone; careful clinical assessment is needed. Extra hydrocortisone dosing is required in labour (see ➔ Box 3.5, p. 305).
  - *Thyroxine:* requirements may increase, particularly in the 1st trimester. Monitor FT_4 each trimester, and increase T_4 dose accordingly (see ➔ The maternal thyroid, p. 470).
  - *GH replacement:* may be required to restore fertility. GH replacement is usually stopped by 20 weeks' gestation, but available data suggest no adverse effect on pregnancy outcomes or fetal abnormalities.

Lymphocytic hypophysitis

(See also ➔ Lymphocytic hypophysitis, pp. 216–17.)
- Rare disorder caused by pituitary infiltration with T- and B-lymphocytes.
- Traditionally associated with late pregnancy or the 1st year post-partum.
- Associated with other autoimmune diseases, particularly Hashimoto's thyroiditis, Graves' disease, Addison's, and T1DM.
- *Symptoms:* mass effect; hypopituitarism; 20% have symptoms of DI.
- *Diagnosis:* MRI shows pituitary enlargement, often with stalk thickening. DI is associated with loss of the posterior pituitary bright spot.
- All pituitary hormones must be checked, being aware of differences in reference ranges in pregnancy. Axes can be variably affected (gonadotrophins and GH levels are usually preserved; PRL levels may be mildly elevated in a third, and low in a third).
- *Management:* pituitary hormone replacement as required—may vary over time.
- Monitor visual fields.
- Surgical decompression if pressure symptoms persist.

Sheehan's syndrome

- Post-partum pituitary infarction/haemorrhage, resulting in hypopituitarism. Because the pituitary is enlarged in pregnancy, a small change in BP can cause a pituitary infarction.
- Increasingly uncommon in developed countries with improvements in obstetric care and management of post-partum haemorrhage.
- *Risk factors:* post-partum haemorrhage, sickle cell disease, T1DM.
- *Symptoms:* symptoms of hypopituitarism—often missed as fatigue/weight loss/amenorrhoea, etc. are seen as normal in the post-partum period; DI is rare.
- *Management:* immediate steroid replacement; subsequently, all deficient pituitary hormones may need replacement.

Diabetes insipidus in pregnancy

- Seen in 4:100,000 pregnancies.
- Placental vasopressinase causes a reduction of plasma osmolality by 10mOsm/kg in normal pregnancy. Plasma sodium is also usually at the lower end of normal.
- *Causes:* central DI, nephrogenic DI, transient DI of pregnancy.
- Transient DI of pregnancy can occur due to placental vasopressinase. Typically presents in the late 2nd/3rd trimester as intense polydipsia and polyuria. This may be associated with hepatic impairment in pre-eclampsia, acute fatty liver of pregnancy, and haemolysis, elevated liver enzymes, and low platelet (HELLP) syndrome.
- *Diagnosis:* water deprivation tests must be used with caution in pregnancy. 1° polydipsia must be excluded through the history. Copeptin concentration in pregnancy has not been validated.
- *Management:* desmopressin should be used, as not degraded by placental vasopressinase. Regular monitoring required, as doses may need to increase during pregnancy. The dose should be reduced in the immediate post-partum period, particularly in transient DI of pregnancy, as vasopressinase levels drop dramatically at delivery. Care must be taken during labour to maintain adequate fluid balance in women with DI without causing hyponatraemia from excessive desmopressin use.

Further reading

Ananthakrishnan S (2016). Diabetes insipidus during pregnancy. *Best Pract Res Clin Endocrinol Metab* **30**, 305–15.

Bernard N, et al. (2015). Severe adverse effects of bromocriptine in lactation inhibition: a pharmacovigilance survey. *BJOG* **122**, 1244–51.

Caimari F, et al. (2017). Cushing's syndrome and pregnancy outcomes: a systematic review of cases. *Endocrine* **55**, 555–63.

Chanson P (2019). Other pituitary conditions and pregnancy. *Endocrinol Metab Clin North Am* **48**, 583–603.

Chanson P, et al. (2019). An update on clinical care for pregnant women with acromegaly. *Exp Rev Endocrinol Metab* **14**, 85–96.

Eschler DC, et al. (2015). Management of adrenal tumours in pregnancy. *Endocrinol Metab Clin North Am* **44**, 381–97.

Higham CE, et al. (2016). Hypopituitarism. *Lancet* **388**, 2403–15.

Huang W, Molitch ME (2019). Pituitary tumours in pregnancy. *Endocrinol Metab Clin North Am* **48**, 569–81.

Jallard RS, et al. (2018). Outcome of pregnancies in a large cohort of women with acromegaly. *Clin Endocrinol (Oxf)* **88**, 896–907.

Karaca Z, et al. (2010). Pregnancy and pituitary disorders. *Eur J Endocrinol* **162**, 453–75.

Lambert K, et al. (2017). Macroprolactinomas and non-functioning pituitary adenomas: pregnancy outcomes. *Obstet Gynecol* **129**, 185–94.

Machado MC, et al. (2018). Pregnancy in patients with Cushing's syndrome. *Endocrinol Metab Clin North Am* **47**, 441–9.

Melmed S, et al. (2011). Diagnosis and treatment of hyperprolactinaemia: an Endocrine Society clinical practice guideline. *J Clin Endocrinol Metab* **96**, 273–88.

Vila G, et al. (2015). Pregnancy outcomes in women with growth hormone deficiency. *Fertil Steril* **104**, 1210–17.

Adrenal disorders

Changes in adrenal physiology

- *Maternal adrenal gland:* cortisol and MC production increases during pregnancy. The progesterone produced by the placenta counteracts the increase in aldosterone, preventing hypertension and hypokalaemia.
- *Placenta:* placental 11β-HSD inactivates most maternal GCs. Maternal androgens are converted to oestrogens by placental aromatase, thus protecting ♀ fetus from virilization.
- Maternal catecholamines are broken down by placental catechol-*O*-methyltransferase and monoamine oxidase activity.
- *Fetal adrenal gland:* produces DHEAS and cortisol in significant amounts; fetal DHEAS is converted by the placenta to oestradiol.

Addison's disease in pregnancy

- *Maternal complications:* Addisonian crises, particularly at delivery.
- *Fetal complications:* intrauterine growth retardation in women with chronic adrenal insufficiency which is poorly managed.
- *Diagnosis:* if required, an SST can be performed. However, due to the increase in cortisol through pregnancy, trimester-specific cut-offs for cortisol must be used in an SST (see Table 5.2).
- *Management:* women need to be clinically assessed for evidence of hypocortisolaemia (fatigue, hypotension, salt craving, vomiting, hyperpigmentation). These can be hard to distinguish from normal pregnancy. If present, increase steroid/MC replacement until delivery.
- *Hydrocortisone:* dose may need to be ↑ by 20–40% in the 3rd trimester, as the increase in CBG will reduce the bioavailability of hydrocortisone; careful clinical assessment is needed. Extra hydrocortisone dosing is required in labour (see ➋ Box 3.5, p. 305).
- If ↑ during pregnancy, hydrocortisone dose should return to normal 2 days post-partum.
- No routine increase in hydrocortisone is required in breastfeeding.
- All pregnant women must be aware of the importance of increasing GC dose when unwell and to cover the stress of labour (sick day rules).

Table 5.2 Trimester-specific minimal cortisol levels to exclude adrenal insufficiency

| | Cortisol level (nmol/L) after short Synacthen® test | |
	0min	30min
1st trimester	300	700
2nd trimester	450	800
3rd trimester	600	900
Non-pregnant state	400	450

Clinical practice point

Management of adrenal insufficiency in labour

- *For women having a vaginal birth:* continue regular oral steroids. When in established 1st stage of labour, start hydrocortisone 50mg IM, and further 50mg every 6h until the baby is born.
- *For women having a Caesarean section:* continue regular oral steroids and give IV hydrocortisone when starting anaesthesia; 50mg should be given if the woman has already had hydrocortisone in labour, and 100mg if she has not. Give further 50mg IM hydrocortisone 6h after the baby is born.

Congenital adrenal hyperplasia

(See ➡ Management of pregnancy in CAH, p. 359.)

- Fertility is reduced, particularly women with the salt wasting form of CAH, due to anovulation 2° to hyperandrogenaemia; adverse effects on the endometrium due to ↑ progestogen levels; abnormal vaginal anatomy; sexual dysfunction.
- However, in those seeking pregnancy and who had spontaneous puberty, pregnancy rates can be normal in adequately treated classic CAH.
- Women with non-classic 21-hydroxylase deficiency often conceive spontaneously without steroid replacement.
- *Preconception:* optimize fertility with adequate androgen suppression; ensure women receive genetic counselling about risk of baby having CAH.
- *Maternal complications:* ↑ risk of miscarriage; ↑ rate of Caesarean section due to cephalopelvic disproportion.
- *Fetal complications:* virilization of ♀ fetus if mother on inadequate steroid replacement.
- *Management of mother with CAH:*
  - Adequate androgen suppression with prednisolone/ hydrocortisone—typically avoid dexamethasone as it crosses the placenta; however, dexamethasone is sometimes used to avoid virilization of a ♀ fetus (see ➡ Management of pregnancy in CAH, p. 359). Monitor serum testosterone and electrolytes every 6–8 weeks, and increase corticosteroids if levels rise.
  - In those on fludrocortisone, ↑ doses may be needed.
  - Ensure women know sick day rules, and follow as for the non-pregnant state.
  - Ensure adequate steroid cover during labour.
- *Management of the fetus:*
  - If partner is a heterozygote for CAH, then the fetus has a 50% risk of CAH.
  - Prenatal treatment with dexamethasone will then be necessary to avoid virilization of a ♀ fetus. However, this needs to be given from 7 weeks' gestation to avoid virilization, i.e. before it is known whether the fetus is ♂ or ♀—this leads to some ethical concerns about early treatment and long-term effects, including impaired neurological and behavioural development.

Phaeochromocytoma

- Rare, but potentially lethal in pregnancy—maternal and fetal mortality up to 8% and 17%, respectively, in undiagnosed cases. Mortality higher if diagnosis made during pregnancy rather than pre-pregnancy.
- Offer high-risk women screening preconception (personal or family history of phaeochromocytoma, MEN2, VHL, SDH mutations).
- *Maternal complications:* hypertensive crisis, stroke, pulmonary oedema, arrhythmia, MI, aortic dissection, heart failure, death.
- *Fetal complications:* placental vasoconstriction may cause intrauterine death, IUGR, and fetal hypoxia.
- *Symptoms:* hypertension, palpitations, sweating, headache, anxiety, dyspnoea, vomiting, hyperglycaemia.
- May present for the 1st time in pregnancy due to ↑ intra-abdominal pressure, mechanical effects of a gravid uterus, uterine contractions, haemorrhage into tumour, stress of labour, etc.
- Symptoms may be assumed to be due to pre-eclampsia, but must suspect in women with early hypertension, i.e. in 2nd/early 3rd trimester, especially if labile or paroxysmal, without proteinuria or other signs of pre-eclampsia.
- *Diagnosis:*
  - Plasma catecholamines (levels fall in normal pregnancy) or 24h urinary catecholamines (normal ranges unaltered in pregnancy). Ensure not taking labetalol or methyldopa, as may cause false +ve results.
  - MRI or US to localize tumour. Avoid CT scans and MIBG scintigraphy.
  - Consider later genetic testing if phaeochromocytoma diagnosed in pregnancy—up to 30% of pregnant women with phaeochromocytomas are found to have a genetic predisposition.

Management of phaeochromocytomas in pregnancy

Medications

- α-*blockade with phenoxybenzamine:* phenoxybenzamine does cross the placenta and may cause transient hypotension and respiratory depression in the neonate. Caution to maintain uterine perfusion—start at 10mg 12-hourly (ensuring adequate hydration), and increase gradually while monitoring BP response. Ideally start 10–14 days prior to surgery. PO prazosin or doxazosin, and IV phentolamine can also be used.
- β-*blockade:* propranolol. Only after adequate α-blockade. Give in a dose of 40mg 8-hourly.
- *Drugs to avoid:* steroids, opioids, antiemetics such as metoclopramide, and some anaesthetics—as can cause catecholamine release and hypertensive crisis. Also avoid methyldopa as may worsen hypertension in phaeochromocytoma.
- *Surgery:* if diagnosed in early pregnancy, aim for surgical removal in 2nd trimester. After 24 weeks' gestation, defer until after delivery. Ensure adequate α-blockade and restoration of intravascular volume prior to surgery.

- *Delivery:* historically, the preferred method of delivery was elective Caesarean section, but increasingly, vaginal deliveries with adequate epidural analgesia are chosen within an MDT setting.
- Magnesium sulfate often given as an adjunct to anaesthetic during delivery.

Breastfeeding
- Limited data about use of phenoxybenzamine in lactation; therefore, breastfeeding is usually avoided.

Further reading

Bancos I, et al. (2021). Maternal and fetal outcomes in phaeochromocytoma and pregnancy: a multicentre retrospective cohort study and systematic review of literature. *Lancet Diabetes Endocrinol* **9**, 13–21.

van der Weerd K, et al. (2017). Endocrinology in pregnancy: Pheochromocytoma in pregnancy: case series and review of literature. *Eur J Endocrinol* **177**, R49–58.

Primary aldosteronism

- *Incidence:* rare; <50 cases of pregnancy with Conn's reported.
- *Causes:* adrenal adenoma, idiopathic bilateral adrenal hyperplasia, GC remedial hyperaldosteronism.
- *Symptoms:* hypertension, hypokalaemia.
- *Maternal complications:* pre-eclampsia, placental abruption, pulmonary oedema, renal failure.
- *Fetal complications:* IUGR, preterm delivery, intrauterine and neonatal death.
- *Diagnosis:*
  - Suppressed renin and raised aldosterone (aldosterone usually raised in pregnancy, so ensure renin suppressed).
  - Do not do captopril or saline suppression tests.
  - MRI and US can localize tumour.
- *Management:*
  - Look for end-organ damage: echocardiography, check urinary protein, retinal screening.
  - Treat as hypertension in pregnancy.
  - May need potassium supplements.
  - Amiloride and eplerenone can also be used; avoid spironolactone, as associated with ambiguous sexual genitalia in ♂ rats.
  - Surgical resection rarely needed, but if necessary, perform in 2nd trimester. Some reports of exacerbation of hypertension post-partum.
  - Breastfeeding: spironolactone can be used; no evidence of safety of eplerenone or amiloride.

Further reading

Biggar MA, Lennard TW (2013). Systematic review of phaeochromocytoma in pregnancy. *Br J Surg* **100**, 182–90.

Casteras A, et al. (2009). Reassessing fecundity in women with classical congenital adrenal hyperplasia (CAH): normal pregnancy rate but reduced fertility rate. *Clin Endocrinol (Oxf)* **70**, 833–7.

Dorr HG, et al. (2018). Miscarriages in families with an offspring that have classic congenital adrenal hyperplasia and 21-hydroxylase deficiency. *BMC Pregnancy Childbirth* **18**, 456.

Gunganah K, et al. (2015). Eplerenone use in primary aldosteronism during pregnancy. *Clin Case Rep* **4**, 81–2.

Landau E, Amar L (2016). Primary aldosteronism and pregnancy. *Ann Endocrinol (Paris)* **77**, 148–60.

Lebbe M, Arlt W (2013). What is the best diagnostic and therapeutic management strategy for an Addison patient during pregnancy? *Clin Endocrinol (Oxf)* **78**, 497502.

Livadas S, Bothou C (2019). Management of the female with non-classical congenital adrenal hyperplasia (NCCAH): a patient-oriented approach. *Front Endocrinol (Lausanne)* **10**, 366.

Morton A (2015). Primary aldosteronism and pregnancy. *Pregnancy Hypertens* **5**, 259–62.

National Institute of Health and Care Excellence (2019). *Intrapartum care for women with existing medical conditions or obstetric complications and their babies.* NICE Guideline [NG121]. ℘ https://www.nice.org.uk/guidance/ng121

Natrajan PG, et al. (1982). Plasma noradrenaline and adrenaline levels in normal pregnancy and in pregnancy-induced hypertension. *BJOG* **89**, 1041–5.

Quartermaine G, et al. (2018). Hormone-secreting adrenal tumours cause severe hypertension and high rates of poor pregnancy outcome: a UK Obstetric Surveillance System study with case control comparisons. *BJOG* **125**, 719–27.

Rainey WE, *et al.* (2004). Fetal and maternal adrenals in human pregnancy. *Obstet Gynecol Clin North Am* **31**, 817–35.

Riester A, Reincke E (2015). Progress in primary aldosteronism: mineralocorticoid receptor antagonists and management of primary aldosteronism in pregnancy. *Eur J Endocrinol* **172**, R23–30.

Speiser PW, *et al.* (2018). Congenital adrenal hyperplasia due to steroid 21-hydroxylase deficiency: an Endocrine Society clinical practice guideline. *J Clin Endocrinol Metab* **103**, 1–46.

Tingi E, *et al.* (2016). Recurrence of phaeochromocytoma in pregnancy in a patient with multiple endocrine neoplasia 2A: a case report and review of literature. *Gynecol Endocrinol* **32**, 875–80.

van der Weerd K, *et al.* (2017). Endocrinology in pregnancy: pheochromocytoma in pregnancy: case series and review of literature. *Eur J Endocrinol* **177**, R49–58.

Van't Westeinde A, *et al.* (2020). First-trimester prenatal dexamethasone treatment is associated with alterations in brain structure at adult age. *J Clin Endocrinol Metab* **105**, dgaa340.

Calcium and bone metabolism

Neil Gittoes and Richard Eastell

Calcium and bone physiology

Bone turnover

In order to ensure that bone can undertake its mechanical and metabolic functions, it is in a constant state of turnover (see Fig. 6.1).

- *Osteoclasts*—derived from cells of the monocyte–macrophage line; resorb bone under control of osteoblasts, with key regulation through the RANK/RANKL pathway.
- *Osteoblasts*—derived from mesenchymal stem cells that lay down bone.
- *Osteocytes*—buried osteoblasts; sense mechanical strain in bone.

Bone mass during life

(See Fig. 6.2.)

Bone is laid down rapidly during skeletal growth at puberty under the influence of GH. Following this, there is a period of stabilization of bone mass in early adult life. After the age of ~40, there is a gradual loss of bone in both sexes. This occurs at a rate of ~0.5% annually. However, in ♀ after the menopause, there is a period of rapid bone loss. The accelerated loss is maximal in the first 2–5 years after the cessation of ovarian function and then gradually declines until a gradual rate of loss is once again established. The excess bone loss associated with the menopause is of the order of 10% of skeletal mass. This menopause-associated loss, coupled with higher peak bone mass acquisition in ♂, largely explains why osteoporosis and its associated fractures are commoner in ♀.

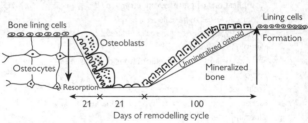

Fig. 6.1 Bone turnover during remodelling cycle.

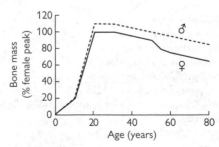

Fig. 6.2 Bone mass across life.

Roles of calcium

- Skeletal strength.
- Neuromuscular conduction.
- Stimulus–secretion coupling.
- Ca concentration is tightly regulated (see Fig. 6.3 for a schema of relationships.)

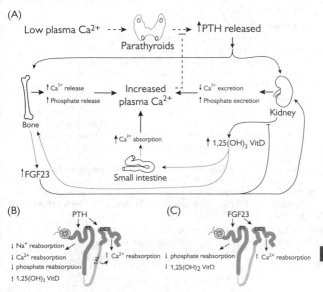

Fig. 6.3 Hormonal regulation of renal function.

Calcium in the circulation

Circulating Ca exists in several forms (see Fig. 6.4); only a proportion of total Ca has biological action:

- Ionized—biologically active.
- Complexed to citrate, PO_4, etc.—biologically active.
- Bound to protein, mainly albumin—inactive.

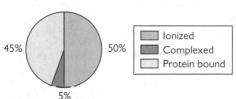

Fig. 6.4 Forms of circulating calcium.

Investigation of bone

Bone turnover markers

May be useful in:
- Assessing overall risk of osteoporotic fracture and accelerated bone loss.
- Identifying response to treatments for osteoporosis, and hence poor adherence to therapy.

Resorption markers

- *Collagen crosslinks*. These are products of collagen degradation. The small fragments of the ends of the collagen molecule are known as *telopeptides* (NTX and CTX), and the measurement of these in urine and blood (respectively) are the preferred biochemical measure of bone resorption.

Formation markers

- *Total ALP* is not specific to bone and is also found in the liver, intestine, and placenta. It is also insensitive to small changes in bone turnover and is only of general use in monitoring the activity of Paget's disease.
- *Bone-specific ALP* is a more specific and reliable measure of bone formation.
- *Osteocalcin* is a component of bone matrix, and the serum level of osteocalcin reflects osteoblast activity; it is the most specific marker.
- *P1NP* is a procollagen fragment released from the N terminal as type I collagen is laid down. When measured in serum, it is the most sensitive marker of bone formation.

Bone turnover markers are recommended by the IOF for monitoring osteoporosis treatment with oral bisphosphonates.

Bone imaging

Skeletal radiology

- Useful for:
  - Diagnosis of fracture.
  - Diagnosis of specific diseases (e.g. Paget's disease and osteomalacia). Osteomalacia is characterized by pseudofractures (Looser's zones) which appear like fractures, but without any displacement of the bone contour.
  - Diagnosis of bone metastases; these may appear lytic (common in breast cancer) or sclerotic (common in prostate cancer).
  - Identification of bone dysplasia.
- Not useful for assessing bone density.

Isotope bone scanning

Bone-seeking isotopes, particularly ^{99m}technetium-labelled bisphosphonates, are concentrated in areas of localized ↑ bone cell activity. Isotope bone scans are useful for identifying localized areas of bone disease such as fracture, metastases, or Paget's disease. Lesions can be better identified by combining the scan with CT in SPECT.

However, isotope uptake is not selective, and so ↑ activity on a scan does not indicate the nature of the underlying bone disease. Hence, subsequent radiology of affected regions is needed to establish the diagnosis.

Isotope bone scans are particularly useful in Paget's disease to establish the extent and sites of skeletal involvement and the underlying disease activity.

CT is very helpful in bone imaging and is useful in identifying focal lesions such as tumour and fibrous dysplasia and can be used to guide the biopsy needle. MRI does not usually produce a +ve signal from bone, but the bone marrow changes are very helpful; for example, after a vertebral fracture, there is ↑ marrow signal on the T_2 image for up to a year.

Bone mass measurements

(See Table 6.1.)

Interpretation of results

- Bone mass is quoted in terms of the number of standard deviations
  (SD) from an expected mean. The most useful way of expressing this
  is as T scores. T scores represent observed bone mass in comparison
  to a sex-matched young, healthy population. Z scores are sometimes
  quoted and relate to bone density, according to a sex- and an age-
  matched group. It is usual to report Z scores for children and young
  adults (up to the age of 40 years). We usually use T scores in older
  adults.
- A reduction of one SD in bone density will approximately double the
  risk of fracture.
- The WHO has established criteria for the diagnosis of osteoporosis in
  post-menopausal ♀ (see ➲ Table 6.8).
- No similar criteria have been set in ♂, but the same thresholds are
  generally accepted.
- For some 2° causes of osteoporosis, particularly GC use, a less
  stringent criterion of T score <−1.5 should be used as a bone density-
  determined treatment intervention threshold.

Table 6.1 Measurement of bone density

Technique	Site	Measures	Radiation	Reproducibility
DXA	Spine* Femur* Whole body Forearm	Areal bone mineral density (g/cm²)	15 microsieverts for spine, 9 μSv for hip	1.6% at spine 1.5% at total hip
Quantitative CT (QCT)	Spine Forearm	Volumetric BMD (g/cm³)	980 microsieverts at spine	2–8%

* Accepted as gold standard measurement.

Bone biopsy

Bone biopsy is occasionally necessary for the diagnosis of patients with
complex metabolic bone diseases. This is usually in the context of suspected osteomalacia or renal osteodystrophy. Bone biopsy is not indicated
for routine diagnosis of osteoporosis. *It should only be undertaken in highly
specialist centres with appropriate expertise.*

Investigation of calcium, phosphate, and magnesium

Blood concentration

Calcium
- Serum Ca:
  - Non-fasting, but important to adjust for serum albumin (see Box 6.1).
- Ionized Ca:
  - In most clinical situations, direct measurement of ionized Ca concentration is unnecessary.
  - Consider use of ionized Ca measurement if concern that total serum Ca concentration does not reflect ionized Ca, e.g.:
    - When albumin is very low, the formula in Box 6.1 is not reliable.
    - In critical illness, factors such as metabolic acidosis can affect Ca binding to proteins.

PTH

Phosphate and magnesium
- Serum PO_4:
  - PO_4 measurements vary with time of day and fasting status.
  - Blood for measurement of PO_4 level should ideally be collected after an overnight fast.
- Plasma Mg:
  - Non-fasting.
  - Measurement is a poor indicator of total body stores.
  - Only ~1% of magnesium (Mg) is in the blood; the majority (~50%) is within the skeleton.

Box 6.1 Adjustment of measured calcium concentration

Adjusted Ca = measured Ca + 0.02 × (40 − albumin)

(where Ca is in mmol/L, and albumin in g/L)

Tips
- When albumin is very low, this formula is not reliable.
- In critical illness, factors such as metabolic acidosis can affect Ca binding to proteins.
- If doubt whether total serum Ca reflects ionized Ca, ionized levels should be measured directly.

Urine excretion

Calcium

- Measurement of 24h urinary excretion of Ca provides some measure of risk of renal stone formation or nephrocalcinosis.
- Helpful in assessment of causes of hypercalcaemia and monitoring of treatment of some causes of hypocalcaemia such as hypoparathyroidism.
- An estimate of the ratio of renal clearance of Ca to that of creatinine (Cr) in the fasting state is also of value in differentiating familial hypocalciuric hypercalcaemia (FHH) from PHPT (see Box 6.2).
  - If all values are in mmol/L, the ratio is typically >0.02 in PHPT; values <0.01 are suggestive of hypocalciuric hypercalcaemia. (Exclude other causes of hypercalciuria, including renal insufficiency and vitamin D deficiency.)

Tips
- Genetic panel testing for FHH can also be used to help differentiate from PHPT.
  - It may shorten the diagnostic odyssey and may prove a cost-effective approach, especially if biochemical tests are not immediately definitive.

Phosphate

- 24h collection:
  - Little clinical utility—reflects dietary PO_4 intake.

Box 6.2 Calculation of calcium/creatinine excretion ratio

CaE = [Urine Ca (mmol)/urine Cr (mmol)]
× [(plasma Cr (micromol)/1000)/plasma Ca (mmol)]
= <0.01 in FHH
= >0.02 in PHPT

These numeric parameters are not fully sensitive or specific and genetic testing should also be considered in the diagnostic pathway.

Calcium-regulating hormones

Parathyroid hormone

- Indications for testing:
  - Abnormality of Ca or PO_4 homeostasis.
  - Chronic renal disease.
  - Vitamin D deficiency.
  - Osteoporosis.
- Reference ranges depend on assay employed, but typical values are 10–60ng/L (1–6pmol/L).

Vitamin D and its metabolites

25-hydroxyvitamin D (25OHD)

- Main storage form of vitamin D.
- Measurement of 'total vitamin D' is the most clinically useful measure of vitamin D status.
- Internationally, there remains controversy around a 'normal' or 'optimal' concentration of vitamin D. Levels over 50nmol/L are generally accepted as satisfactory, and values <25nmol/L represent deficiency. True osteomalacia occurs with vitamin D values <15nmol/L.
- Low levels of 25OHD can result from a variety of causes (see ➜ Vitamin D deficiency, p. 537).
- Unlikely to see serious toxicity with 25OHD concentrations of <200nmol/L.
- Indications for testing:
  - Investigation of vitamin D deficiency, osteomalacia, and rickets.
  - Investigation of 2° causes of osteoporosis.

1,25-dihydroxyvitamin D (1,25(OH)₂D)

- Active form of vitamin D.
- Under physiological conditions, 1α hydroxylase in renal parenchyma catalyses conversion of 25OHD to $1,25(OH)_2D$.
- Indications for testing:
  - Measurement very rarely indicated.
  - Sometimes useful diagnostically in rare conditions of extrarenal synthesis of $1,25(OH)_2D$ such as sarcoidosis and lymphoma.

Parathyroid hormone-related peptide

- Indications for testing:
  - Very rarely indicated.
  - *In exceptional circumstances, may aid in clarifying the cause of hypercalcaemia.*

Calcitonin

- Indications for testing:
  - Calcitonin assays are available, but their utility is confined to the diagnosis and monitoring of MTC.
  - There is no role for calcitonin measurements in the routine investigation of Ca and bone metabolism.

Hypercalcaemia

Epidemiology

Hypercalcaemia is found in 5% of hospital patients and in 0.5% of the general population.

Causes

Many different disease states can lead to hypercalcaemia. These are listed by order of importance in hospital practice in Box 6.3. In asymptomatic community-dwelling subjects, the vast majority of hypercalcaemia is the result of PHPT.

Clinical features

Notwithstanding the underlying cause of hypercalcaemia, the clinical features are similar. With adjusted serum Ca levels <3.0mmol/L, significant classical hypercalcaemia-related symptoms are unlikely. With progressive increases in Ca concentration, the likelihood of symptoms increases rapidly.

The clinical features of hypercalcaemia are well recognized (see Table 6.2). Unfortunately, they are non-specific and may relate to an underlying illness.

Clinical signs of hypercalcaemia are rare. With the exception of band keratopathy, these are not specific. It is important to seek clinical evidence of underlying causes of hypercalcaemia, particularly malignant disease.

In addition to specific symptoms of hypercalcaemia, symptoms of long-term consequences of hypercalcaemia should be sought. These include the presence of bone pain or fracture and renal stones. These indicate the presence of chronic hypercalcaemia.

Investigation of hypercalcaemia

Confirm the diagnosis
- Serum Ca (adjusted for albumin).

Determine the mechanism
- ↑ *PTH*. Parathyroid overactivity (1° or tertiary hyperparathyroidism but can also occur in FHH and lithium therapy due to faulty Ca-sensing).
- ↓ *PTH*. PTH-independent cause.
- *Normal PTH:*
  - May imply parathyroid overactivity—incomplete suppression.
  - May imply altered Ca-sensing—FHH—Ca/Cr excretion ratio low.
- Urine Ca to quantify excretion and to determine Ca/Cr excretion ratio (not directly correlated with risk of stones).
- Consider genetic panel testing.

Seek underlying illness (where indicated)
- History and examination.
- Chest X-ray (CXR).
- FBC and ESR.
- Biochemical profile (renal and liver function).
- TFTs (exclude thyrotoxicosis).
- 25OHD (rarely 1,25(OH)$_2$D if considering possibility of granulomatous disease and extrarenal synthesis of 1,25(OH)$_2$D).
- Plasma and urine protein electrophoresis (exclude myeloma).
- Serum cortisol (SST—exclude Addison's disease).

To determine end-organ damage

- 24h urine Ca (± urine creatinine for reproducibility).
- Renal tract US (calculi, nephrocalcinosis).
- BMD by DXA to include distal radius; consider performing vertebral morphometry for vertebral fractures.

Box 6.3 Causes of hypercalcaemia

Common

- Hyperparathyroidism:
  - 1°.
  - Tertiary.
- Malignancy:
  - Humoral hypercalcaemia.
  - Multiple myeloma.
  - Bony metastases.

Uncommon

- FHH.
- Sarcoidosis and other granulomatous diseases.
- Thiazide diuretics.
- Lithium.
- Immobilization.
- Vitamin D intoxication.
- Hyperthyroidism.
- Renal failure.
- Addison's disease.
- Vitamin A intoxication.

Table 6.2 Clinical features of hypercalcaemia

Renal	GI	CNS	Other
Polyuria	Anorexia	Confusion	Pruritus
Polydipsia	Vomiting	Lethargy	Sore eyes
	Constipation	Depression	
	Abdominal pain		

Source: data from Shine B *et al* (2015) "Long-term effects of lithium on renal, thyoid, and parathyroid function: a restrospective analysis of laboratory data" *The Lancet* 386(9992):461–468.

Primary hyperparathyroidism

Present in up to 1 in 500 of the general population where it is predominantly a disease of post-menopausal ♀ (14/100,000 ♂, 28/100,000 ♀). The normal physiological response to hypocalcaemia is an increase in PTH secretion. This is termed 2° *hyperparathyroidism* and is not pathological in as much as the PTH secretion remains under feedback control. Continued stimulation of the parathyroid glands can lead to autonomous production of PTH. This, in turn, causes hypercalcaemia which is termed *tertiary hyperparathyroidism*. This is usually seen in the context of renal disease.

Pathology

- 85% single adenoma.
- Overexpression of cyclin D1, a key cell cycle regulator, is implicated in the pathogenesis of 20–40% of sporadic parathyroid adenomas.
- 14% hyperplasia (may be associated with other endocrine abnormalities, particularly MEN1 and 2 (see ➲ MEN type 1, pp. 674–5; ➲ MEN type 2, pp. 684–5).
- <1% carcinoma.

Clinical features

- Often detected incidentally on biochemistry testing.
- Majority of patients have few or no symptoms.
- Significance of chronic undifferentiated symptoms such as fatigue and brain fog is unclear.
- Normocalcaemic PHPT now recognized and probably represents early expression of PHPT—role of parathyroidectomy controversial (see ➲ Treatment of hyperparathyroidism, p. 514).
- Features of hypercalcaemia.
- End-organ damage (see Box 6.4).

Natural history

- In the majority of patients without end-organ damage, disease is not rapidly progressive over months.
- A significant minority (~25%) will develop new indications for surgery over a 15-year follow-up, and thus long-term monitoring in non-operated patients is required.
- Excess mortality associated with PHPT is probably linked to CVD and possibly malignancy, but there is no evidence that parathyroidectomy reverses any excess risk.

Investigation

(See Boxes 6.5 and 6.6.)
   Potential diagnostic pitfalls:
- Concomitant vitamin D deficiency is common. Supplementation with vitamin D to correct deficiency is important. Risk of worsening of hypercalcaemia of PHPT is low, but monitoring of plasma Ca is required.
- FHH—differentiate with assessment of urine Ca excretion, including 24h urine collection and Ca/Cr excretion ratio (see ➲ Familial hypocalciuric hypercalcaemia, p. 522) (<0.01 in FHH; >0.02 in hyperparathyroidism); genetic testing for FHH.

Tips
- Measurement of urine Ca excretion may be low if there is significant untreated vitamin D deficiency, even in the presence of PHPT. This can be misleading. Replace vitamin D and repeat measurement of urine calcium excretion.
- Drugs associated with hypercalcaemia:
  - Thiazides—ideally discontinue and reassess Ca.
  - Lithium—potentially complex and requires specialist assessment as probable potential to induce parathyroid hyperplasia or adenoma, as well as reversible 'lithium-induced' hypercalcaemia.

Box 6.4 End-organ damage in hyperparathyroidism

Bone
- Osteoporosis:
  - Common.
  - Affects all sites, but predominant loss in peripheral cortical bone.
- Osteitis fibrosa cystica:
  - Rare.
  - Usually with tertiary hyperparathyroidism.

Kidneys
- Seen in 15–20% cases.
- Renal calculi.
- Nephrocalcinosis.
- Renal impairment.

Pancreatitis

Box 6.5 Diagnosis of primary hyperparathyroidism
- Ca > reference range (2.60mmol (adjusted) × 2).
- Urea and electrolytes (U&E), Cr normal.
- Not on lithium or thiazide diuretic.
- PTH > midpoint reference range (20% patients have PTH within reference range).
- Urine Ca excretion over 24h not low.
- Vitamin D within reference range.

Box 6.6 Other causes of raised PTH
- Renal insufficiency.
- Vitamin D deficiency.
- Hypercalciuria.
- Drugs (e.g. lithium, thiazides).

Exclusion of associated underlying condition
- PHPT can be associated with genetic abnormalities, especially MEN1 and 2, as well as familial hyperparathyroidism.
- Conditions of genetic susceptibility should be sought in patients presenting with PHPT and a family history in ≥1 1st-degree relatives, a young age (<40 years), or multigland parathyroid disease.

Localization of abnormal parathyroid glands

(See Boxes 6.7.and 6.8.)

This is not part of the initial diagnostic work-up of PHPT but is per-formed to assist surgical approach.

- Co-localization with two separate techniques (usually US and ^{99m}Tc-sestamibi or four-dimensional (4D)-CT) is usually required for focused parathyroidectomy.
- Otherwise, open bilateral neck exploration by an experienced surgeon (>20 operations per year) is optimal in the 1st instance.
- Point to note—once a decision for parathyroidectomy has been made, −ve or non-concordant imaging does not provide a reason for not operating; open bilateral neck exploration should be performed by an appropriately experienced surgeon.
- After failed neck exploration, other localizing techniques are required, which include:
  - ^{99m}Tc-sestamibi.
  - 4D-CT.
  - ^{18}F-choline PET/CT in specialist centres.
- Angiography with selective venous sampling may be employed in difficult cases but should be confined to specialist centres with experience in this technique.

Box 6.7 Normocalcaemic primary hyperparathyroidism (NPHPT)

- Formally recognized as part of the disease spectrum of PHPT in 2008.
- Defined as persistently elevated PTH in the setting of persistently normal serum Ca concentration, after recognized 2° causes of elevated PTH have been excluded.
- Pathogenesis of NPHPT is unclear and may be an early or biochemically mild expression of PHPT. It is feasible that NPHPT represents a heterogeneous diagnosis with multiple causes.
- Population prevalence data are very variable, from 0.1% to 6%. With long-term follow-up, the prevalence falls significantly, suggesting NPHPT may be reversible in some instances.
- The natural history of NHPT remains unknown. NPHPT only rarely progresses to PHPT.
- Classical and non-classical clinical features of PHPT are seen in cases of NPHPT, but numbers in studies of NPHPT are small.
- There are few data on the outcomes of parathyroidectomy or medical management in NPHPT.
- In NHPT, there is a higher prevalence of multigland disease, smaller gland size, and lower surgical cure rates.
- Caution should be used in recommending surgery for NPHPT, and an individualized assessment is advocated.
  (See ➔ Chapter 10.)

Box 6.8 Atypical parathyroid adenomas

- <1% parathyroid tumours.
- Uncertain malignant potential.
- Characterized by histological features which can be difficult to differentiate from carcinoma (solid growth pattern, cellular atypia, but absence of local invasion and/or metastasis).
- Sporadic/hereditary.
- Germline mutation *CDC73* commonly found, suggesting a variant of hyperpararathyroidism–jaw tumour syndrome.
- Clinical features are of hyperparathyroidism, although occasionally, there is a palpable nodule.
- Biochemistry is characterized by moderate hypercalcaemia and elevated PTH.
- A family history should be checked.
- Close annual follow-up is recommended, as there is a low risk of recurrence, although others suggest close follow-up is only necessary if there is loss of parafibromin expression or in large tumours.

Source: data from Cetani F. et al. (2019) "Atypical parathyroid adenomas: challenging lesions in the differential diagnosis of endocrine tumors" *Endocrine-Related Cancer* 27(7): R441–R464.

Treatment of hyperparathyroidism

Parathyroid surgery

(Aspects of parathyroid surgery are also covered in → Indications for surgery in primary hyperparathyroidism, p. 515.)

- Parathyroidectomy is the only potentially curative treatment for PHPT.
- For indications, see Table 6.3.
- By experienced surgeon (suggested >20 procedures per year):
  - *Adenoma.* Remove affected gland—often by focused surgery.
  - *Multigland disease, including hyperplasia.* Partial parathyroidectomy (perhaps with reimplantation of tissue in more accessible site with 4-gland hyperplasia).

Observation

- Consider parathyroidectomy in all, but observation may be suitable for some patients with 'mild' disease with no evidence of end-organ damage.
- Most such patients have stable disease over many years but do require monitoring:
  - *Annual* serum Ca and renal function, cardiovascular risk assessment.
  - *Every 2–3 years*—BMD, renal US if suspicion of renal stone.
- Any significant biochemical or symptomatic deterioration is an indication for reconsideration of surgery, as is development of end-organ damage.

Medical management

- Bisphosphonates:
  - Given PO, have clinically inconsequential effect on plasma and urine Ca.
  - Preserve bone mass and can be considered at all stages in management.
- Ca-sensing receptor agonists:
  - Only indicated in certain patients if not suitable for surgery or after failed parathyroid surgery.
  - Cinacalcet (starting dose from 30mg od or bd) reduces serum, but not urine, Ca concentration. It increases sensitivity of Ca-sensing receptor, decreasing PTH secretion. It is licensed for patients with PHPT in whom parathyroid surgery is contraindicated or clinically inappropriate, and parathyroid carcinoma. It may also be used following unsuccessful parathyroid surgery.
  - Cinacalcet does not prevent renal stones or bone loss and thus should not be seen as equivalent to parathyroidectomy in offering 'cure'.

Indications for surgery in primary hyperparathyroidism

It is generally accepted[1,2] that all patients with symptomatic hyperparathyroidism, evidence of end-organ damage, or significantly and consistently elevated serum Ca should be referred for consideration of parathyroidectomy. This would include:

- Definite symptoms of hypercalcaemia. There is less good evidence that non-specific symptoms, such as abdominal pain, tiredness, or mild cognitive impairment, benefit from surgery.
- Impaired renal function.
- Renal stones (symptomatic or on radiograph).
- Parathyroid bone disease, including osteoporosis and fragility fractures.
- Pancreatitis.
- Adjusted serum Ca concentration >2.85mmol/L.

Guidelines for the management of hyperparathyroidism have been produced for the UK by NICE. NICE Guideline 132[1] also recommends to 'consider' referral for parathyroidectomy in all patients with a confirmed diagnosis of PHPT, even if they do not have the features listed above. This takes into account patients with less classical symptoms and promotes a more overarching and individualized assessment of benefits and potential risks of parathyroidectomy for patients, irrespective of age.

Table 6.3 Table comparing indications for parathyroidectomy in patients with what has been termed asymptomatic PHPT according to UK (NICE Guideline 132)[1] vs USA (Fourth International Workshop)[2] opinion

	UK	USA
Serum Ca	2.85mmol/L	2.85mmol/L
Urine Ca	No threshold defined	>10mmol/day
Cr clearance	No threshold estimated glomerular filtration rate (eGFR)	eGFR <60mL/min
BMD	Osteoporosis or fragility fracture	T score <−2.5 or fragility fracture
Age	No threshold	<50

Source: data from Hyperparathyroidism (primary): diagnosis, assessment and initial management; NICE guideline [NG132], Published date: May 2019, ℘ https://www.nice.org.uk/guidance/NG132 and Silverberg SJ, et al. (2014) Current issues in the presentation of asymptomatic primary hyperparathyroidism: proceedings of the Fourth International Workshop. *J Clin Endocrinol Metab.* 99,3580–94.

Conservative management

- Patients not managed with surgery require regular follow-up.
- There are again some differences between recommendations in the UK[1] and USA[2] (see Table 6.4).

NICE Guideline 132[1] also recommends that all patients with PHPT should be assessed regularly for cardiovascular and fracture risk.

Table 6.4 Table comparing management recommendations for patients in the USA and the UK

	UK	USA
Serum Ca	12 months	12 months
eGFR	12 months	12 months
24h urine	Not recommended	If suspected stones
BMD	24–36 months	12–24 months
US kidneys	If suspected stone	If suspected stone

References

1. National Institute for Health and Care Excellence (2019). *Hyperparathyroidism (primary): diagnosis, assessment and initial management.* NICE guideline [NG132]. ℘ https://www.nice.org.uk/guidance/NG132
2. Silverberg SJ, et al. (2014). Current issues in the presentation of asymptomatic primary hyperparathyroidism: proceedings of the Fourth International Workshop. *J Clin Endocrinol Metab* **99**, 3580–94.

Further reading

Caldwell M, et al. (2019). Persistently elevated PTH after parathyroidectomy at one year: experience in a tertiary referral center. *J Clin Endocrinol Metab* **104**, 4473–80.

Ejlsmark-Svensson H, et al. (2019). Effect of parathyroidectomy on cardiovascular risk factors in primary hyperparathyroidism: a randomized clinical trial. *J Clin Endocrinol Metab* **104**, 3223–32.

Leere JS, et al. (2020). Denosumab and cinacalcet for primary hyperparathyroidism (DENOCINA): a randomised, double-blind, placebo-controlled, phase 3 trial. *Lancet Diabetes Endocrinol* **8**, 407–17.

Lundstam K, et al. (2017). Effect of surgery versus observation: skeletal 5-year outcomes in a randomized trial of patients with primary HPT (the SIPH Study). *J Bone Miner Res* **32**, 1907–14.

Parathyroid UK (formerly Hypopara UK). [Support for patients with hypoparathyroidism and hyperparathyroidism]. ℘ http://hypopara.org.uk/

Rubin MR, et al. (2008). The natural history of primary hyperparathyroidism with or without parathyroid Surgery after 15 years. *J Clin Endocrinol Metab* **93**, 3562–70.

Walker MD, Silverberg SJ (2018). Primary hyperparathyroidism. *Nat Rev Endocrinol* **14**, 115–25.

Complications of parathyroidectomy

Mechanical
- Vocal cord paresis:
  - May be permanent, particularly with repeated surgery.

Metabolic (hypocalcaemia)
- Transient:
  - Due to suppression of remaining glands.
  - May sometimes require oral therapy with Ca ± vitamin D metabolites.
- Severe:
  - Due to hungry bones—rare and tricky to manage. Treatment with calcitriol 1 microgram/day (sometimes higher doses required) and PO (and IV) Ca may be required for several weeks.
  - Occurs in patients with pre-existing bone disease.
  - Minimize risk by pretreatment of any vitamin D deficiency for several weeks. Risk of significant worsening of hypercalcaemia is very low, but monitoring of serum Ca is recommended.
  - Acute severe hypocalcaemia requires initial IV Ca to stabilize metabolic status.
- Permanent:
  - Hypoparathyroidism due to irreversible damage to all parathyroid glands. Rare after focused surgery, but may ensue after 'subtotal' parathyroidectomy for multigland disease.

Outcome after surgery
- <5% fail to become normocalcaemic, and these should be considered for a 2nd operation.
- Monitoring for residual/recurrent PHPT by checking serum Ca.
- PTH measurement helpful post-operatively in managing hypocalcaemia, but not in longer term as monitoring tool if Ca normal.
- One-third of cases have elevated PTH despite successful surgery. The clinical meaning and importance of this observation is unclear.
- All patients with hyperplasia (including MEN) identified on histopathology should have long-term monitoring of serum Ca to detect recurrent PHPT.
- Patients rendered permanently hypoparathyroid by surgery require lifelong supplements of active metabolites of vitamin D with Ca. This can lead to hypercalciuria, and the risk of stone formation is present in these patients. Target serum Ca in these patients towards the low end of the reference range to minimize hypercalciuria. PTH 1-84 is available in some countries as an adjunctive treatment for chronic hypoparathyroidism.

Tricky situations post-parathyroid surgery
- Not cured despite 'four glands removed'.
- Utilize experienced MDT.
- Review all imaging modalities available as described in ⊃ Localization of abnormal parathyroid glands, p. 512.
- Consider extended imaging, potentially at another centre with expertise in F18-choline PET/CT, selective venous sampling, and angiography.

Atypical parathyroid adenoma

(See also Box 6.8.)

Hyperplasia and one gland removed
- If Ca normalized, no requirement to surgically pursue other glands, unless persistent/recurrent hypercalcaemia.
- Maintain appropriate follow-up to detect ↑ likelihood of recurrent PHPT.
- Consider genetic panel testing.
- Consider operative approach if recurrent PHPT—3.5 gland parathyroidectomy or total parathyroidectomy with reimplantation.

Candidates for genetic screening
(See also ➲ Chapters 10 and 13.)
- <40 years with PHPT.
- Other clinical features of syndromes associated with PHPT.
- PHPT gene panel.

Other causes of hypercalcaemia

Hypercalcaemia of malignancy

Mechanism
(See Table 6.5.)

Clinical features
Hypercalcaemia is usually a late manifestation of malignant disease, and the 1° lesion is usually evident by the time hypercalcaemia is apparent (50% of patients die within 30 days). One exception to this is in small endocrine tumours, such as carcinoids and islet cell tumours, which can produce humoral mediators of hypercalcaemia (PTHrP) in the absence of significant spread. Symptoms of hypercalcaemia may be non-specific and difficult to distinguish from those of the underlying disease.

Investigation
(See investigation of hypercalcaemia in ➜ Clinical features, p. 508.)
   Factors suggesting hypercalcaemia of malignancy include:
- ↑ Ca.
- ↓ PTH.
- Other features of malignant disease.
- ↑ PTHrP—do not routinely measure in clinical practice.

Steroid suppression tests are rarely indicated. May suppress Ca with malignancy, but not with PHPT.

Treatment
Patients requiring treatment will often have severe symptomatic hypercalcaemia and emergency treatment is necessary to stabilize the patient. In such circumstances, the principles of management are the same as those of severe hypercalcaemia from any cause (see Box 6.9).

Table 6.5 Types of hypercalcaemia associated with cancer

Type	Frequency (%)	Bone metastases	Causal agent	Tumour type
Local	20	Common	Cytokines	Breast
Osteolysis		Extensive	Chemokines PTHrP	Myeloma Lymphoma
Humoral	80	Minimal	PTHrP	Squamous carcinoma Renal Ovarian Endometrial Breast HTLV Lymphoma
1,25OHD	<1	Variable	1,25(OH)$_2$D	Lymphoma
Ectopic PTH	<1	Variable	PTH	Variable

Box 6.9 Management of severe hypercalcaemia

- Vigorous rehydration—0.9% saline 4–6L in 24h.
- Monitor for fluid overload if renal impairment or elderly.
- Loop diuretics rarely used and only if fluid overload develops; not effective for reducing serum Ca.
- If further treatment required, consider zoledronic acid 4mg IV or pamidronate 30–90mg IV.
- Ca falls within 12h, nadir 2–4 days.
- Duration of effect is variable, but usually 1–6 weeks.
    1. Stabilize the level of hypercalcaemia, and prevent any further decline in renal function using volume expansion with large quantities of 0.9% saline in first 24h. This should take place before considering use of an IV bisphosphonate.
    2. Once the patient is volume-replete and if still significant hypercalcaemia, consider IV bisphosphonate— zoledronic acid (4mg) or pamidronate (30–90mg) are the most frequently used. Repeat doses may be required. Even patients who are acutely hypercalcaemic can rarely develop hypocalcaemia following IV bisphosphonate therapy, especially if they are vitamin D-deficient.
    3. In very severe hypercalcaemia with renal impairment, dialysis may be of value.
    4. Calcitonin, GCs, and cinacalcet are not routinely used in the acute management of hypercalcaemia.
    5. Denosumab should only be considered under strict specialist supervision.

Source: data from Walsh J, *et al.* (2016) Society for Endocrinology Endocrine Emergency Guidance: Emergency management of acute hypercal-caemia in adult patients. *Endocr Connect* 5, G9–G11.

Familial hypocalciuric hypercalcaemia

FHH is a very rare AD syndrome associated with hypercalcaemia and relative hypocalciuria that is most often due to heterozygous inactivating mutations of the *CASR* gene encoding the Ca-sensing receptor.

- Rare—incidence ~1:80,000, compared to PHPT ~1:1000.
- AD, with virtually complete penetrance, but may also rarely be AR.
- Mutation in the Ca-sensing receptor that reduces its sensitivity such that the body behaves as if it were experiencing normocalcaemia, even though the serum Ca level is elevated.
- Characteristic biochemical features:
  - Hypercalcaemia.
  - Hypocalciuria.
  - PTH within reference range or mildly elevated.
- Important to differentiate from PHPT, as does not usually show any benefit from parathyroidectomy.
- Genetics:
  - The homozygous state produces severe life-threatening hypercalcaemia soon after birth (neonatal severe hyperparathyroidism). In such cases, total parathyroidectomy is lifesaving.
  - The heterozygous state is generally benign and unassociated with symptoms or adverse effects such as renal stones or bone disease.
- Management—none specific usually required.

(See Box 6.9 for management of hypercalcaemia.)

Patients have low urine Ca excretion (24h <2.5mmol, fasting Ca/Cr excretion ratio <0.01) (see Box 6.2).

Further reading

Hannan FM, et al. (2018). The calcium-sensing receptor in physiology and in calcitropic and noncalcitropic diseases. *Nat Rev Endocrinol* **15**, 33–51.

Vitamin D intoxication

- Overt vitamin D toxicity manifests through chronic hypercalciuria and hypercalcaemia.
- It is rarely seen clinically unless the vitamin D dose is very high.
- Doses below 10,000 IU/day are rarely associated with toxicity,
- >50,000 IU/day for several weeks or months are associated with toxicity, including hypercalcaemia.[1]
- Diagnosis:
  - Greatly elevated concentrations of 25OHD (there is no universally accepted threshold, but hypercalcaemia is very rarely seen unless 25OHD >200nmol/L) and 1,25(OH)$_2$D.
  - Suppressed PTH.

NB. If calcitriol or alfacalcidol is the offending compound causing hypercalcaemia, then 25OHD levels will not be elevated, but 1,25-dihydroxycholecalciferol may be helpful in delineating the cause of the hypercalcaemia.

- Management:
  - In mild cases, particularly when the active vitamin D metabolites are involved, the only treatment necessary is to withdraw the offending treatment and to allow Ca to settle.
  - If longer-acting vitamin D metabolites are involved, then active treatment may be necessary.
  - Patients should first be stabilized with a saline infusion (see Box 6.9).
  - Following this, traditional management has been high-dose PO GCs such as prednisolone 40mg daily.
  - IV bisphosphonates should also be considered in the acute setting.

References

1. Francis RM, et al. (2015). National Osteoporosis Society practical clinical guideline on vitamin D and bone health. Maturitas **80**, 119–21.

Sarcoidosis and other granulomatous diseases

- Mechanism of hypercalcaemia—extrarenal production of $1,25(OH)_2D$ in granulomata.
- The process is not under feedback inhibition but is substrate-regulated. The hypercalcaemia is therefore dependent on vitamin D supply. Patients may present with hypercalcaemia in summer or following foreign holidays when endogenous production of vitamin D is maximal.
- Investigations:
  - Normal 25OHD.
  - Raised $1,25(OH)_2D$.
  - Suppressed PTH.
  - Other markers of sarcoid activity, such as raised ACE activity, may also be present.
- Treatment:
  - GCs to control sarcoid activity and minimize the effects of excess $1,25(OH)_2D$ and hypercalcaemia.

Further reading

Bollerslev J, et al. (2019). Management of endocrine disease: Unmet therapeutic, educational and scientific needs in parathyroid disorders. *Eur J Endocrinol* **181**, P1–19.

Cetani F, et al. (2018). Non-surgical management of primary hyperparathyroidism. *Best Pract Res Clin Endocrinol Metab* **32**, 821–35.

Cristina EV, Alberto F (2018). Management of familial hyperparathyroidism syndromes: MEN1, MEN2, MEN4, HPT-jaw tumour, familial isolated hyperparathyroidism, FHH, and neonatal severe hyperparathyroidism. *Best Pract Res Clin Endocrinol Metab* **32**, 861–75.

Crowley RK, Gittoes NJ (2016). Elevated PTH with normal serum calcium level: a structured approach. *Clin Endocrinol (Oxf)* **84**, 809–13.

Cusano NE, et al. (2018). Management of normocalcemic primary hyperparathyroidism. *Best Pract Res Clin Endocrinol Metab* **32**, 837–45.

Goltzman D (2019). Nonparathyroid hypercalcemia. *Front Horm Res* **51**, 77–90.

Hannan FM, et al. (2019). Genetic approaches to metabolic bone diseases. *Br J Clin Pharmacol* **85**, 1147–60.

Hypocalcaemia

Causes

Although hypocalcaemia can result from failure of any of the mechanisms by which serum Ca concentration is maintained, it is usually the result of either failure of PTH secretion or because of the inability to release Ca from bone. These causes are summarized in Box 6.10.

Clinical features

The clinical features of hypocalcaemia are largely as a result of ↑ neuromuscular excitability. In order of ↑ severity, these include:

- Tingling—especially of fingers, toes, or lips.
- Numbness—especially of fingers, toes, or lips.
- Cramps.
- Carpopedal spasm.
- Stridor due to laryngospasm.
- Seizures.

The symptoms of hypocalcaemia tend to reflect the severity and rapidity of onset of the metabolic abnormality.

Clinical signs of hypocalcaemia depend upon the demonstration of neuromuscular irritability before this necessarily causes symptoms:

- *Chvostek's sign* is elicited by tapping the facial nerve in front of the ear. A +ve result is indicated by twitching of the corner of the mouth. Slight twitching is seen in up to 15% of normal ♀, but more major involvement of the facial muscles is indicative of hypocalcaemia or hypomagnesaemia.
- *Trousseau's sign* is produced by occlusion of the blood supply to the arm by inflation of a sphygmomanometer cuff above the arterial pressure for 3min. If +ve, there is carpopedal spasm, which may be accompanied by painful paraesthesiae.

In addition, there may be clinical signs and symptoms associated with the underlying condition:

- *Vitamin D deficiency* may be associated with generalized bone pain, proximal myopathy, or fractures (see ➜ Vitamin D deficiency, p. 537).
- *Hypoparathyroidism* can be accompanied by clouded thinking and personality disturbances, as well as extrapyramidal signs, cataracts, and rarely papilloedema.
- If *hypocalcaemia* is present during the development of permanent teeth, these may show areas of enamel hypoplasia. This can be a useful physical sign, indicating that the hypocalcaemia is long-standing.

Pseudohypoparathyroidism

- Resistance to PTH action.
- Due to defective signalling of PTH action via cell membrane receptor.
- Also affects TSH, LH, FSH, and GH signalling.
- Most commonly caused by AD mutation of *GNAS1* gene.
- Significant imprinting:
  - Maternal transmission leads to full blown syndrome of hormone resistance.
  - Paternal transmission causes only phenotypic features of Albright's hereditary osteodystrophy.

Box 6.10 Causes of hypocalcaemia

Hypoparathyroidism
- Destruction of parathyroid glands:
  - Surgical.
  - Autoimmune.
  - Radiation.
  - Infiltration.
- Failure of parathyroid development:
  - Isolated, e.g. X-linked.
  - With other abnormalities, e.g. di George syndrome (with thymic aplasia, immunodeficiency, and cardiac anomalies).
- Failure of PTH secretion:
  - Mg deficiency.
  - Overactivity of Ca-sensing receptor.
- Failure of PTH action:
  - Pseudohypoparathyroidism—due to G protein abnormality.

Failure of release of calcium from bone
- Osteomalacia:
  - Vitamin D deficiency.
  - Vitamin D resistance.
  - Renal failure.
- Inhibition of bone resorption:
  - Drugs linked to hypocalcaemia, e.g. cisplatin, calcitonin, PO PO_4, IV bisphosphonates, denosumab.
- ↑ uptake of Ca into bone:
  - Osteoblastic metastases (e.g. prostate).
  - Hungry bone syndrome.
  - Imatinib mesylate

Complexing of calcium from the circulation
- ↑ albumin-binding in alkalosis.
- Acute pancreatitis:
  - Formation of Ca soaps from autodigestion of fat.
  - Abnormal PTH and vitamin D metabolism.
  - PO_4 infusion.
- Multiple blood transfusions—complexing by citrate.

Albright's hereditary osteodystrophy

Patients with the commonest type of pseudohypoparathyroidism (type Ia) have a characteristic set of skeletal abnormalities, known as Albright's hereditary osteodystrophy. This comprises:
- Short stature.
- Obesity.
- Round face.
- Short metacarpals.

Some individuals with Albright's hereditary osteodystrophy do not have a disorder of Ca metabolism. The term *pseudopseudohypoparathyroidism* has been used to describe this phenomenon. However, it is now clear that these reflect different manifestations of the same underlying genetic defect as a result of imprinting. In the light of the same underlying aetiology, there has been a tendency to avoid the more cumbersome designations and to refer to all such patients as having Albright's hereditary osteodystrophy.

Investigation of hypocalcaemia

(See Table 6.6.)

Table 6.6 Investigation of hypocalcaemia

	ALP	PO$_4$	PTH	Vitamin D	U&E	Mg
Vitamin D deficiency	↑	↓	↑	↓	N	N
Hypoparathyroidism	N	↑	L	N	N	N/↓
Pseudohypoparathyroidism	N	↑	↑↑	N	N	N
PPI-induced hypomagnesaemia/ hypocalcaemia	N	N	N	N	N	↓↓

- Serum Ca.
- PTH—the presence of a low, or even normal, PTH concentration implies failure of PTH secretion in the presence of hypocalcaemia.
- U&E.
- Total vitamin D.
- PO$_4$.
- Mg.
- The Ellsworth–Howard test can be performed if pseudohypoparathyroidism is suspected (measurement of serum and urine phosphorus after IV administration of PTH).

Further reading

Bilezekian JP (2020). Hypoparathyroidism. *J Clin Endocrinol Metab* **105**, 1722–36.
Cianferotti L, Brandi ML (2018). Pseudohypoparathyroidism. *Minerva Endocrinol* **43**, 156–67.

Treatment of hypocalcaemia

- *Acute symptomatic hypocalcaemia* is a medical emergency and demands urgent treatment whatever the cause (see Box 6.11).[1]
- Treatment of *chronic hypocalcaemia* is more dependent on the cause.

Chronic hypocalcaemia

Hypoparathyroidism

- Target serum Ca should be at the low end of the reference range, because the renal retention of Ca brought about by PTH has been lost. Thus, any attempt to raise the plasma Ca well into the reference range is likely to result in unacceptable hypercalciuria, with the risk of nephrocalcinosis and renal stones in the long term. Monitoring 24h urine Ca excretion is an important tool to avoid prolonged hypercalciuria.
- Vitamin D analogues, such as alfacalcidol (long half-life) or calcitriol, to maintain acceptable plasma Ca levels are required by the majority.
- The dose of vitamin D analogues is determined by the clinical response but usually lies in the range of 0.5–2 micrograms daily.
  - Tip: the calcaemic effect of calcitriol is ~100% greater than alfacalcidol.
  - In those who have swallowing problems, e.g. radiotherapy, neck dissection, liquid preparations are available.
- Routine biochemical monitoring of serum levels of Ca, PO_4, Mg, and Cr (eGFR), as well as assessment of symptoms of hypocalcaemia and hypercalcaemia, should be conducted at regular time intervals (e.g. every 3–6 months). Closer monitoring should occur at around times of dose adjustments (recheck biochemistry within 1–2 weeks).
- Supplemental Ca salts are sometimes co-prescribed, but in many patients, adequate dietary Ca intake can suffice as long as the dose of activated vitamin D analogue is adequate.
- PTH (1-84) treatment is available in some countries as an adjunct (not sole therapy) to conventional therapies in hypoparathyroidism. It is as yet unclear whether PTH treatment improves QoL and renal and bone outcomes.
- Thiazide diuretics can sometimes be helpful in mitigating hypercalciuria.

Pseudohypoparathyroidism

- The principles underlying the treatment of pseudohypoparathyroidism are the same as those underlying hypoparathyroidism.

> NB. Patients with the commonest form of pseudohypoparathyroidism may have resistance to the action of other hormones that rely on G protein signalling. They therefore need to be assessed for thyroid and gonadal dysfunction (because of defective TSH or gonadotrophin action). If these deficiencies are present, they should be treated in the conventional manner.

Vitamin D deficiency

Treatment of osteomalacia and vitamin D deficiency is described in ➲ Vitamin D deficiency, p. 537.

Box 6.11 Treatment of acute hypocalcaemia

- Patients with tetany or seizures require urgent IV treatment with calcium gluconate (less irritant than calcium chloride).
  - This is a 10% weight/volume (w/v) solution (10mL = 2.25mmol elemental Ca).
  - The solution should always be further diluted to minimize the risk of phlebitis or tissue damage if extravasation occurs.
- Initially, 10–20mL of 10% calcium gluconate diluted in 50–100mL of 5% glucose and infused over about 10min.
- Repeat if symptoms not resolved.
- Care must be taken if the patient has heart disease, especially if taking digoxin, as too rapid elevation of plasma Ca can cause arrhythmias. Cardiac monitoring is advisable.
- In order to maintain the plasma Ca, a Ca infusion is required; 100mL of 10% calcium gluconate (ten vials) should be added to 1L of saline or glucose solution and infused at 50–100mL/h.
- The plasma Ca should be checked regularly (not less than 6-hourly), and the infusion rate adjusted in response to the change in concentration.
- Failure of plasma Ca to respond to infused calcium should raise the possibility of underlying hypomagnesaemia. This can be rapidly ascertained by plasma Mg estimation and, if appropriate, an Mg infusion commenced (see ➲ Hypomagnesaemia, pp. 542–3).
- Treat the underlying cause.
- Once PO or NG tube intake is possible, Ca, vitamin D, and active vitamin D metabolites should be substituted according to the underlying cause.

Source: data from Turner J, et al. (2016) Society for Endocrinology Endocrine Emergency Guidance: Emergency management of acute hypocalcae-mia in adult patients. *Endocr Connect* 5:G7–G8.

Overactivity of calcium-sensing receptor
This leads to a condition known as AD hypocalcaemia where there is hypocalcaemia and relative hypercalciuria. It is a benign condition in which hypocalcaemia is usually asymptomatic. Treatment with Ca supplementation should be avoided in the absence of symptoms, as elevation of Ca levels, even to within the reference range, may cause renal dysfunction.

References

1. Turner J, et al. (2016). Society for Endocrinology Endocrine Emergency Guidance: Emergency management of acute hypocalcaemia in adult patients. *Endocr Connect* **5**, G7–8.

Further reading

Bollerslev J, et al. (2015). European Society of Endocrinology Clinical Guideline: Treatment of chronic hypoparathyroidism in adults. *Eur J Endocrinol* **173**, G1–20.

Brandi ML, et al. (2016). Management of hypoparathyroidism: summary statement and guidelines. *J Clin Endocrinol Metab* **101**, 2273–83.

Cooper MS, Gittoes NJ (2008). Diagnosis and management of hypocalcaemia. *BMJ* **336**, 1298–302.

Gafni RI, Collins MT (2019). Hypoparathyroidism. *N Engl J Med* **380**, 1738–47.

Mannstadt M, et al. (2017). Hypoparathyroidism. *Nat Rev Dis Primers* **3**, 17055. Erratum in: *Nat Rev Dis Primers* **3**, 17080.

Parathyroid UK (formerly Hypopara UK). [Support for patients with hypoparathyroidism and hyperparathyroidism]. ℜ http://hypopara.org.uk/

Siggelkow H, et al. (2020). Burden of illness in not adequately controlled chronic hypoparathyroidism: findings from a 13-country patient and caregiver survey. *Clin Endocrinol (Oxf)* **92**, 159–68.

Tay YD, et al. (2019). Therapy of hypoparathyroidism with rhPTH (1-84): a prospective eight year investigation of efficacy and safety. *J Clin Endocrinol Metab* **104**, 5601–10.

Rickets, osteomalacia, and hypophosphataemia

Definitions and mechanism

- *Osteomalacia* occurs when there is inadequate mineralization of mature bone.
  - In most instances, osteomalacia leads to build-up of excessive unmineralized osteoid within the skeleton.
- *Rickets* is a disorder of the growing skeleton where there is inadequate mineralization of bone as it is laid down at the epiphysis.
  - There is build-up of unmineralized osteoid in the growth plate. This leads to the characteristic radiological appearance of rickets, with widening of the growth plate and loss of definition of the ossification centres.

(See Box 6.12 for vitamin D resistance, and Box 6.13 for abnormal vitamin D metabolism.)

Clinical features

Osteomalacia

- Bone pain.
- Deformity.
- Fracture.
- Proximal myopathy.
- Hypocalcaemia (late manifestation in vitamin D deficiency).

Rickets

- Growth retardation.
- Bone pain and fracture.
- Skeletal deformity:
  - Bowing of the long bones.
  - Widening of the growth plates, widening of the wrists, 'rickety rosary' (costochondral junctions enlarged).

Diagnosis

- The diagnosis of osteomalacia is usually based on the appropriate biochemical findings (see Table 6.7).
- The majority of patients with osteomalacia will show no specific radiological abnormalities.
- The most characteristic abnormality is the *Looser's zone* or pseudofracture. If these are present, they are virtually pathognomonic of osteomalacia.
- In clinical practice, bone biopsy is rarely indicated.

Box 6.12 Vitamin D resistance

- Several different kindreds shown to have defective vitamin D receptor.
- Inherited as an AR condition.
- Produces hypocalcaemia and osteomalacia, with elevated serum levels of $1,25(OH)_2D$.
- Approximately two-thirds of affected individuals have total alopecia.
- Known as vitamin D-dependent rickets (VDDR) type II. If alopecia is present, it is often termed type IIA, in contrast to type IIB where hair growth is normal.
- Treatment usually requires administration of large doses of active vitamin D metabolites, sometimes reaching doses of 60 micrograms of calcitriol daily.

Box 6.13 Abnormal vitamin D metabolism

- The commonest cause of failure of 1α-hydroxylase is renal failure.
- Congenital absence of this enzyme leads to a condition known as VDDR type I.
- AR inheritance.
- Leads to profound rickets, with myopathy and enamel hypoplasia.
- Very large doses of calciferol are needed to heal the bone lesions which, in contrast, will respond to physiological doses of alfacalcidol or calcitriol.

(In practice, liver disease seldom results in clinical problems of vitamin D metabolism.)

Table 6.7 Diagnosis of osteomalacia

	Ca	PO₄	ALP	25OHD	1,25(OH)2D	PTH	Other
Vitamin D deficiency	↓	↓	↑	↓	↓	↑	
Renal failure	↓	↑	↑	N	↓	↑	↓ GFR
VDDR type I (deficient 1α-hydroxylase)	↓	↓	↑	N	↓	↑	
VDDR type II (deficient vitamin D receptor)	↓	↓	↑	N	↑	↑	
X-linked hypophosphataemia (vitamin D-resistant rickets)	N	↓	↑	N	N	N or ↑	
Oncogenic	N or ↓	↓	↑	N	↓	N	May have aminoaciduria, proteinuria
PO₄ depletion	N	↓	↑	N	↑	N	↑ urine Ca
Fanconi syndrome	↓ or N	↓	↑	N	↑	N	Acidosis, aminoaciduria, glycosuria
Renal tubular acidosis	↓ or N	↓	↑	N	N or ↓	N	Acidosis
Toxic (etidronate, fluoride)	N	N	N	N	N	N	Diagnosed on biopsy

Vitamin D deficiency

Causes

- Poor sunlight exposure:
  - Elderly housebound.
  - Extensive skin coverage with clothes.
  - Darker skin pigmentation.
- Poor diet (especially vegetarians):
  - Malabsorption.
  - ↑ catabolism of vitamin D.
- 2° hyperparathyroidism:
  - Malabsorption.
  - Post-gastrectomy.
  - Enzyme-inducing drugs, e.g. phenytoin.

Investigation

- Characteristic biochemical abnormalities (see Box 6.13).
- Frank osteomalacia is usually associated with very low levels of 25OHD (<15nmol/L).
- Elevated PTH (2° hyperparathyroidism).
- Associated 2° hyperparathyroidism frequently results in normal, or even elevated, concentrations of $1,25(OH)_2D$.

Treatment

- Calciferol is preferred (not active metabolites of vitamin D) to restore body stores, correct biochemical abnormalities, and heal bony abnormalities.
- In adults, treatment can be given as a daily dose of calciferol (800 (20 micrograms)–4000IU (100 micrograms)). This can be administered in combination with a Ca supplement. Alternative oral regimens with less frequent dose administration can also be considered. IM injections of vitamin D are rarely advised; absorption is very variable. If obese, the dose can be ↑ 2- to 3-fold.
- In severe deficiency, 50,000IU can be given weekly for 8 weeks.
- Following treatment, there is usually a steady improvement in myopathy and bone pain, and biochemical abnormalities may not fully settle for several months.
- Following the onset of therapy, markers of bone turnover, such as ALP, might even show a transient increase, as the osteoid is mineralized and remodelled. (The BP directs that when calciferol is prescribed or demanded, colecalciferol or ergocalciferol should be dispensed or supplied.)

Further reading

Bouillon R (2020). Safety of high-dose vitamin D supplementation. *J Clin Endocrinol Metab* **105**, 1290.

Hypophosphataemia

- PO_4 is important for normal mineralization of bone.
- In the absence of sufficient PO_4 in the long term, osteomalacia can occur.
- Clinically, osteomalacia is usually indistinguishable from other causes, although there may be features that will help distinguish the underlying cause of hypophosphataemia.
- PO_4 is important in its own right for neuromuscular function, and profound hypophosphataemia can be accompanied by encephalopathy, muscle weakness, and cardiomyopathy.
- As PO_4 is primarily an intracellular anion, low plasma PO_4 does not necessarily represent actual PO_4 depletion.
- Fasting levels of PO_4 give a more accurate idea of hypophosphataemia.
- Several different causes of hypophosphataemia are recognized (see Box 6.14).

X-linked hypophosphataemia

- X-linked dominant genetic disorder.
- Severe rickets and osteomalacia.
- Mutation of an endopeptidase gene (*PHEX*).

Clinical features

- Abnormal PO_4 levels are often detected early in infancy, but skeletal deformities are not apparent until walking commences.
- Typical severe rickets, with short stature and bony deformity.
- Continues into adult life, with bone pain, deformity, and fracture in the absence of treatment.
- Proximal myopathy is absent.
- Adults suffer from excessive new bone growth, particularly affecting entheses and the longitudinal ligaments of the spinal canal. This can cause spinal cord compression which may need surgical decompression.

Oncogenic osteomalacia

- Certain tumours produce fibroblast growth factor 23 (FGF23), which is phosphaturic.
- Rare and usually occurs with mesenchymal tumours (such as haemangiopericytomas, haemangiomata, or osteoid tumours) but has also been reported with a variety of adenocarcinomas (particularly prostatic cancer) and haematological malignancies (e.g. myeloma and chronic lymphocytic leukaemia). A similar picture can also be seen in some cases of NF.
- Clinically, such patients usually present with profound myopathy, as well as bone pain and fractures.
- Biochemically, the major abnormality is hypophosphataemia, but this is usually accompanied by marked reduction in $1,25(OH)_2D$ concentrations.
- In some patients, other abnormalities of renal tubular function, such as glycosuria or aminoaciduria, are also present.

- FGF23 levels are elevated and fall with tumour removal. Causal tumours are potentially difficult to localize, but CT, MRI, PET, and nuclear medicine approaches such as DOTATATE PET/CT have all been employed successfully to identify the underlying causal tumour. Selective venous catheterization for FGF23 may also a play role. Medical treatment can help symptoms while seeking an underlying cause and may include supplemental PO_4 with activated vitamin D analogues. Complete removal of the tumour results in rapid resolution of the biochemical and skeletal abnormalities. If this is not possible or if a causal tumour is not identified, treatment with vitamin D metabolites and PO_4 supplements (as for X-linked hypophosphataemia; see ➔ X- linked hypophosphataemia, p. 538) may help the skeletal symptoms.

Fanconi syndrome

- Fanconi syndrome is a combination of renal tubular defects that can result from several different pathologies.
- In particular, there is renal wasting of PO_4, bicarbonate, glucose, and amino acids.
- The combination of hypophosphataemia with renal tubular acidosis means that osteomalacia is a frequent accompaniment. This can be exacerbated by defective 1α-hydroxylation of vitamin D to its active form.
- The osteomalacia is treated by correction of the relevant abnormalities. This might involve the administration of PO_4, alkali, or $1,25(OH)_2D$ (calcitriol), depending on the precise circumstances.

Treatment of hypophosphataemia

The mainstay is PO_4 replacement, usually Phosphate-Sandoz®—each tablet provides 500mg of PO_4. Ideally, patients should receive 2–3g of PO_4 daily between meals, but this is not easy to achieve. PO_4 preparations are unpalatable and are osmotic purgatives, causing diarrhoea. Slow uptitration can be helpful to mitigate this effect. Long-term administration of PO_4 supplements stimulates parathyroid activity.

This can lead to hypercalcaemia and a further fall in PO_4, with worsening of bone disease due to the development of hyperparathyroid bone disease, which may necessitate parathyroidectomy. To minimize parathyroid stimulation, it is usual to give one of the active metabolites of vitamin D in conjunction with PO_4. Typically, alfacalcidol or calcitriol in a dose of 1–2 micrograms daily is used. Patients receiving such supraphysiological doses of vitamin D metabolites are at continued risk of hypercalcaemia and require regular monitoring of plasma Ca, preferably at least every 3 months. In adults, active treatment for X-linked hypophosphataemia is probably confined to symptomatic bone disease.

- There is little evidence that it will improve the long-term outcome.
- Some evidence suggests that treatment might accelerate new bone formation.
  - In children, conventional treatment is usually given in the hope of improving final height and minimizing skeletal abnormality—the evidence that it is possible to achieve these goals is conflicting.
  - Most recently, burosumab, a monoclonal antibody drug that targets and inhibits FGF23, has been shown to be effective in children in improving renal tubular PO_4 reabsorption, serum PO_4, linear growth, and physical function, with a reduction in pain and severity of rickets.[1]

Box 6.14 Causes of hypophosphataemia

Decreased intestinal absorption
- PO_4-binding antacids.
- Malabsorption.
- Starvation/malnutrition.

Increased renal losses
- Hyperparathyroidism:
  - 1°.
  - 2°, e.g. in vitamin D deficiency.
- Renal tubular defects:
  - Fanconi syndrome.
- X-linked hypophosphataemia.
- Tumour-induced osteomalacia.
- Alcohol abuse.
- Poorly controlled DM.
- Acidosis.
- Drugs:
  - Intravenous iron infusion
  - Diuretics.
  - Corticosteroids.
  - Calcitonin.

Shift into cells
- Septicaemia.
- Insulin treatment.
- Glucose administration.
- Salicylate poisoning.
- Catecholamine.
- Hyperventilation.

References

1. Carpenter TO, et al. (2018). Burosumab therapy in children with X-linked hypophosphatemia. *N Engl J Med* **378**, 1987–98.

Further reading

Christov M, Jüppner H (2018). Phosphate homeostasis disorders. *Best Pract Res Clin Endocrinol Metab* **32**, 685–706.

Hassan-Smith ZK, et al. (2017). Effect of vitamin D deficiency in developed countries. *Br Med Bull* **122**,79–89.

Metabolic Support UK. [Charity for patients with rare inherited metabolic disorders]. ℳ https:// www.metabolicsupportuk.org/

Rayamajhi SJ, et al. (2019). Tumor-induced osteomalacia: current imaging modalities and a systematic approach for tumor localization. *Clin Imaging* **56**, 114–23.

Royal Osteoporosis Society. [UK charity supporting patients with osteoporosis and promoting bone health for all]. ℳ https://theros.org.uk/

XLH Network. [Support network for those with X-linked hypophosphataemic rickets]. ℳ https:// xlhnetwork.org/

Yuzamp N, et al. (2020). The game is afoot. *N Engl J Med* **382**, 2249.

Hypomagnesaemia

- Low plasma Mg levels are common in acutely ill patients. Clinical manifestations of this are not common.
- In the presence of Mg deficiency, PTH secretion is inhibited and the peripheral action of PTH is also attenuated.
- Symptoms:
  - Neuromuscular excitability, muscular weakness, which is virtually indistinguishable from that associated with hypocalcaemia, which frequently coexists. Arrhythmias can also occur, as can coma.
- Signs:
  - +ve Chvostek's and Trousseau's signs are seen.
- Biochemistry:
  - Associated with hypocalcaemia and hypokalaemia.
  - Hypomagnesaemia-induced hypocalcaemia will not respond to Ca treatment unless the Mg deficiency is corrected first.
  - Hypokalaemia is also frequently seen in association with hypomagnesaemia. Treatment with potassium supplementation is often unsuccessful, unless Mg is replaced at the same time.

(See Box 6.15 for causes.)

Tip

PPI-induced hypomagnesaemia is now well recognized and usually presents with serum Mg <0.3mmol/L, and sometimes profound hypocalcaemia on a background of longer-term PPI use and a possible intercurrent diarrhoeal illness. Once established as a diagnosis, PPIs should be avoided as future use will almost inevitably result in recurrent hypomagnesaemia.

Treatment

Symptomatic Mg deficiency, especially if associated with hypocalcaemia or hypokalaemia, requires parenteral treatment.

- Magnesium sulfate 50% solution contains ~2mmol Mg/mL. This should be administered IV, although IM is feasible but painful. An initial 4–8mmol should be given over 15min, followed by a slow infusion of 1mmol/h. The rate of infusion can be adjusted in light of the response in plasma Mg.
- In the presence of renal impairment, plasma Mg can rise quickly, so care must be undertaken if Mg infusion is contemplated in the presence of renal failure.
- After repletion has been achieved IV, or in less severe cases, treatment can be continued PO.
- Various salts of Mg have been used, including chloride, oxide, and glycerophosphate. Dosing is frequently limited by the purgative properties of Mg salts.

Box 6.15 Causes of hypomagnesaemia

- GI losses:
  - Vomiting.
  - Diarrhoea.
  - Losses from fistulae.
  - Malabsorption.
- Renal losses:
  - Chronic parenteral therapy.
  - Osmotic diuresis.
  - Gitelman's syndrome (see ➲ Gitelman's syndrome, p. 284)
- DM.
- Drugs:
  - Alcohol.
  - Loop diuretics.
  - PPIs.
  - Aminoglycosides.
  - Cisplatin.
  - Ciclosporin.
  - Amphotericin.
- Metabolic acidosis.
- Hypercalcaemia.
- Other causes:
  - PO_4 depletion.
  - Hungry bone syndrome.

Further reading

Ayuk J, Gittoes NJ (2014). Contemporary view of the clinical relevance of magnesium homeostasis. *Ann Clin Biochem* **51**, 179–88.

Osteoporosis

Introduction

- Osteoporosis:
  - Refers to reduction in the amount of bony tissue within the skeleton.
  - Generally associated with a loss of structural integrity of the internal architecture of the bone.
  - Combination of both these changes leads to high risk of fracture, even after trivial injury.
- Commonest osteoporotic fractures:
  - Hip.
  - Wrist (Colles').
  - Compression fractures of vertebral bodies.
  - Patients who fracture ribs, the upper humerus, leg, and pelvis also have a higher incidence of osteoporosis.

Over recent years, there has been a change in focus in the treatment of osteoporosis.

- Historically: 1° reliance on BMD as a threshold for treatment.
- Currently: greater emphasis on assessing individual patients' risk of fracture that incorporates multiple clinical risk factors, as well as BMD.

Causes

(See Box 6.16.)

Box 6.16 Underlying causes of osteoporosis

- Gonadal failure:
  - Premature menopause (age <45).
  - Hypogonadism in men.
  - Turner syndrome.
- Conditions leading to amenorrhoea, with low oestrogen (persisting >6 months):
  - Hyperprolactinaemia.
  - Anorexia nervosa.
  - HA.
- Endocrine disorders:
  - Cushing's syndrome.
  - GH deficiency.
  - Hyperparathyroidism.
  - Acromegaly with hypogonadism.
  - Hyperthyroidism (within 3 years).
  - DM.
- GI disorders:
  - Malabsorption.
  - Post-gastrectomy.
  - Coeliac disease.
  - Crohn's disease.
- Liver disease:
  - Cholestasis.
  - Cirrhosis.

- Neoplastic disorders:
  - Multiple myeloma.
  - Systemic mastocytosis.
- Inflammatory conditions:
  - Rheumatoid arthritis.
  - CF.
- Nutritional disorders:
  - Parenteral nutrition.
  - Lactose intolerance.
- Drugs:
  - Systemic GCs.
  - Heparin (when given long term, particularly in pregnancy).
  - Chemotherapy (primarily through gonadal damage).
  - GnRH agonists.
  - Ciclosporin (high PTH).
  - Anticonvulsants (long-term).
  - Aromatase inhibitors for breast cancer.
  - Androgen deprivation therapy (prostate cancer).
  - PPIs.
  - SSRIs.
- Metabolic abnormalities:
  - Homocystinuria.
- Hereditary disorders.
  - Osteogenesis imperfecta.
  - Marfan's syndrome.
  - Hajdu–Cheney syndrome (AD), with marked bone loss (acroosteolysis with osteoporosis and changes in skull and mandible).

Pathology of osteoporosis

Osteoporosis may arise from failure of the body to lay down sufficient bone during growth and maturation, an earlier than usual onset of bone loss following maturity, or an ↑ rate of that loss.

(See Table 6.8 for definitions, and Box 6.17 for causes.)

Peak bone mass

- Mainly genetically determined:
  - Racial effects (bone mass higher in Afro-Caribbeans and lower in Caucasians).
  - Family influence on the risk of osteoporosis—may account for 70% of variation.
  - So far, >15 separate genetic associations with fracture described.
- Also influenced by environmental factors:
  - Exercise—particularly weight-bearing.
  - Nutrition—especially Ca.
- Exposure to oestrogen is also important:
  - Early menopause or late puberty (in ♂ or ♀) is associated with ↑ risk of osteoporosis.

Early onset of loss

- Early menopause (= 45 years).
- Conditions leading to bone loss, e.g. GC therapy.

Increased net loss

- Ageing:
  - Vitamin D insufficiency.
  - Declining bone formation.
  - Declining renal function.
- Underlying disease states (see Box 6.16).

Lifestyle factors affecting bone mass

Increase

- Weight-bearing exercise.

Decrease

- Smoking.
- Excessive alcohol.
- Nulliparity.
- Poor Ca nutrition.

Table 6.8 WHO definitions for osteoporosis and low bone mass

T score	Fragility fracture	Diagnosis
−1		Normal
<−1 but >−2.5		Low bone mass (osteopenia)
≤−2.5	No	Osteoporosis
≤−2.5	Yes	Established (severe) osteoporosis

Box 6.17 Causes of increased bone mineral density

Artefacts
- Excess skeletal Ca.
- Extraskeletal Ca.
- Vertebral fracture.
- Radiodense material.

Generalized increase
- Acquired osteosclerosis, e.g. renal osteodystrophy, fluorosis, mastocytosis, myelofibrosis, acromegaly.

Focal increase in bone
- Paget's.
- Tumours.

Genetic
- Sclerosing bone dysplasias.
- ↓ absorption, e.g. osteopetrosis.
- ↑ absorption, e.g. sclerosteosis, *LRP5* mutation.

Epidemiology of osteoporosis

- Age: ↑ risk of osteoporotic fracture with age.
- Sex: fracture rates in ♂ are approximately half of those seen in ♀ of the same age.
- A ♀ aged 50 has ~1:2 chance of sustaining an osteoporotic fracture in the rest of her life.
- A ♂ aged 50 has ~1:5 chance of sustaining an osteoporotic fracture in the rest of his life.
- In the UK, each year, in ♀:
  - >25,000 vertebral fractures come to clinical attention.
  - >40,000 wrist fractures.
  - >50,000 hip fractures—these are a particular health challenge, as they invariably result in hospital admission.
  - One-fifth of hip fracture victims will die within 6 months of the injury, and only 50% will return to their previous level of independence.
- Estimated overall cost of osteoporotic fractures in the UK is £2.1 billion annually.

(See Box 6.18 for investigations.)

Box 6.18 Investigations to consider an underlying cause of osteoporosis

Useful in most patients
- FBC.
- ESR.
- Ca, PO₄, ALP.
- Cr and eGFR.
- Liver function (gamma glutamyl transferase (GGT)).
- Thyroid function (TSH).
- Testosterone and LH (only in ♂).
- Vitamin D.
- PTH.

Useful in specific instances
- Oestradiol and FSH (in ♀ where menopausal status not clear).
- Serum and urine electrophoresis (if raised ESR or plasma globulin elevated).
- Anti-tissue transglutaminase antibodies (if any suggestion of coeliac disease).
- 24h urine Ca excretion (to detect idiopathic hypercalciuria).
- Other investigations for specific diseases.

Low-trauma fractures associated with osteoporosis
Any fracture, other than those affecting the fingers, toes, or face, which is caused by a fall from standing height or less, is called a fragility (low-trauma) fracture, and underlying osteoporosis should be considered. Patients suffering such a fracture should be considered for investigation and/or treatment for osteoporosis.

Presentation of osteoporosis

- Usually clinically silent until an acute fracture.
- Two-thirds of vertebral fractures do not come to clinical attention.
- Typical vertebral fracture:
  - Sudden episode of well-localized pain.
  - May, or may not, have been related to injury or exertion.
  - May be radiation of the pain in a girdle distribution.
  - Pain may initially require bed rest but gradually subsides over 4–8 weeks; even after this time, there may be residual pain at the fracture site.
  - Osteoporotic vertebral fractures only rarely lead to neurological impairment.
- Any evidence of spinal cord compression should prompt a search for malignancy or other underlying cause.
- Following vertebral fracture, a patient may be left with persistent back pain, kyphosis, or height loss.
- Although height loss and kyphosis are often thought of as being indicative of osteoporosis, they are more frequently the result of degenerative disease, including disc disease. These changes cannot be attributed to osteoporosis in the absence of vertebral fractures.
- Peripheral fractures are common in osteoporosis.
- If a bone breaks from a fall from less than standing height, this represents a low-trauma fracture which might indicate underlying osteoporosis.
- Osteoporosis does not cause generalized skeletal pain.

Investigation of osteoporosis

Establish the diagnosis

- Plain radiographs are useful for determining the presence of fracture. Apart from this, they are of little utility in the diagnosis of osteoporosis. Bone density cannot be assessed reliably from a plain radiograph.
- *Bone densitometry.* In order to identify the presence of T score-defined osteoporosis, it is important to measure BMD appropriately. This is usually carried out at the hip and lumbar spine, using DXA. The presence of degenerative disease or arterial calcification can elevate the apparent bone density of the spine without adding to skeletal strength. ↑ reliance is therefore being placed on measurements derived from the hip. The diagnostic criteria for osteoporosis have been derived through the WHO (see Table 6.8).
- Biochemical markers of bone turnover may be helpful in the calculation of fracture risk and in judging the response to drug therapies, but they have no role in the diagnosis of osteoporosis.
- Use of fracture risk algorithms is now available to determine individuals' fracture risk (e.g. ℘ http://www.shef.ac.uk/FRAX). Such an approach can help tune therapies to those patients at heightened risk of fracture.

Exclude underlying causes

An underlying cause for osteoporosis is present in ~10–30% of women and up to 50% of men with osteoporosis. Many of the underlying causes (see Box 6.18) should be apparent from a careful history and physical examination. A few basic investigations are useful to exclude the commoner underlying conditions. Other investigations may be needed to exclude other specific conditions.

It is helpful to target investigations at those people who have a significantly lower than expected bone mass for their age (Z score <−2).

Monitoring therapy

- Repeat bone densitometry is helpful for monitoring.
- Minimum time interval should be 2 years between scans.
- Effective treatment leads to modest rise (~5% at spine) in bone density.
- Biochemical markers of bone turnover may be helpful (e.g. P1NP, CTX, and NTX), usually taken at baseline and after 3–6 months (see Table 6.9).

(See Table 6.10 for efficacy for types of treatments.)

Table 6.9 Biochemical markers and their expected decrease with satisfactory treatment

Measurement	Matrix	Reflects	Desired decrease
PINP	Serum	Formation	>25%
CTX	Plasma	Resorption	>25%
NTX	Urine	Resorption	>25%

Table 6.10 Grade of evidence of anti-fracture efficacy of approved treatments for post-menopausal women with osteoporosis (when given with calcium + vitamin D)

Treatment	Vertebral fracture	Non-vertebral fracture	Hip fracture
Alendronic acid	A	A	A
Ibandronic acid*	A	A	NAE
Risedronate	A	A	A
Zoledronic acid	A	A	A
Denosumab	A	A	A
Calcitriol	A	B	NAE
Raloxifene	A	NAE	NAE
Teriparatide	A	A	NAE
HRT	A	A	A

A, grade level of evidence A (high-quality evidence); B, grade level of evidence B (moderate-quality evidence); HRT, hormone replacement therapy; NAE, not adequately evaluated.

* In subsets of patients only.

Treatment of osteoporosis

Treatments should be considered according to their effect on fracture risk reduction and side effect profile.

In addition to pharmacological treatments aimed at reducing fracture risk, it must be remembered that non-pharmacological measures are also important. Thus, it is prudent to minimize the risk of falling by adjusting the home environment and reviewing the need for medications, such as hypnotics and antihypertensives, for instance.

Lifestyle measures

- Stop smoking.
- Avoid alcohol excess.
- Encourage weight-bearing exercise:
  - Lower-impact exercise, e.g. walking outdoors for 20min three times weekly, may reduce fracture risk.
- Encourage well-balanced diet.
- Ensure adequate Ca and vitamin D intake.
- If necessary, give supplements to achieve Ca intake of ~1g daily.

Choice of therapy and who to treat

The Endocrine Society guidelines propose that we treat patients who have had a prior hip or spine fracture, patients with a BMD T score of −2.5 or less at the spine or hip, and patients with a high 10-year risk of major or hip fractures. The latter information can be obtained by going to the FRAX website (𝕊 https://www.sheffield.ac.uk/FRAX/).

The commonest treatment is alendronic acid given as 70mg once a week before breakfast, with a full glass of water, with a recommendation not to eat for at least 30min. This can give rise to dyspepsia and so might need to be changed to another bisphosphonate, e.g. risedronate, or to a different route of administration (e.g. IV zoledronic acid) or a different class (e.g. denosumab). If a fracture occurs during treatment or if monitoring shows no response, then again consider an alternative agent. If the fracture is a vertebral fracture, then consider teriparatide. If the oral bisphosphonate is well tolerated and the patient has completed 5 years, then it is usual to check the fracture risk; if it is relatively low (e.g. T score >−2.5), then a drug holiday of up to 5 years is recommended.

In premenopausal women, we are careful not to use bisphosphonates unless there have been fractures, as these drugs can cross the placenta. There is no upper age limit to the use of these drugs.

(See Box 6.19 for vertebroplasty.)

Glucocorticoid-induced osteoporosis

GC treatment is one of the major 2° causes of osteoporosis. Not all patients receiving steroid treatment do lose bone, and it is not clear what determines this. Patients who sustain fractures while taking GCs do so at higher bone density levels than in post-menopausal women, leading to the assertion that such patients should be treated at a higher bone density (T score <−1.5) than would be the case for post-menopausal osteoporosis. The risk is assessed using FRAX, with minor adjustments if the dose of prednisolone is >7.5mg daily.

Box 6.19 Vertebroplasty

- Percutaneous injection of bone cement into the fractured vertebral body.
- Effective at resolving pain in the short and longer term.
- Best for patients with acute fractures and persistent pain (>6 weeks).

Complications of therapy for osteoporosis

(See Boxes 6.20 and 6.21 for special considerations.)

HRT

- Because of adverse effects (breast cancer, VTE, coronary disease, and stroke), HRT is no longer regarded as a 1° treatment for osteoporosis in post-menopausal ♀.
- When a woman is receiving HRT for climacteric symptoms, however, there will be a beneficial effect on fracture risk reduction.
- Skeletal protection is rapidly lost on cessation of HRT.
- In ♀ with premature menopause, HRT remains the most appropriate means of preventing bone loss in the absence of other contraindications.

Bisphosphonates

- Weekly (PO), daily (PO), monthly (PO), 3-monthly (IV), and annual (IV) preparations are available.
- Drugs work by inhibiting the enzyme farnesyl pyrophosphate synthase and inhibiting osteoclasts; hence, there is a reduction in bone turnover and bone loss is prevented.
- Oral preparations require patients to follow strict dosing instructions. Oral bisphosphonates should be taken on an empty stomach, and 30–60min (dependent on drug) should pass prior to additional oral intake.
- GI disturbance, including nausea and oesophagitis, are common.
- Osteonecrosis of the jaw is a very rare side effect of bisphosphonates in doses given to treat osteoporosis (<0.5%).
- Flu-like symptoms occur in 20–30%, following IV administration of zoledronate (acute phase response commoner in younger patients).
- There is an association with atypical femoral fractures (affecting the shaft and subtrochanteric regions of the femur) in patients who have taken bisphosphonates for >5 years (3.2–5/100,000 person-years).
- If treated for 5 years, consider therapeutic holiday, unless T score worse than –2.5 at the hips or with existing history of vertebral fractures.

Calcium and vitamin D

- Constipation.
- Recent reports have raised queries of a link between exogenous Ca supplementation and ↑ risk of CVD.

Raloxifene

- Similar increase in risk of venous thrombosis as HRT.
- May induce/worsen climacteric symptoms.
- Reduces risk of breast cancer.
- Reduces the risk of vertebral fractures only, not other fractures.

Denosumab

- Effective for at least 10 years. It is an effective alternative to bisphosphonates.
- Drugs work by inhibiting RANK (receptor activator of nuclear factor kappa-B) ligand, and thus inhibiting osteoclasts; hence, there is a reduction in bone turnover and bone loss is prevented.
- Skin infections/eczema.
- Hypocalcaemia (ensure Ca and vitamin D levels normal prior).
- Always follow treatment with an alternative, otherwise an ↑ risk of multiple vertebral fractures.

Teriparatide

- Contraindications: hypercalcaemia, renal impairment, unexplained elevation of ALP—Paget's disease, prior irradiation.
- The drug works by stimulating bone formation with only a small increase in bone resorption; hence, there is a large increase in BMD.
- It is used in patients who have low or very low BMD and who have had vertebral fractures on treatment with alendronic acid.
- Risk of hypercalcaemia is not great, and no specific monitoring of treatment is recommended.
- Vomiting.
- Leg cramps.
- ↑ risk of osteosarcoma seen in rats given teriparatide for most of their life. It should be avoided in patients with ↑ risk of bone tumours (Paget's disease, raised ALP, previous skeletal radiotherapy).
- Always follow treatment with an antiresorptive drug such as bisphosphonates, denosumab, or raloxifene; otherwise, the improvement is reversed.

Romosozumab

- This drug works by inhibiting sclerostin and, as a result, is both anabolic (↑ formation) and antiresorptive.
- The drug has been licensed, but at the time of writing, it has not been considered by NICE.
- It is used for a 1-year course and is followed by an antiresorptive drug such as alendronic acid or denosumab.
- It increases the risk of MI and stroke and so should not be used in patients who have already suffered from these illnesses.

Box 6.20 Special considerations in men

- 2° causes of osteoporosis are commoner in ♂ and need to be excluded in all ♂ with osteoporotic fracture.
- Bisphosphonates benefit bone mass in ♂ in a similar way to post-menopausal ♀.
- Hypogonadal ♂ show an improvement in bone mass on testosterone replacement. However, hypogonadal ♂ respond to bisphosphonates as do those with normal testosterone levels. Replacement testosterone, along with bisphosphonate therapy, is appropriate.

Box 6.21 Special considerations in premenopausal women

- 'Osteoporosis' in premenopausal ♀ is rare, but well recognized.
- Younger women have a lower risk of fracture.
- It is important to exclude underlying causes of accelerated rates of bone loss.
- Osteoporosis can very rarely occur in conjunction with pregnancy or lactation. This is frequently self-limiting and usually requires little treatment other than Ca supplementation.
- In the absence of a pre-existing fracture, fracture risk is low. Advice regarding +ve lifestyle factors is always prudent. Further assessment should be made around the age of natural menopause.
- In other situations, particularly where low-trauma fractures have occurred, other therapies may be carefully considered, recognizing there are no data to support the use of anti-fracture drugs in premenopausal women.
- Some caution needs to be exercised over the use of bisphosphonates in younger people:
  - Teratogenic in animals.
  - Long skeletal retention time.
  - In such patients, it may be worth considering alternative agents such as calcitriol.

In general, the management of premenopausal women with osteoporosis and high fracture risk should be assessed by a clinician with a specialist interest in metabolic bone diseases.

Further reading

Barrionuevo P, et al. (2019). Efficacy of pharmacological therapies for the prevention of fractures in postmenopausal women: a network meta-analysis. *J Clin Endocrinol Metab* **104**, 1623–30.

Black DM, et al. (2018). Atypical femur fractures: review of epidemiology, relationship to bisphosphonates, prevention, and clinical management. *Endocr Rev* **40**, 333–68.

Black DM, et al. (2020). Atypical femur fracture risk versus fragility fracture prevention with bisphosphonates. *N Engl J Med* **383**, 743–53.

Bone HG, et al. (2017). 10 years of denosumab treatment in postmenopausal women with osteoporosis: results from the phase 3 randomised FREEDOM trial and open-label extension. *Lancet Diabetes Endocrinol* **5**, 513–23.

Compston J, et al.; National Osteoporosis Guideline Group (NOGG) (2017). UK clinical guideline for the prevention and treatment of osteoporosis. *Arch Osteoporos* **12**, 43.

Compston JE, et al. (2019). Osteoporosis. *Lancet* **393**, 364.

Cosman F, et al.; National Osteoporosis Foundation (2014). Clinician's guide to prevention and treatment of osteoporosis. *Osteoporos Int* **25**, 2359–81.

Cosman F, et al. (2016). Romosozumab treatment in postmenopausal women with osteoporosis. *N Engl J Med* **375**, 1532.

Eastell R, et al. (2016). Postmenopausal osteoporosis. *Nat Rev Dis Primers* **2**, 16069.

Eastell R, et al. (2018). Diagnosis of endocrine disease: bone turnover markers: are they clinically useful? *Eur J Endocrinol* **178**, R19–31.

Eastell R, et al. (2019). Pharmacological management of osteoporosis in postmenopausal women: an Endocrine Society clinical practice guideline. *J Clin Endocrinol Metab* **104**, 1595–622.

Khan AA, et al. (2015). Diagnosis and management of osteonecrosis of the jaw: a systematic review and international consensus. *J Bone Miner Res* **30**, 3–23.

Marom R (2020). Osteogenesis imperfecta: an update on clinical features and therapies. *Eur J Endocrinol* **183**, R95–106.

Rachner T, *et al.* (2019). Novel therapies in osteoporosis: PTH-related peptide analogs and inhibitors of sclerostin. *J Mol Endocrinol* **62**, R145–54.

Saag KG, *et al.* (2017). Romosozumab or alendronate for fracture prevention in women with osteoporosis. *N Engl J Med* **377**, 1417–27.

Shoback D, *et al.* (2020). Pharmacological management of osteoporosis in postmenopausal women: an Endocrine Society guideline update. *J Clin Endocrinol Metab* **105**, 587–94.

Tsourdi E, *et al.* (2017). Discontinuation of denosumab therapy for osteoporosis: a systematic review and position statement by ECTS. *Bone* **105**, 11–17.

Paget's disease

Paget's disease is the result of greatly ↑ local bone turnover, which occurs particularly in the elderly but can affect younger people.

Pathology

- The 1° abnormality in Paget's disease is gross overactivity of the osteoclasts, resulting in greatly ↑ bone resorption. This secondarily results in ↑ osteoblastic activity. The new bone is laid down in a highly disorganized manner and leads to the characteristic pagetic abnormality, with irregular packets of woven bone being apparent on biopsy and a disorganized internal architecture of the bone on plain radiographs.
- Paget's disease can affect any bone in the skeleton but is most frequently found in the pelvis, vertebral column, femur, skull, and tibia. In most patients, it affects several sites, but in about 20% of cases, a single bone is affected (monostotic disease). Typically, the disease will start in one end of a long bone and spread along the bone at a rate of about 1cm per year. Although it can spread within an affected bone, it appears that the pattern of disease is fixed by the time of clinical presentation and it is exceedingly rare for new bones to become involved during the course of the disease.
- Paget's disease alters the mechanical properties of the bone. Thus, pagetic bones are more likely to bend under normal physiological loads and are thus liable to fracture. This can take the form of complete fractures, which tend to be transverse, rather than the commoner spiral fractures of long bones. More frequently, fissure or incremental fractures are seen on the convex surface of bowed pagetic bones. These may be painful in their own right but are also liable to proceed to complete fracture. Pagetic bones are also larger than their normal counterparts. This can lead to ↑ arthritis at adjacent joints and to pressure on nerves, leading to neurological compression syndromes and, when it occurs in the skull base, sensorineural deafness.

Aetiology

Unclear. There are two major theories:
- Familial:
  - Some genetic associations, especially with a sequestasome-1 mutation.
  - These are not invariable.
- Viral:
  - Inclusion bodies, similar to those seen in viral infections, have been identified in osteoclasts from patients with Paget's.
  - Some workers have found paramyxoviral (measles or canine distemper) protein or nucleic acid in pagetic bone; others have not been able to replicate this.

Epidemiology

Paget's disease is present in about 2% of the UK population over the age of 55. Its prevalence increases with age, and it is commoner in ♂ than in ♀. Only about 10% of affected patients will have symptomatic disease. It is commonest in the UK or in migrants of British descent in North America and Australasia, but rare in Africa. Studies in the UK and New Zealand have suggested that the prevalence may be declining with time.

Clinical features

- 90% asymptomatic.
- Most notable feature is pain. This is frequently multifactorial:
  - ↑ metabolic activity of the bone.
  - Changes in bone shape.
  - Fissure fractures.
  - Nerve compression.
  - Arthritis.
- Pagetic bones tend to increase in size or become bowed (16% of cases)—bowing can be so severe as to interfere with function.
- Fractures (either complete or fissure) present in 10%.
- Risk of osteosarcoma is ↑ in active Paget's disease but is a very rare finding.

Investigation

The diagnosis of Paget's disease is primarily radiological.

Radiological features

- Early disease—primarily lytic:
  - V-shaped 'cutting cone' in long bones.
  - Osteoporosis circumscripta in skull.
- Combined phase (mixed lytic and sclerotic):
  - Cortical thickening.
  - Loss of corticomedullary distinction.
  - Accentuated trabecular markings.
- Late phase—primarily sclerotic:
  - Thickening of long bones.
  - Increase in bone size.
  - Sclerosis.

An isotope bone scan is frequently helpful in assessing the extent of skeletal involvement with Paget's disease. It is particularly important to identify Paget's disease in a weight-bearing bone because of the risk of fracture. The uptake of tracer depends on the disease activity, and isotope bone scans can also be used to assess the response to therapy.

In active disease, plasma ALP activity is usually (85%) elevated. An exception to this is in monostotic disease when there may be insufficient bone involved to raise the enzyme levels above normal. ALP activity responds to successful treatment. There is little advantage in using the more modern markers of bone turnover over total ALP activity for the monitoring of pagetic activity, except in mild disease (monostotic Paget's) or else concomitant liver disease.

Complications

- Deafness is present in up to half of cases of skull base Paget's.
- Other neurological complications are rare. These can include:
  - Compression of other cranial nerves with skull base disease.
  - *Spinal cord compression.* Commonest with involvement of the thoracic spine and is thought to result as much from a vascular steal syndrome as from physical compression. It frequently responds to medical therapy without the need for surgical decompression.
  - Platybasia which can lead to obstructive hydrocephalus that may require surgical drainage.

- Osteogenic sarcoma:
  - Very rare complication of Paget's disease.
  - Rarely amenable to treatment.
  - Presents with ↑ pain/radiological evidence of tumour, mass, and very elevated ALP.
- Any increase of pain in a patient with Paget's disease should arouse suspicion of sarcomatous degeneration. A commoner cause, however, is resumption of activity of disease.

Pagetic sarcomas are most frequently found in the humerus or femur but can affect any bone involved with Paget's disease.

Treatment

It is usual to treat a patient who suffers from pain as a result of Paget's disease. Treatment is also effective for patients with neurological complications of Paget's disease such as spinal steal syndrome.

Treatment with agents that decrease bone turnover reduces disease activity, as indicated by bone turnover markers and isotope bone scans. Bisphosphonates are the most commonly used drugs, and the most effective of these is zoledronic acid. There is evidence to suggest that such treatment leads to deposition of histologically normal bone. Although such treatment has been shown to help pain, there is little evidence that it benefits the other consequences of Paget's disease. In particular, the deafness of Paget's disease does not regress after treatment. Guidelines recommend that bisphosphonates are effective in patients suffering from bone pain.

Goals of treatment
- Minimize symptoms.
- Prevent long-term complications.
- Normalize bone turnover.
- ALP in normal range.
- No actual evidence that treatment achieves these goals.

Monitoring therapy

- Plasma ALP every 6–12 months.
- Clinical assessment.

Re-treat if symptoms recur with objective evidence of disease recurrence (ALP or +ve isotope scan). There is no evidence that treating raised ALP in the absence of symptoms affects the outcome in Paget's.

Further reading

Albagha OM, et al. (2011). Genome-wide association identifies three new susceptibility loci for Paget's disease of bone. *Nat Genet* **43**, 685–9.

Ralston SH, et al. (2019). Diagnosis and management of Paget's disease of bone in adults: a clinical guideline. *J Bone Miner Res* **34**, 579–604.

Singer FR, et al. (2014). Paget's disease of bone: an Endocrine Society clinical practice guideline. *J Clin Endocrinol Metab* **99**, 4408.

Inherited disorders of bone

Osteogenesis imperfecta

- Osteogenesis imperfecta is an inherited form of osteoporosis.
- Vast majority of cases due to a genetic defect in one of the two genes COLIA1 and COLIA2 encoding the α-chain of collagen type I. Several different mutations are recognized, and these produce different clinical pictures; these are generally separated into at least four types (see Table 6.11).

Clinical features

- Osteoporosis and easy fracture.
- ± abnormalities of the teeth (dentinogenesis imperfecta).
- Blue sclerae.
- Hearing loss.
- Hypermobility.

Cardiac valvular lesions

Radiological features include:
- Generalized osteopenia.
- Multiple fractures with deformity.
- Abnormal shape of long bones.
- Wormian bones in skull (accessory skull bones completely surrounded by a suture line).

Diagnosis

- Features described in ➲ Clinical features, p. 562 and family history.
- Analysis of collagen type I genes (detect 90%).
- Three criteria:
  - Three fragility fractures aged <20 years.
  - At least one of: blue sclerae, scoliosis, hearing loss, joint laxity, dentinogenesis imperfecta, and family member.
  - Osteoporosis.

Management

Recent studies have demonstrated that infusions of pamidronate lead to ↑ bone mass and reduced fracture incidence in affected children. Patients with milder disease might only be recognized in adulthood. There is no established role for bisphosphonates in young adults with osteogenesis imperfecta, although each case should be assessed on balance of risk factors for fracture. It is also noteworthy that fracture risk increases steeply with ageing in patients with osteogenesis imperfecta, and thus consideration should be given to interventions, including use of anti-fracture drugs.

Prenatal diagnosis of severe types is possible, and genetic counselling should be offered to all at-risk families.

Further reading

Etich J, et al. (2020). Osteogenesis imperfecta: pathophysiology and therapeutic options. Mol Cell Pediatr **7**, 9.

Marom R, et al. (2020). Osteogenesis imperfecta: an update on clinical features and therapies. Eur J Endocrinol **183**, R95–106.

Table 6.11 Classification of osteogenesis imperfecta

Type	Inheritance	Stature	Teeth	Sclerae	Hearing	Genetic defect
I	AD (mild)	Normal	Normal	Blue	Variable loss	Substitution for glycine in COL1A1
II	AD/AR	Lethal deformity				Rearrangement of COL1A1 and COL1A2
III	AD/AR (progressive deforming)	(Very short, severe scoliosis)	Abnormal	Variable	Loss common	Glycine substitution in COL1A1 and COL1A2
IV	AD	Mild	Abnormal	Normal	Occasional loss	Point mutations in a2(I) or a1(I)

Paediatric endocrinology

Ken Ong and Emile Hendriks

Growth

Regulation of growth

Normal human growth can be divided into three overlapping stages (the Karlberg model), each under the control of different factors:

- *Infancy*. Growth is largely under nutritional regulation, and wide inter-individual variation in rates of growth is seen. Many infants show significant 'catch-up' or 'catch-down' in weight and length, and by 2 years, length is much more predictive of final adult height than at birth.
- *Childhood*. Growth is regulated by GH and thyroxine. It is characterized by alternating periods of mini-growth spurts with intervening stasis, each phase lasting several weeks. However, over years, a child will tend to maintain the same centile position on height charts, with a velocity between the 25th and 75th centiles on height velocity charts.
- *Puberty*. The combination of GH and sex hormones promotes bone maturation and a rapid growth acceleration or 'growth spurt'. In both sexes, oestrogen eventually causes epiphyseal fusion, resulting in the attainment of final height.

Sex differences

Adult heights differ between ♂ and ♀ by, on average, 13cm. However, during childhood, onset of the pubertal growth spurt is earlier in ♀ who are therefore, on average, taller than ♂ between the ages of 10 and 13 years.

Tempo

Within each sex, there may also be marked inter-individual differences in *tempo* of growth (or rate of attainment of final height) and the timing of puberty. Delay or advance of bone maturation is linked with timing of puberty. Constitutional delay in growth and puberty often runs in families, reflecting probable genetic factors. Comparison of *bone age* (estimated from a hand radiograph) with chronological age is therefore an important part of growth assessment.

Final height

Final height is estimated as the height reached when growth velocity slows to <2cm/year and can be confirmed by finding epiphyseal fusion on hand radiograph. Final height is usually largely genetically determined, and a child's target height can be estimated from their parents' heights.

Assessment of growth

Measurement

- From birth to 2 years old, supine length is measured ideally using a measuring board (e.g. Harpenden neonatometer) and two adults to ensure that the child is lying straight with the legs extended.
- From 2 years old, standing height is measured against a wall-mounted or free-standing stadiometer, with the measurer applying moderate upward neck traction and the child looking forward in the horizontal plane.
- To minimize error in the calculation of height velocity (cm/year), height measurements should be taken at least 6 months apart, using the same equipment and ideally by the same person.
- Measurement of *sitting height* and calculation of *leg length* (*standing height − sitting height*) allows an estimate of body proportion.

Growth charts
(See Figs. 7.1 and 7.2.)

Height and weight should be compared to age- and sex-appropriate reference data by plotting values on standard growth charts. This allows identification of the child's height and weight *percentiles*, as well as visualization of the child's growth trajectory based on repeated measurements over time. The Royal College of Paediatrics and Child Health (RCPCH) and the UK government recommend the UK-WHO growth charts, which are based on a combination of international and UK-specific growth data, for use in the UK for children of all backgrounds (℞ https://www.rcpch.ac.uk/resources/growth-charts). Other charts exist for BMI, head circumference, height velocity, sitting height, and leg length, as well as growth in certain disorders (e.g. Turner syndrome).

Mid-parental height
Mid-parental height (MPH) is an estimate of a child's genetic height potential and is calculated as:

[(Mother's height + father's height)/2] + 7cm (for boys) *or* − 7cm (for girls).

MPH is used to estimate a child's expected final height, but there is a wide target range (MPH ± 10cm for boys and ± 8.5cm for girls), and it is more commonly used to assess whether the child's current height percentile is consistent with their genetic expectation. Caveats include the presence of a growth disorder in the parent(s) and families from settings with marked secular trends in growth.

Bone age
Skeletal maturation proceeds in an orderly manner from the 1st appearance of each epiphyseal centre to the fusion of the long bones. From chronological age 3–4 years, bone age may be quantified from radiographs of the left hand and wrist by comparison with standard photographs (e.g. Greulich and Pyle method) or by an individual bone scoring system (e.g. Tanner–Whitehouse method). The difference between bone age and chronological age represents the tempo of growth. Puberty onset occurs approximately at a bone age of 10.5–11 years in girls and 11–11.5 years in boys. Girls reach skeletal maturity at a bone age of 15 years, and boys when bone age is 17 years. Thus, bone age estimates the remaining growth potential.

Final height prediction
Predictions of final height can be derived from information on current height, age, pubertal status, and bone age, using calculations described by Tanner and Whitehouse or Bayley and Pinneau, among others.[1]

Secular trends

Children's height ↑ by >1cm in England and by >2cm in Scotland during the period from 1972 to 1994, and similar trends are seen in many other Western countries. Marked secular trends have been seen in some countries, such as China, Japan, and South Korea. Nutrition in early life is considered a key factor. Population growth references may occasionally need to be updated.

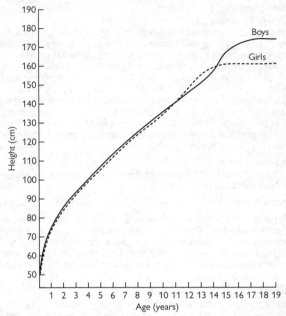

Fig. 7.1 Typical individual height-attained curves for boys and girls (supine length to the age of 2; integrated curves of Fig. 7.2).

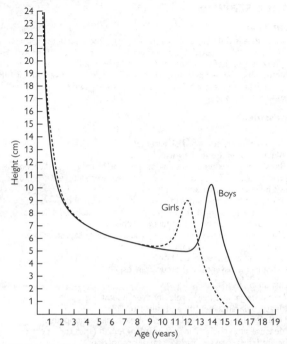

Fig. 7.2 Typical individual velocity curves for supine length or height in boys and girls. These curves represent the velocity of the typical boy and girl at any given instant.

References

1. De Waal WJ, et al. (1996). Accuracy of final height prediction and effect of growth-reductive therapy in 362 constitutionally tall children. *J Clin Endocrinol Metab* **81**, 1206–16.

Short stature

Definition

Short stature is defined as height (or length) <2nd centile for age and sex on the UK-WHO growth chart. However, abnormalities of growth may be present long before attained height falls below this level and may be detected much earlier by assessing the child's height relative to their MPH percentile, plotting serial height measurements on a growth chart, and calculating height velocity.

Assessment

History
- Who is concerned—child or parents?
- What are the parental heights?
- Has the child always been small or does the history suggest recent growth failure? Try to obtain previous measurements (e.g. from parents, GP, health visitor, school).
- Ask about maternal illness in pregnancy, gestation at delivery, size at birth (weight/length/head circumference), childhood illnesses, medication, and developmental milestones.
- Systematic enquiry for headaches, visual disturbance, asthma/respiratory symptoms, abdominal symptoms, and diet.
- Is there a family history of short stature or pubertal delay?
- Any adverse psychosocial circumstances?

Examination
- Assess height and height velocity over at least 6 months.
- Measure parents' heights, and calculate MPH.
- Look for dysmorphic features and signs of endocrinopathy.
- Measure sitting height, and calculate leg length (standing height − sitting height (cm)) to assess for skeletal disproportion.
- Assess for the presence and severity of chronic disease. Low weight for height suggests a nutritional issue, GI disorder, or other chronic disease.
- Pubertal stage using Tanner's criteria (see ➔ Table 7.2).

Investigations

- Baseline laboratory tests include: FBC, ESR, CRP, urea, Cr, electrolytes, thyroid function, Ca, PO_4, ALP, tissue transglutaminase antibodies, IGF-1, PRL, karyotype, blood gas (in infants), and urinalysis.
- Left hand and wrist radiograph for bone age.
- These tests may be clinically indicated: GH provocation testing (e.g. arginine, glucagon, or ITT) (see Table 7.1), with other anterior pituitary function tests, MRI scan with specific reference to the hypothalamus and pituitary, skeletal survey (for bone dysplasia), and, very rarely, an IGF-1 generation test (for GH resistance, see Box 7.1).

Causes

Idiopathic short stature
- Familial short stature.
- Constitutional delay in growth and puberty—these first two causes together account for ~40% of cases.

Table 7.1 Comparison of GH provocation tests

	Insulin (IV)	Arginine (IV)	Glucagon (IM)
Age	>5 years	Any	Any, including neonates
Advantages	Gold standard Also tests ACTH–cortisol axis	Safe Consistent response	Safe Also tests ACTH–cortisol axis
Disadvantages	Risk of severe hypoglycaemia, but good safety record in supervised experienced centres	Occasional nausea and vomiting Can cause skin irritation	Nausea may last 3–4h Beware of late hypoglycaemia

Other agents (e.g. L-dopa or clonidine) are less commonly used. Measurement of GH levels after exercise has poor sensitivity and specificity for detecting GH deficiency.

Primary growth disorders
- Dysmorphic syndromes (e.g. Turner syndrome (short stature, congenital heart defects, webbed neck), Noonan syndrome, Down's syndrome).
- Small-for-gestational age (SGA), including IUGR (7.5%).
- Skeletal dysplasia (e.g. achondroplasia, hypochondroplasia, short stature homeobox-containing (*SHOX*) gene haploinsufficiency).
- Metabolic bone disease (e.g. hypophosphataemic rickets, osteogenesis imperfecta).

Secondary growth disorders
- Chronic illness (including untreated coeliac disease, congenital heart disease, CRF, inflammatory bowel disease).
- Psychosocial deprivation (may be associated with reversible GH deficiency; see ➋ Psychosocial deprivation, p. 574).
- Malnutrition (rare in the UK).
- GH deficiency (8%):
  - Idiopathic (including those with mild abnormal pituitary morphology on MRI).
  - Congenital malformation in the hypothalamus/pituitary (HP) (e.g. septo-optic dysplasia), rare mutations in the *GH1* or GHRH receptor gene or in transcription factors controlling pituitary development (see ➋ Primary GH deficiency, p. 573).
  - Acquired HP disorders (e.g. craniopharyngioma, after cranial irradiation or trauma).
- GH resistance (rare genetic mutations in the GH receptor or GH-signalling molecules).
- Other endocrine disorders (e.g. hypothyroidism, hypoparathyroidism, Cushing's syndrome).
- Medication (e.g. systemic or inhaled GCs).

Familial short stature

Stature is a highly polygenic trait determined by thousands of genetic variants and with a high heritability of ~80%. Therefore, most children fall within their MPH target range. It should be remembered that some short parents may themselves have an unidentified genetic disorder (e.g. hypochondroplasia or *SHOX* gene defect).

Constitutional delay of growth and puberty

Clinical features

- This is a common condition, especially in ♂, which often presents in adolescence but may also be recognized in earlier childhood.
- Characteristic features include short stature and delay in pubertal development by >2 SD and/or bone age delay in an otherwise healthy child. In the adolescent years, short sitting height percentile, compared to leg length, is typical.
- There is often a family history of delayed puberty.
- Bone age delay may also develop in a number of other conditions, but in constitutional delay, bone age delay usually remains consistent over time and height velocity is normal for the bone age.
- GH secretion is usually normal, although provocation tests should be primed by prior administration of exogenous sex hormones if bone age in boys aged >10 years with testicular volumes of <6ml and girls aged >9 years with breast stage 2 or less (see Box 7.1).

Management

Often only reassurance is necessary. Short-course, low-dose exogenous sex steroids can be used to induce pubertal changes in adolescents with difficulty coping with short stature or delayed sexual maturation.

- Boys (>13–14 years): *testosterone* (50–100mg IM, monthly for 6 months; alternatively, 10mg transdermal gel, daily for 6 months).
- Girls (>13 years): *ethinylestradiol* (2 micrograms/day PO, for 6 months) OR *estradiol* (5 micrograms/day transdermal, for 6 months).

(See Box 7.1 for GH assessment.)

Box 7.1 GH assessment

GH is normally secreted overnight in regular pulses (pulse frequency 180min). Frequently sampled overnight GH profiles are costly and laborious, and therefore standardized stimulation tests are more commonly used. Peak GH <10 micrograms/L indicates GH deficiency (values >5 and <10 micrograms/L indicate partial GH deficiency). However, there can be large variation between different assay methods, and exact cut-offs must be locally validated. In late prepuberty, there is physiological blunting of GH secretion, and when boys aged >10 years with testicular volumes of <6ml or girls aged >9 years with breast stage 2 or less, sex steroid priming (17β-oestradiol e.g. estradiol valerate, 1mg daily (<20kg), 2mg daily (>20kg) orally for 3 days before GH test in both sexes) is necessary.

A number of different agents may be used to stimulate GH secretion (arginine, insulin, or glucagon; see Table 7.1). All tests should be performed in the morning following an overnight fast, and serial blood samples are collected over 90–180min.

An IGF-1 level should also be measured in the baseline sample, as an additional marker of GH status.

IGF-1 generation test

In short children with high basal and stimulated GH levels, but low IGF-1 levels, measurement of IGF-1 levels before (day 1) and following (day 5) administration of GH (30 micrograms/kg/day) SC for 4 days allows an assessment of GH sensitivity/resistance. This test is rarely necessary.

Primary GH deficiency

Primary GH deficiency is usually sporadic, but rarely it may be inherited as AD, AR, or X-linked recessive and may be associated with other pituitary hormone deficiencies. Mutations in the *GH1* and GHRH receptor (*GHRHR*) genes are causes of familial isolated GH deficiency. Congenital multiple pituitary hormone deficiencies arise from defects in homeobox genes which control HP development (e.g. *Pit1* (leading to GH, TSH, and PRL deficiencies), *Prop1* (leading to GH, TSH, PRL, gonadotrophin, and later ACTH deficiencies), or *Hesx1*). Mutation in *Hesx1* is associated with midline defects such as optic nerve hypoplasia and corpus callosum defects (i.e. 'septo-optic dysplasia'). In combined pituitary hormone deficiencies, GH deficiency usually arises because of failure of release of GHRH from the hypothalamus.

Clinical features

- *Infancy.* GH deficiency may present with hypoglycaemia. Coexisting ACTH, TSH, and gonadotrophin deficiencies may cause prolonged hyperbilirubinaemia and micropenis. Size may be normal, as fetal and infancy growth is more dependent on nutrition and other growth factors than on GH.
- *Childhood.* Typical features include slow growth velocity, short stature, ↓ muscle mass, and ↑ SC fat. Underdevelopment of the mid-facial bones, relative protrusion of the frontal bones because of mid-facial hypoplasia, delayed dental eruption, and delayed closure of the anterior fontanelle may be seen. These children have delayed bone age and delayed puberty.

Secondary GH deficiency

Brain tumours and cranial irradiation

Pituitary or hypothalamic tumours may impair GH secretion, and deficiencies of other pituitary hormones may coexist. Cranial irradiation, used to treat intracranial tumours, facial tumours, and acute leukaemia, may also cause GH deficiency. Risk of HP damage is related to total dose administered, fractionation (single dose more toxic than divided), location of the irradiated tissue, and age (younger children are more sensitive to irradiation damage).

GH secretion is most sensitive to irradiation damage, followed by gonadotrophins, TSH, and ACTH. Central precocious puberty may also occur and may mask GH deficiency by promoting growth, but at the expense of rapidly advancing bone age, and will compromise final height if untreated. At-risk children should be screened regularly by careful examination and multiple pituitary hormone testing.

These survivors of childhood cancer may also have other endocrine problems, including gonadal damage related to chemotherapy or irradiation scatter, 1° hypothyroidism related to spinal irradiation, or glucose intolerance related to total body irradiation. It is recommended that all such patients should undergo endocrine surveillance.

Psychosocial deprivation

Severe psychosocial deprivation may cause reversible GH insufficiency and growth failure. GH secretion improves within 3 weeks of removal from the adverse environment, and catch-up growth is often dramatic (see Fig. 7.3), although these children may continue to exhibit other features of emotional disturbance.

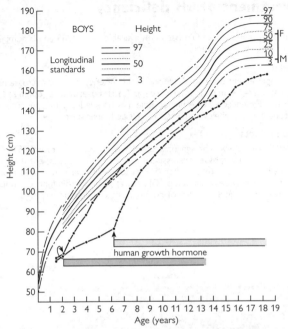

Fig. 7.3 Height of a child with psychosocial short stature, compared to a child with GH deficiency. Note catch-up on removal from parental home, marked by curved arrow.

Reproduced from Brook C (2001). *Brook's Clinical Pediatric Endocrinology*, Blackwell Publishing, with permission from Wiley Blackwell.

Treatment of GH deficiency

(See Fig. 7.4.)

Recombinant human GH has been available since 1985 and is administered by daily SC injection.

Dose

The replacement dose for childhood GH deficiency is 25–50 micrograms/kg/day (0.7–1.4 micrograms/m²/day). Catch-up growth is optimized if GH is commenced early. A higher dose may be needed during puberty, reflecting the normal elevation in GH levels at Tanner stages 3–4.

Side effects

Local lipoatrophy and benign intracranial hypertension occur rarely. Slipped upper femoral epiphyses are associated with GH deficiency, but the incidence is similar before and after GH treatment. Other pituitary hormone deficiencies may be unmasked by GH therapy, and thyroid function should be checked within 4–6 weeks of commencing GH therapy.

Monitoring GH therapy

Children receiving GH therapy should be monitored 6-monthly for efficacy (if poor, consider administration issues, compliance, and dose adjustments) and side effects. Check IGF-1 and thyroid function ~12-monthly.

Retesting in adulthood

Once final height is achieved (height velocity <2cm/year), GH secretion should be retested, as many children with GH deficiency (especially if isolated and idiopathic) have normal GH secretion in adulthood. In those with confirmed GH deficiency, continuation of GH treatment (at a dose of 0.2–0.5mg/day) during the late adolescent years into early adulthood (the transition phase) will promote somatic development (increasing bone density, lean body mass and muscular strength, reducing fat mass, and promoting a healthy lipid and metabolic profile). GH treatment may need to be continued beyond this phase as adult GH replacement.

The transition from paediatric to adult care is an important time, not only to re-evaluate GH status, but also to reassess other pituitary function and management of any underlying disorder.

It is also recommended that assessment of BMD, body composition, fasting lipid profile, and QoL by questionnaire should be undertaken at this time and repeated at 3- to 5-yearly intervals for those continuing on GH treatment.

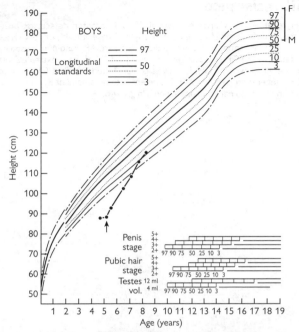

Fig. 7.4 Height of one brother with isolated GH deficiency treated with human GH from age 5 years. Catch-up is partly by high velocity and partly by prolonged growth, and so is incomplete at age 8. F and M, parents' height centiles; vertical thick line, range of expected heights for family.

Reproduced from Brook C (2001). *Brook's Clinical Pediatric Endocrinology*, Blackwell Publishing, with permission from Wiley Blackwell.

GH resistance

GH resistance may arise because of 1° GH receptor defects or post-receptor defects, or 2° to malnutrition, liver disease, T1DM, or very rarely circulating GH antibodies. *Laron syndrome* is a rare AR condition caused by mutation of the GH receptor gene. Affected individuals have extreme short stature, high levels of GH, low levels of IGF-1, and impaired GH-induced IGF-1 generation (see Box 7.1). Treatment with recombinant IGF-1 is available and leads to partial improvements in growth.

Hypothyroidism

(See Fig. 7.5.)
- Congenital 1° hypothyroidism is detected by neonatal screening.
- Hypothyroidism presenting in childhood is usually autoimmune in origin and is more common in girls and those with personal or family history of other autoimmune disease.
- In childhood, hypothyroidism may present with growth failure alone, and bone age is often disproportionately delayed. Rarely, early puberty timing and pituitary hyperplasia may occur.
- Investigations show low T_4 and T_3, high TSH, +ve TgAb and TPOAb (microsomal).
- Replacement therapy with PO levothyroxine (100 micrograms/m²/day, titrated with thyroid function) results in catch-up growth, unless diagnosis is late.

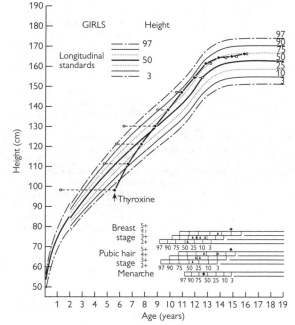

Fig. 7.5 Growth response of a hypothyroid child treated with thyroxine. Solid circles, height for age; open circles, height for bone age.

Reproduced from Brook C (2001). *Brook's Clinical Pediatric Endocrinology*, Blackwell Publishing. With permission from Wiley Blackwell.

Coeliac disease

Short stature, with or without delayed puberty, may be 2° to undernutrition and GI disorders, including inflammatory bowel disease and coeliac disease. The latter is more common in children with other autoimmune disorders. The classical childhood presentation is an irritable toddler with poor weight gain, diarrhoea, and abdominal pain and distension. However, poor height growth with bone age delay, and delayed puberty in older children, may be the presenting feature. Measurement of tissue transglutaminase antibodies is a valuable screening test, assuming the child is being exposed to gluten, but diagnosis should be confirmed by small bowel biopsy. Catch-up growth usually follows commencement of, and adherence to, a gluten-free diet.

Skeletal dysplasias

- This heterogeneous group of rare and mostly dominantly inherited disorders includes *achondroplasia* and *hypochondroplasia*.
- This group also includes *SHOX* haploinsufficiency. *SHOX* encodes a transcription factor which plays a key role in long bone growth. Haploinsufficiency (e.g. due to *SHOX* gene mutations or deletions) leads to mesomelic short stature (shortening of forearms and lower legs) and Madelung's wrist deformity (radius stops growing early). It is inherited in a pseudo-AD manner.
- Children with skeletal dysplasia usually have disproportionate short stature and a +ve or suspicious family history. However, *SHOX* haploinsufficiency can present with only mildly disproportionate short stature.
- Sitting height measurement is a very useful clinical tool to identify mildly disproportionate patients. UK reference charts for sitting height and leg length are available.
- Radiological assessment by skeletal survey and candidate gene sequencing often allow a specific diagnosis to be made.
- High-dose GH therapy (45–50 micrograms/kg/day) has been used in these disorders, with often a reasonable growth response in patients with *SHOX* haploinsufficiency (overall height gain ~7 cm), but with variable success in other skeletal dysplasias. Surgical leg lengthening before and/or after puberty is an additional option.

Small-for-gestational age and intrauterine growth restriction

- SGA is defined as birthweight and/or length at least 2 SD below the mean for gestational age. IUGR is defined as growth failure on serial antenatal US scans and usually leads to SGA. However, IUGR in late gestation may result in a baby who is within 2 SD of the mean for birthweight or length.
- Ninety per cent of infants born SGA show spontaneous catch-up growth by age 3 years; 8% of individuals born SGA will remain small (i.e. short) at 18 years of age. Catch-up growth is more common in those SGA infants who are thin with relative sparing of birth length and head circumference (>10th centile).
- In severe IUGR, length and head circumference are also reduced. Severe IUGR may be due to maternal factors such as hypertension in pregnancy, placental dysfunction, or a wide range of chromosomal or genetic conditions in the fetus.
- Silver–Russell syndrome is characterized by severe IUGR and SGA, lateral asymmetry (hemihypotrophy), triangular facies, clinodactyly (curved 5th finger), and poor infancy feeding and postnatal weight gain.
- Children with severe IUGR/SGA who do not show catch-up growth may have early-onset puberty, despite bone age delay, and therefore achieve a poor final height.
- Numerous epidemiological studies have shown a relationship between low birthweight and an ↑ risk of a number of disorders in later life, including hypertension, IHD, cerebrovascular disease, metabolic syndrome, and T2DM. The risk is ↑ with rapid postnatal weight gain and is associated with higher childhood BMI and adiposity.

Management

GH therapy is indicated for the SGA/IUGR child who has failed to show catch-up growth by age 4 years (height <−2.5 SD for age and sex). GH (35–67 micrograms/kg/day) increases growth velocity and final height. HbA1c should be monitored because GH therapy increases insulin resistance, but studies show no long-term ↑ risk of T2DM or adverse cardiometabolic profiles in previously treated young adults.

Turner syndrome

(See also Box 4.7.)

Turner syndrome should always be considered in a girl who is short for her parental target, as the classical dysmorphic features may be difficult to identify, especially at young ages. The diagnosis is made by karyotype. Sufficient cells (>30) should be examined to exclude the possibility of mosaicism.

Clinical features

There may be a history of lymphoedema in the newborn period, or an early diagnosis of congenital cardiac defects, e.g. coarctation of the aorta.

Typically, growth velocity starts to decline from age 3–5 years (see Fig. 7.6), and gonadal failure, combined with a degree of skeletal dysplasia, results in loss of the pubertal growth spurt. Final height is ~20cm below the MPH (on average 143–146cm). GH secretion is normal, although IGF-1 levels may be low. Puberty (breast development) may start spontaneously in 30% but rarely progresses to menarche and ovulatory cycles.

Management

- High-dose *GH therapy* (45 micrograms/kg/day) increases childhood and final height, although individual responses are variable. The height gained is greater when GH therapy is commenced early, ideally from age 3–5 years.
- *Oestrogen therapy* should be commenced at around 12–14 years (when LH and FSH levels rise in the absence of spontaneous puberty) to promote 2° sexual development and pubertal growth. It should be started in low dose preferably via the transdermal route (transdermal estradiol 5 micrograms/day or, if unavailable, PO ethinylestradiol 2 micrograms/day) and gradually ↑ with age. *Cyclical progesterone* (e.g. medroxyprogesterone acetate 5mg/day on days 15–25) should be added if breakthrough bleeding occurs or after 3 years of unopposed oestrogen therapy.
- A multidisciplinary approach of Turner syndrome patients includes cardiology review, renal US, ENT and audiology review, ophthalmology review, and regular screening of associated conditions such as autoimmune hypothyroidism and coeliac disease. Common educational and psychological issues require regular input from neuropsychology and allied behavioural health services.

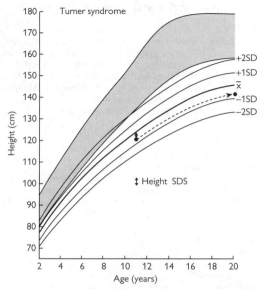

Fig. 7.6 Turner syndrome height reference chart (the normal population range in shaded grey).

Reproduced from Brook C (2001). *Brook's Clinical Pediatric Endocrinology*, Blackwell Publishing. With permission from Wiley Blackwell.

Further reading

Gravholt CH, *et al.* (2017). Clinical practice guidelines for the care of girls and women with Turner syndrome: proceedings from the 2016 Cincinnati International Turner Syndrome Meeting. *Eur J Endocrinol* **177**, G1–70.

Tall stature and rapid growth

Definition

Although statistically as many children have heights >2 SD above the mean as those who have heights >2 SD below the mean, referral for evaluation of tall stature is much less common than for short stature. Socially, for boys, heights of up to 200cm are often acceptable, whereas for many girls, heights >182cm may be distressing. However, tall stature, and particularly accelerated growth rates in early childhood, may indicate an underlying hormonal disorder such as precocious puberty. (For causes, see Box 7.2.)

Assessment

History
- Is tall stature long-standing or does the history suggest recent growth acceleration? Try to obtain previous measurements.
- Enquire about size at birth, infancy weight gain, intellectual development, and neurological development.
- Enquire about headaches, visual disturbance, and evidence of puberty.
- Is there a family history of tall stature or early puberty?

Examination
- Assess height and height velocity over at least 4–6 months.
- Measure sitting height (↑ sitting height/height ratio seen in skeletal dysplasias) and arm span (arm span/height ratio >1.05 indicative of Marfan's syndrome).
- Pubertal stage?
- Dysmorphic features? Eunuchoid habitus?
- Measure parents' heights, and calculate MPH (see ➔ Assessment of growth, pp. 566–7).

Investigations
The following investigations may be clinically indicated:
- Wrist radiograph for bone age.
- Sex hormone levels (testosterone, oestrogen, androstenedione, DHEAS), baseline and GnRH-stimulated LH and FSH levels.
- Karyotype.
- Serum IGF-1 levels.
- OGTT—GH levels normally suppress to low or undetectable levels (<0.5 microgram/L).
- Specific molecular tests for overgrowth syndromes, either targeted testing of specific genes if specific dysmorphic features are present (Marfan's: *FBN1*; Sotos: *NSD1*; Beckwith–Wiedemann: epigenetic changes of chromosome 11p15; Weaver: *EZH2*; and fragile X: *FMR1* CGG repeat length) or an unbiased approach such as array comparative genomic hybridization (CGH) or whole exome sequencing.

Management of tall stature

After excluding abnormal pathology, often only reassurance and information on predicted final height are necessary. In younger children, early induction of puberty, using low-dose sex steroids, advances the pubertal growth spurt and promotes earlier epiphyseal fusion. In older boys who are peripubertal or already in puberty, high-dose testosterone may be used to induce rapid skeletal maturation. High-dose oestrogen therapy was previously used similarly in girls. However, due to recent evidence of reduced fertility in women treated with high-dose oestrogen, this treatment is no longer used. Epiphysiodesis is an alternative option for tall girls and boys. High-dose testosterone-treated men appear to have normal fertility.

Box 7.2 Causes of tall stature in childhood

Normal variants
- Familial tall stature.
- Early maturation (largely familial, but also promoted by early childhood nutrition and obesity; height is not excessive for bone age which is advanced).

Hormonal
(See ➜ Precocious puberty, pp. 592–5.)
- GH or GHRH excess ('pituitary gigantism'), resulting from pituitary adenoma or ectopic adenomas, is a very rare cause of tall stature (see ➜ Acromegaly, p. 168).
- Other hormonal excess, e.g. hyperthyroidism, CAH (associated with signs of virilization), familial GC deficiency.
- Rarely, oestrogen receptor or aromatase deficiencies delay puberty and epiphyseal fusion, resulting in tall adult height.

Chromosomal abnormalities
- XXY (Klinefelter's syndrome) (see ➜ Primary hypogonadism, pp. 418–20).
- XYY, XYYY (each 'extra Y' confers, on average, 13cm of additional height).

Other rare syndromes
Overgrowth and dysmorphic features are seen in Marfan syndrome, homocystinuria, Sotos syndrome (early excessive growth ± autism), Beckwith–Wiedemann syndrome (overgrowth disorder and ↑ risk of childhood cancer), and Weaver syndrome (typical facial appearances with hypertelorism and retrognathia plus variable intellectual disability)

Further reading

Ahmid M, et al. (2018). Childhood-onset growth hormone deficiency and the transition to adulthood: current perspective. *Ther Clin Risk Manag* **14**, 2283–91.

Allen DB, Cuttler L (2013). Clinical practice. Short stature in childhood: challenges and choices. *N Engl J Med* **368**, 1220–8.

Clayton PE, et al. (2007). Management of the child born small for gestational age child (SGA) through to adulthood: a consensus statement of the International Societies of Paediatric Endocrinology and the Growth Hormone Research Society. *J Clin Endocrinol Metab* **92**, 804–10.

Collett-Solberg PF, et al. (2019). Diagnosis, genetics, and therapy of short stature in children: a Growth Hormone Research Society international perspective. Horm Res Paediatr **92**, 1–14.

Conway GS (2009). Adult care of pediatric conditions: lessons from Turner's syndrome. J Clin Endocrinol Metab **94**, 3185–7.

De Waal WJ, et al. (1996). Accuracy of final height prediction and effect of growth-reductive therapy in 362 constitutionally tall children. J Clin Endocrinol Metab **81**, 1206–16.

Hendriks AEJ, et al. (2011). Fertility and ovarian function in high-dose estrogen treated tall women. J Clin Endocrinol Metab **96**, 1098–105.

Kelly WH, et al. (2012). Effect of inhaled glucocorticoids in childhood on adult height. N Engl J Med **367**, 904–12.

Latronico AC, et al. (2016). Causes, diagnosis, and treatment of central precocious puberty. Lancet Diabetes Endocrinol **4**, 265–74.

Richmond E, Rogol AD (2016). Treatment of growth hormone deficiency in children, adolescents and at the transitional age. Best Pract Res Clin Endocrinol Metab **30**, 749–55.

Saenger P, et al. (2000). Recommendations for the diagnosis and management of Turner's syndrome. J Clin Endocrinol Metab **86**, 3061–9.

Normal puberty

Puberty is the sequence of physical and physiological changes that occur at adolescence, culminating in sexual maturity and adult body size.

Age at onset

Average age at onset of puberty is earlier in girls (~11 years) than in boys (~12 years) but varies widely (~ ± 2 years from the mean age of onset) and is influenced by a number of factors:
- *Historical.* Mean age of menarche in Europe has ↓ from 17 years in 1900 to 12.8 years today, presumably due to improved childhood nutrition and growth.
- *Genetic.* Age at onset of puberty is a polygenic trait with estimated heritability of ~50–60%.
- *Ethnicity.* Afro-Caribbean and South Asian girls tend to have earlier puberty than Caucasians.
- *Weight gain.* Earlier puberty is more common in overweight girls, whereas girls who engage in regular physical activity and are thin often have delayed puberty.

Hormonal changes prior to and during puberty

- Mini-puberty is a physiological process in normal infants aged 3–6 months old. LH, FSH, and sex hormone levels may transiently reach adult levels during this period, without 2° sexual development. This axis is then actively suppressed until puberty onset.
- Adrenal androgens (DHEAS and androstenedione) start to rise 2 years before puberty onset ('adrenarche'). This usually causes no physical changes but occasionally results in mild pubic hair, body odour, and acne ('premature adrenarche').
- Pulsatile secretion of LHRH from the hypothalamus at night is the 1st step in the initiation of puberty. This results in pulsatile secretion of LH and FSH from the pituitary, and the gonadotrophin response to GnRH administration changes from prepubertal FSH predominance to a higher response in LH levels.

Physical changes

The 1st indication of puberty is breast development in girls and an increase in testicular size in boys. Puberty then progresses in an orderly or 'consonant' manner through distinct stages (see Table 7.2). Puberty rating by an experienced observer involves identification of the pubertal stage—particularly, breast development in girls and testicular volume (using an orchidometer) in boys.

Pubertal growth spurt

↑ oestrogen levels in both boys and girls leads to ↑ GH secretion. Peak height velocity occurs at puberty stages 2–3 in girls and occurs later in boys at stages 3–4 (testicular volume 10–12mL).

Table 7.2 The normal stages of puberty ('Tanner stages')

Boys

Stage	Genitalia	Pubic hair	Other events
I	Prepubertal	Vellus not thicker than on abdomen	TV* <4mL
II	Enlargement of testes and scrotum	Sparse, long, pigmented strands at base of penis	TV 4–8mL Voice starts to change
III	Lengthening of penis	Darker, curlier, and spreads over the pubis	TV 8–10mL Axillary hair
IV	Increase in penis length and breadth	Adult-type hair, but covering a smaller area	TV 10–15mL Upper lip hair Peak height velocity
V	Adult shape and size	Spreads to medial thighs (stage 6: spreads up linea alba)	TV 15–25mL Facial hair spreads to cheeks Adult voice

Girls

Stage	Breast	Pubic hair	Other events
I	Elevation of papilla only	Vellus not thicker than on abdomen	
II	Breast bud stage: elevation of breast and papilla	Sparse, long, pigmented strands along labia	Peak height velocity
III	Further elevation of breast and areola together	Darker, curlier, and spreads over pubis	
IV	Areola forms a 2nd mound on top of breast	Adult-type hair, but covering a smaller area	Menarche
V	Mature stage: areola recedes and only papilla projects	Spreads to medial thighs (stage 6: spreads up linea alba)	

* TV, testicular volume—measured by size comparison with a Prader orchidometer.

Source: data from Tanner JM (1962) *Growth at adolescence*, 2nd edn. Blackwell Scientific Publications, Oxford.

Precocious puberty

Definition

- Precocious puberty is defined as onset at <8 years in girls and <9 years in boys.
- Gonadotrophin-dependent ('central' or 'true') precocious puberty is characterized by early breast development in girls and testicular enlargement in boys.
- Gonadotrophin-independent ('peripheral') puberty occurs due to abnormal peripheral sex hormone secretion, resulting in isolated development of specific 2° sexual characteristics.

Assessment of precocious puberty

History

- Age when 2° sexual features first noted.
- What features are present and in what order did they appear? For example, virilization (pubic, axillary, or facial hair; acne; body odour), genital or breast enlargement, galactorrhoea (very rare), menarche, or cyclical mood changes?
- Recent growth acceleration?
- Family history of early puberty?
- Past history of rapid early life weight gain, adoption or migration from a poorer social setting, or prior CNS abnormality or insult (e.g. irradiation)?

Examination

- Breast or genital and testicular size; degree of virilization (clitoromegaly in girls indicates abnormal androgen levels).
- Neurological examination, including visual fields and fundoscopy.
- Abdominal or testicular masses?
- Unusual skin pigmentation? (café-au-lait patches—McCune–Albright (see ⊃ McCune–Albright syndrome, pp. 654–5) or NF type 1 (NF-1) (see ⊃ Neurofibromatosis, pp. 658–60)).
- Assess height and BMI, and height velocity over 4–6 months.

Investigations

The following investigations may be indicated:

- Hand radiograph to detect and quantify bone age advance.
- Thyroid function.
- Sex hormone levels (testosterone, oestrogen, androstenedione, DHEAS).
- LH and FSH levels (random, or baseline and 30 and 60min post-IV GnRH). Central puberty is indicated by LH level >4–6IU/L.
- 17αOHP levels (random, or baseline and 30 and 60min post-IV Synacthen®) (see ⊃ Congenital adrenal hyperplasia, pp. 606–8).
- Tumour markers (aFP, β-hCG).
- 24h urine steroid profile.
- Abdominal US scan (adrenal glands, ovaries).
- MRI scan (cranial, adrenal glands).

Central (gonadotrophin-dependent) precocious puberty

This is due to premature activation of pulsatile GnRH secretion from the hypothalamus. The normal progression in physical changes ('consonance') is maintained but may be accelerated. As precocious puberty is defined as age at onset 2 SD before the average age, with ongoing secular trends to earlier puberty, this may be physiological in an increasing number of children, especially in girls with a family history of early puberty. By contrast, boys with precocious puberty have a greater risk of intracranial or other pathology.

Causes
- Idiopathic or familial.
- Intracranial tumours (in particular, optic nerve glioma and hypothalamic germinoma), hypothalamic hamartoma, hydrocephalus, and non-specific brain injury (e.g. cerebral palsy).
- Post-cranial irradiation or trauma.
- May also be triggered by long-standing elevation in sex hormones resulting from any peripheral source (e.g. late-presenting simple virilizing CAH or inadequately treated CAH).
- 1° hypothyroidism (long-standing elevated TRH and/or TSH are conjectured to stimulate FSH release and/or FSH receptors).
- Gonadotrophin-secreting tumours (e.g. pituitary adenoma or hepatoblastoma) are rare.

Treatment
Aims of treatment are:
- To avoid psychological distress for the child.
- To avoid reduced final height due to premature bone maturation and early epiphyseal fusion. A *final height prediction* is often helpful when considering treatment. Significant improvement in adult height is only likely to be achieved if treatment is started ≤6 years of age.

Pituitary LH and FSH secretion is inhibited by continuous exposure to GnRH analogues, e.g. *goserelin* 3.6mg SC monthly or 10.8mg SC 3-monthly, or *triptorelin* 3.75mg monthly (lower doses if weight <30kg) or 11.25mg 3-monthly SC or deep IM every 2 weeks for the first three injections, then 3- to 4-weekly thereafter. Treatment efficacy should be monitored regularly by clinical observation and ensuring that pre-dose LH, FSH, and sex hormone levels remain at low prepubertal levels. The dosing intervals may need to be reduced if there is evidence of inadequate suppression of pubertal development.

Peripheral (gonadotrophin-independent) precocious puberty

In the following conditions, sex hormones are secreted autonomously by peripheral tissues. Hence, levels of LH and FSH are initially suppressed by feedback inhibition. However, prolonged exposure to sex hormones may also trigger central precocious puberty.

McCune–Albright syndrome

(See also ➔ McCune–Albright syndrome, pp. 654–5.) This is a sporadic condition due to a somatic activating mutation of the GSα protein subunit which affects bones (polyostotic fibrous dysplasia), skin (café-au-lait spots), and may potentially cause multiple endocrinopathies.

Several hormone receptors share the same G protein-coupled cyclic adenosine monophosphate (AMP) signalling system. In addition to abnormal activation of gonadotrophin receptors, hyperthyroidism, hyperparathyroidism, or GH excess may also be present.

All cells descended from the mutated embryonic cell line are affected, while cells descended from non-mutated cells develop into normal tissues. Thus, the phenotype is highly variable in physical distribution and severity.

Testotoxicosis

This is a rare familial condition, due to an activating LH receptor gene mutation, resulting in precocious puberty only in boys. The testes show only little increase in size, and on biopsy, Leydig cell hyperplasia is characteristic. Treatment is with androgen receptor-blocking agents (CPA or flutamide) and aromatase inhibitors.

Congenital adrenal hyperplasia

(See also ➔ Congenital adrenal hyperplasia, pp. 606–8.) Classical CAH presents at or soon after birth with virilized genitalia (in girls), salt wasting, and GC insufficiency (in both sexes). Non-classical ('late-onset') CAH presents in childhood with rapid growth, advanced bone age, and moderate to severe virilization in the absence of testicular or breast development.

Sex hormone-secreting tumours

Peripheral androgens may be secreted by adrenal, testicular, or ovarian tumours. Affected children usually have severe features of virilization. (NB. A testicular tumour may cause asymmetrical enlargement.)

Peripheral oestrogen production from an ovarian tumour is a very rare cause of precocious breast development in girls.

Other variants of early puberty

Premature thelarche

Premature breast development, in the absence of other signs of puberty, may present at any age from infancy. Breast size is often asymmetrical, fluctuates with time, and is usually self-limiting. The cause is unknown, although typically FSH levels (and oestradiol, but not LH) are transiently elevated, and US may reveal a single large ovarian cyst. Bone maturation, growth rate, and final height are unaffected.

Thelarche variant

This is an intermediate condition between premature thelarche and central precocious puberty. The aetiology is unknown. These girls demonstrate ↑ height velocity and rate of bone maturation. Ovarian US reveals a multicystic appearance, as in true puberty. Decision to treat should take into account height velocity and final height prediction, as well as the severity and rate of physical maturation.

Premature adrenarche and premature pubarche

Adrenal androgen secretion ('adrenarche') starts to rise 1–2 years before the onset of puberty. 'Premature' adrenarche is due to ↑ androgen production and/or sensitivity and presents with mild features of virilization, such as mild pubic hair ('pubarche'), axillary hair, body odour, or acne before age 8 years in girls and 9 years in boys, in the absence of other features of puberty. It is more common in girls, with a history of low birthweight and a family history of early puberty timing or PCOS. (NB. Clitoromegaly in girls suggests a more severe pathology with excessive androgen production, e.g. CAH or androgen-secreting tumour.)

The management of premature adrenarche usually involves only reassurance after exclusion of other causes of virilization, as there is no significant impact on final height and onset/progression of puberty.

Isolated premature menarche

This term describes young girls with prepubertal physical appearances who present with a single or repeated episodes of vaginal bleeding (usually mild spotting or staining of underwear). This condition is uncommon and idiopathic, and is hypothesized to be due to high sensitivity to low levels of oestradiol. It is usually self-limiting and does not progress to precocious puberty. Management involves exclusion of precocious puberty and localized sources of bleeding (including local trauma, foreign bodies, and sexual abuse), possibly requiring gynaecology referral for genital examination under anaesthesia (EUA).

Delayed/absent puberty

Definition

Delayed puberty is defined as lack of puberty at >2 SD older than the average age, i.e. >13 years in girls and >14 years in boys. Although by definition, it affects 2% of boys and girls, boys present much more commonly than girls (by contrast, precocious puberty presents more commonly in girls). In addition, some children present with >2 years of 'arrested progression' from one pubertal stage to the next.

Affected individuals may be distressed by their short stature and/or lack of 2° sexual characteristics. In the long term, severe delay is a risk factor for ↓ BMD and osteoporosis.

Causes

General

- Constitutional delay of growth and puberty is the most common cause (see ➋ Constitutional delay of growth and puberty, p. 572).
- Chronic childhood disease, malabsorption (e.g. coeliac disease, inflammatory bowel disease), or undernutrition.

Primary (hypergonadotrophic) hypogonadism

Gonadal failure may be:

- Chromosomal (e.g. Turner syndrome in girls (see ➋ Turner syndrome, pp. 584–5), Klinefelter syndrome in boys (see ➋ Primary hypogonadism, pp. 418–20)).
- Acquired (e.g. following chemotherapy, radiotherapy, infection, testicular torsion).

In these conditions, basal and stimulated gonadotrophin levels are raised once the child has reached adolescence.

Hypogonadotrophic hypogonadism

- Kallmann syndrome (including anosmia).
- HP lesions (tumour, post-radiotherapy or surgery, dysplasia).
- Rare inactivating mutations of genes encoding LH, FSH, or their receptors.

These conditions may also present in the newborn period with micropenis and undescended testes in boys.

Investigation

The following investigations may be indicated:

- LH and FSH levels (random or basal and post-IV GnRH stimulation).
- Plasma oestrogen or testosterone levels.
- Anti-Müllerian hormone (in boys) and inhibin levels (in both sexes) are circulating markers of functioning gonadal tissue.
- Karyotype.
- Pelvic US in girls to assess ovarian morphology.
- Measurement of androgen levels before and after IM hCG administration (initially 1500–2000U/day for 3 days; sometimes followed by 1500–2000U twice weekly for 3 weeks) to indicate presence of functional testicular tissue in boys.
- US or MRI to detect intra-abdominal testes in boys.

- Cranial MRI in HH.
- For those with HH, mutation screening for a monogenic cause may be indicated.

It is often difficult to distinguish adolescents with constitutional delay (temporary ↓ gonadotrophin levels) and those with permanent HH, as the latter is often only confirmed by ongoing low levels at age 18 years. In these cases, induction of puberty may be indicated, with regular assessment of testicular growth in boys (which is independent of testosterone therapy), followed by withdrawal of treatment and biochemical reassessment when final height is reached.

Management

Depending on the age and concern of the child and parents, short-course, low-dose exogenous sex steroids can be used to induce pubertal changes (see ◑ Constitutional delay of growth and puberty, p. 572).

For permanent 1° hypogonadism or HH, gradually increasing doses of exogenous sex steroids are required to induce, progress, and maintain pubertal development (see Table 7.3).

Table 7.3 Pubertal induction and maintenance in boys and girls

Testosterone dose	Testosterone interval	Ethinylestradiol dose (daily)	Estradiol 25-microgram matrix patch	Duration
50mg	4 weeks	2 micrograms	1/4 patch for 3–4 days per week	6 months
100mg	4 weeks	4 micrograms	1/4 patch changed every 3–4 days	6 months
150mg	4 weeks	6 micrograms	1/2 patch 3–4 days then 1/4 patch 3–4 days	6 months
200mg	4 weeks	8 micrograms	1/2 patch changed every 3–4 days	6 months
250mg	3–4 weeks	10 micrograms (+ progesterone when bleed)	1 patch changed every 3–4 days	6 months
		20- to 30-micrograms 'pill'	Combined oestrogen and progestogen patch	Onwards

Long-term treatment

Boys

Testosterone (by IM injection) 50mg 4-weekly, gradually ↑ to 250mg 3- to 4-weekly. Transdermal gel is an alternative option.

- Monitor penis enlargement, pubic hair, height velocity, and adult body habitus.
- Side effects include severe acne and, rarely, priapism.

Girls

Oestrogen (PO or transdermal). Start at low dose and gradually ↑ dose.

- Promotes breast and uterus development and adult body habitus.
- *Progesterone* (PO) should be added if breakthrough bleeding occurs or after 3 years of unopposed oestrogen therapy.

Further reading

British Society for Paediatric Endocrinology and Diabetes (2016). *Hormone supplementation for pubertal induction in girls.* ℬ https://www.bsped.org.uk/clinical-resources/guidelines/

British Society for Paediatric Endocrinology and Diabetes (2019). *Testosterone replacement guidelines.* ℬ https://www.bsped.org.uk/clinical-resources/guidelines/

Palmert MR, Dunkel L (2012). Clinical practice. Delayed puberty. *N Engl J Med* **366**, 443–53.

Wei C, Crowne EC (2016). Recent advances in the understanding and management of delayed puberty. *Arch Dis Child* **101**, 481–8.

Normal sexual differentiation

Gonadal development

- In the ♂ or ♀ embryo, the bipotential gonad develops as a thickening of mesenchymal cells and coelomic epithelium around the primitive kidney. This *genital ridge* is then colonized by primordial germ cells which migrate from the yolk sac to form the *gonadal ridge*. In the absence of a Y chromosome, the gonad develops into an ovary.
- In the presence of a normal Y chromosome, immature Sertoli cells, germs cells, and seminiferous tubules can be recognized by 7 weeks, and testis differentiation is complete by 9 weeks. The *SRY* gene is an essential 'sex-determining region' on the Y chromosome which signals for testis differentiation.

Internal genitalia

- Embryonic *Müllerian* structures form the uterus, Fallopian tubes, and upper third of the vagina.
- In ♂, AMH is secreted by immature Sertoli cells in the testis by 6 weeks, and this causes regression of the Müllerian structures. Leydig cells appear in the testis at around day 60 and produce *testosterone* under placental hCG stimulation. Testosterone promotes growth and differentiation of the *Wolffian ducts* to form the epididymis, vas deferens, and seminal vesicles.

External genitalia

- In the absence of any androgen secretion, the labia majora, labia minora, and clitoris develop from the embryonic genital swelling, genital fold, and genital tubercle, respectively.
- Development of normal ♂ external genitalia requires testosterone production from the testis and its conversion to *DHT* by the enzyme *5α-reductase*. In the presence of DHT, the genital tubercle elongates to form the corpora cavernosa and glans penis; the urethral fold forms the penile shaft, and the labioscrotal swelling forms the scrotum. This process commences at around 9 weeks and is completed by 13 weeks. Testicular descent in ♂ occurs in the later two-thirds of gestation under the control of fetal LH and testosterone.

Assessment of ambiguous genitalia

Most cases of ambiguous genitalia present at birth. Involvement of an experienced paediatric endocrinologist and a urological surgeon should be sought as early as possible.

History

- Any maternal medication during pregnancy?
- Are parents consanguineous or is there a family history of ambiguous genitalia?
- Is there a neonatal history of hypoglycaemia or prolonged jaundice?

Examination

- Assess clitoris/phallus size, degree of labial fusion, and position of the urethra/urogenital sinus (anterior or posterior).
- Are the gonads palpable? Check along the line of descent.
- Are there any signs indicating panhypopituitarism, e.g. midline defects/hypoglycaemia/hypocortisolaemia/prolonged jaundice?
- Dysmorphic features of Turner syndrome may be seen in XO/XY mosaicism (mixed gonadal dysgenesis).

Investigations

- Karyotype, electrolytes, blood glucose, 17αOHP.
- US of pelvis and labial folds (for Müllerian structures and gonads).
- Clinical photographs.
- After 48h old, when the neonatal hormonal surge has ↓, repeat bloods for 17αOHP, cortisol, LH, FSH, and androgen levels. Collect a 24h urine sample to measure the steroid profile.
- EUA and cystogram may be required.

Specific tests

- SST in a virilized XX (when CAH is suspected).
- A 3-day hCG test in an undervirilized '♂' (testes present or 46,XY) assesses stimulated gonadal production of androgens. May identify androgen biosynthesis defects or androgen insensitivity.
- GnRH test to assess pituitary gonadotrophin secretion (this test is only informative in the neonatal period).
- Glucagon test to assess cortisol and GH secretion.
- Androgen receptor function can be tested in cultured fibroblasts from a genital skin biopsy.
- DNA analysis for androgen receptor mutation, CAH mutations, and androgen biosynthesis mutations.

Disorders of sex development

♂ and ♀ internal and external genitalia develop from common embryonic structures. In the absence of ♂ differentiating signals, normal ♀ genitalia develop. Genital ambiguity may therefore occur as a result of chromosomal abnormality, gonadal dysgenesis, biochemical defects of androgen synthesis, inappropriate exposure to external androgens, or androgen receptor insensitivity. (See Box 7.3 for definitions.)

46,XX DSD

Biochemical defects leading to androgen oversecretion

CAH, most commonly due to 21-hydroxylase deficiency, is the most common cause of ambiguous genitalia in 46,XX.

Disorders of ovarian development

Abnormal ♂ differentiation can occur if the *SRY* gene has been translocated onto an autosome.

Maternal hyperandrogenism

- A ♀ fetus may be virilized if maternal androgen levels exceed the capacity of placental aromatase to convert these to oestrogen.
- This may occur due to maternal disease (e.g. CAH, adrenal and ovarian tumours) or use of androgenic medication in pregnancy or, very rarely, placental aromatase deficiency.

46,XY DSD

Disorders of testis development

- XY gonadal dysgenesis can be caused by mutations in a number of genes controlling ♂ sexual differentiation, including *SRY*, *SF-1*, *WT-1*, and *SOX*. Affected individuals show apparently normal ♀ external and internal genitalia.
- Early-gestation testicular failure resulting from torsion or infarction.

Biochemical defects of androgen synthesis

Rare deficiencies of the enzymes 5α-reductase, 17β-hydroxysteroid dehydrogenase, or 3β-hydroxysteroid dehydrogenase (also associated with GC and MC deficiencies); are autosomal recessively inherited and may result in variable degrees of undervirilization.

Androgen receptor insensitivity syndrome

Defects of the androgen receptor gene on the X chromosome or autosomal post-receptor signalling genes may result in complete or partial androgen insensitivity.

- *Complete androgen insensitivity*. Results in apparently normal ♀ external genitalia and usually presents with testicular prolapse in childhood or 1° amenorrhoea in adolescence.
- *Partial androgen insensitivity*. Presentation may vary from mild virilization to micropenis, hypospadias, undescended testes, or in adult life with ↓ spermatogenesis.

Box 7.3 Definitions

Chromosomal disorders

Include:
- 45,X Turner syndrome and variants.
- 47,XXY Klinefelter syndrome and variants.
- 45,X/46,XY mixed gonadal dysgenesis.
- 46,XX/46,XY gonadal chimera.

46,XX DSD

Include:
- Disorders of gonadal (ovarian) development.
- Androgen excess.
- Structural disorders, e.g. cloacal exstrophy, vaginal atresia.

46,XY DSD

Include:
- Disorders of gonadal (testicular) development.
- Disorders in androgen synthesis and action.
- Structural disorders, e.g. severe hypospadias, cloacal exstrophy.

Gonadotrophin defects
- Gonadotrophin deficiency may occur in *hypopituitarism* or may be associated with anosmia (*Kallmann syndrome*). It usually presents with absent puberty but is an occasional cause of micropenis and undescended testes.
- LH receptor gene defects are rare and result in complete absence of virilization, as the testes are unable to respond to placental hCG.

Anti-Müllerian hormone deficiency or insensitivity

The testes are usually undescended, and the uterus and Fallopian tubes are present.

Management of ambiguous genitalia

In the newborn period, the infant should be monitored in hospital for:
- Hypoglycaemia (until hypopituitarism is excluded).
- Salt wasting (until CAH is excluded).

Explain to the parents that the infant appears to be healthy but has a defect that interferes with determining sex. It is helpful to show the parents the physical findings as you explain this. Advise them to postpone the registration of the birth due to the delay in sex assignment until after investigations, and discuss what they will say to relatives and friends.

Sex assignment

Decision on the sex of rearing should be based on the optimal expected outcome in terms of psychosexual and reproductive function. Parents should therefore be encouraged to have discussions with an endocrinologist, a surgeon specializing in urogenital reconstruction, a psychologist, and a social worker. Following the necessary investigations and discussions, agreement on sex assignment as early as possible optimizes the psychosexual outcome.

Further management
- If ♀ sex is assigned, any testicular tissue should be removed.
- Reconstructive surgery may include clitoral reduction, gonadectomy, and vaginoplasty in girls, and phallus enlargement, hypospadias repair, and orchidopexy in boys. In both sexes, multiple-stage procedures may be required. The optimal timing of these procedures is debated and recent guidelines recommend postponing surgery until the patient is old enough to be actively involved in decision-making wherever possible.
- IM testosterone esters or topical *DHT* may enhance phallus size in ♂ infants, and a trial of therapy is sometimes useful before sex assignment.
- HRT may also be required from adolescence into adulthood.
- Continuing psychological support for the parents and children is very important.

Congenital adrenal hyperplasia

(See also ➔ Congenital adrenal hyperplasia in adults, pp. 354–5.)

A number of autosomally inherited enzyme deficiencies result in cortisol deficiency, excess pituitary ACTH secretion, and adrenal gland hyperplasia.

21-hydroxylase deficiency (>90%)

The most common cause of CAH results in cortisol and MC deficiency, while the build-up of precursor steroids is channelled into excess adrenal androgen synthesis. Different defects in the 21-hydroxylase gene (e.g. deletion, splice site or point mutation) result in different degrees of enzyme deficiency, and thus a wide variation in phenotypes.

Clinical features

- Virilization of ♀ fetuses may result in clitoromegaly and labial fusion at birth; 75% have MC deficiency resulting in renal salt wasting. Because ♂ have normal genitalia at birth, they may present acutely ill in the neonatal period with vomiting, dehydration, collapse, hyponatraemia, and hyperkalaemia. Non-salt-wasting boys present in childhood with early genital enlargement, pubarche, and rapid growth.
- If untreated or poorly treated, both sexes may develop pubic hair, acne, rapid height velocity, advanced bone maturation, and precocious puberty, which may result in very short adult height.
- 'Non-classical CAH' is due to milder 21-hydroxylase deficiencies. Affected girls present in childhood or adulthood with hirsutism, acne, premature/exaggerated adrenarche, menstrual irregularities, and/or infertility.

11β-hydroxylase deficiency (~5%)

This enzyme converts 11-deoxycortisol to cortisol and is the final step in cortisol synthesis. In addition to excess adrenal androgens, the over-produced precursor corticosterone has MC activity. Thus, in contrast to salt wasting in 21-hydroxylase deficiency, affected individuals may have hypernatraemia and hypokalaemia. Hypertension is rare in infancy but may develop during childhood and affects 50–60% of adults.

Specific investigations for CAH

(See also ➔ Assessment of ambiguous genitalia, p. 601.)

- *Plasma 17αOHP.* An elevated level indicates 21-hydroxylase deficiency. It may be difficult to distinguish this from the physiological hormonal surge which occurs in the first 2 days of life. This test should therefore be repeated (together with 11-deoxycortisol) after 48h of age.
- 24h urine steroid profile (also collected after 48h of age) to confirm the diagnosis and to detect rarer enzyme defects.
- Synacthen® stimulation test may be required to discriminate between enzyme deficiencies.
- Plasma and urine electrolytes should be regularly monitored during the first 2 weeks of life.
- Plasma renin level to assess salt wasting in those with normal serum Na and relatively mild 21-hydroxylase deficiency.

Other rare enzyme deficiencies

- *17α-hydroxylase deficiency*. Impairs cortisol, androgen, and oestrogen synthesis, but overproduction of MCs leads to hypokalaemia and hypertension.
- *3β-hydroxysteroid dehydrogenase deficiency*. Impairs cortisol, MC, and androgen biosynthesis. ♂ have hypospadias and undescended testes; however, excess DHEA, a weak androgen, may cause mild virilization in ♀.

Steroid acute regulatory protein

- *STAR* mutation: 46,XY sex reversal and severe adrenal failure. Heterozygous defects. Extremely rare.
- CYPIIAI (P450: side chain cleavage cytochrome enzyme): 46,XY sex reversal and severe adrenal failure. Heterozygous defects. Extremely rare.
- P450 oxidoreductase deficiency: biochemical picture of combined 21-hydroxylase/17α-hydroxylase/17,20 lyase deficiencies. Wide spectrum of presentation from ambiguous genitalia, adrenal failure, and Antley–Bixler skeletal dysplasia (complex craniosynostosis) syndrome through to mildly affected individuals with PCOS.

Management

- *Hydrocortisone* (10–15mg/m²/day PO in three divided doses). In addition to treating cortisol deficiency, this suppresses ACTH and thereby reduces excessive production of adrenal androgens. Occasionally, higher doses are required to achieve adequate androgen suppression; however, overtreatment may suppress growth and promote excessive appetite and weight gain.
- In *salt wasting*, initial *IV fluid resuscitation* (10–20mL/kg normal saline) may be required to treat circulatory collapse. Long-term MC replacement (*fludrocortisone* 0.05–0.3mg/day) may have incomplete efficacy, particularly in infancy, and *NaCl* supplements are also needed. Up to 10mmol/kg per day may be needed in infancy.
- *Reconstructive surgery* (clitoral reduction, vaginoplasty) by an experienced surgeon. Used to be performed in infancy, with further procedures sometimes required at puberty. However, recent guidelines recommend postponing surgery until the patient is old enough to be actively involved in decision-making wherever possible.
- Patients and families need to be aware of the need for extra hydrocortisone during intercurrent illness or significant stress. Instructions on what to do for mild, moderate, and severe illnesses ('sick day rules') and for operative procedures should be made available. Patients and families should have parenteral hydrocortisone available to give in emergency situations.

Monitoring of hormonal therapy

- *Height velocity and bone age.* If hydrocortisone therapy is insufficient, growth rate will be above normal and bone age will be advanced. Conversely, if hydrocortisone therapy is excessive, growth rate is suppressed.
- *17αOHP.* Blood levels should be assessed several times each year. Levels should be measured before and after each hydrocortisone dose; these may be collected at home by the parents, using capillary bloodspot samples. In girls and prepubertal boys, androgen levels (testosterone and androstenedione) are informative if there is concern about poor control and/or virilization.
- *MC and Na replacement.* Regularly monitor BP, plasma electrolytes, and renin levels.

Genetic advice

- The inheritance of CAH is AR, and parents should be informed of a 25% risk of recurrence in future offspring.
- If the mutation is identifiable on DNA analysis in the child and parents, chorionic villus sampling may allow prenatal diagnosis.
- Maternal *dexamethasone* therapy from around 5–6 weeks of pregnancy prevents virilization of the ♂ fetus without significant maternal complications (see ➋ Congenital adrenal hyperplasia, p. 493).

Further reading

Ahmed SF, *et al.* (2021). Society for Endocrinology UK guidance on the initial evaluation of an infant or an adolescent with a suspected disorder of sex development (revised 2021). *Clin Endocrinol (Oxf)* **84**, 771–88. DOI: 10.1111/cen.14528

Cools M, *et al.* (2018). Caring for individuals with a difference of sex development (DSD): a consensus statement. *Nat Rev Endocrinol* **14**, 415–29.

Dattani MT, Brook CGD (eds.) (2019). *Brook's Clinical Paediatric Endocrinology*, 7th edn. Wiley-Blackwell, Oxford.

Hochberg Z (ed.) (1998). Practical Algorithms in Pediatric Endocrinology. Karger, Basel.

Hughes IA (1989). *Handbook of Endocrine Investigations in Children*. John Wright & Sons, Bristol.

Speiser PW, *et al.* (2010). Congenital adrenal hyperplasia due to steroid 21-hydroxylase deficiency: an Endocrine Society clinical practice guideline. *J Clin Endocrinol Metab* **95**, 4133–60.

Chapter 8

Transitional endocrinology

Helena Gleeson

Overview

- Young people (aged 10–24) access endocrine care with a range of concerns.
- Some have presentations that are similar to those seen in older adults, but some are unique to this age group.
- Differentiating what is normal physiology from pathology is important to prevent over-investigation, e.g. in young people with delayed puberty, menstrual irregularity, or gynaecomastia.
- Engaging the young person presenting for the 1st time with signs and symptoms of PCOS, or the growing number of young people with long-term endocrine conditions, including those with DM and survivors of childhood cancer, could influence outcomes in adult life.
- Care and services should be designed to meet the needs of young people, with a focus on making services accessible, emphasizing confidentiality, improving the environment and staff training, offering joined-up working and advice on health issues, and involving young people in designing and evaluating the service.
- Useful guidance on principles, planning, and infrastructure is available (ℜ https://www.nice.org.uk/guidance/ng43).

Biopsychosocial development

- Adolescence is a time of rapid biological, psychological, and social change and continues into young adulthood (see Fig. 8.1).
- Biopsychosocial development is an interdependent process, and there are a number of factors, including cultural and socioeconomic, that may alter the rate of progression through adolescence and into young adulthood.
- The bidirectional relationship between 'normal' development and having an endocrine condition is significant.
- Different aspects of development can be affected by having an endocrine condition, which may lead to difficulty in having peer relationships and social isolation, failing to achieve financial independence, and an increase in risky health behaviours and mental health problems.
- Conversely, 'normal' development can affect a young person with an endocrine condition from the perspective of engagement with healthcare and adherence with medication and the adoption of health behaviours.
- Understanding biopsychosocial development and the potential complex interplay is invaluable for all clinical interactions between healthcare professionals and young people.
- These should be addressed as part of routine care.

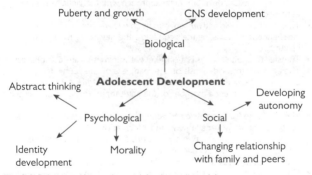

Fig. 8.1 Bidirectional biopsychosocial development in adolescence.

Aspects of healthcare

Developmentally appropriate healthcare

All young people require an approach which is developmentally appropriate to address their varied needs. It should contain the following elements:
- Biopsychosocial development and holistic care.
- Acknowledgement of young people as a distinct group.
- Adjustment of care as the young person develops.
- Empowerment of the young person by prioritizing health education and health promotion.
- Interdisciplinary and inter-organizational work.
- Recognition of importance of appropriate parental involvement as indicated by the young person.

Transition

- Transition is part of developmentally appropriate healthcare for this age group.
- Transition is a multifaceted active process that attends to the medical, psychosocial, and educational/vocational needs of adolescents as they move from child into adult care.
- This process should begin in early adolescence (11–13 years of age) and continue into young adulthood (23–25 years of age).
- This broad age range allows for a structured transition programme, adopting a flexible developmental approach with individuals progressing at their own speed.
- The process should actively encourage the young person to become independent in managing their condition and navigating their own healthcare.
- Transfer to adult services is a single event *within* the transition process.
- The age of transfer depends on the readiness of the young person, control of the condition, whether other aspects of life are stable, and opportunity to meet a member of the adult team providing care after transfer.
- The challenge for paediatric and adult endocrine services is to provide continuity of staff, management, and information.
- Good links between the two services are essential, with an agreed transition policy and mechanisms to reduce the number of young people getting lost during the transfer.
- Components of care that have shown +ve benefit in transition include patient education and skills training, transition care coordinators, joint and young adult clinics, and enhanced follow-up and out-of-hours support.

Consultation skills for adolescents and young adults

- Healthcare professionals should adapt their consultation style, screening for psychosocial issues and health behaviours.
- Young people should be asked who they have brought with them to establish they are the centre of the consultation.
- Young people should be encouraged, if appropriate, to be seen for part or all of the consultation without their parents, while recognizing and encouraging the parents' important role in supporting the young person.

HEEADDSS: a psychosocial interview

The HEEADDSS (Home, Education and employment, Exercise and eating, Activity and peers, Drugs, Depression, Sexuality and sexual health, Sleep, Safety) screening tool is useful at identifying issues that require attention.
- If areas that require attention are identified, it is important that they are addressed, employing the 5As (Ask, Advise, Agree, Assist, Arrange).
- The tool should ideally only be used if the young person is on their own, and going through the meaning and limitation of confidentiality is important.

(See Box 8.1.)

Specific areas to be covered in consultations with young people

Exploratory and risk-taking behaviours
- During adolescence, it is normal to explore behaviours that healthcare professionals consider risky.
- Substance use, including smoking, drugs, and alcohol, will commonly be tried for the 1st time during adolescence.
- Ninety-five per cent of adult smokers have usually started by age 25 years, which indicates that health choices made during adolescence translate into longer-term habits and adverse health outcomes.
- In consultations with young people with endocrine conditions, consideration should be given to whether these exploratory behaviours are occurring, potentially at a higher rate than in healthy peers, and that such behaviours may have more serious consequences for some young people, e.g. childhood cancer survivors.
- Therefore, there needs to be a non-judgemental and open approach to discussing these issues.
- This is also a real opportunity to consider health promotion elements of consultations, as these behaviours often translate into adult life.

Sexual and reproductive health
- The average age of 1st sexual intercourse is 16 years, which falls in the middle of this development phase.
- There is a duty to consider sexual health issues in consultations with young people in an endocrine clinic.
- Young people may have questions regarding sex and intimacy that they do not have the opportunity to discuss with other healthcare providers; indeed many young people will see the endocrine clinic as their main healthcare point of contact and will not attend their GP much, if at all.

Box 8.1 HEEADDSS: a psychosocial interview

- H, Home—where do you live and who lives there with you? How do you get along with each member? Who could you go to if you needed help with a problem?
- E, Education and employment—what do you like about school/work? What are you good and not good at? How do you get along with teachers and other students/work colleagues? Inquire about bullying. What are your future plans?
- E, Exercise and eating, including body image—are you happy with your weight? If you were going to lose weight, how would you do it?
- A, Activities and peers—what sort of things do you do in your spare time? Are most of your friends from school/work? Do you have one best friend, a few friends or lots of friends?
- D, Drugs, including smoking and alcohol—many young people at your age are starting to experiment with cigarettes or alcohol. Have you or your friends tried these or other drugs? How do you pay for them? Do any members of your family smoke or drink?
- D, Depression, including suicide—what sort of things do you do if you are feeling sad/angry/hurt? Some people who feel really down often feel like hurting themselves or even killing themselves. Have you ever felt this way? Have you ever tried to hurt yourself?
- S, Sexuality and sexual health—some young people are getting involved in sexual relationships. Have you had a sexual experience with a boy or girl, or both? Inquire about contraception and avoidance of sexually transmitted infections.
- S, Sleep—inquire about sleep. Adolescents who are depressed and anxious have difficulty falling asleep.
- S, Safety—inquire about driving and Internet safety.

Cohen, E, MacKenzie, R.G., Yates, G.L. (1991). HEADSS, a psychosocial risk assessment instrument: Implications for designing effective intervention programs for runaway youth. *Journal of Adolescent Health* 12 (7): 539–544.

- There is an opportunity to address safe sex, sexually transmitted infections (STIs), and contraception.
- Some endocrine conditions may generate questions around the ability to have sex, fertility, and whether there is a need for contraception— this needs to be openly addressed and questions should be welcomed.
- These areas often need revisiting at subsequent appointments, as the young person often needs time to reflect, question, and explore.

Overweight and underweight
- One in five children aged 11–15 years is obese in England.
- It is now the commonest disorder in childhood and adolescence.
- Teenagers consume eight times the recommended daily sugar allowance, and exercise levels are decreasing—by age 13–15 years, only 19% of boys and 7% of girls achieve 1h of exercise per day, and only one in 12 young people aged 11–18 years eat five portions of fruit and vegetables per day.
- Some young endocrine clinic attenders have particular issues with appetite and weight gain such as those with hypothalamic disorders.

- The sequelae of obesity in adolescence are multifactorial and include psychosocial issues, development of T2DM, and ↑ cardiovascular risk, asthma, musculoskeletal problems, and liver disease.
- At the opposite extreme, eating disorders, including anorexia nervosa, bulimia nervosa, and binge eating, can also present in adolescence.
- Factors influencing their development include biological, psychological, and cultural factors. Being underweight during adolescence or exercising too vigorously can impact on normal endocrine development with poor pubertal progression or cessation of menses, poor growth, and poor bone development.

Sleep and fatigue
- Sleep disorders can be both a cause of problems and the result of other issues in adolescence.
- The normal circadian rhythm slows during adolescence, meaning that young people are awake for longer, and it can be normal to be unable to sleep until after 11 p.m.
- Eight to 10 hours are needed per night for optimal functioning during adolescence, but many do not achieve this.
- It is also more likely that sleep patterns will vary day to day, which can disrupt sleep quality.
- Treatable sleep disorders can also occur, including insomnia, narcolepsy, sleep apnoea, and restless legs.
- Fatigue is also a common problem in adolescence and could be considered normal for many young people.
- It is defined as abnormal exhaustion after normal activities.
- There are increasing demands during adolescence as a result of physical changes, growth, and increasing social and academic demands, all of which are compounded by reduced sleep time.
- Most young people will still manage to engage in usual activities despite experiencing fatigue.
- But for a minority, this fatigue is significant and leads to reduced school attendance, impaired academic performance, and reduced social interaction, and impacts on relationships.
- When fatigue is persistent and impacting on function over a period of >3 months, consideration should be given to investigation for underlying medical causes, psychological causes, and also the possibility of chronic fatigue syndrome (CFS).
- CFS (see ➔ Clinical practice point: chronic fatigue syndrome, p. 772) is reported to occur in 0.2–0.6% of young people in the UK, a much higher rate than in the adult population. CFS is the commonest cause of school absence in the UK.

Self-harm and mental health issues
- Seventy-five per cent of mental health issues start before 24 years of age, with 10% of young people experiencing a mental health disorder at any one time.
- A quarter of young women aged 16–24 years exhibit symptoms of anxiety or depression.
- There may be concurrent issues that point towards mental health problems such as trouble at school, violence, and substance use.
- Long-term conditions increase the likelihood of mood disorder in young people, as well as in adults, including endocrine conditions.

Concordance/adherence
- Young people may not reliably take their medications, and if catastrophic consequences do not occur, it is difficult to convince young people to take their medications solely on the premise that bad things may happen.
- This relates most often to the concrete thinking of early adolescence, having yet to progress to abstract thought processes and an understanding of consequences.
- Other factors include lack of practice at looking after their own medications, differing priorities, and psychological problems.
- This is a challenge in some endocrine disorders, the prime example being adrenal insufficiency, where healthcare providers must ensure safety education highlights that GC replacement is vital for a healthy life (see ➔ Treatment of primary adrenal insufficiency, p. 303).
- Concordance, or the establishment of a therapeutic alliance between the young person and the healthcare provider, is the key to improving adherence with a long-term medication regimen for a long-term condition.
- The emphasis is on a shared approach to the condition and its treatment, rather than a judgemental, paternalistic approach, which is likely to be ineffective.
- Where there are cognitive impairments limiting adherence to treatment regimens, e.g. in some congenital/genetic disorders, or after brain radiotherapy, there needs to be collaboration with families and caregivers to develop practical solutions to the problem.

Common clinical endocrine presentations of young people during adolescence

Delayed puberty or interrupted puberty

(See **◆** Constitutional delay of growth and puberty, p. 572.)
- Puberty represents the biological change seen during adolescence and heralds the development of 2° sexual characteristics, the growth spurt, and eventually fertility.
- Puberty normally starts between the ages of 8 and 13 in girls with breast development, advancing to menarche by the age of 16. In boys, puberty starts between the ages of 9 and 15 with testicular enlargement (≥4mL).
- Delayed or interrupted puberty is defined as follows:
  - ♀: no signs of breast development by the age of 13, or no periods by the age of 15.
  - ♂: no signs of testicular enlargement (<4mL) by the age of 14.
- Delayed puberty is more frequently seen in ♂.
- A minority of adolescents will have evidence of HH, the prevalence of which is estimated to be at 13%. The remainder have impaired secretion and/or action of hypothalamic GnRH. The majority of these patients will have constitutional delay.
- History and examination need to look for indications of the following causes of HH:
  - Functional causes (chronic illness, medication, excessive exercise, malnutrition, or stress).
  - Pathology-related causes (hypothalamic and pituitary tumours, especially craniopharyngiomas).
  - Genetic causes (congenital abnormalities—indicated by midline defects, microphallus, cryptorchidism, cleft lip/palate, and scoliosis; anosmia—Kallmann's syndrome).
- A +ve family history is relevant in constitutional delay and congenital GnRH deficiency, which has a significant genetic basis, often with an AD inheritance pattern.
- Investigation depends on history and examination and should be tailored accordingly.
- Imaging of the HP axis is only required if history, examination, and investigations suggest a central lesion or if other symptoms/signs such as anosmia need further exploration.
- Distinguishing constitutional delay from HH and its causes is challenging, particularly as 10–15% of adolescents with well-documented isolated HH undergo spontaneous reversal.
- A trial of low-dose testosterone (50 mg) monthly for 3–6 months with reassessment of testicular volumes is a pragmatic approach.
- The psychological and social impact of having delayed puberty, particularly in boys, needs to be recognized and addressed.

Abnormal uterine bleeding in adolescence

- During the first 2 years after menarche, there is considerable cycle variability due to anovulatory cycles. In the 1st year, 50% of cycles are anovulatory, with 80% of cycles occurring at 21–45 days and lasting 2–7 days.

- Abnormal uterine bleeding is therefore defined in adolescence as:
  - A period of bleeding with a duration >7 days.
  - A period of bleeding with a flow >80mL/cycle (>6 pads/tampons a day).
  - Periods of bleeding that occur more frequently than every 21 days (19 days if 1st year after menarche) or less frequently than every 45 days (or 90/60 days if 1st/2nd year after menarche).
  - Intermenstrual bleeding or post-coital bleeding.
- If abnormal uterine bleeding is identified, history, examination, and appropriate investigations should be performed.
- Excluding pregnancy and enquiring about sexual history and counselling about sexual health are essential.
- When alternative diagnoses have been excluded, a diagnosis of abnormal uterine bleeding due to anovulatory cycles can be made and managed appropriately.

PCOS in adolescence

(See ➋ Polycystic ovary syndrome, pp. 340–3.)

- Symptoms and signs of PCOS frequently begin in adolescence; however, the anovulatory cycles following menarche are just one reason why diagnosing PCOS in adolescence is challenging.
- Experts have cautioned against over-diagnosing the condition in this age group, and a recent collaboration has suggested that the following two criteria should be present before considering a diagnosis of PCOS:
  - Oligomenorrhoea (>35 days) for 2 years since menarche or 1° amenorrhoea at age 16 (>199 days).
  - Moderate severe hirsutism or acne or evidence of biochemical hyperandrogenaemia on measuring serum testosterone and SHBG, with calculation of the free androgen index, androstenedione, and DHEAS.
- The psychological and social impact of having PCOS needs to be recognized and addressed.
- The approach to young people with PCOS depends on presentation and concerns, and includes identifying opportunities to discuss lifestyle in young people who are a healthy weight, overweight, or obese, to prevent the long-term consequences associated with the condition of reduced fertility and T2DM; recognizing the burden of hirsutism and offering options for management; discussing the importance of contraception while on antiandrogens; and reassuring young people about future fertility options.

Gynaecomastia in adolescence

(See ➋ Gynaecomastia, p. 430.)

- Gynaecomastia is common in adolescence (40–69%) due to an imbalance of oestradiol and testosterone production during puberty.
- Pubertal gynaecomastia is usually most obvious between 13 and 14 years of age and resolves by the age of 17, although in some instances it may persist.
- Persistent pubertal gynaecomastia accounts for 25% of gynaecomastia presenting in adulthood.
- Reassurance is often all that is required.

Young people with endocrine conditions undergoing transition

The approach to a young person with an endocrine condition depends on the condition and the timing of the presentation and includes the following aims:

- To ensure the young person who presented earlier in childhood has all the information previously shared with their parents about their diagnosis, previous investigations, and management.
- To address the priorities of the young person presenting later in adolescence, particularly in respect of delayed puberty and short stature.
- To revisit the diagnosis or degree of hormone deficiency/excess, e.g. GHD (see ➔ Management of young people with hypopituitarism and growth hormone deficiency, pp. 624–5).
- To discuss investigations and management with the young person regarding cardiovascular, bone, and reproductive health, as well as QoL.
- To raise awareness of maintaining safety for those on hydrocortisone and desmopressin and recognizing ill health and what to do and when to seek help.
- To identify the level of endocrine care required in adult life and whether care can be provided by the family doctor, e.g. in congenital hypothyroidism, or whether transfer to adult services is required.

In addition, more generic approaches are also important.

- To encourage increasing independence on healthcare, including organizing medication and prescriptions, arranging appointments at times suitable to them, coming in for part or all of the consultation independently of their parents, and contacting the hospital in between appointments to seek information and advice.
- To address barriers to engagement with healthcare, including adherence.
- To discuss useful resources to get health information and support, including patient support groups.
- To address concerns about venepuncture or injections, particularly around transfer to adult services.
- To highlight benefits and ways of disclosure about the condition to friends, teachers, and employers.
- Through psychosocial screening (see ➔ HEEADDSS: a psychosocial interview, p. 614) to address broader issues such as psychological, social, and educational/vocational issues and health behaviours by identifying risk and protective factors.
- To deliver health promotion, including discussion about sexual health and contraception.

Ongoing management of congenital and acquired conditions diagnosed in childhood

Who needs re-evaluation?

The completion of linear growth is an opportunity to review current endocrine status and adequacy of endocrine replacement, and for some to revisit the diagnosis, and screen for health conditions commoner in adult life. Agreement would be required between paediatric and adult endocrine teams and the young person and their carers where it is most appropriate for these evaluations to take place.

This is the case for:

- Patients where the underlying diagnosis made in childhood was unclear and establishing that the endocrine issues persist is important.
- Patients with hypopituitarism, particularly isolated hormone deficiencies which may recover, e.g. GHD (see ➔ Management of young people with hypopituitarism and growth hormone deficiency, pp. 624–5) and HH (10–20% exhibit spontaneous recovery).
- Patients at risk of evolving hypopituitarism: post-radiotherapy and those with congenital hypopituitarism associated with structural abnormalities in the HP area (e.g. ectopic posterior pituitary), midline brain and optic nerve abnormalities, and genetic defects (e.g. in the *GH-1* or *POU1F1* genes; see ➔ Management of young people with hypopituitarism and growth hormone deficiency, pp. 624–5).
- Patients with HP lesions that require ongoing serial imaging with MRI.
- Patients with CAH; an SST to assess cortisol status may assist in those with non-classical CAH as alternative management could be considered at this age and, on occasion, in those who are poorly compliant with GCs by providing further information to support discussion with the young person.
- Patients who require assessment of reproductive health, e.g. testicular US for testicular adrenal rest tumours in boys with CAH and assessment by gynaecology for some girls with CAH (see ➔ Congenital adrenal hyperplasia in adults, pp. 354–5).
- Patients who require comprehensive health screening, e.g. in young people with Turner syndrome (requirement for cardiovascular and hearing assessment) and in childhood cancer survivors (monitoring for non-endocrine late effects).

Who needs to be part of the wider MDT involved in transition in endocrinology?

Involvement of the MDT is important at this time; paediatric and adult endocrinologists and endocrine nurses need to liaise with each other. Young people should have access to the following people (dependent on the condition):

- Psychologists (although not always available within the service) can provide much needed support for all young people with endocrine conditions as they make the transition from childhood to adulthood.
- Clinical geneticist should be a key member of the transition team from several perspectives: to provide information about those with a clear or potential genetic diagnosis that may have previously been shared with parents, to explain the potential implications of genetic mutations for future offspring (as in CAH).
- A urologist/gynaecologist is essential for many patients with a DSD who may require a physical assessment and a discussion about sexual function and future pregnancy.
- A fertility specialist is essential for those focused on understanding more about options for fertility at this time, particularly if there may be opportunities for fertility preservation, e.g. in ♀ with Turner syndrome with a menstrual cycle, ♀ childhood cancer survivors at risk of POI, ♂ with Klinefelter's syndrome, ♂ with CAH who have testicular adrenal rest tumours.
- A cardiologist is important for ♀ with Turner syndrome and cancer survivors previously treated with anthracyclines or chest irradiation.

- Neuro-rehabilitation specialists, neurologists, and neurosurgeons for young people are required for those with a past history of a brain tumour who require ongoing surveillance or have neurological sequelae from the tumour or its treatment.
- ENT/audiology are key for groups of young people with endocrine conditions associated with reduced hearing which, in turn, reduces QoL, e.g. Turner syndrome, CHARGE syndrome (coloboma of the eye, heart defects, atresia of the nasal choanae, restriction of growth, genital and/or urinary abnormalities, and ear abnormalities or deafness), and some childhood cancer survivors.

The focus of care in late adolescence is related to QoL and cardiovascular, bone, and reproductive health from the perspective of monitoring and optimizing hormone replacement. In adolescents, after the achievement of adult height, there is a change in the management approach in some conditions from that in paediatrics to reflect adult practice, e.g. management of sex steroid deficiency or GC replacement in CAH in adolescents who have completed puberty. However, adolescence and young adulthood are seen as a distinct treatment period for young people with GHD.

Management of young people with hypopituitarism and growth hormone deficiency

(See ➡ Hypopituitarism, pp. 138–9.)

- Young people with childhood-onset GHD that is persistent have a deficit in muscle and bone mass.
- GH replacement reduces this deficit and, in addition, for some young people, improves energy levels/QoL, one of the 1° indications for GH replacement in adult life.
- Young people treated with GH replacement for GHD during childhood require reassessment when growth rate falls to <2cm/year.
- This is necessary, as a high percentage of young people with GHD will retest as normal and could discontinue treatment and be discharged.
- Some patient groups who are at risk of evolving pituitary dysfunction, e.g. those who have undergone radiation treatment, those with structural abnormalities affecting the pituitary gland, and those with other pituitary hormone deficiencies, should not be discharged, even if found to be normal at reassessment.
- Reassessment strategies are based on whether the young person has three or more additional pituitary hormone deficiencies or whether they have a high or low likelihood of GHD. Peak GH level during provocative testing in childhood should also be considered.
- Of note, other indications for GH treatment in childhood, such as Turner syndrome, do not require assessment of GH status at the end of growth.

High likelihood of persistent growth hormone deficiency

Indications that there is a high likelihood of persistent GHD are as follows:
- For congenital/idiopathic GHD:
  - Septo-optic dysplasia and other midline defects.
  - A defined genetic mutation.
  - Structural abnormalities that are located in the HP axis and affect positioning of the posterior pituitary gland or the pituitary stalk, or are associated with three or more pituitary hormone deficits.
- For acquired GHD:
  - A destructive lesion affecting the HP axis.
  - Cranial irradiation (high dose).

Low likelihood of persistent growth hormone deficiency

Indications that there is a low likelihood of persistent GHD are as follows:
- For idiopathic GHD: isolated GHD or GHD with two or less pituitary hormone deficits in the absence of structural abnormalities located in the HP axis and affecting positioning of the posterior pituitary gland or the pituitary stalk.
- For acquired GHD: cranial irradiation (low dose).

Reinitiation of growth hormone replacement

- In those with persistent GHD (IGF-1 <−2 SD or peak GH (depending on consensus document or guidance being followed) <3, 5, or 6 micrograms/L (for ITT)), GH replacement should be offered to the young person and restarted at the lower dose of 0.2–0.3mg, with titration to IGF-1 levels similar to practice in adults.

Summary

- Care for adolescents in endocrinology should include a developmental approach focusing on psychosocial and educational and vocational, as well as medical, outcomes; transition is part of this.
- Transition should begin in early adolescence and, to be successful, requires close working between paediatric and adult endocrine teams.
- Knowledge of normal physiology in adolescence relating to puberty and the menstrual cycle allows tailoring of investigations and appropriate management.
- Young people with long-term endocrine conditions require a change of focus in their care in late adolescence and a start on screening for issues relevant in adult life.

Further reading

Clayton PE, et al. (2005). Consensus statement on the management of the GH-treated adolescent in the transition to adult care. *Eur J Endocrinol* **152**, 165–70.

Crowley R, et al. (2011). Improving the transition between paediatric and adult healthcare: a systematic review. *Arch Dis Child* **96**, 548–53.

Derbyshire Children and Young People's Health Promotion Programme. *You're Welcome Quality Criteria: young people friendly health services.* ℘ http://www.dchs.nhs.uk/assets/public/dchs/dchs_health_promo_service/cyph/youre_welcome/YWGettingStartedFlier.pdf

Goldenring JM, Rosen DS (2004). Getting into adolescent heads: an essential update. *Contemp Pediatr* **21**, 64–90.

National Institute for Health and Care Excellence (2016). *Transition from children's to adults' services for young people using health or social care service.* NICE guideline [NG43]. ℘ https://www.nice.org.uk/guidance/ng43

Peacock A, et al. (2012). Period problems: disorders of menstruation in adolescents. *Arch Dis Child* **97**, 554–60.

Sklar CA, et al. (2018). Hypothalamic-pituitary and growth disorders in survivors of childhood cancer: an Endocrine Society clinical practice guideline. *J Clin Endocrinol Metab* **103**, 2761–84.

Wales JK (2012). Disorders pubertal development. *Arch Dis Child Educ Pract Ed* **97**, 9–16.

Neuroendocrine disorders

Karin Bradley

The neuroendocrine system

- Neuroendocrine cells are found in many sites throughout the body. These cells have the ability to synthesize, store, and release peptide hormones.
- Due to the prevalence of neuroendocrine cells, the majority of NETs occur within the gastroenteropancreatic axis but may also be found in other areas, including the lungs and thymus.
- The incidence of NETs globally has steadily risen over the last 50 years. For example, a 5-fold increase in the annual age-adjusted incidence of NETs from 1.09/100,000 in 1973 to 5.25/100,000 in 2004 was observed in the United States. Other studies across many countries show a similar trend. This may, in part, be related to an ↑ awareness and improved diagnosis of this tumour group.
- NETs encompass a spectrum from benign to malignant and may be functional (hormone-secreting) or non-functional (see Table 9.1).
- This chapter focuses on gastroenteropancreatic (GEP) NETs.
- NETs most commonly occur as sporadic (non-inherited) tumours, but a minority (up to 10%) may occur as part of an inherited syndrome. For inherited syndromes associated with NETs, see Table 9.2.

Table 9.1 NET classification

NET	Secretory products
Non-functioning	Nil
Carcinoid syndrome	Serotonin, tachykinins, bradykinins, histamine
Insulinomas	Insulin
Gastrinomas	Gastrin
Glucagonomas	Glucagon
VIPomas	VIP
Somatostatinomas	Somatostatin
Rare NETs	ACTH, PTHrP, GHRH, renin

- There are various systems with proven prognostic significance (e.g. Ki67) for staging and grading NETs and tumour classification.
- Tumours localized to the rectum or appendix have a good prognosis (5-year survival >80%), whereas pancreatic NETs (pNETs) have the least good outcomes (5-year survival 45%).
- ~50% of NET patients overall present with operatively incurable metastatic disease at the time of diagnosis and so treatment strategies frequently need to extend beyond surgery.
- Endocrinologists are often primarily responsible for functioning NETs, those that result in systemic carcinoid syndrome, or functioning pNETs such as insulinomas, gastrinomas, VIPomas, and glucagonomas. More rarely, functional NETs may secrete other biologically active peptides such as ACTH, GHrH, PTHrP, somatostatin, or renin.

Table 9.2 Inherited syndromes associated with NETs

Inherited syndrome	Possible associated NETs
MEN1	Gastrinomas (duodenal or pancreatic)
	Other pancreatic NETs (typically functional, secreting glucagon, insulin, or pancreatic polypeptide)
	(Rarely phaeochromocytomas)
VHL	Pancreatic NETs (usually non-functioning)
	(Phaeochromocytomas)
NF-1	GEP NETs
	(Phaeochromocytomas)
Tuberous sclerosis	Pancreatic NETs (most commonly insulinomas)

- Treatment strategies should be delivered via an experienced NET MDT comprising medical oncologists, endocrinologists, surgeons, radiologists, gastroenterologists, histopathologists, and nurse specialists.

Further reading

Association for Multiple Endocrine Neoplasia Disorders (AMEND). ℜ https://www.amend.org.uk

Caplin ME, et al.; the CLARINET Investigators (2014). Lanreotide in metastatic enteropancreatic neuroendocrine tumors. *N Engl J Med* **371**, 224–33.

Davar J, et al. (2017). Diagnosing and managing carcinoid heart disease in patients with neuroendocrine tumours. *J Am Coll Cardiol* **69**, 1288–304.

Falconi M, et al. (2016). ENETS consensus guidelines. *Neuroendocrinology* **103**, 153–71.

Hofland J, et al. (2018). Role of biomarker tests for the diagnosis of neuroendocrine tumours. *Nat Rev Endocrinol* **14**, 656–69.

Hofland J, et al. (2019). Management of carcinoid syndrome: a systematic review and meta-analysis. *Endocr Relat Cancer* **26**, 145–56.

Neuroendocrine Cancer UK (formerly NET Patient Foundation). ℜ https://www.neuroendocrinecancer.org.uk/about-ncuk/

Raymond E, et al. (2011). Sunitinib malate for the treatment of pancreatic neuroendocrine tumors. *N Engl J Med* **364**, 501–13.

Rinke A, et al. (2009). Placebo-controlled, double-blind, prospective, randomized study on the effect of octreotide LAR in the control of tumor growth in patients with metastatic neuroendocrine midgut tumors: a report from the PROMID Study Group. *J Clin Oncol* **27**, 4656–63.

Strosberg J, et al. (2017). NETTER 1, phase III trial of 177Lu dotatate for midgut neuroendocrine tumors. *N Engl J Med* **376**, 125–35.

Yao JC, et al. (2008). One hundred years after 'carcinoid': epidemiology of and prognostic factors for neuroendocrine tumors in 35,825 cases in the United States. *J Clin Oncol* **26**, 3063–72.

Yao JC, et al. (2011). Everolimus for advanced pancreatic neuroendocrine tumors. *N Engl J Med* **364**, 514–23.

Yao JC, et al. (2016). Everolimus for the treatment of advanced, non-functional neuroendocrine tumours of the lung or gastrointestinal tract (RADIANT-4): a randomised, placebo-controlled, phase 3 study. *Lancet* **387**, 968–77.

Neuroendocrine tumours

Diagnostic investigations

Pathology

- The WHO 2010 and European Neuroendocrine Tumor Society (ENETS) systems are used to grade and stage NETs.
- A measure of the nuclear protein Ki67, which is a marker of cellular proliferation, is included and may be prognostic.
- Tumours are graded 1 (well differentiated, low grade), 2 (well differentiated, intermediate grade), or 3 (poorly differentiated, high grade).

Biochemical investigations

- Chromogranin A is a glycoprotein found in neuroendocrine cells. The sensitivity of this test varies widely (32–92%) and is influenced by tumour type, functionality, and disease extent. False +ves occur in renal failure, liver failure, PPIs, atrophic gastritis, and inflammatory bowel disease. False −ves occur with levodopa or phenothiazine therapy.
- Chromogranin B is typically unhelpful, apart from possibly in patients taking PPIs as these drugs do not affect chromogranin B in the same way as chromogranin A.
- A fasting plasma gut hormone profile is important to identify NETs causing secretory hormone syndromes.
- Liver biochemistry is an unreliable marker of hepatic involvement.
- A subset of NETs (most commonly small intestinal NETs) may secrete serotonin (5-hydroxytryptamine). When secretion is in sufficient amounts and when it bypasses the portal venous system (non-GI 1° tumour (e.g. thymus) or in the presence of liver metastases directly accessing the systemic circulation), carcinoid syndrome may develop.
- 5-hydroxyindoleacetic acid (5-HIAA) is the main metabolite of serotonin and can be measured in urine or plasma. The test has limited sensitivity, but better specificity, provided that dietary (e.g. bananas, avocados, tomatoes, walnuts, pecan nuts, aubergines, kiwis, plums, pineapples, coffee, tea, and chocolate) or medication (see Box 9.1) influences on serotonin are avoided 3 days prior to, and for the duration of, the test (72h). False +ves may result in the context of coeliac disease, CF, and small cell lung cancer.

Box 9.1 Drugs causing increase or decrease in 5-HIAA

Drugs that increase:

- Caffeine
- Diazepam
- Ephedrine
- Fluorouracil
- Guaifenesin
- Naproxen
- Nicotine
- Paracetamol
- Phenobarbital
- Phentolamine
- Reserpine
- Aspirin
- Chlorpromazine
- Imipramine
- Levodopa
- MAO inhibitors
- Heparin
- Isoniazid
- Methyldopa
- Perchloperazine
- Phenothiazine
- Promazin
- Promethazine
- Tricyclic antidepressants

Exclude associated inherited syndromes
- NETs may be associated with MEN1 and, more rarely, with VHL, NF-1, and tuberous sclerosis (see Table 9.2).

Tumour localization and staging
- Cross-sectional imaging with CT/MRI, in combination with PET/CT with gallium-68 (^{68}Ga)-labelled SSAs, aims to both localize the 1° tumour and assess the extent of metastatic spread.
- Imaging modalities are outlined in Table 9.3.

Table 9.3 Imaging modalities for NETs

Imaging modality	Main utility
CT	Often initial imaging technique
	Useful for disease staging and surgical planning due to excellent anatomical detail
MRI	Provides excellent information regarding hepatic metastases
	CT typically better at locating 1° tumour, except in pNETs
^{18}FDG-PET	NETs typically −ve unless high grade
Octreoscan	Functional whole body imaging which confirms presence of somatostatin receptor expression by tumour and therefore aids diagnostically and potentially therapeutically
	Can be fused with CT to improve anatomical localization
^{68}Ga PET/CT	As for octreoscan, except superior sensitivity
	Most sensitive imaging modality overall for 1° tumour and metastases

Box 9.2 Monitoring treatment
- Imaging modalities are the mainstay for essential monitoring of tumour burden and documenting response to treatment intervention according to RECIST (response evaluation criteria in solid tumours).
- Serum chromogranin A, urinary 5-HIAA, or other biomarkers can be useful to monitor response to therapy if those markers were elevated at diagnosis.
- Non-functioning NETs of ≤2cm do not change size in 50–80%.

Treatment
- A multidisciplinary approach to treatment of these tumours is essential. Care should be delivered under the supervision of an experienced NET MDT.
- Monitoring treatment is shown in Box 9.2.

Surgical treatment
- In patients with local disease or limited hepatic metastases, surgery can be curative.
- Non-curative debulking surgery may be appropriate in selected cases, e.g. size >10–20mm or >5mm increase in size in 6 months.
- Surgery may be required to alleviate obstructive intestinal disease.

Symptomatic medical treatment
- Certain symptom-specific medical agents can be useful such as loperamide or codeine for diarrhoea or, more specifically, telotristat ethyl (serotonin synthesis inhibitor).
- SSAs.

Somatostatin analogues
- The SSAs octreotide or lanreotide reduce the level of biochemical tumour markers in the majority of patients and typically ameliorate symptoms in patients with well-differentiated grade 1 and 2 and metastatic NETs.
- However, the efficacy of these agents in also offering control of tumour growth has only been recognized since 2009. Two landmark trials (PROMID and CLARINET) have led to these agents becoming routine treatment for grade 1 NETs (see Table 9.4).
- A continuous IV infusion of octreotide is the most effective treatment for a carcinoid crisis and is generally given at a rate of 50–100 micrograms/h. A similar approach is used prophylactically for patients with carcinoid syndrome undergoing procedures/surgery.

Everolimus
- Everolimus (an inhibitor of the mTOR pathway) can offer benefits in tumour control and overall survival in progressive well-differentiated, unresectable, or metastatic NETs (grades 1 and 2) originating from the pancreas, lung, GI tract, or where the 1° site is unknown (RADIANT trial data). Adverse events include anaemia, hyperglycaemia, and pneumonitis.

Table 9.4 Landmark NETs studies

Study	Summary findings
PROMID (2009)	Octreotide LAR® significantly lengthens time to tumour progression, compared with placebo, in patients with functionally active and inactive metastatic midgut (no pancreatic) NETs; 66% reduction in risk of disease progression
CLARINET (2014)	Lanreotide Autogel® significantly lengthens time to tumour progression, compared with placebo, in patients with metastatic grade 1/2 non-functioning GEP NETs; 53% reduction in risk of disease progression
RADIANT 1–4 (2010–2016)	Everolimus significantly lengthens time to tumour progression, compared with placebo, in patients with advanced, progressive grade 1/2 non-functioning and functioning GEP and lung NETs

Sunitinib

- Sunitinib (a TKI) can offer benefits in tumour control and overall survival in progressive well-differentiated, unresectable, or metastatic NETs (grades 1 and 2) originating from the pancreas. Adverse effects incude anaemia, hyperglycaemia, and pneumonitis.

Liver targeted therapies

- Data are confounded by the myriad of different ablative options which may or may not incorporate chemotherapy or radiotherapy.
- These are essentially palliative procedures which may offer symptomatic relief by decreasing tumour bulk.
- The duration of improvement may be short-lived and, occasionally, significant side effects, such as hepatorenal syndrome, may occur.

External beam radiotherapy

- May provide palliation in those with symptomatic bone metastases or spinal cord compression.

Chemotherapy

- Cytotoxic chemotherapy may be considered in patients with advanced, progressive, or uncontrolled symptomatic disease, as it has been shown to offer a survival advantage over best supportive care.
- In clinical practice, chemotherapy is mainly utilized in people with a high disease burden and with grade 3 tumours (Ki67 >20%) which have poor survival rates.
- Cisplatin and etoposide are one of the most widely used regimens, although data supporting other options also exist (e.g. streptozotocin-based regimens).
- Side effects remain the greatest limitation to the use of chemotherapy.

Immunotherapy

- Interferon alfa has been shown to offer biochemical and radiological improvements for patients with progressive disease and has been shown to be helpful in combination with SSAs, but is actually rarely used due to its high toxicity rates.

Peptide receptor radionuclide therapyy (PRRT)

- PRRT using ^{177}Lu-DOTATATE was approved by NICE in 2018 as a treatment option for unresectable or metastatic, progressive, well-differentiated (grade 1 or 2) somatostatin receptor +ve GEP NETs in adults.
- The NETTER-1 trial data demonstrate that this treatment modality improves progression-free and overall survival, as well as offers good QoL in this patient group.
- Treatment is typically well tolerated, and renal, hepatic, and bone marrow risks appear to be low.

Prognosis

- The site of origin of the 1° tumour, together with any functionality subtype and the extent of metastatic disease, largely determines prognosis, which may be highly variable and unpredictable.
- Many NETs are indolent and may be incidental findings or even postmortem diagnoses.
- For grade 1 and 2 NETs where the disease at diagnosis is confined locally to the region of the 1° tumour, 5-year survival is typically >70%.
- The 5-year survival rate for grade 1 and 2 NETs when hepatic metastases are present ranges from 14% to 54%, dependent upon the 1° site.
- Both survival time and QoL for NET patients are typically improved by the use of more interventional therapies.
- In carcinoid syndrome specifically, prognosis is greatly influenced by the development of carcinoid heart disease and whether it is then amenable to treatment by heart valve replacement.

Further reading

Caplin ME, et al.; for the CLARINET Investigators (2014). Lanreotide in metastatic enteropancreatic neuroendocrine tumors. *N Engl J Med* **371**, 224–33.

European Neuroendocrine Tumor Society. *Current ENETS guidelines.* ℬ https://www.enets.org/current_guidelines.html

Harper S, Harrison B (2015). First surgery for pancreatic neuroendocrine tumours in a patient with MEN1: enucleation versus disease-modifying surgery. *Clin Endocrinol (Oxf)* **83**, 618–21.

Hofland J, et al. (2018). Role of biomarker tests for the diagnosis of neuroendocrine tumours. *Nat Rev Endocrinol* **14**, 656–69.

Maxwell J, et al. (2015). Imaging in neuroendocrine tumours: an update for the clinician. *Int J Endocrinol Oncol* **2**, 159–68.

Pavel M, et al. (2012). ENETs consensus guidelines for the management of patients with liver and other distant metastases from NETs of foregut, midgut, hindgut and unknown primary. *Neuroendocrinology* **95**, 157–76.

Raymond E, et al. (2011). Sunitinib malate for the treatment of pancreatic neuroendocrine tumors. *N Engl J Med* **364**, 501–13.

Rinke A, et al. (2009). Placebo-controlled, double-blind, prospective, randomized study on the effect of octreotide LAR in the control of tumor growth in patients with metastatic neuroendocrine midgut tumors: a report from the PROMID Study Group. *J Clin Oncol* **27**, 4656–63.

Strosberg J, et al. (2017). NETTER-1, phase III trial of 177Lu-dotatate for midgut neuroendocrine tumors. *N Engl J Med* **376**, 125–35.

UK and Ireland Neuroendocrine Tumour Society. *Clinical practice.* ℬ https://www.ukinets.org/net-clinics-clinical-practice/

Yao JC, et al. (2011). Everolimus for advanced pancreatic neuroendocrine tumors. *N Engl J Med* **364**, 514–23.

Yao JC, et al. (2016). Everolimus for the treatment of advanced, non-functional neuroendocrine tumours of the lung or gastrointestinal tract (RADIANT-4): a randomised, placebo-controlled, phase 3 study. *Lancet* **387**, 968–77.

Carcinoid syndrome

(See Boxes 9.3 and 9.4.)

- Occurs in a small subset of patients typically with NETs where the 1°
  arises in the small intestine.
- Symptoms develop when sufficient vasoactive substances are released
  into the systemic circulation and therefore are typically seen in the
  context of liver metastases.
- The predominant peptide secreted is serotonin (5-hydroxytryptamine),
  but tachykinins, bradykinins, and histamine may also be implicated.
- Symptoms include flushing (~94%), diarrhoea (~80%), and dyspnoea/
  wheezing (~10%) 2° to bronchospasm. These symptoms have multiple
  aetiologies, and careful gastroenterological or respiratory specialist
  assessments may be useful.
- The carcinoid flush may be precipitated by spicy food, hot drinks,
  alcohol, exercise, and postural changes. Patients should be given
  relevant lifestyle advice to minimize these precipitants.
- Acute attacks typically cause a diffuse erythematous flush affecting the
  face and upper thorax, whereas long-standing carcinoid syndrome may
  be associated with a violacious flush and facial telangiectasia.
- Pellagra (niacin deficiency) may occur (~5%) and is characterized by
  dermatitis, diarrhoea, and dementia.
- Symptoms are improved with SSA therapy in the majority of patients
  (>70%). In resistant patients, antidiarrhoeal agents, antihistamines, or
  telotristat ethyl (serotonin synthesis inhibitor) may be trialled. The
  latter is reported to be effective in around one-third of patients with
  previously uncontrolled diarrhoea.
- Longer-term, patients with carcinoid syndrome may develop fibrosis
  within the gut mesentery and affecting the structure and function of the
  cardiac valves (typically the right-sided tricuspid and pulmonary valves).

Box 9.3 Perioperative management of NETs causing carcinoid syndrome and carcinoid crisis

- It is useful to give IV octreotide (50–100 micrograms/h) in the
  perioperative period, as both anaesthesia and surgery may be associated
  with the release of vasoactive peptides which can result in hypotension
  and bronchospasm, leading to a potentially fatal carcinoid crisis.
- A carcinoid crisis refers to the situation where cardiovascular
  instability results from excessive release of vasoactive peptides from
  a functioning NET. IV octreotide is the mainstay of treatment and IV
  fluids, antihistamines, and bronchodilator agents may be helpful.

Box 9.4 Carcinoid heart disease

- Occurs in the majority of patients with carcinoid syndrome.
- The mechanism is poorly understood, but consequent on chronic over-exposure to high plasma serotonin levels.
- Pathologically, the lesions are characterized by fibrous thickening of the endocardium in plaques.
- The right side of the heart is more typically involved and is the predominantly affected side in >90% of cases. Thickening and retraction of the tricuspid and pulmonary valve leaflets lead to tricuspid regurgitation in nearly all, and less commonly pulmonary regurgitation, tricuspid stenosis, and pulmonary stenosis.
- Carcinoid heart disease is a major source of morbidity and mortality for carcinoid syndrome patients.
- Measurement of urine or plasma 5-HIAA levels and plasma N-terminal pro-B-type natriuretic peptide levels, and transthoracic echocardiography may all be useful tools in the assessment of patients at risk from or with carcinoid heart disease. The exact approach to screening will be centre-dependent, but some form of assessment should be completed annually.
- Medical management of heart failure, lowering of 5-HIAA levels, and cardiac valve replacement may all be therapeutic strategies that improve QoL and length of life, and patients should be managed in a centre experienced in assessing patients with carcinoid heart disease.

▶ Tricky issue: Who to investigate for carcinoid syndrome?

- Patients with persistent classical carcinoid symptoms unexplained by other diagnoses should be screened for carcinoid syndrome, initially with urinary or plasma 5-HIAA (sensitivity 73%, specificity 100%) and serum chromogranin A (sensitivity 63%, specificity 98%).
- Imaging may be considered in the context of −ve biochemistry if clinical suspicion remains high (decision by experienced NET clinician).
- Avoid: bananas, plums, tomatoes, walnuts, pineapples, pecan nuts, and drugs, e.g. phenacetin for 3 days prior (see Box 9.1).

Further reading

Davar J, et al. (2017). Diagnosing and managing carcinoid heart disease in patients with neuroendocrine tumours. *J Am Coll Cardiol* **69**, 1288–304.

Hart EA, et al. (2017). Carcinoid heart disease. *Neth Heart J* **25**, 471–8.

Hofland J, et al. (2019). Management of carcinoid syndrome: a systematic review and meta-analysis. *Endocr Relat Cancer* **26**, 145–56.

Insulinomas

Definitions

- An insulinoma is a tumour of the endocrine pancreas that causes hypoglycaemia through its inappropriate secretion of insulin.
- Unlike other endocrine tumours of the pancreas where malignancy is common, >90% of insulinomas are benign.
- The vast majority of insulinomas are <2cm in size, solitary, benign, and sporadic, but up to 5% occur in the context of MEN1.
- Insulinomas are found with equal frequency throughout the head, body, and tail of the pancreas.

Incidence

- The annual incidence of insulinomas is recognized to be in the order of 1–32 per million population.

Clinical presentation

- Symptoms of hypoglycaemia may include both adrenergic (e.g. pallor, sweating, tremor, and tachycardia) and neuroglycopenic (e.g. irritability, confusion, aggression, seizures, and coma) symptoms.
- Whipple's triad should be confirmed as part of the diagnostic work-up, but be aware that, over time, hypoglycaemia unawareness may develop and potentially confound the clinical picture.
- Symptoms are typically precipitated by fasting or with exercise, but a minority present with postprandial hypoglycaemia as the only symptom.
- Weight gain is often seen.

Biochemical investigations

- A laboratory glucose measurement after three separate 15h fasts is a reliable initial screening test for insulinoma. If these glucose results are normal and clinical suspicion is low, then the diagnosis can often be excluded. These can be completed as an outpatient, unless there is concern regarding severe hypoglycaemia or hypoglycaemia unawareness.
- The presence of sulfonylurea metabolites in the urine or plasma should be excluded, and abuse of exogenous insulin considered.
- In those rare cases where the 15h fasts fail to reveal hypoglycaemia and a diagnosis of insulinoma remains strongly suspected, then the gold standard test remains the inpatient supervised 72h fast. The patient must remain active and exercise normally throughout the test. The criteria to confirm the diagnosis are symptomatic hypoglycaemia (<2.2mmol/L) in association with inappropriately elevated insulin (>5 microunits/mL in 91%), proinsulin, and C-peptide levels.
- Chromogranin A is not a helpful diagnostic test. β-hydroxybutyrate levels are low.
- A prolonged OGTT may be required to diagnose those cases presenting as postprandial hypoglycaemia (other differential diagnoses of postprandial hypoglycaemia will then need excluding).

Tumour localization

(See Table 9.5.)

- Islet cell tumours are often small and may not be detected by any imaging technique. The available radiological modalities have a wide reported range of sensitivity which is frequently dependent on the equipment and the operator.
- Cross-sectional imaging with CT (sensitivity 16–73%) or MRI (sensitivity 7–45%) is important to complete in order to identify the less common large or metastatic tumours and to facilitate preoperative planning.
- Endoscopic US (sensitivity 37–94%) is recommended if no lesions are visible on CT/MRI. It is more effective at identifying lesions in the head vs the tail of the pancreas.
- Arterial calcium stimulated venous sampling (sensitivity 90–100%) is an invasive technique and typically is reserved for the situation of multiple lesions (especially in MEN1). It can also be utilized in a minority (<10%) of insulinomas that are not localizable by conventional techniques prior to proceeding to surgery. A +ve result is a 2-fold increase in right hepatic vein insulin from baseline and/or 60s after injection; false −ves may be seen if glucose-sensitive insulinoma or on diazoxide treatment.
- Intraoperative US (sensitivity 75–100%) using a transducer applied directly to the pancreas may be extremely helpful and experienced surgeons can frequently identify the lesions intraoperatively by palpation alone, and the risk of multiple tumours makes a thorough examination of the whole pancreas essential at operation.
- Conventional somatostatin receptor scintigraphy is +ve in a minority of cases since most insulinomas do not express somatostatin receptors and even PET/CT with ⁶⁸Ga-labelled SSAs is only +ve in up to 30% of insulinomas.
- For the future, glucagon-like peptide-1 (GLP-1) receptor scintigraphy shows potentially encouraging results.

Table 9.5 Radiological localization of pancreatic insulinomas

Localization technique	Reported sensitivity (%)
CT	16–73
MRI	7–45
Endoscopic US	37–94
Intraoperative US	75–100
⁶⁸Ga-labelled PET/CT	Up to 30
Venous sampling	90–100

Treatment

- The treatment of choice in all but very elderly or debilitated patients is surgical removal, preferably by enucleation or limited resection. This approach yields extremely high cure rates.
- A laparoscopic approach is recommended for patients with a sporadic isolated lesion.
- The perioperative mortality rates are <1% in the hands of an experienced surgeon. Mortality is largely influenced by the incidence of acute pancreatitis and peritonitis.
- Postoperative hyperglycaemia may occur, even following partial pancreatectomy.
- Ablative therapy has also been reported to be a successful therapeutic option.
- Medical improvement of hypoglycaemia may be achieved by dietary modifications and the use of diazoxide in the 1st instance. Octreotide may be helpful, but via GH and glucagon suppression, it may actually exacerbate hypoglycaemia in some patients.
- Treatment strategies for those with malignant insulinomas (<10%) may include debulking surgery, peptide receptor radionuclide therapy (PRRT), liver targeted therapies, systemic chemotherapy, or use of everolimus or sunitinib. It is worth noting that the common side effect of hyperglycaemia with everolimus may be advantageous in this patient group.

Prognosis

- Following removal of a solitary insulinoma, life expectancy is restored to normal.
- Malignant insulinomas, with metastases usually to the liver, have a natural history of years, rather than months (49–66% 5-year survival).

Further reading

Bernard V, et al. (2013). Efficacy of everolimus in patients with metastatic insulinoma and refractory hypoglycemia. *Eur J Endocrinol* **168**, 665.

Dauben L, et al. (2019). Comparison of the diagnostic accuracy of the current guidelines for detecting insulinoma. *Eur J Endocrinol* **180**, 381

Dimitriadis G, et al. (2016). Medical management of secretory syndromes related to GEP NETs. *Endoc Relat Cancer* **23**, 423–36.

Guettier JM, et al. (2013). The role of proinsulin and insulin in the diagnosis of insulinoma: a critical evaluation of the Endocrine Society clinical practice guideline. *J Clin Endocrinol Metab* **98**, 4752.

Wexler DJ, et al. (2018). Case 23-2018: a 36-year-old man with episodes of confusion and hypoglycemia. *N Engl J Med* **379**, 376–85.

Gastrinomas

Definitions

- Gastrin, synthesized in G cells situated predominantly in the gastric antrum, is the principal gut hormone stimulating gastric acid secretion.
- Zollinger–Ellison (gastrinoma) syndrome (ZES) is due to excessive release of gastrin by NETs of the GI tract and pancreas.
- Twenty-five per cent of gastrinomas are located in the pancreatic islets, while 70% arise from gastrin-producing cells in the duodenum; 5% occur at other sites.
- Gastrinomas have extremely high malignancy rates (60–90%).
- They are associated with MEN1 in 20–25% of cases.

Incidence

- The annual incidence of gastrinoma is recognized to be in the order of 0.5–21.5 per million population.

Clinical presentation

- Patients typically present with peptic and/or oesophageal ulcers that are multiple and refractory to standard medical treatment.
- Complications of peptic ulcer disease, such as perforation, haemorrhage, and pyloric stenosis, are frequently seen.
- Pain (79–100%), diarrhoea (90–100%), oesophageal symptoms (31–56%), and malabsorption (due to acid-related inactivation of enzymes and mucosal damage in the upper small bowel) are all common presentations.

Biochemical investigations

- The diagnosis rests on finding an inappropriately elevated fasting plasma gastrin in the presence of ↑ gastric acid secretion.
- A clear diagnosis (~40% of ZES patients) comprises a very elevated serum gastrin (>10× ↑) in the context of an acidic gastric pH <2.0.
- If the gastric pH is <2.0, but the fasting serum gastrin is only mildly elevated, then a provocation test such as the secretin test may be utilized to confirm a gastrinoma diagnosis. A +ve result is when serum gastrin rises >100pg/mL from baseline following an IV injection of secretin (0.4 micrograms/kg).
- If the gastric pH is >2.0 and the patient is on PPIs, then a diagnosis will require these to be weaned (potentially replaced with H_2 receptor antagonists) before reassessment of the biochemistry. Care and monitoring are required with this approach, as it may precipitate severe disease complications.
- If the gastric pH is >2.0 and the patient is not on PPIs, then hypergastrinaemia due to another cause needs to be considered (see Table 9.6).
- Chromogranin A is not a reliable diagnostic test.

Tumour localization

- Very small tumours or duodenal tumours can be very hard to localize and even small tumours are frequently associated with local lymph node disease.
- The tumour localization techniques described for insulinomas are also relevant for gastrinomas (see ➔ Tumour localization, p. 639).
- The modality of choice for localizing all pNETs (excluding insulinomas) is PET/CT with ^{68}Ga-labelled SSAs.

Table 9.6 Causes of hypergastrinaemia

Low or normal gastric acid production (gastric pH >2)	Elevated gastric acid production (gastric pH <2)
H₂ blockers	Gastrinoma
PPIs	G cell hyperplasia
Vagotomy	
Hypochlorhydria (2° to conditions such as pernicious anaemia, atrophic gastritis, or *Helicobacter pylori* infection)	
Short gut syndrome	
Renal failure	
Hypercalcaemia	

Treatment

- The treatment of choice for ZES in MEN1 −ve patients is complete surgical tumour removal (including adjacent lymph nodes), aiming for long-term cure. Historically, this was usually only considered after the tumour had been identified on preoperative imaging, but survival outcomes have been shown to be improved regardless, with high rates of tumour identification being achieved at the time of surgery.
- In patients with ZES in the context of MEN1, management is less well defined—the usual policy being to enucleate when a well-defined tumour >2cm can be identified and otherwise to opt for medical management. More extensive surgery for multiple lesions has been shown to yield good outcomes but remains controversial due to the risks along with the good survival rates from medical management alone.
- PPIs typically offer safe, long-term control of excess acid secretion (check biannually).
- SSAs, chemotherapy, and PRRT have all been shown to potentially be of benefit in metastatic disease. Everolimus patient outcome data are lacking, but it has been shown to significantly lower serum gastrin levels in pNET patients. Sunitinib is also licensed for progressive pNETs, but data specific for gastrinomas are lacking.

Prognosis

- Tumour size and the development and extent of liver metastases are determinants of poor prognosis.
- 5-year survival without liver metastases is 90%.
- 5-year survival with liver metastases is 20–30%.

Further reading

Dimitriadis G, et al. (2016). Medical management of secretory syndromes related to GEP NETs. *Endocr Relat Cancer* **23**, 423–36.

Simmons LH, et al. (2013). Case records of the Massachusetts General Hospital. Case 6-2013. A 54-year-old man with recurrent diarrhea. *N Engl J Med* **368**, 757–65.

Yu F, et al. (1999). Prospective study of the clinical course, prognostic factors, causes of death, and survival in patients with long-standing Zollinger–Ellison syndrome. *J Clin Oncology* **17**, 615–30.

Glucagonomas

Definitions

- Glucagonomas are pNETs arising from α cells of the pancreatic islets.
- The classical glucagonoma syndrome is consequent on the secretion of glucagon and other peptides derived from the preproglucagon gene.
- The majority of glucagonomas (50–80%) are malignant and many patients will have lymph node or liver metastases at the time of presentation.
- Up to 20% of glucagonoma patients will have associated MEN1.

Incidence

- The annual incidence of glucagonomas is recognized to be in the order of 0.01–0.1 per million population.

Clinical presentation

- The characteristic rash necrolytic migratory erythema occurs in 67–90% of cases and usually manifests initially as a well-demarcated area of erythema in the groin before migrating to the limbs, buttocks, and perineum.
- Mucous membrane involvement is common, with stomatitis, glossitis, vaginitis, and urethritis being frequent features.
- Glucagon antagonizes the effects of insulin, particularly in hepatic glucose metabolism, and glucose intolerance is a frequent association (>38–87%).
- Sustained gluconeogenesis also causes amino acid deficiencies and results in protein catabolism which can be associated with unrelenting weight loss (66–96%).
- Glucagon has a direct suppressive effect on the bone marrow, resulting in normochromic normocytic anaemia in almost all patients.

(See Table 9.7.)

Table 9.7 Clinical features of the glucagonoma syndrome

Site	Clinical features
Skin	Necrolytic migratory erythema
Mucous membranes	Angular stomatitis Atrophic glossitis Vulvovaginitis Urethritis
Nails	Onycholysis
Eyes	Conjunctivitis
Scalp	Alopecia
Metabolism	Glucose intolerance Protein catabolism and weight loss
Haematological	Anaemia Venous thromboses
Psychiatric	Depression Psychosis

Biochemical investigations

- The diagnosis is confirmed on finding raised plasma glucagon levels in the context of symptoms consistent with the glucagonoma syndrome.
- Mildly elevated plasma glucagon levels may be seen in other conditions.
- A gut hormone profile may also show elevated neuroendocrine markers such as pancreatic polypeptide.
- IGT and hypoaminoacidaemia may be present.

Tumour localization

- At the time of diagnosis, many glucagonomas will have metastasized to the liver and most 1° tumours will be >3cm in diameter and visible with conventional cross-sectional imaging.
- Small tumours may require more sophisticated imaging techniques. The modality of choice for localizing all pNETs (excluding insulinomas) is PET/CT with ⁶⁸Ga-labelled SSAs.

Treatment

- Surgery is the only curative therapeutic option, but the potential for a complete cure may be very low. Hyperglycaemia should be controlled preoperatively.
- Glucagonoma patients have a high risk of thromboembolic disease.
- SSAs are the treatment of choice, with excellent response rates in treating necrolytic migratory erythema. They are less effective at reversing the weight loss and have an inconsistent effect on glycaemic control such that DM may need to be managed with insulin therapy.
- Amino acid infusions may also help relieve symptoms.
- SSAs, liver targeted therapies, systemic chemotherapy, and PRRT may all offer potential benefit in surgically incurable disease.
- Everolimus and sunitinib are licensed for progressive pNETs, but tumour subtype-specific data are lacking.

Further reading

Dimitriadis G, et al. (2016). Medical management of secretory syndromes related to GEP NETs. *Endocr Relat Cancer* **23**, 423–36.
Kindmark H, et al. (2007). Endocrine pancreatic tumours with glucagon hypersecretion. *Med Oncol* **24**, 330–7.

VIPomas

Definitions

- In 1958, Verner and Morrison first described a syndrome consisting of refractory watery diarrhoea and hypokalaemia associated with a NET of the pancreas.
- The syndrome of watery diarrhoea (90–100%), hypokalaemia (80–100%), and dehydration (>80%) is due to secretion of VIP.
- >90% of VIPomas originate from the pancreas and the majority are solitary lesions.
- Forty to 70% of VIPomas have metastasized at presentation.
- ~5% of VIPoma patients will have associated MEN1.

Incidence

- The annual incidence of VIPomas is recognized to be in the order of 0.05–0.2 per million population.

Clinical presentation

(See Box 9.5.)

- The most prominent symptom in most patients is profuse watery diarrhoea which is secretory in nature and therefore rich in electrolytes. The diarrhoea is typically large volume and persists with fasting.
- Other causes of secretory diarrhoea should be considered in the differential diagnosis (see Box 9.6).

Biochemical investigations

- Elevated levels of plasma VIP are found in all patients with VIPoma syndrome, although false +ves may occur in dehydrated patients due to diarrhoea from other causes.
- A gut hormone profile may identify other raised tumour markers, such as pancreatic polypeptide, and aid detection of some other causes of watery diarrhoea, e.g. gastrinomas.
- It is important to note that VIP-secreting phaeochromocytomas have been described.

Box 9.5 Clinical features of the VIPoma syndrome

- Watery diarrhoea
- Hypokalaemia
- Achlorhydria
- Metabolic acidosis
- Hypercalcaemia
- Hyperglycaemia
- Hypomagnesaemia
- Muscle cramps 2° to electrolyte imbalance
- Facial flushing
- Nausea
- Weight loss

Box 9.6 Differential diagnosis of secretory diarrhoea
- Infection, e.g. *Escherichia coli* or cholera toxins
- Crohn's disease
- Stimulant laxatives
- Colorectal villous adenoma
- Other gut NETs, e.g. those causing carcinoid syndrome or gastrinomas
- Chronic alcohol ingestion
- MTC
- Systemic mastocytosis
- Immunoglobulin A deficiency
- Eosinophilic gastroenteritis

Tumour localization
- At the time of diagnosis, most VIPomas are >3cm and are consequently typically visible with conventional cross-sectional imaging.
- The modality of choice for localizing all pNETs (excluding insulinomas) is PET/CT with ^{68}Ga-labelled SSAs.

Treatment
- Severe cases require IV fluid replacement and careful correction of electrolyte disturbances.
- Surgery to remove the tumour is the treatment of 1st choice if technically possible and may be curative. Surgical debulking may also be of palliative benefit.
- SSAs may produce effective symptomatic relief from diarrhoea, as well as offer antiproliferative benefit.
- GCs in high doses have been shown to provide good relief of symptoms.
- Potential therapies for progressive unresectable disease include liver targeted therapies, systemic chemotherapy, and PRRT.
- Everolimus and sunitinib are licensed for progressive pNETs, but tumour subtype-specific data are lacking.

Further reading
Dimitriadis G, *et al.* (2016). Medical management of secretory syndromes related to GEP NETs. *Endocr Relat Cancer* **23**, 423–36.
Song S, *et al.* (2009). Diagnosis and treatment of pancreatic VIP endocrine tumours. *Pancreas* **38**, 811–14.

Other rare functional pNETs

- Rarely, functional NETs may secrete other biologically active peptides such as ACTH, GHrH, PTHrP, somatostatin (see Box 9.7), or renin.
- The clinical features will be largely dependent upon the nature of the secreted peptide.
- The modality of choice for localizing all pNETs (excluding insulinomas) is PET/CT with ^{68}Ga-labelled SSAs (see Box 9.8).
- Curative surgery (if possible) is the treatment of choice.
- The 1st-line medical therapy for symptoms and tumour control is a SSA.
- Potential therapies for progressive unresectable disease include liver targeted therapies, systemic chemotherapy, and PRRT.
- Everolimus and sunitinib are licensed for progressive pNETs, but tumour subtype-specific data are lacking.
- End-of-life care should be personalized (see Box 9.9).

Box 9.7 Somatostatinoma

- Rare—true incidence unknown.
- May be associated with NF-1 or MEN1.
- Results in glucose intolerance, gallstones, diarrhoea, weight loss, anaemia, and hypochlorhydria.
- Diagnosed by raised somatostatin levels ± elevations in other hormones such as ACTH or calcitonin.

Box 9.8 Somatostatin analogues: key issues

- These agents have proven benefit in symptom reduction in secretory NETs.
- They also have evidence for reducing time to tumour progression in functional and non-functional unresectable NETs across multiple sites of tissue origin.
- Octreotide IV can be used for perioperative stability or in the event of a carcinoid crisis.
- Octreotide SC may be used by patients for symptom breakthrough.
- Long-acting somatostatin analogues in routine clinical use for NET management are octreotide LAR® and lanreotide. There are five somatostatin receptor subtypes 1–5 and these agents particularly target receptor subtype 2 commonly expressed by NETs.
- Tachyphylaxis may be seen with SSA therapy.
- Common side effects of SSA therapy include diarrhoea, abdominal pain, nausea, gallstone development, hyper- or hypoglycaemia, cardiac conduction abnormalities, and hypothyroidism. Rarer side effects include alopecia, pancreatitis, and hepatitis.
- Pasireotide is an SSA with multireceptor high affinity (subtypes 1, 2, 3, and 5). It has no evidence of superior tumour control but does have a more adverse side effect profile and so is typically reserved as a 2nd-line agent and for specific SST receptor subtype progression. One of its key side effects is hyperglycaemia and there are data that it may be beneficial in managing hypoglycaemia in insulinoma patients.

Box 9.9 NETs and end-of-life care
- The risk of moderate to severe symptoms is higher in the last few months prior to death.
- Personalized supportive end-of-life care should be coordinated by an experienced NET MDT to target NET-specific symptoms, along with palliative care support.

Further reading
Dimitriadis G, et al. (2016). Medical management of secretory syndromes related to GEP NETs. *Endocr Relat Cancer* **23**, 423–36.

Hallet J, et al. (2019). Symptom burden at the end of life for NETs. *J Clin Oncol* **37**, 297.

Vitale G, et al. (2018). Pasireotide in the treatment of NETs. *Endocr Relat Cancer* **35**, 351–64.

Inherited endocrine syndromes and MEN

Paul Newey

Genetic testing for monogenic endocrine disorders

- The possibility of a monogenic endocrine disorder should be considered when reviewing patients with relevant clinical manifestations. This is particularly important for endocrine tumours, which are a component of several autosomal dominant (AD) syndromes.
- The diagnosis of these disorders is frequently delayed due to incomplete clinical evaluation or a failure to consider the diagnosis.
- Establishing a genetic diagnosis may have benefits for both the patient and the wider family.
- Once a patient is diagnosed with a genetic diagnosis, cascade genetic testing of 'at-risk' relatives should be organized.
- All genetic testing should be undertaken with access to relevant genetic counselling and with informed consent. A close working relationship with the clinical genetics team is required to ensure appropriate use of diagnostic and predictive genetic testing.
- Specialist input may be required in specific circumstances, including provision of pre-conception genetic counselling and/or access to prenatal genetic diagnosis (PGD).

Identification of monogenic endocrine syndromes

- The indications for genetic testing will vary by specific condition. Potential indicators of a genetic endocrine disorder include:
  - Early age of disease onset.
  - Tumour multiplicity: either combinations of relevant tumours (e.g. pituitary and parathyroid tumours in MEN1) or multiple tumours affecting the same tissue (e.g. bilateral PCCs in MEN2).
  - A relevant family history (e.g. affected 1st-degree relatives for AD disorders).
  - Pathognomonic features of a specific disorder (e.g. marfanoid habitus and mucosal neuromas in MEN2B).

NB. Many monogenic disorders may occur in the absence of a relevant family history. This can be due to:
- The mode of inheritance (i.e. sex-linked/recessive disorders).
- Reduced or variable disease penetrance.
- *De novo* mutations.
- Incomplete clinical evaluation of family members.
- Lack of knowledge of their relatives' medical history.

Genetic testing platforms

(See Chapter 13.)

- The majority of monogenic disorders described in this section are inherited in an AD manner and most frequently arise from small changes in DNA sequence within the coding region of the relevant gene.
- These small DNA changes, including single-nucleotide variants (SNVs) or small insertions or deletions (indels), are detected using direct DNA sequencing methods.

- Diagnostic endocrine genetic testing is now most frequently performed using disease-targeted gene panels and next-generation sequencing methods.
- For some disorders (e.g. MEN1, VHL), a minority of cases result from larger genetic abnormalities (e.g. whole/partial gene deletions) and require alternate methods of detection (e.g. multiplex ligation-dependent probe amplification (MLPA)).
- DNA sequence variants are reported according to standardized criteria (e.g. American College of Medical Genetics and Genomics (ACMG) guidelines). Variants reported as 'pathogenic' or 'likely pathogenic' are usually assumed to be disease-causing but need to be interpreted in the context of clinical features. Variants failing to meet criteria for either a benign/likely benign or pathogenic/likely pathogenic interpretation are categorized as 'variants of uncertain significance' (VUS). The decision to report such variants is dependent on whether additional clinical or genetic testing may allow a more definitive categorization, or following MDT discussion assessing the potential utility of the result.

Further reading

Ellard S, et al. (2019). *ACGS best practice guidelines for variant classification 2019.* ℘ https:// www.acgs.uk.com/media/11285/uk-practice-guidelines-for-variant-classification-2019-v1-0-3.pdf

Newey PJ (2019). Clinical genetic testing in endocrinology: current concepts and contemporary challenges. *Clin Endocrinol (Oxf)* **91**, 587–607.

Richards S, et al. (2015). Standards and guidelines for the interpretation of sequence variants: a joint consensus recommendation of the American College of Medical Genetics and Genomics and the Association for Molecular Pathology. *Genet Med* **17**, 405–24.

McCune–Albright syndrome

Definitions

The syndrome is characterized by:
- Polyostotic fibrous dysplasia.
- Café-au-lait pigmented skin lesions.
- Autonomous function of multiple endocrine glands.

A clinical diagnosis requires two of these three pathologies.

Epidemiology

The condition is rare, affecting 1:100,000 to 1:1,000,000 people.

Genetics

- A genetic, but not inherited condition due to post-zygotic somatic activating mutations of the *GNAS* gene (location 20q13.32) that encodes the α-chain of the heterotrimeric cyclic adenosine monophosphate (cAMP)-associated stimulatory G protein (Gsα).
- The proportion and distribution of affected tissues are determined by the precise developmental stage at which the mutation occurred.
- The majority of patients harbour activating missense *GNAS* mutations affecting either Arg201 (>95%) or Gln227 (<5%) of Gsα, which are critical sites for GTPase activity.
- These mutations result in activation of adenylyl cyclase and constitutive activity of the cAMP-dependent protein kinase A pathway.
- A genetic diagnosis may be established by undertaking *GNAS* mutational analysis of affected tissues. Next-generation sequencing may increase sensitivity of testing. Analysis of leucocyte DNA may be helpful, but a −ve test does not exclude the diagnosis.

Clinical features

Polyostotic fibrous dysplasia
- Solitary or multiple bony lesions, which can cause fracture deformities and/or nerve entrapment, typically develop at <5 years of age.
- Thorough clinical, biochemical, and radiological evaluation are required to evaluate the extent of bone disease.
- The femur and pelvic bones are most frequently affected.
- The vast majority of lesions are benign, although occasionally they undergo malignant transformation.

(For treatment, see Box 10.1.)

Café-au-lait pigmentation
The lesions are characterized by a jagged, irregular border ('Coast of Maine' appearance) and have a tendency to occur or reflect around the midline of the body, and are usually ipsilateral to the bone lesions.

Endocrinopathies
(See Table 10.1.)

Involvement of other organs
- Hepatobiliary complications, such as neonatal jaundice, elevated transaminases, and cholestasis, are relatively common.
- Cardiomegaly, tachyarrhythmias, and sudden cardiac death may occur.

- GI polyps, splenic hyperplasia, and pancreatitis are reported complications.
- Recognized CNS associations include microcephaly, failure to thrive, and developmental delay.

Prognosis

- Most patients live well beyond reproductive age.
- Bone deformities may reduce life expectancy.
- Sudden cardiac death, although recognized, is uncommon.

Box 10.1 Treatment of polyostotic fibrous dysplasia

- Lifestyle advice: adequate dietary Ca intake, and ensure 25-OHD replete. Physical therapy to optimize bone health.
- PO_4 replacement if required.
- Simple analgesia (paracetamol, NSAIDs) for bone pain.
- IV bisphosphonates (pamidronate, zoledronic acid) for moderate to severe bone pain, although impact on local bone density or preventing fracture is not established.
- Requirement for surgery determined by site(s) of bone involvement and disease severity (may be complicated by bleeding).

Further reading

De Castro LF, et al. (2020). Diagnosis of endocrine disease: Mosaic disorders of FGF23 excess: fibrous dysplasia/McCune–Albright syndrome and cutaneous skeletal hypophosphatemia syndrome. *Eur J Endocrinol* **182**, R83–99.

Medline Plus Genetics. *McCune–Albright syndrome.* ℘ https://medlineplus.gov/genetics/condition/mccune-albright-syndrome/

Javaid MS, et al. (2019). Best practice management guidelines for fibrous dysplasia/McCune–Albright syndrome: a consensus statement from the FD/MAS international consortium. *Orphanet J Rare Dis* **14**, 139.

Pepe S, et al. (2019). Germline and mosaic mutations causing pituitary tumours: genetic and molecular aspects. *J Endocrinol* **240**, R21–45.

Robinson C, et al. (2016). Fibrous dysplasia/McCune-Albright syndrome: clinical and translational perpectives. *Curr Osteoporos Rep* **14**, 178–86.

Salenave S, et al. (2014). Acromegaly and McCune-Albright syndrome. *J Clin Endocrinol Metab* **99**, 1955–69.

Salpea P, Stratakis CA (2014). Carney complex and McCune Albright syndrome: an overview of clinical manifestations and human molecular genetics *Mol Cell Endocrinol* **386**, 85–91.

Table 10.1 Endocrinopathies in McCune–Albright syndrome

Condition	Presentation	Investigation and treatment
Precocious puberty	Frequently the initial presentation Typically aged 1–9 years Evidence of gonadotrophin-independent sex steroid production—oestrogen from ovarian cysts in ♀, and testosterone from testicular lesions in ♂ Adults fertile	Review of growth/pubertal status Where indicated, measurement of LH, FSH, and sex steroids, and appropriate imaging (e.g. ovarian or testicular US) Treatment: ♀: letrozole (tamoxifen or fulvestrant 2nd line) ♂: testosterone receptor blockers + aromatase inhibitors (surgery of testicular lesions generally avoided)
Thyroid nodules, goitre, and non-autoimmune thyrotoxicosis	Thyroid nodules present in almost all patients 50% of patients have evidence of thyrotoxicosis (raised T_3 due to ↑ deiodinase activity)	TFTs and thyroid US ATDs, radioiodine, surgery
GH-secreting pituitary tumours and prolactinomas (20–30% of patients)	Mean age of onset 24 years (may occur in early childhood) Invariably associated with skull base fibrous dysplasia Coexisting hyperprolactinaemia in ~80% of those with acromegaly Pituitary adenomas observed in majority (mostly macroadenomas). A minority have hyperplasia or no overt abnormality Clinical features of acromegaly or hyperprolactinaemia, although typical features of acromegaly may be absent due to coexisting bone disease	Growth assessment—but may be confounded by bone disease and/or other endocrinopathy (e.g. precocious puberty) IGF-1, GH, PRL, OGTT ± pituitary MRI Medical therapy is 1st-line treatment with somatostatin analogues, GH receptor antagonists (e.g. pegvisomant). Surgery when medical therapy inadequate but is challenging due to coexisting craniofacial fibrous dysplasia. Radiotherapy ideally avoided due to risk of malignant transformation of skull base fibrous dysplasia
Neonatal hyper cortisolism	Hypercortisolism presents exclusively in 1st year of life due to adrenal hyperplasia or adenoma Patients may occasionally present with adrenal insufficiency reflecting resolved hypercortisolism	24h UFC, low-dose dexamethasone suppression test, midnight cortisol; adrenal CT Medical therapy for short-term management, adrenalectomy (Consider observation for mild disease, as may resolve spontaneously in ~30%)

Condition	Presentation	Investigation and treatment
Hypo phosphataemic rickets	Associated with ↑ FGF23 production Hypophosphataemia associated with ↑ fracture risk and bone pain Reduced PO_4, 1,25 vitamin D ↑ ALP Normal Ca, 25OHD, and PTH	Measure baseline Ca, PO_4, and PTH, renal USS, urinary Ca/Cr ratio Treatment with: calcitriol or alfacalcidol, PO_4 supplements

Neurofibromatosis

Definitions

- NF-1 is characterized by the occurrence of multiple neurofibromas, café-au-lait spots, and Lisch nodules of the iris (pigmented hamartoma nodules of aggregated dendritic melanocytes).
- Specific clinical diagnostic criteria are outlined in Box 10.2.
- NF-1 is associated with several endocrine manifestations, most notably disorders of growth and puberty, PCC, and NETs.
- NF-2 is typically characterized by the presence of bilateral acoustic neuromas occurring in adolescence or early adulthood. Other features include posterior subcapsular cataracts, retinal gliomas, pigmented retinopathy, and gaze palsies. No common endocrinopathies are reported.
- NF-2 is rare, with an estimated frequency of 1 in 30–40,000 live births due to a mutation of the *NF2* gene.

NF-1

Epidemiology

- NF-1 is common, with an incidence of 1:3000 of the population.
- Although highly penetrant, NF-1 is associated with marked variability in clinical expression, even within the same family.

Genetics

- NF-1 is a highly penetrant AD condition due to germline mutation of the *NF1* gene located on chromosome 17.
- ~50% of NF-1 cases are familial (i.e. inherited), while the other ~50% occur sporadically due to *de novo* *NF1* mutations.
- A minority of patients have clinical features restricted to one part of the body ('segmental' NF-1) due to somatic mosaicism.
- *NF1* encodes the tumour suppressor protein neurofibromin, expressed in several cell types, e.g. neuronal, glial, chromaffin cells.
- Neurofibromin is a GTPase-activating protein that acts as a −ve regulator of the *RAS* proto-oncogene.
- NF-1-associated tumours demonstrate biallelic *NF1* inactivation, resulting in *RAS* activation and cell growth/proliferation.
- Although diagnosis is usually clinical, genetic testing is increasingly recommended to avoid misdiagnosis that may arise from alternate disorders with overlapping clinical features (e.g. other causes of NF such as NF-2, schwannomatosis) or conditions with café-au-lait patches (e.g. McCune–Albright syndrome; see ➲ McCune-Albright syndrome, pp. 654–5).
- Genetic testing and interpretation may be challenging due to the large size of the gene (60 exons spanning >350kb DNA) and diversity of pathogenic mutations reported (>1000 different mutations identified).
- The genetic testing strategy may involve analysis of genomic DNA and messenger ribonucleic acid (mRNA), and analysis for partial/whole gene deletions.

Clinical features
- Diagnosis is dependent on clinical characteristics (see Box 10.2).
- The café-au-lait spots are visible shortly after birth (95%), enlarge with age, and may merge with a linear edge ('Coast of California' appearance).
- Seventy per cent of NF-1 patients have axillary or inguinal freckling.
- The multiple cutaneous and SC neurofibromas appear around puberty (>95%). The deeper plexiform neurofibromas may undergo malignant change to malignant peripheral nerve sheath tumours (MPNSTs) later in life (8–12% of NF-1 patients).
- Lisch nodules, affecting the iris, typically appear in early childhood (95%).
- Optic gliomas occur in ~15% of patients, while brainstem gliomas occur in ~5% of patients. These occasionally develop into high-grade tumours.
- Skeletal dysplasias (e.g. sphenoid wing dysplasia, tibial pseudoarthrosis) occur in 2–5% of children, while 20–50% have evidence of scoliosis.
- Cognitive dysfunction/learning disability are reported in a proportion of children, while attention-deficit/hyperactivity disorder and autism spectrum disorder occur in 30–50%.
- Vascular dysplasia may occur, most commonly affecting the renal vasculature, resulting in renovasclar hypertension (3%).
- Macrocephaly (16%), seizures (5%), and short stature (6%) are all reported.
- ↑ risk of specific malignancies, including juvenile myelomonocytic leukaemia, embryonal rhabdomyosarcoma, and GI stromal tumours; ↑ risk of additional common cancers, compared to general population (e.g. breast cancer).

The endocrine features are detailed in Box 10.3.

Box 10.2 1987 National Institutes of Health (NIH) diagnostic criteria for NF-1

Two or more of:
- Six or more café-au-lait macules (≥5mm prepuberty or ≥15mm after puberty).
- Axillary or inguinal freckling,
- ≥2 dermal neurofibromas or ≥1 plexiform neurofibroma.
- ≥2 iris hamartomas (Lisch nodules).
- Optic pathway glioma.
- A characteristic long bone dysplasia (e.g. sphenoid dysplasia or pseudoarthrosis).
- A 1st-degree relative with NF-1.

Source: data from Neurofibromatosis. NIH Consensus Statement 1987 Jul 13–15;6(12):1–19.

Box 10.3 Endocrine features of NF-1

- Hypothalamus and pituitary:
  - Optic pathway gliomas may impinge on hypothalamic and/or pituitary function.
  - Central precocious puberty, GH excess, and GHD are each reported.
  - Short stature is common in children with NF-1 but may be independent of GH deficiency (e.g. due to skeletal changes).
- PCC:
  - Reported in 0.1–6.0% of NF-1 patients.
  - Mean age of diagnosis ~40 years (uncommon <20 years).
  - 80–90% solitary adrenal tumour, 10–15% bilateral tumours; ~5% extra-adrenal PGL (e.g. abdominal sympathetic chain, bladder).
  - ~10% malignant.
- Gastropancreatic NETs:
  - Occur in ~1% of NF-1 patients.
  - Typically located in duodenum in peri-ampullary region.
  - Occasional reports of gastrinoma, insulinoma, and non-functioning pNETs.
- Parathyroid tumours and thyroid C cell hyperplasia are also very rarely reported in NF-1.

Prognosis

- Life expectancy in patients with NF-1 is reduced, on average, by 8–21 years.
- Malignant neoplasms are the leading cause of premature death; cumulative risk of 20–40% by 50 years, with lifetime risk of ~60%.

Screening and surveillance

- Provision of education to patients and family regarding potential disease complications.
- Annual clinical assessment in childhood to assess development and growth and to evaluate for associated clinical manifestations.
- Continued awareness of risk of complications in adulthood, with clinical assessment and investigation as appropriate.

Further reading

Evans DGR, et al. (2017). Cancer and central nervous system tumor surveillance in paediatric neurofibromatosis type 1. *Clin Cancer Res* **23**, e46–52.

Medline Plus Genetics. *Neurofibromatosis type 1.* ℅ https://medlineplus.gov/genetics/gene/nf1/

Gruber LM, et al. (2017). Pheochromocytoma and paraganglioma in patients with neurofibromatosis type 1. *Clin Endocrinol (Oxf)* **86**, 141–9.

Gutmann DH, et al. (2017). Neurofibromatosis type 1. *Nat Rev Dis Primers* **3**, 17005.

von Hippel–Lindau disease

Definitions

The syndrome is characterized by:
- Haemangioblastomas of the retina and CNS.
- Renal cysts and renal cell carcinoma (RCC).
- PCC or rarely PGL.
- Pancreatic abnormalities, including multiple cysts and, less commonly, NETs.
- Endolymphatic sac tumours (ELSTs).

A clinical diagnosis is established by one of the following:
- ≥2 retinal/CNS haemangioblastomas.
- One haemangioblastoma and one typical visceral manifestation (i.e. RCC, PCC, ELST).
- One haemangioblastoma or visceral manifestation and a family history of VHL.
- VHL is further subdivided into two main types:
  - Type 1 VHL is the commoner form, characterized by retinal/CNS haemangioblastomas and RCC, but not PCC.
  - Type 2 VHL describes forms in which PCC occurs:
    - Type 2A: PCC and retinal/CNS haemangioblastoma.
    - Type 2B: PCC, retinal/CNS haemangioblastomas, and RCC.
    - Type 2C: PCC only.
- This categorization is of limited clinical utility and does not impact upon surveillance recommendations for patients.

Epidemiology

- Incidence ~1:36,000 live births.
- Average age of presentation ~26 years.
- Highly penetrant: ≥95% of patients manifest disease by age 65 years.

Genetics

- VHL is an AD condition due to germline mutation of the *VHL* gene located at chromosome 3p25.
- ~80% of VHL cases are inherited, with ~20% occurring sporadically due to a *de novo* *VHL* mutation.
- The *VHL* gene encodes the pVHL tumour suppressor protein, which forms part of an E3 ubiquitin ligase complex that targets hypoxia-inducible factor (HIF)-1 and HIF-2 transcription factors for proteosomal degradation. In the absence of functioning pVHL, HIF-1/HIF-2 accumulate, activating hypoxic target genes and promoting tumourigenesis.
- A wide variety of different *VHL* mutations are reported, including: truncating mutations (i.e. nonsense, frameshift, splice site), missense mutations, and large-scale deletions of one or more exons of the *VHL* gene.
- PCC is typically associated with missense mutations affecting surface residues of the pVHL protein (type 2 VHL), while truncating mutations or large deletions result in type 1 VHL.

- Genetic testing following appropriate genetic counselling is recommended in patients with any of the main VHL-associated tumours and in 1st-degree relatives of known *VHL* mutation carriers.
- Predictive genetic testing is recommended in early childhood due to the potential for early-onset clinical manifestations.

Clinical features

- Retinal angiomas (haemangioblastomas) are the most frequent presenting feature, although uncommon before age 10 years. In ~50% of cases, they are multiple and bilateral. They tend to be peripheral in the retina, and bleeding and retinal detachment may occur. Treatment is usually with laser or cryotherapy.
- CNS haemangioblastomas are the initial presenting feature in 40% of patients and, in total, occur in 60–80% of cases. Most commonly occurring in the cerebellum, spinal cord, and brainstem, the lesions are benign, with variable growth rates. Conservative management of asymptomatic lesions may be appropriate. Where indicated, treatment is with surgery or radiotherapy.
- Clear cell RCC is the commonest cause of death in VHL patients. In those with the commonest forms (types 1 and 2B), the penetrance of RCC is ~70% by 60 years, with a mean age of presentation of 40 years. The lesions tend to be multifocal. Tumours >3cm have an ↑ risk of metastases. The management of choice is surgical resection.
- PCC/PGL occur in 10–25% of VHL families, with a mean age of presentation of ~30 years (but may occur in childhood). The majority of tumours occur within the adrenal gland and bilateral disease is common, and the vast majority secrete normetanephrine. Extra-adrenal PGL is also reported, but rare. The majority of PCCs are benign (≤5% malignant), and 1st-line treatment is surgical removal (see ➲ Surgical, p. 326).
- Pancreatic lesions are common in VHL and are most commonly asymptomatic multiple cyst adenomas. Non-functioning pNETs occur in ~10–15% of VHL patients, while functioning NETs with VIP, insulin, glucagon, or calcitonin secretion occur rarely. An ↑ rate of malignancy is observed in VHL-associated pNETs, with surgery recommended for tumours >2–3cm.
- ELSTs occur in ~10–15% of patients and are often bilateral. Frequently asymptomatic, but may result in hearing loss and tinnitus.

Screening and surveillance

- Patients with VHL (including asymptomatic *VHL* mutation carriers identified by predictive genetic testing) are recommended to undergo periodic surveillance to facilitate early tumour detection.
- A suggested surveillance strategy is provided in Table 10.2.

Table 10.2 Suggested tumour surveillance in patients at risk of VHL

Condition	Screening test
Retinal angiomas	Annual ophthalmic examination from infancy/early childhood
CNS haemangioblastomas	Annual neurological evaluation commencing in childhood
	MRI head ± spine every 12–36 months, starting in adolescence
RCC	MRI or US 12-monthly from age of 16 years
PCC/PGL	Annual BP monitoring and annual urine or plasma metanephrines (to commence in early childhood in those at high risk of PCC)
	Imaging if biochemical abnormalities detected

Prognosis

- Until recently, the median survival for a VHL patient was 40–50 years of age, with the majority of deaths attributable to RCC.
- Currently, the prognosis for individual patients depends upon the location and complications of the associated tumours.
- Overall, the prognosis is improving due to the institution of screening programmes and earlier therapeutic interventions.

Further reading

Dombos D 3rd, *et al*. (2018). Review of the neurological implications of von Hippel–Lindau disease. *JAMA Neurol* **75**, 620–7.

Medline Plus Genetics. *Von Hippel-Lindau syndrome*. ♫ https://medlineplus.gov/genetics/condition/von-hippel-lindau-syndrome/

Gossage L, *et al*. (2015). VHL, the story of a tumour suppressor. *Nature Rev Cancer* **15**, 55–64.

Maher RM, *et al*. (2011). Von Hippel–Lindau disease: a clinical and scientific review. *Eur J Hum Genet* **19**, 617–23.

Rednam SP, *et al*. (2017). Von Hippel–Lindau and hereditary pheochromocytoma/paraganglioma syndromes: clinical features, genetics, and surveillance recommendations in childhood. *Clin Cancer Res* **23**, e68–75.

Carney complex

Definitions

- Carney complex is a multiple neoplasia syndrome characterized by:
  - Pigmented skin lesions.
  - Cardiac or cutaneous myxomas.
  - A variety of endocrine and non-endocrine tumours.

Epidemiology

- A rare disorder with unknown incidence.
- >750 cases reported worldwide.
- Median age of diagnosis ~20 years.

Genetics

- AD disorder with high penetrance.
- Most commonly due to germline inactivating mutation of the *PRKAR1A* gene located on chromosome 17q2 (70–80% of cases).
- ~70–80% of cases with *PRKAR1A* mutations are inherited, while ~20–30% occur due to *de novo* *PRKAR1A* mutations.
- The majority of *PRKAR1A* mutations involve nonsense or frameshift variants, with missense mutations occurring less frequently.
- A minority of patients harbour large-scale deletions involving the 17q24.2-q24.3 locus that includes *PRKAR1A* and may manifest a more severe phenotype.
- *PRKAR1A* encodes the regulatory subunit type 1α of PKA, a cAMP-dependent protein kinase. Inactivation of *PRKAR1A* results in ↑ cAMP PKA activity, promoting tumourigenesis.
- A minority of patients with Carney complex do not harbour *PRKAR1A* mutations. A 2nd genetic locus has been identified at chromosome 2p16, but the causative gene is not known.
- Genetic testing should be offered to those with clinical features suggestive of Carney complex, as well as to 1st-degree relatives of those with a known *PRKAR1A* mutation.

Clinical features

- Pigmented skin lesions: most commonly lentigines (~70% of patients), occurring as <0.5cm brown/black macules around the eyelids, mouth, ears, and genitals. Epithelioid blue naevi also occur.
- Myxomas: cardiac myxomas are observed in ~30% of patients and can occur in any of the four heart chambers, and may be multiple and recurrent. Cardiac myxomas result in significant morbidity and mortality (e.g. stroke, sudden death) and surgical removal is required. Cutaneous myxomas are found in ~30–50% of patients.
- For endocrine manifestations, see Box 10.4.
- Breast lesions: a variety of benign breast lesions reported, although no clear ↑ risk of breast cancer established.
- Psammomatous melanotic schwannoma (PMS) occur in ~10% of patients and can occur anywhere in the CNS or peripheral nervous system. Most frequently found in the GI tract and paraspinal sympathetic chain. Malignant transformation may occur.
- Adrenal, hepatocellular, pancreatic, and bone cancers have also been reported but are rare.

Box 10.4 Endocrine manifestations associated with Carney complex

- PPNAD (see also ➲ Table 3.5):
  - Results in ACTH-independent Cushing's syndrome.
  - Occurs in 25–60% of patients ($♀ > ♂$), with mean age of diagnosis of <30 years.
  - Characterized by small (<10mm) pigmented nodules in both adrenals.
  - 'Paradoxical' rise in 24h UFC/17-hydroxysteroids during a prolonged dexamethasone suppression text (Liddle's test).
  - Bilateral adrenalectomy is the most effective treatment.
- Pituitary abnormalities:
  - Elevations in IGF-1 and GH are common, although only ~10% of patients manifest acromegaly, usually by the 3rd decade.
  - Acromegaly is most commonly associated with pituitary mammosomatotroph hyperplasia, although GH/PRL-secreting pituitary adenomas are also reported.
- Thyroid abnormalities:
  - Thyroid nodules (75% of patients).
  - DTC (<10% of patients).
- Testicular tumours:
  - Benign large cell calcifying Sertoli cell tumour (LCCSCT).
  - ~40% of affected ♂ (usually occurring before puberty).
  - Testicular adrenal rest tumours.
- Ovarian lesions:
  - 15% of ♀ have ovarian lesions, including cysts, cystadenomas, and teratomas.

Screening and surveillance

Patients with Carney complex should undergo at least annual clinical evaluation to assess for associated clinical manifestations. Suggested clinical follow-up may include:

- In children/adolescents, regular monitoring of growth/puberty.
- Annual echocardiography beginning in infancy.
- Regular IGF-1, OGTT + GH, and PRL beginning in adolescence, with additional investigation (e.g. MRI pituitary) as indicated.
- Regular biochemical evaluation for Cushing's syndrome (e.g. UFC); additional investigation as indicated.
- Thyroid US.
- Ovarian or testicular US.
- Baseline MRI brain, spine, chest, abdomen, and pelvis to detect PMS, and repeated if clinical neurological features suggest disease.

Further reading

Bertherat J, et al. (2009). Mutations in regulatory subunit type 1A of cyclic adenosine 5'-monophosphate-dependent protein kinase (PRKAR1A): phenotype analysis in 353 patients and 80 different genotypes. *J Clin Endocrinol Metab* **94**, 2085–91.

Correa R, et al. (2015). Carney complex: an update. *Eur J Endocrinol* **173**, M85–97.

Espiard S, et al. (2020). Frequency and incidence of Carney complex manifestations: a prospective multicenter study with a three-year follow-up. *J Clin Endocrinol Metab* **105**, dgaa002.

Medline Plus Genetics. *Carney complex*. https://medlineplus.gov/genetics/condition/carney-complex/

Pepe S, et al. (2019). Germline and mosaic mutations causing pituitary tumours: genetic and moelcular aspects. *J Endocrinol* **240**, R21–45.

Salpea P, et al. (2014). Deletions of the PRKAR1A locus at 17q24.2-q24.3 in Carney complex: genotype-phenotype correlations and implications for genetic testing. *J Clin Endocrinol Metab* **99**, E183–8.

Cowden syndrome

Clinical presentation and diagnosis

- The condition is characterized by multiple hamartomas and ↑ lifetime risk of several cancer types.
- The clinical diagnosis of Cowden syndrome is based on the presence of pathognomonic major and minor criteria.
- Pathognomonic criteria include mucocutaneous lesions (i.e. trichilemmomas, acral keratosis, and papillomatous papules).
- Major criteria include macrocephaly (>97th centile) and breast, thyroid, or endometrial cancer.
- Minor criteria include learning difficulties, benign thyroid disease, GI hamartomas, renal cell cancer, lipomas, fibromas, and uterine fibroids.
- Details of endocrine manifestations are provided in Box 10.5.

Epidemiology

- Estimated to affect 1 in 200,000 individuals.
- The true prevalence may be higher, as likely to be underdiagnosed due to variable clinical expression.

Genetics

- AD inheritance.
- Inactivating germline mutations of the tumour suppressor gene *PTEN* are identified in ~25–80% of affected probands, depending on the criteria used to establish the clinical diagnosis.
- Cowden syndrome due to *PTEN* mutations is categorized under the group of PTEN hamartoma tumour syndromes.
- Other disorders in this group include Bannayan–Riley–Ruvalcaba syndrome (characterized by macrocephaly, intestinal hamartomatous polyposis, lipomas, and genital freckling), and *Proteus* syndrome (characterized by overgrowths of multiple tissues of all germ layers).
- Some patients with Cowden syndrome without *PTEN* mutations have been reported to harbour mutations of alternate genes, including *KLLN*, *SDHB*, *SDHD*, *PIK3CA*, and *AKT1*.

Cancer risk

- Cancer types and lifetime risk:
  - Breast cancer: 65–85%.
  - Thyroid cancer: 6–38%.
  - Endometrial cancer: 21–28%.
  - Renal cell cancer: 2–34%.
  - Colon cancer: 9–17%.
  - Melanoma: 2–6%.

Box 10.5 Endocrine features of Cowden syndrome

- Thyroid involvement:
  - Benign thyroid disease, including multinodular goitre and follicular adenomas, occur in ~75% of patients.
  - DTC occurs in ~35%, with mean age of onset of 35–40 years.
  - Ratio of follicular to papillary thyroid cancer: 1:2 (i.e. marked over-representation of follicular lesions, compared to the general population).
- Other endocrine manifestations appear to very rare.

Screening and surveillance

- Patients with Cowden syndrome should undergo regular clinical surveillance for early detection of associated cancers.
- A suggested surveillance schedule may include:
  - Regular breast examination from age 18 years and annual mammography (or MRI) from age ~30 years.
  - Annual thyroid US.
  - Colonoscopy every 2–5 years from age 35 years.
  - Renal US every 2 years from age 40 years.
  - Consider screening for endometrial cancer from age 30 years (e.g. annual biopsy or transvaginal US).
  - Annual skin check for melanoma.

Further reading

Medline Plus Genetics. *Cowden syndrome.* https://medlineplus.gov/genetics/condition/cowden-syndrome/

Mester J, Eng C (2015). Cowden syndrome: recognizing and managing a not-so-rare hereditary cancer syndrome. *J Surg Oncol* **111**, 125–30.

Pilarski R, et al. (2013). Cowden syndrome and the PTEN hamartoma tumor syndrome: systematic review and revised diagnostic criteria. *J Natl Cancer Inst* **105**, 1607–16.

Yehia L, Eng C (2018). 65 years of the double helix: One gene, many endocrine and metabolic syndromes: PTEN-opathies and precision medicine. *Endocr Relat Cancer* **25**, T121–40.

Yehia L, et al. (2019). PTEN-opathies: from biological insights to evidence-based precision medicine. *J Clin Invest* **129**, 452–64.

POEMS syndrome

Definitions

- POEMS syndrome is a rare paraneoplastic syndrome characterized by progressive polyneuropathy, organomegaly, endocrinopathy, M-protein, and skin changes (POEMS). Diagnosis is made by the presence of mandatory criteria of polyneuropathy and monoclonal plasma cell proliferation, and at least one additional major and one minor clinical feature. Several major and minor criteria are not included in the POEMS acronym.

Epidemiology

- Rare, with estimated prevalence of 1:300,000.

Pathogenesis

- A paraneoplastic disorder due to underlying monoclonal plasma cell proliferation/neoplasm.
- The pathogenesis of the disorder is poorly understood but characterized by high levels of VEGF and other cytokines.
- In comparison to multiple myeloma, POEMS is almost always associated with lambda clones and overall prognosis is generally better. In addition, symptoms related to bone pain, renal failure, or marked bone marrow infiltration are not usually a feature.

Clinical feature and diagnosis

- Median age of onset is in 6th decade, with slight ♂ predominance.
- Progressive polyneuropathy is often the 1st presentation. It is typically a painful symmetrical distal sensorimotor neuropathy.
- The plasma cell dyscrasia is typically IgA or IgG lambda restricted, and a paraprotein is usually detectable on protein electrophoresis.
- Major diagnostic criteria include Castleman's disease (giant lymph node hyperplasia), sclerotic bone lesions, and elevated VEGF levels.
- Minor criteria include organomegaly (hepatosplenomegaly, lymphadenopathy), extravascular volume overload (i.e. oedema, pleural effusion, ascites), endocrinopathy (see below), skin changes (e.g. angiomas, hyperpigmentation, hypertrichosis), papilloedema, and thrombocytosis/polycythaemia.
- Other clinical features are diverse and may include clubbing, weight loss, thrombotic disease, pulmonary hypertension, and diarrhoea.
- Endocrinopathies are common (reported in >80%) and are often multiple, although the pathogenesis is poorly understood.
- Endocrine features include:
  - Hypogonadism (70%).
  - Hypothyroidism (60%).
  - Hypoadrenalism (60%).
  - DM (50%).
  - Hyperprolactinaemia (20%).
  - Gynaecomastia (common).

Treatment

- Most successful treatments have resulted from targeting the underlying abnormal plasma cell population, rather than solely targeting elevated VEGF levels (i.e. with anti-VEGF antibodies).
- Potential therapies include alkylating chemotherapy, irradiation, autologous stem cell transplant, thalidomide, and lenalidomide.
- Studies of anti-VEGF monoclonal antibodies (e.g. bevacizumab) have shown mixed results and their role in treatment is unclear.

Further reading

Brown R, Ginsberg L (2019). POEMS syndrome: clinical update. *J Neurol* **266**, 268–77.

Dispenzieri A (2017). POEMS syndrome: 2017 update on diagnosis, risk stratification, and management. *Am J Hematol* **92**, 814–29.

Multiple endocrine neoplasia type 1 (MEN1)

Definitions
Characterized by the combined occurrence of
- Parathyroid tumours/hyperplasia.
- Anterior pituitary adenomas.
- Duodenopancreatic NETs.

Additional endocrine tumours include thymic/bronchial NETs and adrenal tumours (functioning and non-functioning). Several non-endocrine tumours also occur (see Box 10.6).

Diagnosis
A clinical diagnosis of MEN1 is established in an individual who manifests ≥2 of the three main tumour types. A genetic diagnosis is established by the identification of a *MEN1* mutation in an individual who may be asymptomatic and without biochemical or radiological evidence of tumour development.

Epidemiology
- The population prevalence of MEN1 is ~1 in 30,000.
- Estimated age-related penetrance of clinical manifestations: by 10 years, 7% penetrance; 20 years, 52%; 30 years, 87%; 40 years, 98%.
- Biochemical and/or radiological evidence of associated tumours often precedes symptomatic presentations.
- Clinical features are unusual in early childhood (e.g. <10 years), but occasional clinical presentations (e.g. prolactinoma, insulinoma) have been reported in children as young as 5 years old.
- Occasional malignant tumours (e.g. ACC) have also been reported in early childhood.

Genetics
- MEN1 is an AD disorder due to loss-of-function mutations of the *MEN1* gene.
- The *MEN1* gene is located on the long arm of chromosome 11 (11q13) and encodes the multifunctional scaffold protein menin, which is involved in transcriptional and epigenetic regulation, and modulation of several cell signalling pathways.
- In endocrine tissues, menin is a tumour suppressor protein, with MEN1 tumours typically demonstrating biallelic *MEN1* inactivation (i.e. germline mutation of one *MEN1* allele and somatic inactivation of the 2nd allele).
- >1200 germline *MEN1* mutations have been reported (~600 different mutations) and occur throughout the *MEN1* coding region. Somatic mosaicism has also been reported in MEN1.
- *De novo* mutations are reported in 10% of cases (i.e. occur in the absence of a relevant family history).
- Disease-causing *MEN1* mutations include frameshift, nonsense, splice site, and missense mutations, and there is no clear genotype–phenotype correlation.

- ~10% of patients with MEN1 will not have a mutation within the coding region of the *MEN1* gene. A minority of these patients will have large-scale deletions involving the *MEN1* locus, or mutations of other genes (i.e. *CDKN1B*; see ➲ Genetics, p. 693). Some will also represent individuals with a chance occurrence of ≥2 sporadic endocrine tumours.

Genetic testing for *MEN1*

- Genetic testing may be employed in the diagnostic (i.e. in a patient with relevant clinical features) or predictive setting (e.g. in asymptomatic relatives of a known *MEN1* mutation carrier).
- Genetic testing should be undertaken with appropriate genetic counselling and after obtaining informed consent.
- Predictive genetic testing is recommended in early childhood (e.g. by age of 5 years) due to the high penetrance of tumours in childhood (will require parental consent).
- *MEN1* genetic testing is initially undertaken by DNA sequence analysis of the coding region of the *MEN1* gene. Where no mutation is found, further analysis (e.g. MLPA) is recommended to detect large-scale deletions involving the *MEN1* gene.

Indications for *MEN1* genetic testing include:
- All patients with a clinical diagnosis of MEN1 (i.e. ≥2 of the main clinical features).
- All 1st-degree relatives of a known *MEN1* mutation carrier (irrespective of whether asymptomatic or with relevant clinical features).

MEN1 testing should be considered in patients with
- Parathyroid adenoma/hyperplasia <35 years.
- Gastrinoma or multiple pNETs.
- Insulinoma or pituitary adenoma <20 years.
- ≥2 MEN1-associated tumours outwith the classic triad (e.g. parathyroid plus adrenal tumour).
- A MEN1-associated tumour and a 1st-degree relative with a MEN1-associated tumour.

Preconception genetic counselling should be offered to all individuals at risk of transmitting *MEN1* to their offspring. Preimplantation genetic diagnosis is available in some settings in the UK to avoid transmission of *MEN1*.

Box 10.6 Clinical features in MEN1 (estimated penetrance)

PHPT (>95%)
- Parathyroid adenoma/hyperplasia (>95%).
- Parathyroid carcinoma (very rare).

Pancreatic NETs (30–80%)
- Gastrinoma (30–40%)—majority occurring in duodenum.
- Insulinoma (10–30%).
- Glucagonoma (<3%).
- VIPoma (very rare).
- Non-functioning NETs (30–60%).

Pituitary adenoma (30–40%)
- Prolactinoma (20%).
- Somatotropinoma (<10%).
- Corticotropinoma (<5%).
- Non-functioning adenoma (10–25%).

Foregut NETs (5–15%)
- Thymic NET (2–8%).
- Bronchial NET (5–15%).
- Gastric NET (10%).

Adrenocortical tumours (20–40%)
- Conn's adenoma (~1%).
- Cortisol-secreting adenoma (~1%).
- PCC (very rare).
- Non-functioning adenoma (10–20%).
- ACC (~1%).

Miscellaneous tumours
- Lipomas (30%).
- Angiofibromas (85%)—>3 shows a sensitivity in MEN1 of 75% and a specificity of 95%.
- Collagenomas (70%).
- Meningiomas (~5%).
- Ependymomas (<5%).
- Breast cancer (↑ relative risk reported).

Clinical features and management of MEN1

- The clinical features of MEN1 are related to the specific sites of tumour development and/or the consequences of hormone hypersecretion.
- Early detection of tumours through regular clinical, biochemical, and radiological surveillance is recommended, with the aim of improving clinical outcomes and prognosis.
- Thorough clinical evaluation is required and the possibility of multiple synchronous tumours affecting the same tissue (e.g. pancreas) or different tissues should be considered.
- The aim of treatment should be to minimize disease-associated morbidity and mortality, while preserving the patient's QoL.
- Investigation and treatment require a multidisciplinary approach, with patients playing an active role in decision-making.

Primary hyperparathyroidism

(See ⊃ Primary hyperparathyroidism, pp. 510–12.)
- PHPT is the commonest feature of MEN1, occurring in >95% of patients (equal ♂:♀).
- The degree of hypercalcaemia is often mild and patients are frequently asymptomatic, although symptomatic presentations may occur due to marked hypercalcaemia or end-organ damage (e.g. renal stones, osteitis fibrosa cystica).
- Synchronous or asynchronous involvement of all parathyroid glands is typically observed, with histopathological evidence of hyperplasia or adenoma(s). Parathyroid carcinoma is very rare.
- Surgical management is the gold standard, although timing and extent of surgery remain controversial. Potential indications for surgery include: evidence of end-organ damage (e.g. renal stones, reduced BMD/ fracture), symptomatic hypercalcaemia, coexisting gastrinoma, or if pregnancy is being considered.
- Most centres advocate open neck exploration with subtotal (≥3.5 glands) parathyroidectomy. Concurrent transcervical thymectomy is recommended to remove ectopic parathyroid tissue embedded in the thymus.
- Minimally invasive approaches are not usually recommended due to high likelihood of recurrence, although some advocate ipsilateral clearance in select cases in the knowledge that future contralateral surgery may be required.
- Cinacalcet has been used where surgery has failed or in those deemed to be at high operative risk.

Pituitary tumours

- Occur in 30–50% of MEN1 patients (micro- and macroadenomas).
- Prolactinomas, non-functioning adenomas, and GH-secreting tumours occur most frequently.
- Presentations in late teens or early adulthood are common, and early childhood presentations are also reported.

- The diagnosis and clinical management of MEN1-associated pituitary tumours is similar to that employed for their sporadic counterparts (see ➜ Pituitary tumours, pp. 154–6).

Duodenopancreatic NETs

(See ➜ The neuroendocrine system, pp. 628–9.)
- Leading cause of premature death in MEN1 patients.
- Clinically apparent tumours occur in 30–80% of patients, although microscopic islet tumours are virtually universal.
- Clinical features are related to local mass effects or a consequence of hormone hypersecretion.
- Although many MEN1-associated pNETs display indolent behaviour, some run an aggressive disease course with metastases to local lymph nodes, the liver, and other distant sites.
- Surgery provides the only curative approach (i.e. for localized disease) but may be associated with significant morbidity. It may also be complicated by the presence of ≥1 synchronous tumour.
- All decisions regarding the treatment of pNETs should be undertaken by an MDT with experience in MEN1 management.

Gastrinoma

(See ➜ Gastrinomas, pp. 642–3.)
- Untreated, gastrin-secreting tumours result in gastric acid hypersecretion and recurrent peptic ulceration (i.e. ZES), resulting in considerable morbidity and mortality.
- Occur in 20–60% of MEN1 patients, with the majority occurring as multiple, small (<5mm) lesions in the duodenal mucosa, and are often malignant with metastases to local lymph nodes. Macroscopic pancreatic gastrinomas are unusual in MEN1.
- Diagnosis is made by demonstrating ↑ fasting serum gastrin in association with ↑ basal acid secretion. Raised serum gastrin levels are also observed in achlorhydria, G-cell hyperplasia, *Helicobacter pylori* infection, renal failure, and PPI therapy.
- Localization of gastrinoma may be undertaken by endoscopic US, CT, MRI, somatostatin receptor scintigraphy, selective angiography, or Ca stimulation tests.
- High-dose PPI therapy (e.g. omeprazole 20–60mg bd) is effective at reducing basal acid secretion. H_2 receptor blockade can be added for symptom control.
- The role of surgery for multiple small duodenal gastrinomas is controversial. Although several approaches have been reported (e.g. duodenotomy with peripancreatic lymph node removal, pancreas-preserving duodenectomy, partial pancreaticoduodenectomy), the benefits on long-term survival are unknown.

Insulinoma

(See ➜ Insulinomas, pp. 638–40.)
- Occur in 10–30% of MEN1 patients and may occur in childhood (reported as young as 5 years).
- Majority occur as single lesions in the body or tail of the pancreas, although multicentric insulinoma may occur.

- Clinical features and diagnosis do not differ from sporadic insulinoma, although the potential for synchronous pancreatic tumours may complicate localization studies.
- Surgical removal is the treatment of choice, with several surgical approaches available, dependent on the number/location of the tumours.

Non-functioning NETs

- Clinically significant non-functioning NETs occur in 30–60% of patients and represent the commonest cause of premature death.
- Can present at any age, including childhood (reported as young as 12 years), with penetrance of ~10–30% by 21 years.
- Most commonly detected by surveillance imaging, although may be associated with minor elevation of pancreatic hormones (e.g. pancreatic polypeptide, glucagon).
- Imaging modalities for detection/evaluation of tumours include:
  - Endoscopic US: sensitive technique for detection or monitoring of small tumours, but invasive and user-dependent.
  - MRI (and CT) retain good sensitivity for detection of clinically significant tumours.
  - Somatostatin receptor scintigraphy: reduced specificity for detection of NETs, but useful for detecting metastases. Modalities such as ^{68}Ga-DOTATATE PET/CT may have ↑ sensitivity.
- Disease course related to tumour size, with ↑ risk of metastases for larger tumours (~4% for <1cm, ~10% for 1–2cm, ~20% for 2–3cm, >40% for >3cm).
- Surgery is recommended for tumours >2cm (or smaller tumours demonstrating rapid growth), although some advocate surgery at lower size thresholds. While the majority of tumours <2cm demonstrate an indolent behaviour on serial imaging, a minority are associated with an aggressive disease course (e.g. development of metastatic disease). All decisions regarding surgery should involve the MDT and take account of the patient's wishes.
- Observational studies of SSA therapy for small (i.e. <2cm) pNETs have demonstrated potential utility but require validation in larger controlled studies.
- For those with advanced disease, treatment options include SSA therapy, tyrosine kinase (TK) receptor inhibitors, mTOR inhibitors, PRRT, chemotherapy, and locoregional treatments.

Thymic carcinoids

- Reported in 2–8% of MEN1 patients (predominantly ♂ in European populations), with median age of diagnosis of 40–45 years.
- Associated with high rates of malignancy and account for 20% of premature deaths (median survival ~8–10 years).
- Symptoms relate to local mass effects (e.g. pain, vena caval obstruction), with features of carcinoid syndrome usually absent.
- Diagnosis reliant on imaging (urinary 5-HIAA unreliable) and several modalities of use (CT, somatostatin receptor scintigraphy, FDG-PET).
- Surgical resection is the treatment of choice, although recurrence rates are high.

Bronchial carcinoids

- Reported in 15–25% of MEN1 patients.
- Single or multiple tumours may occur, often of small size, and present at a median age of ~40 years.
- Majority demonstrate an indolent behaviour, with good prognosis. A minority are malignant and run an aggressive disease course.
- Surgery may be considered for solitary tumours, although potential benefit extrapolated from sporadic cases. Surveillance may be appropriate for small stable lesions.

Adrenal tumours

(See ➔ Treatment of adrenal Cushing's syndrome, pp. 274–7.)

- Reported in ~20–55% of patients, with the majority occurring as non-functional adenomas.
- A minority (≤10%) result in hormonal hypersecretion, most commonly 1° hyperaldosteronism and ACTH-independent Cushing's syndrome. ACC is also reported, while PCC is very rare.
- Radiological surveillance is undertaken simultaneously with pancreatic imaging; biochemical testing is recommended in those with relevant clinical features or those with tumours >1cm.
- Treatment is similar to that of sporadic adrenal tumours. Surgery is considered for functional tumours, those >4cm, or those with imaging features indicative of possible malignancy.

Tumour surveillance in MEN type 1

- Current guidelines recommend that individuals at high risk of disease (e.g. *MEN1* mutation carriers, 1st-degree relatives of patients with clinical MEN1) undergo periodic clinical, biochemical, and radiological screening (see Table 10.3), although high-quality evidence demonstrating improved clinical outcomes is lacking.
- Clinically overt manifestations of MEN1 are quite rare in early childhood (i.e. <10 years), although screening for hyperparathyroidism, insulinoma, and pituitary tumours through clinical and/or biochemical evaluation is recommended from age of 5 years.
- The optimal surveillance schedule (e.g. age to commence, imaging modalities employed, and interval between testing) is yet to be established. This should balance the potential benefits of early tumour detection vs the risks of the respective screening modalities (e.g. cumulative doses of ionizing radiation/gadolinium) and take into account patient acceptability and local availability.
- An illustrative schedule for surveillance is outlined in Table 10.3.

Prognosis

(See Box 10.7.)

Table 10.3 Outline of recommended surveillance in MEN1

MEN1-associated tumour	Age to begin (years)	Biochemical screening test (annually)	Imaging screening test (interval)
Parathyroid	8	Ca, PTH	None
Pancreatic			
Gastrinoma	20	Fasting gastrin	None
Insulinoma	5	Fasting glucose	None
Other PNETs	10	Chromogranin A*, gut hormones	MRI/endocoscopic US (1–2 years)
Pituitary adenoma			
Prolactinoma	5	PRL	None
Somatotropinoma	5	GH, IGF-1	None
Other (e.g. non-functioning NET)	10	Only if relevant symptoms/signs	MRI (3 years)
Adrenocortical	10	Only if relevant symptoms/signs or tumour >1cm	MRI (1–2 years)
Thymic/bronchial carcinoid	15	None	Consider CT or MRI# (1–3 years)

* Although chromogranin A, pancreatic polypeptide, and glucagon concentrations can be elevated with non-functioning NETs, they have low sensitivity and specificity such that their value is debated.

The optimum schedule of screening for thymic and/or bronchial carcinoids is debated, given relatively low penetrance of these tumours and concern over cumulative doses of ionizing radiation with CT scanning.

Box 10.7 Prognosis

MEN1 is associated with a mortality of nearly 50% by the age of 50 years. ~30–70% of patients with MEN1 will die of causes directly related to the disorder, with malignant duodenopancreatic NETs and thymic carcinoids accounting for the greatest risk of premature death.

Further reading

Challis BG, et al. (2019). What is the appropriate management of non-functioning pancreatic neuro-endocrine tumours disclosed on screening in adult patients with multiple endocrine neoplasia type 1? *Clin Endocrinol (Oxf)* **91**, 708–15.

Frost M, et al. (2018). Current and emerging therapies for PNETs in patients with or without MEN1. *Nat Rev Endocrinol* **14**, 216–27.

Medline Plus Genetics. *Multiple endocrine neoplasia.* ⟋ https://medlineplus.gov/genetics/condition/multiple-endocrine-neoplasia/

Goudet P, et al. (2015). MEN1 disease occurring before 21 years old: a 160-patient cohort study from the Groupe d'étude des Tumeurs Endocrines. *J Clin Endocrinol Metab* **100**, 1568–77.

Pieterman CRC, et al. (2017). Long-term natural course of small nonfunctional pancreatic neuro-endocrine tumors in MEN1: results from the Dutch MEN1 Study Group. *J Clin Endocrinol Metab* **102**, 3795–805.

Sadowski SM, et al. (2017). The future: surgical advances in MEN1 therapeutic approaches and man-agement strategies. *Endocr Relat Cancer* **24**, T243–60.

Singh Ospina N, et al. (2016). When and how should patients with multiple endocrine neoplasia type 1 be screened for thymic and bronchial carcinoid tumours? *Clin Endocrinol (Oxf)* **84**, 13–16.

Thakker RV, et al.; Endocrine Society (2012). Clinical practice guidelines for multiple endocrine neo-plasia type 1 (MEN1). *J Clin Endocrinol Metab* **97**, 2990–3011.

Yates CJ, et al. (2015). Challenges and controversies in management of pancreatic neuroendocrine tumours in patients with MEN1. *Lancet Diabetes Endocrinol* **3**, 895–905.

Multiple endocrine neoplasia type 2 (MEN2)

Definitions

MEN2 may be divided into two main forms:
- MEN2A comprises MTC in combination with PCC and parathyroid tumours. MEN2A accounts for nearly 90–95% of all MEN2 cases. Three additional variants of MEN2A include: MEN2A with cutaneous lichen amyloidosis (CLA); MEN2A with Hirschsprung's disease (HD); and familial medullary thyroid cancer (FMTC) only.
- MEN2B is defined as the occurrence of MTC in association with PCC, mucosal neuromas, marfanoid habitus, medullated corneal fibres, and intestinal ganglion dysfunction leading to megacolon. MEN2B comprises 5–10% of MEN2 cases and usually runs a more aggressive disease course due to early-onset MTC.

Epidemiology

- Incidence of MEN2A is reported to be 1:80,000, while MEN2B occurs less frequently.
- Prevalence (and mutation spectrum) may be population-dependent.

Genetics

(See Fig. 10.1.)
- MEN2 is an AD condition due to activating mutations of the *RET* proto-oncogene, located at 10q11.21
- *RET* encodes a TK receptor which is involved in the neural crest and enteric nervous system development.
- The RET receptor comprises an extracellular domain which includes a cysteine-rich region, a transmembrane domain, and an intracellular domain with TK activity.
- >50 different MEN2-associated *RET* mutations are reported, with the majority limited to a small number of exons (10, 11, 13–16).
- The majority of MEN2A *RET* mutations affect the cysteine-rich domain, with Cys634 the most frequently affected residue.
- ~95% of MEN2B cases are due to the Met918Thr mutation in the TK domain, and of these, ~75% occur *de novo* (i.e. without a family history), frequently delaying diagnosis.
- MEN2 *RET* mutations result in ligand-independent receptor activation either via dimerization of unpaired cysteine residues (i.e. due to mutations in the cysteine-rich domain) or as monomers with autonomous TK activity (e.g. TK domain mutations).
- Loss-of-function *RET* mutations are associated with HD. Notably, a minority of MEN2 patients have paradoxical features of both MEN2 and HD.
- The population frequency of some MEN2-associated *RET* mutations is higher than the prevalence of disease, indicating that such variants are likely associated with reduced penetrance (e.g. Val804Met).

Genotype–phenotype correlation

- MEN2 demonstrates a strong genotype–phenotype correlation, whereby specific *RET* mutations predict the timing of MTC onset and the wider clinical features.
- For high penetrance variants, nearly all patients (~95%) develop MTC, while the risk of PCC (≤50%) and PHPT (≤30%) is dependent on the specific *RET* mutation.
- *RET* mutations predict the age of onset of MTC and are categorized according to the American Thyroid Association (ATA) risk groups:
  - *Highest*: comprising the Met918Thr MEN2B variant.
  - *High*: Cys634 and Ala883Phe variants.
  - *Moderate*: all other MEN2A-associated variants.
- Surveillance and treatment guidelines for MEN2 are based on these ATA risk categories, including timing of 'prophylactic' thyroidectomy in asymptomatic mutation carriers.

Genetic testing

- Implementation of *RET* genetic testing has transformed the management of MEN2 by allowing identification and treatment of those at risk of disease.
- Identification of an index case with MEN2 should prompt testing of the wider family (e.g. all 1st-degree relatives initially).
- Predictive genetic testing should be performed as soon as feasible, due to the potential for early-onset MTC (e.g. testing in infancy/early childhood for highest-/high-risk ATA mutations).
- *RET* genetic testing should be considered in the following settings:
  - Patients with a clinical diagnosis of MEN2 (e.g. MTC + PCC) or associated features of MEN2B.
  - All 1st-degree relatives of a known *RET* mutation carrier.
  - Patients with MEN2 tumours and relevant family history.
  - Patients with apparently sporadic MTC.
  - Patients with bilateral PCC (or solitary PCC at an early age).

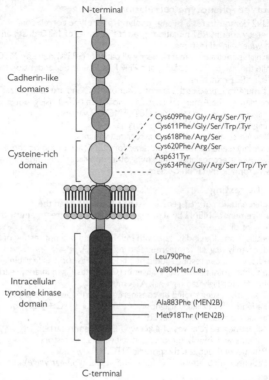

Fig. 10.1 RET receptor structure and location of common MEN2-associated *RET* mutations.

Adapted from Newey PJ. Multiple Endocrine Neoplasia. *Medicine.* 2017;45(9);538–542, with permission from Elsevier.

Clinical features and management of MEN2

Medullary thyroid cancer

(See ➔ Medullary thyroid carcinoma, p. 116.)

Clinical features and diagnosis

- MTC is the leading cause of premature mortality in MEN2.
- MTC occurs in the majority of MEN2 patients (70–100% by 70 years) and is frequently the 1st manifestation of disease.
- The timing of MTC onset is related to the ATA risk category of mutation, with the highest risk Met918Thr associated with MTC as early as the 1st year of life (earliest reported onset: 9 weeks of age).
- High- and moderate-risk *RET* mutations have a median age of MTC diagnosis of 20–25 years and ~40 years, respectively, although early childhood presentations are reported.
- Symptomatic presentations are usually with a neck lump, with or without diarrhoea and flushing (due to high calcitonin levels).
- Rarely, MTC causes ectopic ACTH secretion/Cushing's syndrome.
- Diagnosis is based on cytology/histology (e.g. from FNA/biopsy), together with high basal serum calcitonin levels. Elevated calcitonin levels can also occur in renal failure, thyroiditis, lung or prostate cancer, and other NETs, reducing specificity. Additional tumour markers of MTC include CEA.
- Preoperative staging includes neck US with cross-sectional imaging (e.g. CT, MRI, FDG-PET/CT) in those in whom metastatic disease is suspected (e.g. based on symptoms/calcitonin levels).
- Tumour spread is commonest to cervical and mediastinal lymph nodes, but distant metastases may occur (e.g. bone, lung, liver).

Treatment

- Surgery with total thyroidectomy and dissection of cervical lymph node compartments (by an experienced surgeon) is the recommended treatment and offers the best chance of cure. The extent of lymph node resection is debated and guided by preoperative imaging and calcitonin levels.
- PCC should be excluded prior to MTC surgery.
- Post-operative calcitonin levels provide prognostic information and indicate the extent of residual disease.
- Monitoring of calcitonin levels (e.g. every 6 months) and 'calcitonin doubling time' informs prognosis and further management.
- The management of advanced disease may require a multimodal approach. Local treatments include further surgery, chemoembolization, external beam radiotherapy, and RFA.
- Systemic therapies for metastatic disease include targeted therapy with receptor tyrosine kinase (RTK) inhibitors (vandetanib, cabozantinib). Conventional chemotherapy is associated with poor response rates.
- RTK inhibitors are reported to improve progression-free survival and an objective tumour response is seen in ≤50% of patients with advanced disease. Drug resistance usually develops, such that benefits are usually short to medium term.

Prophylactic thyroidectomy

- Prophylactic thyroidectomy should be considered in asymptomatic individuals harbouring *MEN2* mutations and has the potential to prevent the morbidity and mortality associated with MTC.
- The timing of surgery is guided by the ATA risk category of *RET* mutations, together with imaging features and calcitonin levels (see Table 10.4). Surgery should be undertaken before there is a significant risk of metastatic disease.
- For highest- and high-risk mutations, thyroidectomy is recommended before the age of 1 year and 5 years, respectively. A more nuanced approach may be taken for moderate-risk mutations, based on calcitonin levels, neck US features, and patient/parent preferences (see Table 10.4).

Phaeochromocytoma

(See also → Phaeochromocytomas and paragangliomas, pp. 314–17.)

- Usually presents later than MTC, although the presenting feature in ~10% of MEN2 cases. Childhood presentations are rare, although occasional cases aged <12 years.
- Highest penetrance with Cys634 mutations, as well as the MEN2B Met918Thr and Ala883Phe variants.
- 50% of PCCs occur bilaterally (especially codon 634 mutations), either synchronously or metachronously.
- Almost all occur within the adrenal medulla; extra-adrenal disease (i.e. PGL) is very rare.
- The vast majority of MEN2 PCCs are benign; malignancy in <5%.
- Clinical features and diagnosis are as for sporadic PCC, although the possibility of multifocal/bilateral disease should be considered.
- Up to 50% of MEN2 patients with PCC are asymptomatic, and thus PCC must be excluded prior to any surgery or pregnancy.
- Surgical resection is the treatment of choice.
- Unilateral surgery is recommended for single tumours, accepting that further disease may occur in the contralateral gland.
- Patients undergoing bilateral adrenalectomy require lifelong GC/MC replacement.
- Adrenal-sparing surgery (i.e. subtotal adrenalectomy) may be considered for those with bilateral disease to avoid the need for lifelong steroid replacement. This may not be feasible with multifocal disease, and higher recurrence rates are to be expected.

Primary hyperparathyroidism

(See also → Primary hyperparathyroidism, pp. 510–12.)

- Variable penetrance dependent on genotype; most frequent in those with Cys634 mutations (10–30%). Not observed in MEN2B.
- Parathyroid hyperplasia and/or adenoma(s) affect one or more parathyroid glands.
- Diagnosis is made in a similar manner to sporadic disease. Patients are frequently asymptomatic with mild hypercalcaemia.
- Indications for surgery are broadly similar to that of sporadic disease.
- Treatment recommendations favour surgical removal of only enlarged and/or abnormal parathyroid glands.

- The role of preoperative imaging and localization studies is dependent on timing relative to that of MTC surgery; if diagnosed concurrently with MTC, all four glands should be explored at the time of surgery; if diagnosed subsequent to thyroidectomy, preoperative imaging may help localize abnormal glands.

MEN2A variant disorders

- *FMTC only:* describes kindreds in which MTC is the sole manifestation of MEN2, although differentiating from MEN2A is difficult due to reduced penetrance of other features. When strict diagnostic criteria are applied, FMTC is very rare.
- *MEN2A with CLA:* CLA is reported in ~30% of patients with codon 634 mutations and typically presents with pruritus and rash in the interscapular region of the T2–T6 dermatome region.
- *MEN2A with HD:* <10% of MEN2A patients manifest features of HD shortly after birth with inability to pass stool and megacolon. Only reported in those with exon 10 variants affecting cysteine residues 609, 611, 618, and 620. These mutations are hypothesized to result in both *RET* activation and reduced cell surface expression leading to abnormal enteric neural development.

Additional clinical features associated with MEN2B

- Recognition of MEN2B features, which may be evident early in life, can facilitate timely diagnosis but are often overlooked.
- Features include a marfanoid habitus, mucosal neuromas on the tongue, lips, and oral cavity, conjunctival neuromas, upper GI tract symptoms and signs (e.g. swallowing difficulty, vomiting, feeding intolerance), and lower GI manifestations, including constipation/impaired colonic motility and megacolon.

Screening and intervention in MEN2

- Establishing a genetic diagnosis of MEN2 prior to the onset of clinical features enables appropriate monitoring and treatment.
- Patients already diagnosed with clinical features of MEN2 also require lifelong surveillance for additional manifestations.
- The majority of individuals at risk of MEN2 (i.e. *RET* mutation carriers) are recommended to undergo prophylactic thyroidectomy.
- The recommended schedule of tumour surveillance and timing of prophylactic thyroidectomy is guided by the ATA risk category of the *RET* mutation (see Table 10.4).

Prognosis

(See Box 10.8.)

Table 10.4 Surveillance schedule and timing of prophylactic thyroidectomy in MEN2

	ATA 'highest' risk	ATA 'high' risk	ATA 'moderate' risk
RET mutation(s)	Met918Thr	Codon 634 + Ala883Phe	All other pathogenic RET mutations
Age to undertake RET genetic testing	<1 year	<3 years	<3–5 years
MTC			
Age to begin calcitonin/US monitoring	<0.5–1 year	3 years	5 years
Age to undertake prophylactic thyroidectomy	<1 year	5 years or earlier	>5 years (based on US/calcitonin)
Age to begin screening for PCC	11 years	11 years	16 years
Age to begin screening for PHPT	NA	11 years	16 years

Risk category of RET mutation and screening and treatment schedule based on data from the Revised American Thyroid Association Guidelines for the Management of Medullary Thyroid Carcinoma; Wells et al Thyroid 2015; 25: 567–610.

Box 10.8 Prognosis

- MTC is responsible for the majority of morbidity and premature mortality in MEN2. The major predictor of premature mortality is metastatic MTC.
- The prognosis for MEN2 patients is improving with early genetic diagnosis and the ability to undertake tumour screening and prophylactic thyroidectomy.
- In some countries, cascade genetic testing and prophylactic thyroidectomy have reduced the number of patients presenting with MEN2-associated MTC.
- Clinical outcomes in MEN2B are less favourable due to earlier age of MTC onset and delays in diagnosis because of the high rate of de novo mutations.

Further reading

Castinetti F, et al. (2014). Outcomes of adrenal-sparing surgery or total adrenalectomy in phaeochromocytoma associated with multiple endocrine neoplasia type 2: an international retrospective population-based study. *Lancet Oncol* **15**, 648–55.

Castinetti F, et al. (2019). Natural history, treatment, and long-term follow up of patients with multiple endocrine neoplasia type 2B: an international, multicentre, retrospective study. *Lancet Diabetes Endocrinol* **7**, 213–20.

Machens A, Dralle H (2015). Therapeutic effectiveness of screening for multiple endocrine neoplasia type 2A. *J Clin Endocrinol Metab* **100**, 2539–45.

Machens A, Dralle H (2018). Advances in risk-oriented surgery for multiple endocrine neoplasia type 2. *Endocr Relat Cancer* **25**, T41–5.

Plaza-Menacho I (2018). Structure and function of RET in multiple endocrine neoplasia type 2. *Endocr Relat Cancer* **25**, T79–90.

Romei C, et al. (2016). A comprehensive overview of the role of the RET proto-oncogene in thyroid carcinoma. *Nat Rev Endocrinol* **12**, 192–202.

Waguespack SG, et al. (2011). Management of medullary thyroid carcinoma and MEN2 syndromes in childhood. *Nature Rev Endocrinol* **7**, 596–607.

Wells SA, et al. (2015). Revised American Thyroid Association guidelines for the management of medullary thyroid carcinoma. *Thyroid* **25**, 567–610.

Wirth LJ, et al. (2013). Case records of the Massachusetts General Hospital. Case 5-2013. A 52-year-old woman with a mass in the thyroid. *N Engl J Med* **368**, 664–73.

Multiple endocrine neoplasia type 4 (MEN4)

Definitions

- A disorder with a similar clinical phenotype to MEN1, although parathyroid and pituitary tumours appear to predominate.

Epidemiology

Rare disorder with only ~20 index cases reported to date.

Genetics

- AD inheritance due to mutation of the *CDKN1B* gene located on chromosome 12p13.
- *CDKN1B* encodes the cyclin-dependent kinase inhibitor p27Kip1 which is involved in cell cycle regulation.
- Genetic testing for MEN4 should be considered in those with clinical features of typical or atypical MEN1 in whom *MEN1* genetic testing is −ve, or in 1st-degree relatives of patients with a known *CDKN1B* mutation.

Clinical features

- Due to the rarity of MEN4, a full clinical description of the disease is not available.
- PHPT reported in ~80% of MEN4 cases.
- Pituitary tumours, including somatotropinomas, corticotropinomas, prolactinomas, and non-functioning adenomas reported in 30–40% of cases.
- Duodenopancreatic NETs reported in ~5–30% of cases.
- Additional manifestations include GI, bronchial, and cervical NETs, non-functional adrenal tumours, and thyroid cancer.
- Investigation and treatment of MEN4-associated tumours are similar to MEN1.
- Although guidance regarding tumour surveillance in MEN4 has not been established, a programme similar to MEN1 may be adopted.

Further reading

Alrezk R, et al. (2017). *MEN4* and *CDKN1B* mutations: the latest of the MEN syndromes. *Endocr Relat Cancer* **24**, T195–208.

Frederiksen A, et al. (2019). Clinical features of multiple endocrine neoplasia type 4: novel pathogenic variant and review of published cases. *J Clin Endocrinol Metab* **104**, 3637–46.

Wasserman JD, et al. (2017). Multiple endocrine neoplasia and hyperparathyroid-jaw tumor syndromes: clinical features, genetics, and surveillance recommendations in childhood. *Clin Cancer Res* **23**, e123–32.

Inherited primary hyperparathyroidism

Definitions

- Parathyroid tumours affect 1–4 in 1000 of the population.
- PHPT is inherited in ≤10% of patients.
- In comparison to sporadic hyperparathyroidism, inherited hyperparathyroidism typically has an earlier age of onset (<40 years of age) and an equal sex distribution.
- Hereditary hyperparathyroidism needs to be differentiated from FHH to avoid unnecessary investigation and treatment.

Causes of hereditary hyperparathyroidism

- MEN1.
- MEN2A.
- MEN4.
- Hyperparathyroidism jaw tumour syndrome (HPT-JT).
- Familial isolated hyperparathyroidism (FIHP) may result from mutations of *MEN1*, *CDC73*, *CASR* and *GCM2*.

HPT-JT

- AD condition due to mutation of the *CDC73* gene located on chromosome 1q31.2, which encodes the tumour suppressor protein parafibromin.
- HPT-JT is characterized by:
  - Parathyroid tumours: often the initial presenting feature (may arise in children and adolescents) and occurs with high penetrance. Parathyroid carcinoma occurs in ~15% of cases.
  - Ossifying fibromas of the maxilla and/or mandible, which occur in ~30% of patients.
- Additional manifestations include: renal lesions (cysts, hamartomas, and occasionally Wilms' tumours); benign and malignant uterine tumours; and more rarely pancreatic adenocarcinomas, testicular mixed germ cell tumours, and Hürthle cell thyroid adenomas.
- The ↑ risk of parathyroid carcinoma should lower the threshold for undertaking surgical resection of any significantly enlarged parathyroid gland.

Familial isolated hyperparathyroidism

- FIHP refers to kindreds in which hereditary hyperparathyroidism occurs as an isolated endocrinopathy.
- Differentiating FIHP from other hereditary parathyroid disorders is difficult, as the other disorders often express hyperparathyroidism as the 1st manifestation (e.g. MEN1, HPT-JT), and additional clinical features may occur with reduced penetrance.
- FIHP is a genetically heterogeneous condition. In some kindreds, mutations of the *MEN1* or *CDC73* genes have been identified, which should revise the diagnosis to MEN1 and HPT-JT, respectively. Loss-of-function mutations of *CASR* are also reported in a small number of kindreds with apparent FIHP, although far more commonly, inactivating *CASR* mutations are associated with FHH, which does not benefit from surgical intervention.
- In ~70% of apparent FIHP cases, the genetic cause remains unknown. Recent studies have implicated variants in the *GCM2* gene in 15–20% of these cases.

Genetic testing

(See also ⬌ Table 13.1.)

Genetic testing should be considered where there are clinical features or a family history to suggest a relevant monogenic endocrine tumour syndrome (e.g. MEN1/MEN2, HPT-JT). In addition, genetic testing should be considered in the following settings:

- Multigland parathyroid disease.
- Parathyroid carcinoma, atypical parathyroid adenoma (CDC73).
- Young age of onset (e.g. <35 years).
- Family history of hyperparathyroidism (e.g. 1st-degree relative).

Further reading

Cardoso L, *et al.* (2017). Molecular genetics of syndromic and non-syndromic forms of parathyroid carcinoma. *Hum Mutat* **38**, 1621–48.

Guan B, *et al.* (2016). GCM2-activating mutations in familial isolated hyperparathyroidism. *Am J Hum Genet* **99**, 1034–44.

Marx SJ (2019). New concepts about familial isolated hyperparathyroidism. *J Clin Endocrinol Metab* **104**, 4058–66.

Hereditary paraganglioma-phaeochromocytoma (PGL/PCC)

Background

- ~30–40% of PGL/PCCs are familial (see ➲ Chapter 3).
- The commonest hereditary causes of PGL/PCC include VHL (see ➲ von Hippel-Lindau disease, pp. 662–4), MEN2 (see ➲ Multiple endocrine neoplasia type 2 (MEN2), pp. 684–5), and the hereditary PGL/PCC syndromes due to mutations in subunits of the succinate dehydrogenase enzyme complex (SDHx).
- Genetic testing should be considered in the majority of patients presenting with PGL/PCC. Typically, genetic testing is performed employing a disease-targeted gene panel, which includes the main PGL/PCC-associated genes (see Table 3.5). Specific indications for testing are determined by local/national guidance. These may include patients with one or more of:
  - Sympathetic PGL.
  - Metastatic PGL/PCC.
  - Bilateral PCCs/multiple PGLs.
  - PGL/PCC and RCC.
  - PGL/PCC at any age and ≥1 relative with PGL/PCC or RCC.
  - PGL/PCC with loss of staining for SDH proteins by immunohistochemistry.
  - Clinical features suggestive of a specific disorder (e.g. VHL, MEN2, NF-1).
  - Young age at presentation (e.g. <60 years of age).

Hereditary PGL/PCC syndromes

Definitions

- Hereditary disorder characterized by the occurrence of PGL/PCC.
- Germline mutations of *SDHx* genes account for 30–40% of hereditary PGL/PCC cases.

Epidemiology

- Estimated incidence of PGL/PCC tumours as part of hereditary PGL/PCC syndromes is ~1/1,000,000/year.

Genetics

- AD inheritance with variable disease penetrance.
- At least five genes associated with familial PGL syndromes, including: *SDHD* (PGL syndrome type 1), *SDHAF2* (PGL syndrome type 2), *SDHC* (PGL syndrome type 3), *SDHB* (PGL syndrome type 4), and *SDHA* (PGL syndrome type 5).
- *SDHA*, *SDHB*, *SDHC*, and *SDHD* encode each subunit of the enzyme SDH involved in the Krebs cycle and oxidative phosphorylation. *SDHAF2* encodes an accessory protein required for normal SDH function. Mutations in the SDH subunits result in succinate accumulation in the cell, which activates hypoxia pathways.
- *SDHD* and *SDHAF2* display parent-of-origin effects, such that disease is only expressed when the mutation is paternally inherited (due to a maternal imprinting effect).
- Other genes recently reported in association with familial PGL include *SLC25A11* and *DLST*.

Clinical features
- The clinical presentation and penetrance of tumours are determined by the specific subunit affected. PGL/PCC due to mutations of *SDHB* and *SDHD* are most frequently encountered among the familial PGL syndromes.
- *SDHB* (penetrance ~20% by age 50 years): associated with sympathetic PGL (less commonly adrenal PCC or head/neck PGL). ↑ risk of malignancy.
- *SDHD* (penetrance ~40% by age 50 years): most commonly associated with head and neck (often multiple) PGL; less commonly abdominal PGL or PCC.
- *SDHC* (estimated <10% lifetime penetrance); most commonly associated with head and neck PGL (often multiple); less commonly abdominal PGL or PCC.
- *SDHA* (estimated <5% lifetime penetrance): head and neck PGL, extra-adrenal PGL, or adrenal PCC.
- *SDHx* mutations may also be associated with additional tumours, including RCC and GI stromal tumours.
- Management of SDHx-associated PGL/PCC is similar to that of non-hereditary PGL/PCC but will be dependent on the number and location of tumours, amenability to surgical resection, and presence or absence of metastatic disease. Multidisciplinary management is essential.

Surveillance of *SDHx* mutation carriers
- Surveillance of *SDHx* mutations carriers is generally recommended (particularly for *SDHB* mutation carriers due to ↑ risk of malignancy). The aims are to facilitate early detection of tumours, although evidence of improved outcomes is yet to be established. The value of surveillance in genes with low penetrance (e.g. *SDHA*) is unclear.
- An optimal surveillance strategy for *SDHx* mutation carriers is yet to be established. An example of a possible surveillance programme is provided in Table 10.5.
- When employing interval surveillance with whole body MRI, it is important to acknowledge the potential for incidental findings.

Table 10.5 Possible surveillance schedule for *SDHx* mutation carriers

Screening test	Frequency	Age to begin#
Clinical evaluation for relevant symptoms and clinical examination	Annual	10 years (5 years for SDHB†)
BP monitoring	Annual	10 years (5 years for SDHB†)
Plasma and/or urinary metanephrines	Annual	10 years (5 years for SDHB†)
Whole body MRI (skull base to pelvis)*	Every 2–3 years	15 years (10 years for SDHB†)

* US may be suitable for children in whom MRI is not tolerated.

Earlier imaging may be suitable if clinical or biochemical abnormalities detected or in kindreds where early disease expression reported.

† Age-related penetrance of clinical phaeochromocytoma and paraganglioma in *SDHB* mutations carriers is 1% and 5% at age 10 years, respectively.

Further reading

Andrews KA, et al. (2018). Tumour risks and genotype–phenotype correlations associated with germline variants in succinate dehydrogenase subunit genes *SDHB*, *SDHC* and *SDHD*. *J Med Genet* **55**, 384–94.

Medline Plus Genetics. *Hereditary paraganglioma–pheochromocytoma.* ℘ https://medlineplus.gov/genetics/condition/hereditary-paraganglioma-pheochromocytoma/

Maniam P, et al. (2018). Pathogenicity and penetrance of germline SDHA variants in pheochromocytoma and paraganglioma (PPGL). *J Endocr Soc* **2**, 806–16.

Muth A, et al. (2019). Genetic testing and surveillance guidelines in hereditary pheochromocytoma and paraganglioma. *J Intern Med* **285**, 187–204.

NGS in PPGL (NGSnPPGL) Study Group; Toledo RA, et al. (2017). Consensus statement on next-generation-sequencing-based diagnostic testing of hereditary phaeochromocytomas and paragangliomas. *Nat Rev Endocrinol* **13**, 233–47.

Tufton N, et al. (2019). Can subunit-specific phenotypes guide surveillance imaging decisions in asymptomatic SDH mutation carriers? *Clin Endocrinol (Oxf)* **90**, 31–46.

Wong MY, et al. (2019). Clinical practice guidance: surveillance for phaeochromocytoma and paraganglioma in paediatric succinate dehydrogenase gene mutation carriers. *Clin Endocrinol (Oxf)* **90**, 499–505.

Inherited renal calculi

Definitions

- Renal calculi affect 15% of ♂ and 5% of ♀ by the 7th decade of life.
- Responsible for >80,000 hospital admissions/year in the UK.
- Renal calculi arise due to reduced urine volume or ↑ excretion of stone-forming components such as Ca, oxalate, urate, cystine, xanthine, and PO_4.
- A variety of causes for renal stones are established, but the commonest aetiology is hypercalciuria.
- Ca stones (i.e. calcium oxalate, calcium phosphate) account for ~75% of all renal calculi.
- Other causes include uric acid stones (~15%) and magnesium ammonium phosphate (~10%), but composition varies by geographical location.
- The commonest cause of hypercalciuria is hypercalcaemia, and this, in turn, is most frequently 2° to PHPT.
- Nephrolithiasis is frequently a recurrent condition, with a relapse rate of 50% at 10 years.

Genetics

- Renal calculi represent multifactorial disease resulting from interaction between genetic and environmental factors.
- A family history of nephrolithiasis is present in 35–65% of patients.
- Twin studies indicate heritability to be >45%.
- ~15% of those patients attending specialist kidney stone clinics have a monogenic aetiology.
- In addition, recent genome-wide association studies (GWAS) have identified multiple genetic variants and molecular pathways associated with ↑ risk of stone formation.

Monogenic disorders associated with hypercalciuria/renal stones

- AD idiopathic hypercalciuria: hypercalciuria may be inherited as a monogenic disorder or as part of a polygenic trait. Genes associated with monogenic inheritance include adenylate cyclase 10 (*ADCY10*) and vitamin D receptor (*VDR*).
- AD hypocalcaemia (ADH); due to gain-of-function mutation in the G-protein-coupled receptor (GPCR) calcium-sensing receptor (*CASR*) signalling pathway. Includes ADH1 due to *CASR* mutations, and ADH2 due to *GNA11* mutations (which encodes the G-protein signalling subunit Gα11). ADH patients may manifest hypercalciuria which increases the risk of renal stones.
- Bartter syndrome: renal tubular disorder characterized by hypokalaemic alkalosis, hyperreninaemic hyperaldosteronism, and hypercalciuria. Multiple subtypes result from mutations of different genes with AR, AD, or X-linked recessive (XLR) inheritance, including: *NKCC2/SLC12A1* (type I, AR); *ROMK/KCNJ1* (type II, AR); *CLCNKB* (type III, AR); *BSND* (type IV, AR); *CASR* (type V, AD); and *CLCN5* (type VI, XLR).
- Dent's disease: XLR disorder of proximal renal tubule due to mutations of *CLCN5* (type 1) or *OCRL* (type 2) genes. Characterized by low-molecular weight proteinuria, hypercalciuria, nephrocalcinosis, and progressive glomerular disease resulting in end-stage renal disease in 30–80% of patients by 5th decade.

- Other hereditary disorders associated with hypercalciuria include: distal renal tubular acidosis; hereditary hypophosphataemic rickets; familial hypomagnesaemia with hypercalciuria; and infantile hypercalcaemia.

Disorders associated with non-calcium stones
- Cystinuria: defective amino acid transport in proximal tubule, resulting in ~5% of stone disease in children, but less common in adults. Type A is an AR disorder due to mutations of *SLC3A1*, while type B is AD with incomplete penetrance due to *SLC7A9* mutations.
- Other disorders include: hereditary hyperuricosuria; hereditary xanthinuria; and adenine phosphoribosyltransferase deficiency.

Polygenic risk factors
- GWAS have identified ≥25 loci associated with renal stones. Several of these overlap with loci implicated in monogenic stone disease (e.g. *CASR*) and/or are implicated in Ca homeostasis or renal tubular function.

(See also Boxes 10.9 and 10.10.)

Box 10.9 Causes of renal calculi
- Hypercalciuria.
- Hyperoxaluria.
- Hyperuricosuria.
- Hypocitraturia.
- Urinary tract infection, e.g. *Proteus*, *Pseudomonas*, *Klebsiella*.
- 1° renal disease, e.g. polycystic kidney disease.
- Drugs, e.g. indinavir (PI—antiretroviral), diuretics, salicylates, allopurinol, some chemotherapeutic agents.

Box 10.10 Genetic testing/mutational analysis
- Currently largely a research tool.
- Target testing to those at highest risk of monogenic disease:
  - Paediatric or adult recurrent stone formers.
  - Patients with a strong +ve family history.
  - Those with phenotypic features consistent with a particular monogenic disorder.

As genetic testing moves into the clinical domain, then family screening will become increasingly relevant.

Investigation of renal calculi
Initial investigation aimed at identifying a cause includes
- Blood tests: Ca, chloride, Cr, bicarbonate, K^+, PO_4, uric acid, PTH if Ca high.
- 24h urine volume and urine osmolarity.
- 24h urinary Ca excretion (plus others as indicated, e.g. uric acid, oxalate, citrate, Na, Mg, PO_4, cysteine excretion).
- Urine pH.
- Stone composition, if possible.

Management
- Increase fluid intake.
- Appropriate dietary modifications.
- Treat underlying cause.

Further reading

Howles SA, Thakker RV (2020). Genetics of kidney stone disease. *Nature Rev Urol* **17**, 407–21.

Sakhaee K, *et al.* (2012). Clinical review. Kidney stones 2012: pathogenesis, diagnosis, and management. *J Clin Endocrinol Metab* **97**, 1847–60.

Worcester EM, Coe FL (2010). Clinical practice. Calcium kidney stones. *N Engl J Med* **363**, 954–63.

Endocrinology and ageing

Antonia Brooke and Andrew McGovern

Endocrinology and ageing

Introduction

- Ageing causes changes in many hormonal axes. How much of this change is normal physiology associated with ageing and how much represents true endocrine dysfunction, and thus warrants treatment, is unclear.
- Concomitant disease and polypharmacy are common in the elderly population, with frequent 2° effects upon the endocrine system.

Fluid and electrolyte homeostasis in the elderly

- Elderly patients are particularly prone to fluid and electrolyte disturbances due to changes associated with ageing, concomitant disease, and drug usage.
- Elderly patients have ↓ renal function compared with younger patients:
  - ↓ GFR, with creatinine clearance ↓ by 8mL/min/1.73m² per decade after age 30.
  - ↑ renovascular disease.
  - ↓ renal sensitivity to circulating hormones:
    - ○ Aldosterone.
    - ○ Vasopressin.
    - ○ Atrial natriuretic peptide (probable).
  - ↓ ability to dilute or concentrate urine.
- Elderly patients have ↓ renin levels, with 2° decreases of aldosterone levels (both basal and stimulated levels). Aldosterone levels may be <50% normal by 70 years of age. ↓ renal sensitivity to aldosterone may result in isolated mineralocorticoid deficiency (distal renal tubular acidosis (type 4) with hyponatraemia, hyperkalaemia, hyperchloraemia, and normal anion gap acidosis); this is commoner with DM.

Vasopressin/ADH

- Unlike many other hormones, vasopressin (ADH) responses are potentiated in elderly patients, with ↑ release from the neurohypophysis in response to an osmotic stimulus and less effective suppression. Normal vasopressin release is a balance of inhibitory and stimulatory effects at baroreceptors and osmoreceptors. It may be that loss of inhibition with ageing due to degenerative changes results in relatively unopposed stimulation of ADH and a ↓ ability to suppress ADH release.
- In addition, altered renal sensitivity to vasopressin results in ↓ ability to excrete free water.

Hypernatraemia and dehydration

- Perception of thirst is reduced in elderly persons (in younger people, thirst is perceived at plasma osmolalities >292mOsm/kg, whereas in older people, thirst is perceived at plasma osmolalities >296mOsm/kg). Elderly patients may be less able to ingest fluids due to physical or cognitive disabilities. Medication (e.g. diuretics) may potentiate fluid loss.
- Thus, elderly persons are particularly susceptible to dehydration when there are ↑ fluid losses (e.g. during hot summers). This is exacerbated by impaired renal concentrating ability.

- Dehydration may have atypical features with fatigue, delirium/confusion, cognitive impairment, anxiety, or agitation.
- Hypernatraemia affects around 1% of elderly people in nursing care facilities. In the hospitalized elderly, it is a marker of poor prognosis (42–52% mortality), although it is not usually the cause of death.

Hyponatraemia
- Common. Hyponatraemia affects 7% of healthy elderly people, 15–18% of elderly people in residential care facilities, and 53% of elderly people in nursing care facilities.
- Mortality rates in hospitalized elderly patients with hyponatraemia are high (in patients aged >65 years, 16% mortality in those with hyponatraemia, compared with 8% in those without hyponatraemia).
- Often associated with medication (e.g. diuretics).
- Many causes of SIADH are commoner in the elderly. Hyponatraemia is also the commonest electrolyte disturbance in cancer (see ➔ SIADH due to ectopic vasopressin production, pp. 748–9).
- Elderly people may also have lower sodium intake and reduced renal sodium-conserving ability.
- Symptoms include confusion, lethargy, coma, and seizures.
- Overall approach to investigation and management is similar to that of hyponatraemia in younger patients (see ➔ Hyponatraemia, pp. 236–8).
- Mild idiopathic hyponatraemia is also recognized in elderly patients, without necessarily having a sinister cause or consequence, and is thought to be 2° to altered threshold for ADH secretion.

Further reading

Ayus JC (1996). Abnormalities of water metabolism in the elderly. *Semin Nephrol* **16**, 277–88.
Beck LH (1998). Changes in renal function with ageing. *Clin Geriatr Med* **14**, 199–209.
Koch CA, Fulop T (2017). Clinical aspects of changes in water and sodium homeostasis in the elderly. *Rev Endocr Metab Disord* **18**, 49–66.
Toor MR, et al. (2014). Characteristics, therapies, and factors influencing outcomes of hospitalized hypernatremic geriatric patients. *Int Urol Nephrol* **46**, 1589–94.

Bone disease in the elderly

Osteoporosis

Osteoporosis is not an inevitable part of ageing, but it is a common disease in elderly people and is associated with high morbidity and mortality in both ♂ and ♀ (see ➔ Osteoporosis, p. 544).

Vitamin D deficiency

(See ➔ Vitamin D deficiency, p. 537.)

- Very common in the elderly.
- Vitamin D insufficiency (evidence of 2° hyperparathyroidism, ↑ bone turnover, BMD loss) occurs at levels of 25OH vitamin D <50nmol/L.
- Vitamin D deficiency usually defined as concentrations <25nmol/L.
- Vitamin D deficiency or insufficiency is common, particularly in elderly institutionalized patients, in extreme latitudes, and in fracture patients.
- Supplementation in elderly patients decrease fracture risk.

Primary hyperparathyroidism

- Prevalence of 1° hyperparathyroidism is 10/100,000 in ♀ <40 years old, rising to 190/100,000 in ♀ >65 years old. Half of all cases of 1° hyperparathyroidism occur in ♀ >60 years old.
- Elderly people are more prone to symptoms (weakness, fatigue, confusion) at relatively mild levels of hypercalcaemia (2.8–3.0mmol/L).
- Other causes of hypercalcaemia must be excluded.
- Coexisting vitamin D insufficiency and deficiency are common.
- Management is similar to that described in ➔ Hypercalcaemia, pp. 508–9.
- Surgery is not contraindicated by age alone.

Paget's disease

(See ➔ Paget's disease, pp. 558–60.)

Further reading

Chapuy MC, *et al.* (1992). Vitamin D3 and calcium to prevent hip fractures in elderly women. *N Engl J Med* **327**, 1637–42.

Mosekilde L (2005). Vitamin D and the elderly. *Clin Endocrinol (Oxf)* **62**, 265–81.

GH and IGF-1 in the elderly

- Many of the features of normal ageing resemble those of GH deficiency in younger patients.
- Changes in body composition with ageing include ↓ lean body mass (↓ body water, ↓ muscle mass, and ↓ bone mass) and ↑ total body fat and visceral fat mass, associated with an abnormal lipid profile (↑ total cholesterol (TC) and LDL-C, ↑ TGs), insulin resistance, and ↓ exercise and cardiac capacity.
- Overall, integrated GH concentrations show a decrease with age, with ↓ GH pulse amplitude and duration, but unchanged pulse frequency. For ♂ over 25 years old, GH secretion ↓ by ~50% every 7 years.
- IGF-1 decreases with ↑ age (reflected in age-adjusted normative ranges).
- Insulin-like growth factor-binding protein 3 (IGFBP-3) decreases with ↑ age (and is also GH-dependent).
- The decrease in GH concentration with age is likely to be related to altered hypothalamic regulation, rather than ↓ secretory capacity.
- Other factors may also decrease GH/IGF-1 concentrations with ageing, such as ↓ physical fitness, ↓ production of sex hormones, fragmented sleep (GH is secreted mainly during slow-wave sleep), and malnutrition (inhibiting IGF-1 synthesis).

Treatment of age-related GH decline

- The use of replacement GH therapy in healthy elderly people has been debated and has previously been suggested to have anti-ageing potential.
- A systematic review of the use of GH in healthy elderly patients found fat mass ↓ by 2.1kg and lean body mass ↑ by 2.1kg. There were no clear benefits to serum lipid measurements and bone density. Side effects were frequently observed (oedema, arthralgias, carpal tunnel syndrome, glucose intolerance). Furthermore, no functional benefits have been demonstrated.
- GH is not licensed in the UK for healthy elderly people.

Treatment of GH deficiency

- Older patients with GH deficiency related to pituitary disease are usually easily differentiated from other subjects with age-related decline in IGF-1, using standard provocative testing (GH response to insulin-induced hypoglycaemia, arginine, or glucagon).
- A systematic review of the use of GH in elderly patients (aged 60–80 years) with GH deficiency found ↓ total cholesterol (4–8%), ↓ LDL-C (11–16%), ↓ waist circumference (~3cm), and ↑ quality of life (measured by AGHDA (Adult Growth Hormone Deficiency Assessment) score). No effects have been clearly demonstrated on HDL-C or TG concentrations, BP, or bone density. Data on the effects of GH on body composition were conflicting in studies.
- Few data exist on the benefits of GH in patients with GH deficiency over the age of 80.

Further reading

Bartke A, Darcy J (2017). GH and ageing: pitfalls and new insights. *Best Pract Res Clin Endocrinol Metab* **31**, 113–25.

Kokshoorn N (2011). GH replacement therapy in elderly GH-deficient patients: a systematic review. *Eur J Endocrinol* **164**, 657–65.

Liu H (2007). Systematic review: the safety and efficacy of growth hormone in the healthy elderly. *Ann Intern Med* **146**, 104–15.

Gonadal function in the elderly

Women

- The mean age of menopause is 51 years (range 35–58 years) and is defined retrospectively after 12 months of amenorrhoea as the permanent cessation of menstruation due to loss of ovarian follicular activity.
  - FSH 10–15× higher than premenopausal levels.
  - LH 3–5× higher.
  - Oestrogen 10% of previous level (often lower than ♂ of similar age).
  - Inhibin often undetectable.
- The adrenal gland is the major source of sex steroids post-menopausally, with oestrogen production mainly from aromatization of adrenal androgens (androstenedione) in adipose tissue.
- Low FSH/LH may indicate hypopituitarism, although gonadotrophins may be depressed by serious illness.

(For further discussion, see ➋ Menopause, p. 384.)

Men

- ♂ may remain potent and fertile until their death. However, sexual activity, libido, and potency decline gradually and progressively from midlife.
- As with GH deficiency, there is an overlap between clinical features of hypogonadism and 'normal ageing' (↓ lean body mass and muscle function, ↑ fat mass, ↓ virility, ↓ libido, and ↓ overall well-being). Functional 2° hypogonadism is common in serious chronic illness, especially when associated with malnutrition and debilitation.
- Normal ranges for testosterone in ♂ of different ages have not been well established; 20% of ♂ over 60 and 50% over 80 have total testosterone values below the reference range for young men.
- Free testosterone levels decrease slowly from age 20–80, but there is significant intra- and inter-individual variation. The underlying mechanism is that of ↓ testosterone production, rather than ↑ clearance of testosterone. Testosterone production decrease with ageing, as testicular weight, Leydig cell function, and FSH/LH response to GnRH stimulation decrease.
- The extent to which lower testosterone per se and/or a lower free androgen index explain the age-related decline in sexual function is not clear. Although testosterone concentrations may be lower than in younger ♂, testosterone concentrations are still sufficient for normal libido and sexual function. Profoundly low testosterone concentrations (<8nmol/L in a 9 a.m. blood sample) in the appropriate clinical setting should prompt investigation for hypoandrogenism. Gonadotrophins should be raised in 1° testicular failure, and low levels associated with low testosterone should prompt a search for 2° causes, though gonadotrophins may be low because of other serious disease or medication, e.g. opiates.
- Fat body mass increases more than lean body mass with age; thus, there is ↑ aromatization of androgens to oestrogens. The effects of this are unclear.

- Hypoandrogenism may also result from hyperprolactinaemia due to pituitary/hypothalamic disease, renal dysfunction, hypothyroidism, drugs (psychotropic and anti-dopaminergic agents); all commoner in the elderly population.

Testosterone therapy

- Few small studies in elderly ♂, either as replacement in patients with clear hypogonadism or in healthy ♂.
- Data point towards a +ve effect on well-being, muscle mass and strength, and ↓ fat mass in elderly patients, with greatest effect in patients with clear hypogonadism.
- Risk of 2° polycythaemia, liver dysfunction (particularly if testosterone taken PO), prostatism, exacerbation of prostate adenocarcinoma, and possibly dyslipidaemia. The cardiovascular safety of replacement remains unclear and an individualized approach should be adopted for elderly men with deficiency.

Erectile dysfunction

- Common in elderly ♂; 50% of ♂ >60 have erectile dysfunction; 90% of these ♂ have concurrent medical problems or are on medication potentially causing impotence.
- Aetiology often multifactorial:
  - Atherosclerosis—commonest cause with both macro- and microvascular disease.
  - Penile denervation—autonomic neuropathy (most commonly due to DM); pelvic surgery (including prostatectomy—30% of ♂ >75 develop erectile dysfunction after prostatectomy (compared with 7% of younger ♂ after prostatectomy)).
  - Drugs (β-blockers, calcium channel antagonists, other antihypertensive agents, psychotropic drugs).
  - Psychogenic.

Delayed/absent ejaculation

- Commoner with age due to autonomic nerve dysfunction, drugs, previous surgery, and usually the harbinger of erectile dysfunction.
- Evaluation similar to that of younger patients (see ➲ Evaluation of erectile dysfunction, pp. 438–9).
- Management similar to younger patients, with caveat that PDE inhibitors may interact with nitrates and antihypertensive agents.

Fertility

- Testicular morphology, semen production, and testicular steroidogenesis are maintained into old age.
- There is some evidence for a small increase in specific genetic disorders in the children of older men.

Further reading

Harman SM, *et al* (2001). Longitudinal effects of aging on serum total and free testosterone levels in healthy men. Baltimore Longitudinal Study of Aging. *J Clin Endocrinol Metab* **86**, 724–31.

Adrenal function in the elderly

Cortisol

- Overall, cortisol secretion generally very similar in elderly persons to younger persons.
- Dynamic testing shows more prolonged release of ACTH and cortisol to stress (physiological, insulin-induced hypoglycaemia, and/or CRH administration) and slower inhibition of ACTH secretion by cortisol.
- Adrenal insufficiency is commoner in the elderly primarily due to greater use of long-term glucocorticoids.

Dehydroepiandrosterone sulfate

- DHEA and DHEAS levels peak in humans aged 20–30 years and thereafter decline with age (20% of peak values in ♂ and 30% of peak values in ♀ by age 70 years). Responsiveness to ACTH-stimulated secretion also reduces with age.
- The physiological relevance of the fall of DHEA and DHEAS levels with age is not established.
- Although DHEA therapy is sometimes used in patients with adrenal insufficiency, its use in otherwise healthy elderly patients (who experience an age-related decrease in DHEA) is not recommended; there have been no demonstrated clinical benefits (in terms of longevity, well-being, bone density, cognitive function, body mass composition, or cardiovascular status).

Aldosterone

(See Fluid and electrolyte homeostasis in the elderly, pp. 704–5.)

Thyroid disease in the elderly

Thyroid disease is twice as common in the elderly as in younger patients (see Table 11.1).

Abnormal thyroid function tests

- Concomitant disease and polypharmacy are common in the elderly and may alter the interpretation of results. For example, glucocorticoids (prescribed to 2.5% of the population aged 70–79 years) cause ↓ TSH, ↓ thyroid hormone release, ↓ concentration of thyroid hormone-binding proteins, and ↓ T_4 to T_3 conversion.
- Sick euthyroid syndrome is commoner in the elderly due to frequent concurrent NTI (see ⊃ Non-thyroidal illness (sick euthyroid syndrome), pp. 878–80), with ↓ FT_3), ↑ reverse FT_3, and (less commonly) ↓ FT_4, with inappropriately normal or suppressed TSH levels.

(See Table 1.4 for effects on thyroid function of drugs frequently prescribed for elderly patients.)

Hypothyroidism

(See ⊃ Hypothyroidism, p. 84.)
- Commonest thyroid problem in elderly people.
- 7–17% of elderly people.
- ♂:♀ ratio increases with ageing.
- Commonest causes are autoimmune thyroiditis, previous surgery, or radioiodine therapy (post-ablative hypothyroidism occurs more frequently in people >55 years old than in younger patients).
- 25% present with classical symptoms of hypothyroidism; 50% complain of fatigue and weakness. Elderly patients with hypothyroidism report cold intolerance, weight gain, paraesthesiae, and muscle cramps less frequently than do younger patients with hypothyroidism.
- The elderly are more susceptible to hypothyroid (myxoedema) coma than younger people; it remains rare, however.
- Elderly patients with unrecognized hypothyroidism may be at greater risk of development of perioperative and intraoperative complications (including intraoperative hypotension, heart failure, CHD, and post-operative GI and neuropsychiatric complications).
- Hypothyroidism should be considered in elderly patients with sinus bradycardia, hypothermia, ↑ creatine kinase (CK) or transaminases, ↓ Na, macrocytic anaemia, or dyslipidaemia.
- Thyroid replacement therapy should be done cautiously, as IHD may be unmasked or exacerbated, e.g. 12.5–25 micrograms/day of levothyroxine, ↑ by 12.5- to 25-microgram increments every 3–8 weeks until TSH is normalized.
- Total replacement T_4 dose is lower in the elderly than in younger patients (in younger patients, ~1.6 micrograms/kg is required, but older patients require 20–30% less).
- Compliance may be problematic. Supervised therapy or administration using a multi-compartment compliance aid (e.g. Dosette® box) may help. Alternatively, calculate the total weekly dose of levothyroxine, and give 70% of the total dose once a week or 50% of the total dose twice weekly.

Table 11.1 Changes in thyroid-related investigations with ageing

TSH	No significant change; secretion remains pulsatile, but loss of physiological nocturnal TSH rise is blunted
T_4	Unchanged overall (both secretion and clearance ↓)
T_3	10–50% decrease; occurs at an earlier age in ♀ than in ♂
rT_3	↑
Thyroid antibodies	Prevalence ↑ with age; significance uncertain (2% at age 25, 15–32% at age 75)
24h radioactive iodine uptake	Unchanged

Hyperthyroidism

(See ➋ Thyrotoxicosis—aetiology, pp. 30–1.)
- 0.3–2% of elderly people.
- Presentation is often atypical, often with few signs or symptoms.
- Clinical symptoms of hyperthyroidism are different in the elderly; non-specific symptoms, such as weight loss, depression, or agitation, predominate. Consider the diagnosis with muscle weakness; heart failure, arrhythmias, atrial fibrillation; weight loss; and osteoporotic fracture.
- Toxic multinodular goitre becomes the most common cause in the elderly.
- Treatment options are similar to those in younger patients (see ➋ Medical treatment, pp. 34–7).
- RAI is favoured because it is definitive and avoids risks of surgery. Hypothyroidism is common after radioiodine therapy in elderly people.

Subclinical thyroid disease

- An isolated elevated TSH is common in the elderly (7–12%; ♀ > ♂) and TSH levels rise in the healthy elderly.
- Treatment does not appear to improve symptoms in those >65 years old. A more cautious approach to replacement should be adopted.
- An isolated completely suppressed TSH concentration is associated with ↑ cardiovascular mortality, ↑ heart failure, and a 3-fold higher risk of atrial fibrillation in the next 10 years; 2–24% of elderly patients with atrial fibrillation are hyperthyroid, and 9–35% of elderly patients with hyperthyroidism have atrial fibrillation.
- Evidence for treatment is unclear if TSH is below normal, but not completely suppressed.
- Low threshold for treatment of thyrotoxicosis in the elderly, especially those with cardiac risk factors or osteoporosis.

Goitre

- Diffuse goitre becomes less frequent with age in both ♂ and ♀ (found in 31% of ♀ aged <45 years, compared with 12% of ♀ aged >75 years on clinical examination.
- Multinodular goitre, as assessed by both clinical and US examination, increases with age (incidence of US-detected multinodular goitre 90% of ♀ >70 years, 60% of ♂ >80 years).
- Management similar to that of multinodular goitre in younger patients (see ➲ Multinodular goitre and solitary adenomas, pp. 72–5).

Thyroid cancer

(See ➲ Epidemiology of thyroid cancer, p. 100.)

- Total incidence rate for all thyroid cancers is unchanged, but the relative frequencies are altered.
- PTC is commoner in young and middle-aged patients and accounts for only 50% of thyroid cancers in patients over 60 years old. Older patients have a higher mortality rate.
- FTC: peak incidence in 6th decade of life. Prognosis is poorer in older patients, possibly due to ↑ frequency of extraglandular recurrences in older patients.
- Anaplastic thyroid carcinoma: peak incidence in 7th decade. Two-thirds of all cases occur in patients >65 years. It presents with a rapidly growing hard mass which is often locally invasive and may be associated with metastatic lesions. The prognosis is poor.
- Sarcomas and 1° thyroid lymphomas are commoner in elderly patients.
- MTC: sporadic forms have a mean age at presentation of 47 years; hereditary forms commoner in younger patients. Older age at diagnosis and more advanced stage are independent markers of a poorer prognosis.
- Overall evaluation and treatment are similar to that of younger patients, but accurate preoperative histology is very important, as tumours not treated surgically (e.g. anaplastic carcinoma and lymphoma) are relatively commoner.

Further reading

Michel J-P, et al. (eds.) (2017). *Oxford Textbook of Geriatric Medicine*, 3rd edn. Oxford University Press, Oxford.

Vermeulen A (1997). Endocrinology of ageing. *Ballière's Clin Endocrinol Metab* **11**, 223–50.

Pituitary disease

- Non-functioning pituitary adenomas (NFPAs) are the commonest pituitary adenomas in the elderly (Cushing's rare).
- Surgical outcomes are similar to younger patients, but surgical risks increase with advancing age, especially electrolyte abnormalities (increasing risk over 80 years).
- Transsphenoidal surgery should be considered when there is mass effect.

Further reading

Grossman R, et al. (2010). Complications and death among elderly patients undergoing pituitary tumor surgery. *Clin Endocrinol (Oxf)* **73**, 361–8.

Endocrinology aspects of other clinical or physiological situations

Antonia Brooke, Kagabo Hirwa, Claire Higham, and Alex Lewis

Hypoglycaemia

Definition (Whipple's triad)

- Plasma glucose of <3mmol/L, associated with:
  - Symptoms of neuroglycopenia, *and*
  - Reversal of symptoms with correction of glucose levels.

Epidemiology

Uncommon in adults, apart from patients with DM being treated with certain agents, either alone or in combination (e.g. insulin, sulfonylureas).

Pathophysiology

Physiology of glucose control

Plasma glucose concentrations are usually kept within narrow limits (~3.3–5.6mmol/L), providing an uninterrupted supply of glucose to the brain (which can consume up to 50% of hepatic glucose output).

The liver is the major regulator (80–85%) of circulating blood glucose concentrations in healthy individuals and responds to changes in circulating insulin, GH, cortisol, glucagon, and adrenaline.

- *Postprandial state:* hepatic glucose production is inhibited by ↑ plasma glucose and ↑ insulin concentrations.
- *Fasting state:* plasma glucose ↓↓, with consequent ↓ in insulin secretion, stimulating hepatic glucose efflux (due to ↑ cortisol, GH, and glucagon).

Mechanisms of hypoglycaemia

- *Excessive/inappropriate action of insulin (or IGF-1):* inhibiting hepatic glucose production, despite adequate glycogen stores, while peripheral glucose uptake is enhanced.
- *Impaired neuroendocrine response* with inadequate counter-regulatory response (e.g. cortisol) to insulin.
- *Impairment of hepatic glucose production* due to either structural damage or abnormal liver enzymes.

Classification of hypoglycaemia

Traditionally, hypoglycaemia has been classified as fasting or postprandial.

- *Fasting hypoglycaemia:* occurring several hours (typically >5h) after food (e.g. early morning, following prolonged fasting or exercise).
- *Postprandial (reactive) hypoglycaemia:* occurring 2–5h after food.

Causes of hypoglycaemia can fit into both categories, so another classification has been proposed, based on whether the patient is unwell (see Box 12.1.)

Box 12.1 Causes of hypoglycaemia in adults

Ill or medicated individual

- Drug-induced (common cause; accidental or intentional):
  - Insulin or insulin secretagogue.
  - Alcohol (impairs hepatic gluconeogenesis and is often associated with poor glycogen stores).
  - Others (e.g. pentamidine, quinine, indometacin, glucagon (during endoscopy)).
- Organ failure or critical illness:
  - Liver failure (>80% of the liver needs to be destroyed/removed).
  - CRF.
  - Sepsis, e.g. malaria, Gram −ve, or meningococcal; related to high metabolic requirements, reduced energy intake, and possibly cytokines from the inflammatory process.
- Hormone deficiency:
  - Cortisol deficiency, e.g. Addison's disease, hypopituitarism.
- Non-islet cell tumours:
  - Excessive IGF-2 secretion from large mesenchymal tumours (non-islet cell tumour hypoglycaemia), e.g. fibrosarcoma, mesothelioma (~1/3 retroperitoneal, 1/3 intra-abdominal, and 1/3 intrathoracic).

Seemingly well individual

- Insulinoma by islet cell insulin secretion:
  - Benign 85%, malignant 15%.
  - Occasionally part of MEN1 (~10%).
- Non-islet cell tumours by IGF-2 or precursors:
  - Adrenal carcinoma, PCC.
  - Hepatocellular carcinoma.
  - Lymphoma, myeloma, leukaemia.
  - Advanced metastatic malignancy.
- Functional β-cell disorders (nesidioblastosis):
  - Non-insulinoma pancreatogenous hypoglycaemia (typically after eating).
  - Post-gastric bypass hypoglycaemia (early dumping syndrome and late hyperinsulinaemic hypoglycaemia (rare and mechanism unknown); may require treatment with α-glucosidase inhibitor, diazoxide, octreotide, or dipeptyl peptidase IV (DPP-IV) inhibitor).
- Autoimmune:
  - Antibodies to insulin (antibody-bound insulin dissociates, leading to elevated free insulin; typically associated with late postprandial hypoglycaemia; mainly reported among people of Japanese or Korean descent).
  - Insulin receptor-activating antibodies (rare; may require treatment with plasmapheresis or immunosuppression).
- Accidental or surreptitious hypoglycaemia (e.g. insulin or insulin secretagogue administration).

Source: data from Cryer P. (1997) *Hypoglycaemia: pathophysiology, diagnosis, and treatment* Oxford University Press: New York.

Symptoms of hypoglycaemia

(See Table 12.1 for classification of symptoms.)

- Adrenergic symptoms have been identified at arterialized plasma glucose concentrations of 3.3mmol/L (equivalent to a venous plasma concentration of 3.1mmol/L).
- Neuroglycopenic symptoms have been identified at arterialized plasma glucose concentrations of 2.8mmol/L (equivalent to a venous plasma concentration of 2.6mmol/L).
- Electroencephalographic (EEG) changes occur at 2.0mmol/L.
- The majority of symptoms of acute hypoglycaemia are adrenergic, but neuroglycopenic symptoms occur with subacute and chronic hypoglycaemia.
- The rate of decrease in plasma glucose concentration does not influence the occurrence of symptoms.
- Patients with recurrent hypoglycaemia may not get symptoms until glucose concentrations are very low (so-called 'hypo unawareness'), while patients with poorly controlled DM may experience hypoglycaemic symptoms at 'normal' blood glucose levels.

Table 12.1 Classification of symptoms and signs of hypoglycaemia

Adrenergic (CBG <3.3mmol/L)	Neuroglycopenic (CBG <2.8–3.1mmol/L)
Sweating	Visual disturbance (e.g. diplopia, blurred vision)
Hunger	Poor concentration
Tingling	Drowsiness
Trembling	Lethargy
Palpitations	Unusual behaviour
Anxiety	Personality change
	Confusion
	Focal neurological abnormality
	Seizures
	Coma

Source: data from PE Cryer, in S. Melmed et als (editors): *William Textbook of Endocrinology*, 12th edition, New York, 2012 and PE Cryer, SN Davis. Hypoglycemia in DL. Kasper et als (editors): *Harrison's principles of Internal Medicine*, 19th Edition, 2015, pp2431.

Investigations of hypoglycaemia

- Glucose (capillary blood glucose) strip, unreliable at low glucose concentration.
- Plasma glucose for low glucose confirmation.
- Liver and renal function tests.
- Blood ethanol concentration.
- Early morning cortisol (and Synacthen® test if low).
- Insulin, C-peptide, proinsulin, and glucose during hypoglycaemia (see Table 12.2).
  - Inappropriately elevated insulin in presence of hypoglycaemia and symptoms suggests insulinoma, self-administration of insulin/ sulfonylurea, post-gastric bypass hypoglycaemia, non-insulinoma pancreatogenous hypoglycaemia syndrome, or insulin autoimmune hypoglycaemia.
  - Absence of C-peptide, but presence of insulin during hypoglycaemia suggests exogenous insulin administration or raised IGF-2.
  - Insulinomas often associated with elevated proinsulin:insulin ratio.
- Consider assay for presence of sulfonylureas.
- Fasting β-hydroxybutyrate (elevated in most causes of hypoglycaemia, but suppressed if insulin present, e.g. insulinoma, self-administration of insulin, or sulfonylureas).
- Consider IGF-1 and -2 and pro-IGF-2. IGF-2 may be normal in non-islet cell hypoglycaemia, but this is in association with suppressed IGF-1 and GH; usual IGF-1:IGF-1 ratio 3:1; ratio >10 seen in non-islet cell hypoglycaemia.

Table 12.2 Biochemical features of insulinoma and factitious hypoglycaemia

Plasma marker	Insulinoma	Sulfonylurea	Insulin injection
Glucose	↓ (<3.0mmol/L)	↓ (<3.0mmol/L)	↓ (<3.0mmol/L)
Insulin	↑ (≥3 microunits/mL)	↑ (≥3 microunits/mL)	↑ (>>3 microunits/mL)
C-peptide	↑ (≥0.2nmol/L)	↑ (≥0.2nmol/L)	↓ (<0.2nmol/L)

Source: data from Cryer PE, Axelrod L, Grossman AB, Heller SR, Montori V, Seaquist ER, Service FJ (2009). Evaluation and management of adult hypoglycaemic disorders: an Endocrine Society clinical practice guideline. *J Clin Endocrinol Metab* 94, 709–28.

Chest and abdominal radiographs/CT

- Consider insulin and insulin receptor antibodies.

Further investigation of fasting hypoglycaemia

15h fast

- Measure plasma glucose and insulin after fasting for 15h.
- Plasma glucose <3mmol/L and insulin >3mU/L are inappropriate, although precise definitions vary, depending on sensitivity cut-offs. Typically, β-cell suppression occurs when glucose is <3mmol/L.
- Good screening test if repeated three times.
- 75% of patients with an insulinoma will develop hypoglycaemia within 18h of beginning a fast.

72h fast
- The most reliable test for hypoglycaemia (detects 98% of patients with insulinoma, compared with >70% at 24h), although the majority will be detected by 48h.
- The patient should remain hydrated and active.
- Measure plasma glucose, insulin, C-peptide, and proinsulin 6-hourly (unless the patient is symptomatic or the glucose level is <3.5mmol/L when measurements are made every 1–2h); the test is terminated when the patient demonstrates symptoms and laboratory glucose is <3mmol/L or after 72h.
- β-hydroxybutyrate should be measured at the end of the fast (its presence makes insulinoma unlikely).

Further investigation of postprandial hypoglycaemia

Prolonged OGTT
- Not physiological test.
- 10% of the normal (asymptomatic) population have a +ve response, with blood glucose levels <2.6mmol/L.

Mixed meal test over 5h
- More physiological.
- Uses foods with a medium to low glycaemic index ('hyperglucidic').
- 47% of patients with suspected postprandial hypoglycaemia have a +ve test vs 1% of asymptomatic subjects.
- However, diagnostic criteria not formally agreed for this test.

Ambulatory glucose sampling
- Gaining favour, as it may correlate symptoms with low sugar readings, and improvement of symptoms with recovery from hypoglycaemia.

Other investigations may be indicated if there is clinical and biochemical evidence of an insulinoma (e.g. see ➜ Tumour localization, p. 639).

Management of hypoglycaemia

Acute hypoglycaemia

If conscious

- A total of 15–20g oral carbohydrate (ideally food and a sugary drink) should be administered as soon as possible.
- Dextrogel®/GlucoGel® (formerly known as Hypostop Gel®), a glucose-containing gel which is absorbed by the buccal mucosa, may be used in drowsy, but conscious individuals.

If unconscious

- A volume of 75–80mL of 20% glucose or 150–200mL of 10% glucose IV into a large vein (over 10–15min), followed by a saline flush as the high concentration of glucose is an irritant and may even lead to venous thrombosis. A maintenance infusion of 5% or 10% glucose is often required thereafter, especially if there is an ongoing risk of recurrent hypoglycaemia (e.g. overdose of a long-acting insulin/analogue).
- Glucagon 1mg IM may be administered if there is no IV access. This increases hepatic glucose efflux, but the effect only lasts for 30min, allowing other means of blood glucose elevation (e.g. oral) before the blood glucose falls again. It is ineffective with hepatic dysfunction and if there is glycogen depletion, e.g. ethanol-related hypoglycaemia, and it is relatively contraindicated in patients with known insulinoma, as it may induce further insulin secretion. Glucagon is ineffective if given within 3 days of a previous dose of glucagon.

Secondary cerebral oedema may complicate hypoglycaemia and should be considered in cases of prolonged coma despite normalization of plasma glucose. Mannitol and/or dexamethasone may be helpful.

Recurrent chronic hypoglycaemia

If definitive treatment of the underlying condition is unsuccessful or impossible, symptoms may be alleviated by frequent (e.g. 4-hourly) small meals, including overnight. Diazoxide, administered by mouth, and/or SC octreotide, is useful in the management of patients with chronic hypoglycaemia from excess endogenous insulin secretion due to an insulinoma or islet cell hyperplasia.

Postprandial reactive hypoglycaemia

Definition

Hypoglycaemia following a meal, due to an imbalance between glucose influx into (exogenous from food and endogenous glucose production) and glucose efflux out of the circulation.

Pathophysiology and causes

- Exaggerated insulin response. Related to rapid glucose absorption, e.g. post-gastrectomy dumping syndrome. This results in a delayed insulin peak with respect to the peak blood glucose, probably related to an exaggerated GLP-1 response.
- Incipient DM. Occasionally presents with postprandial hypoglycaemia, possibly related to disordered insulin secretion.
- Insulin resistance-related hyperinsulinaemia, e.g. obese subjects with or without IGT.
- Impaired glucagon sensitivity and secretion. In response to hypoglycaemia; involved in the pathogenesis of postprandial reactive hypoglycaemia (PRH).
- Renal glycosuria. Accounts for up to 15% of patients with PRH.
- Body composition:
  - 20% of very lean people are prone to PRH.
  - Massive weight reduction increases the risk of PRH.
  - Lower body obesity (especially in ♀) associated with high normal insulin sensitivity and PRH.
- Diet:
  - High-carbohydrate, low-fat diet, by ↑↑ insulin sensitivity.
  - Prolonged very low-calorie diets (>2 weeks) by reducing counter-regulatory hormones, especially GH.
- Alcohol:
  - Inhibits hepatic glucose output.
  - Increases insulin secretion in response to glucose and sucrose.
- Idiopathic.

Investigation

- Prolonged OGTT. Not physiological; 10% of the normal (asymptomatic) population have a +ve response with blood glucose levels <2.6mmol/L.
- Hyperglucidic mixed meal test. More physiological; 47% of patients with suspected PRH have a +ve test vs 1% of asymptomatic subjects.
- Ambulatory glucose sampling. Gaining favour, as it may correlate symptoms with low sugar readings, and improvement of symptoms with recovery from hypoglycaemia.

Management

Diet

- Frequent, small, low-carbohydrate, high-protein meals.
- Avoid rapidly absorbed carbohydrates.
- Avoid sugary drinks, especially in combination with alcohol.
- Addition of soluble dietary fibres, e.g. 5–10g guar gum or pectin or hemicellulose per meal, delays absorption and lowers the glycaemic and insulinaemic indices (especially effective in rapid gut transit time).

Drugs

- Acarbose, an intestinal α-glucosidase inhibitor, delays sugar and starch absorption, thus reducing the insulin response to a meal.
- Metformin can be useful, 500mg with meals.
- Supplemental chromium is reported to downregulate β-cell activity and increase glucagon secretion.
- In exceptional cases, with debilitating PRH, diazoxide (side effects: water retention, hypertrichosis, digestive disorders) or SSAs may be required.
- Propranolol, sitagliptin, and calcium antagonists have been used; however, controlled studies are lacking.

Further reading

Brun JF, et al. (2000). Postprandial reactive hypoglycaemia. *Diabetes Metab* **26**, 337–51.

Challis BG, et al. (2017). Adult-onset hyper-insulinaemic hypoglycae-mia in clinical practice: diagnosis, aetiology and management. *Endocr Connect* **6**, 540–8.

Cryer PE (1997). *Hypoglycemia: Pathophysiology, Diagnosis, and Treatment.* Oxford University Press, New York, NY.

Cryer PE (2004). Diverse causes of hypoglycemia-associated autonomic failure in diabetes. *N Engl J Med* **350**, 2272–9.

Cryer PE, et al. (2009). Evaluation and management of adult hypoglycaemic disorders: an Endocrine Society clinical practice guideline. *J Clin Endocrinol Metab* **94**, 709–28.

de Groot, et al. (2009). Non-islet cell tumour-induced hypoglycaemia: a review of the literature including two new cases. *Endocr Relat Cancer* **14**, 979–93.

Gama R, et al. (2003). Clinical and laboratory investigation of adult spontaneous hypoglycaemia. *J Clin Pathol* **56**, 641–6.

Mastocytosis

Background and definitions

- Mastocytosis is a heterogenous group of disorders characterized by the pathological accumulation of mast cells in tissues, which release histamines, leading to clinical features.
- The main types of mastocytoses are:
  - Cutaneous.
  - Systemic.
- Frequently diagnosed, but seldom established as a differential diagnosis in the work-up of flushing (sensation of warmth, usually on the face and neck, due to vasodilation and ↑ cutaneous circulation).
- Flushing due to neurogenic stimuli are likely to be associated with sweating (wet flushing).
- Flushing due to vasodilator substances associated with 'dry' flushing. Systemic mastocytosis usually features in the latter category.

Classification

Mastocytosis is broadly classified into cutaneous and systemic mastocytosis (see Box 12.2).

Clinical features

- Urticaria pigmentosa and dermographism are the usual cutaneous manifestations (exacerbated when rubbed—Darier's sign).
- Systemic manifestations include flushing, anaphylaxis, abdominal pain, and diarrhoea.
- Anaemia, hepatosplenomegaly, peptic ulceration, and steatorrhoea can occur due to mast cell infiltration.

Epidemiology

- It is a rare disorder.
- Affects both sexes equally.
- Children usually have cutaneous mastocytosis, and adults the systemic variety.

Investigations

- Serum tryptase, which is predominantly produced in mast cells, is usually elevated (see Box 12.3 for causes of raised tryptase).
- Skin biopsy stained with Giemsa and immunohistochemical staining for tryptase and c-kit (mast cell growth factor receptor).
- Bone marrow biopsy is warranted for adults with evidence of mastocytosis to diagnose systemic mastocytosis.

Box 12.2 WHO classification of systemic mastocytosis

- Indolent systemic mastocytosis.
- Systemic mastocytosis with clonal haematological non-mast cell lineage disease.
- Mast cell leukaemia.
- Mast cell sarcoma.
- Extracutaneous mastocytosis.

Box 12.3 Causes of raised tryptase level

- Acute myeloid leukaemia.
- Myelodysplastic disorders.
- Hypereosinophilic syndrome.
- Asthma (mild elevation).

Treatment
- Avoidance of triggers (e.g. alcohol, aspirin).
- Treat anaphylaxis as a medical emergency.
- Preparation of patients appropriately before surgery and other medical procedures with antihistamines, GCs, H_2 blockade, and montelukast.
- Antihistamines, such as cetirizine, fexofenadine, can be used to reduce flushing and itching.
- H_2 blockers and PPIs, such as ranitidine and omeprazole, can help with abdominal symptoms such as pain and heartburn.
- In patients who are not intolerant of NSAIDs, aspirin may help reduce flushing.
- Additional antileukotriene agents, such as montelukast, may help some with ongoing symptoms.
- Other treatment options, including TKIs, have been assessed, but their effectiveness is not convincing.

Further reading

Fallahi P. et al. (2021). Endocrine-metabolic effects of treatment with multikinase inhibitors. *Eur J Endocrinol* **184**, R29–40.

Liu AY, et al. (2010). Clinical problem-solving. A rash hypothesis. *N Engl J Med* **363**, 72–8.

Murali MR, et al. (2011). Case records of the Massachusetts General Hospital. Case 9-2011. A 37-year-old man with flushing and hypotension. *N Engl J Med* **364**, 1155–65.

IgG4-related endocrine manifestations

Definition

- IgG4-related disease is a systemic inflammatory disease which consists of lymphoplasmocytic infiltration, with affected organ fibrosis, and it is frequently associated with elevated IgG4 levels in the serum.

Incidence and epidemiology

- Incidence is estimated to be around 0.28–1.08/100,000.
- Men are more affected than women, and the mean age of onset is 50–60 years, but it can also occur at any age.

Pathophysiology and clinical features

- Digestive system (pancreas, bile ducts, and salivary glands) most affected, but also affects lacrimal lymph nodes, retroperitoneal space, respiratory system, genitourinary system, CNS, and blood vessels. The thyroid and pituitary are the most affected endocrine glands. The adrenal glands and pancreas are also very rarely affected. Thyroid gland manifestations of IgG4-related disease are Hashimoto's thyroiditis, Riedel thyroiditis, fibrous variant of Hashimoto's thyroiditis (FVHT), Graves' disease, and GO.
- IgG4-related pituitary hypophysitis (characterized by pituitary and stalk enlargement) is rare. Panhypopituitarism, anterior hypopituitarism, or DI are possible consequences.
- Autoimmune pancreatitis type 1 (IgG4-related pancreatitis) is characterized by constitutional symptoms, obstructive jaundice, carbohydrate imbalance, and DM.

Diagnosis

- Elevated IgG4 common; however, not diagnostic.
- Histopathological findings (dense lymphoplasmacytic infiltrates; fibrosis with a storiform pattern; obliterative phlebitis and eosinophilic infiltration) of the tissue and organ involved.

Treatment

- Organ-specific replacement; levothyroxine, insulin, and pituitary hormone replacement as required.
- High-dose GC.
- Immunosuppression (rituximab, azathioprine, and mycophenolate) or tamoxifen have been used for refractory cases.

Further reading

Leporati P, et al. (2011). IgG4-related hypophysitis: a new addition to the hypophysitis spectrum. *J Clin Endocrinol Metab* **96**, 1971–80.

Rotondi M, et al. (2019). Diagnosis of endocrine disease: IgG4-related thyroid autoimmune disease. *Eur J Endocrinol* **180**, R175–83.

Rzepecka A, et al. (2019). IgG4 related disease in endocrine practice. *Arch Med Sci* **15**, 55–64.

Shikuma J, et al. (2017). Critical review of IgG4-related hypophysitis. *Pituitary* **20**, 282–91.

Cancer

Endocrine dysfunction is a common consequence of cancer therapy.
- Endocrine effects may manifest during treatment or as a late consequence of treatment.
- Much of the evidence for late consequences of cancer therapy is derived from studies on survivors of childhood cancer.
- The number of adult survivors of childhood cancer and survivors of adult cancer is rising and therefore, awareness is required of the late consequences that may be seen, particularly in adults.
- Detailed documentation of cancer treatment regime is imperative, as it defines potential toxicity, screening, and surveillance.

Chemotherapy

There are several types of anticancer chemotherapeutic agents with variable endocrine effects.

Cytotoxics

- Often given in combination, so difficult to isolate if specific therapy has direct endocrine sequelae.
- Alkylating agents (e.g. cyclophosphamide, busulfan, procarbazine, temozolomide) damage DNA in rapidly dividing cancer cells.
  - Associated with azoospermia in $\male$ and ovarian failure in $\female$.
- Vinca alkaloids, topoisomerase inhibitors, and antimetabolites are less frequently associated with direct or late endocrine effects.

Immunomodulators

Systemic

- GCs in excess cause Cushing's syndrome, including IGT, reduced BMD, and ↑ fracture risk. Monitoring of capillary blood glucose, bone health, and fracture risk assessment should be considered at initiation of therapy. Abrupt withdrawal may precipitate AI.
- Rarely, high-dose GCs may cause osteonecrosis of the jaw.
- Cyclophosphamide is associated with POF.
- Thyroid dysfunction has been reported rarely with tacrolimus and interferon therapy.
- Calcineurin inhibitors (ciclosporin, tacrolimus) may induce β-cell failure, causing DM.

Targeted

Immune checkpoint inhibitors (CPIs) are increasingly being used for a wide variety of cancers. Endocrinopathies occur in up to 25% of patients (see ➔ Immune checkpoint inhibitor endocrinopathy, pp. 744–5).

Hormonal therapy

- SERMs (e.g. tamoxifen) cause menopausal symptoms and reduced bone density in premenopausal women. Premenopause, associated with a 75% higher fracture risk. Post-menopause, there is no ↑ fracture risk.
- Aromatase inhibitors:
  - Older drugs (aminoglutethimide) caused AI by non-specific interference with cytochrome P450.
  - Newer triazoles (anastrozole, letrozole) inhibit aromatase by more specific binding to cytochrome P450; increase bone turnover and induce bone loss at sites rich in trabecular bone, resulting in higher fracture risk (see ➔ Bone density and fractures, p. 742).

- Gonadorelin analogues, used for prostatic cancer and breast cancer, cause an initial increase in LH levels and then suppression, resulting in side effects similar to orchidectomy in men and menopause in women. Bone health assessment must be considered.
- Abiraterone inhibits CYP17A1 and is used in treatment of prostate cancer to reduce androgen levels. Adrenal CYP17A1 inhibition results in hypocortisolaemia and hypokalaemia, and fluid retention and hypertension due to MC effect from excess 11-deoxycortisol. Abiraterone is therefore used alongside prednisolone.
- Antiandrogens (e.g. flutamide, bicalutamide, enzalutamide) used in prostatic cancer may cause gynaecomastia, hot flushes, impotence, and impaired libido.

Radiotherapy

Gray is the unit of absorbed dose of ionizing radiation corresponding to 1J/kg.

Endocrine consequences relate to age at radiotherapy, the dose delivered to endocrine tissue, and the method of delivery (e.g. number of fractions). Advances in radiotherapy techniques such as intensity-modulated radiotherapy (IMRT) and proton beam have allowed more targeted therapy, with less effect to surrounding tissues, potentially reducing the likelihood of endocrine sequelae.

For dose dependence, see Table 12.3.

Cranial radiotherapy

This can result in hypopituitarism if the hypothalamus or pituitary is within the radiation field (see ⊃ Chapter 2).

- Risk of hypopituitarism is influenced by radiation dose, radiation schedule, and age and sex of the patient. Other risk factors, such as concurrent chemotherapy use, may also play a part (see Table 12.3).
- Pituitary irradiation may cause hyperprolactinaemia or hypoprolactinaemia. Hyperprolactinaemia can result from hypothalamic damage and reduced dopaminergic tone. Pituitary irradiation and lactotroph damage may result in hypoprolactinaemia.
- The relationship of radiotherapy dose with pituitary and endocrine sequelae has been less well studied in adults. Severe GH deficiency has been seen with 1° tumour radiation doses of 30Gy. Other anterior pituitary hormone deficiencies were only seen with doses >40Gy.
- Endocrine sequelae commonly occur within 5 years of radiotherapy, but some may occur as late as 11–15 years.
- Long-term follow-up with annual pituitary hormone assessment is important.

Neck irradiation

May result in hypothyroidism, thyroid nodules, thyroid cancer, and hyperparathyroidism.

- The thyroid and parathyroid may be irradiated in those with head and neck tumours and posterior fossa CNS tumours, and in those receiving mediastinal radiotherapy.
- Radiation dose and thyroid volume will determine the likelihood of hypothyroidism.
- Onset of hypothyroidism may be delayed.

- Development of benign and malignant thyroid nodules is dependent on patient age and radiation dose. Minimum latency period is 5–10 years, but they may develop as late as 30 years after exposure. Children are at greatest risk.
- There are insufficient data on the superiority of periodic US vs neck palpation to screen for thyroid nodules or malignancy following radiotherapy.
- Hyperparathyroidism is usually 2° to a parathyroid adenoma and should be investigated and treated as per usual clinical practice (see ➋ Primary hyperparathyroidism, pp. 510–12).

Testicular irradiation

May cause azoospermia and hypogonadism.
- Germ cell function and spermatogenesis are affected more than Leydig cell function and androgen synthesis at very low radiation doses.
- Leydig cell function is usually preserved at up to 20Gy in prepubertal boys and 30Gy in sexually mature men.
- Consider sperm preservation.

Ovarian irradiation

May result in POF or 1° amenorrhoea.
- Effects of radiotherapy on ovarian function are amplified with age.
- Hypogonadism may result from doses >10Gy.
- Consider oocyte preservation.

Table 12.3 Dose dependence of radiation-induced pituitary dysfunction

Hormone dysfunction	Radiation dose (childhood)	Radiation dose (adult)
GH deficiency	≥18Gy	≥30Gy
Central precocious puberty	≥18Gy	N/A
FSH/LH deficiency	≥30Gy	≥40Gy
TSH deficiency	≥30Gy	≥40Gy
ACTH deficiency	≥30Gy	≥40Gy

Endocrine sequelae of survivors of childhood cancer

Short stature

Prevalence of short stature ranges from 9% in studies of childhood acute leukaemia survivors to 40% among survivors of childhood brain tumours.

Several factors may influence this, including GHD, 1° hypothyroidism, and radiation-induced impairment of spinal growth.

GHD may result from direct tumour invasion or as a consequence of cranial surgery or radiotherapy involving the HPA axis.

Presentation of GHD may be delayed 5–10 years after radiotherapy.

Clinical assessment
- Growth velocity.
- Weight and BMI (↑ fat mass, reduced lean body mass).
- Sitting height (radiotherapy can cause vertebral dysplasia).
- Arm span.
- Pubertal assessment for evidence of precocious puberty (may result in falsely reassuring growth spurt).

Investigations

The diagnosis is often difficult to make. GHD is suspected when there is a reduction of growth velocity over 6 months. Diagnosis is made using clinical features and investigations.
- In the presence of three other anterior pituitary hormone deficits, dynamic testing is not required.
- ITT is the gold standard investigation. Diagnostic cut-offs depend on the age group being tested, with a lower threshold for intervention in children and young adults (see Table 12.4).
- Tests, including GHRH (GHRH or GHRH-arginine), may be falsely reassuring if damage is primarily hypothalamic.
- Glucagon stimulation testing has not been thoroughly investigated in this population, so reliability is unknown.
- IGF-1 and IGFBP3 are not reliable markers of GH secretion following radiotherapy or in those with CNS lesions.
- Survivors of childhood cancer diagnosed with isolated GHD in childhood should be retested once they reach adult height (growth velocity <2cm/year).

Table 12.4 Suggested cut-offs for diagnosing GHD on ITT

Childhood	<11ng/mL
Teenage young adult	<7ng/mL
Adult	<3ng/mL + QoL-AGHDA ≥11

Treatment
- Observational longitudinal follow-up data suggest no significant change in the risk of tumour recurrence associated with GH therapy. Previous studies suggested ↑ risk of 2° tumour, but recent studies showed no significant association between GH therapy and the development of a 2nd neoplasm of the CNS.
- GH therapy is usually initiated when the patient has been disease-free for 1 year, as there is significantly reduced risk of tumour relapse at this point.

Thyroid dysfunction
- 1° hypothyroidism can develop up to 25 years after radiotherapy to the head and neck.
- 1° hypothyroidism affects up to 20% of childhood cancer survivors.
- Central hypothyroidism is associated with irradiation to the pituitary/hypothalamus at doses >30Gy in childhood and >40Gy in adults.
- It is important to recognize cases of combined 1° and 2° thyroid dysfunction in patients where both the pituitary and the thyroid are at-risk organs.
- There is an ↑ likelihood of developing thyroid nodules after radiotherapy, some of which may develop into DTC.
- Risk of thyroid cancer increases linearly with increasing radiation doses up to 20Gy but declines at high doses (>40Gy) due to destruction of thyroid tissue at higher doses.

Treatment
- Lifelong follow-up with annual assessment of thyroid function and clinical examination.
- There are insufficient data on the utility of periodic US as a screening tool in this population.
- Current consensus based on expert opinion recommends thyroid palpation every 1–2 years or neck US every 3–5 years, depending on a shared decision between patient and clinician.

Central precocious puberty
(See ➲ Precocious puberty, pp. 592–5.)
- Precocious puberty (<8 years for ♀, <9 years for ♂) is caused by premature activation of the hypothalamic–pituitary–gonadal axis.
- It is associated with hydrocephalus, tumours in or near the hypothalamic region, and low-dose hypothalamo-pituitary irradiation (18–24Gy).
- It is more likely in ♀, those who are overweight, and those treated at a younger age.
- Prevalence estimated at 11.9–15.2% in childhood cancer survivors.

Clinical assessment
- Height and weight on growth charts.
- ↑ growth velocity may be an early sign of precocious puberty. This can be masked by GHD or hypothyroidism.
- Bone age >2 SD of chronological age is consistent with precocious puberty.
- Tanner staging.
- Measure serum gonadotrophins, testosterone, and oestradiol.

Diagnosis
- Clinical diagnosis in ♀ relies largely on observation of breast development.
- In girls with elevated gonadotrophins, measurement of oestradiol levels and assessment of uterine length and shape via US can help distinguish between central precocious puberty and 1° gonadal insufficiency.
- In ♂, testicular volume may be misleading due to use of gonadotoxic treatments causing Sertoli cell and germ cell injury.
- Leydig cell function is less frequently affected. Thus, measurement of testosterone and LH in ♂ may aid diagnosis.

Treatment
- GnRH agonists delay the progression of puberty and may result in better outcomes for adult height (see ➡ Precocious puberty, pp. 592–5).

Hypogonadotrophic hypogonadism
- Less common than GHD and dependent on radiation dose (see Table 12.3).
- Estimated prevalence of 10.8% in childhood cancer survivors.

Clinical findings
- Delayed puberty (absence of puberty >13 years in girls, >14 years in boys).
- Interrupted puberty (failure of progression through Tanner stages).

Treatment
(See ➡ Delayed/absent puberty, pp. 596–8.)

Male gonadal dysfunction
(See also ➡ Male hypogonadism, p. 410.)
- Leydig cells are vulnerable to radiation damage, but relatively tolerant of chemotherapy due to their slow turnover. Children who receive >24Gy for testicular relapse in acute lymphoblastic leukaemia (ALL) have a high risk of developing testosterone deficiency.
- Germ cells are more vulnerable to effects of chemotherapy (e.g. cyclophosphamide, chlorambucil, cisplatin, doxorubicin) and radiotherapy.
- Spermatogenesis is impaired in 40–60% of ♂ survivors of childhood cancer.
- Alkylating agents are associated with the highest risk in terms of chemotherapeutic agents.
- Relatively low doses, such as 0.15Gy, are associated with ♂ subfertility.
- Sperm cryopreservation should be offered for adolescent ♂ prior to cancer treatment.

Further reading
Gebauer J, et al. (2019). Long-term endocrine and metabolic consequences of cancer treatment: a systematic review. *Endocr Rev* **40**, 711–67.

Female gonadal dysfunction

- Ovarian failure can occur either acutely or as a delayed effect following treatment of cancer.
- Delayed puberty or 1° amenorrhoea may occur if ovarian dysfunction predates puberty.
- Ovarian failure during puberty can result in arrested pubertal development, 2° amenorrhoea, and menopausal symptoms.
- Alkylating agents are associated with a high risk of developing ovarian failure.
- Abdominopelvic irradiation increases the risk of ovarian failure. This risk is higher when used in conjunction with alkylating agents.
- Women with ovarian failure are at a higher risk of osteoporosis and CVD if untreated.

Bone density and fractures

- Survivors of childhood cancers are at risk of osteopenia and osteoporosis, and at ↑ risk of fractures.
- During cancer treatment, patients often develop cachexia, nutritional deficiencies, and reduced mobility, all of which can contribute to low BMD and fracture risk.
- Treatment for cancer during childhood or adolescence may prevent or delay attainment of peak bone mass, thus increasing fracture risk in later life. Childhood survivors have smaller-volume bones and therefore, DXA results need to be corrected for volume.
- ↑ fracture risk is dependent on 1° disease and treatment modalities used.
- Use of GCs, chemotherapy, and the presence of hypogonadism or GHD all contribute to fracture risk.
- Focal radiotherapy in children and adults is associated with ↑ fracture risk within the radiation field, typically at doses >40Gy.
- DXA scans should be interpreted with caution, taking into consideration age, pubertal stage, and height.

Obesity and metabolic dysfunction

- Hypothalamic damage can result in hyperphagia and obesity (e.g. craniopharyngiomas, CNS tumours).
- GHD and steroids may contribute to obesity in childhood cancer survivors.
- Insulin resistance is common and T2DM risk is ↑.
- These metabolic factors may contribute to the recent epidemiological finding of raised medium- and long-term risk for CVD and cerebrovascular disease in adult survivors of cancer.

Further reading

Carroll JS, et al. (2017). Deciphering the divergent roles of progestogens in breast cancer. *Nature Rev Cancer* **17**, 54–64.

Chemaitilly W, et al. (2015). Anterior hypopituitarism in adult survivors of childhood cancers treated with cranial radiotherapy: a report from the St Jude Lifetime Cohort study. *J Clin Oncol* **33**, 492–500.

Clement SC, et al. (2018). Balancing the benefits and harms of thyroid cancer surveillance in survivors of childhood, adolescent and young adult cancer: recommendations from the international Late Effects of Childhood Cancer Guideline Harmonization Group in collaboration with the PanCareSurFup Consortium. *Cancer Treat Rev* **63**, 28–39.

Felice FD, et al. (2019). Radiation effects on male fertility. *Andrology* **7**, 2–7.

Gebauer J, et al. (2019). Long-term endocrine and metabolic consequences of cancer treatment: a systematic review. *Endocr Rev* **40**, 711–67.

Howell SJ, Shalet SM (2005). Spermatogenesis after cancer treatment: damage and recovery. *J Natl Cancer Inst Monogr* **2005**, 12–17.

International Guideline Harmonization Group for Late Effects of Childhood Cancer. ℘ http://www.ighg.org/

Kyriakakis N, et al. (2016). Pituitary dysfunction following cranial radiotherapy for adult-onset nonpituitary brain tumours. *Clin Endocrinol (Oxf)* **84**, 372–9.

Sfeir JG, et al. (2018). Diagnosis of GH deficiency as a late effect of radiotherapy in survivors of childhood cancers. *J Clin Endocrinol Metab* **103**, 2785–93.

Sklar CA, et al. (2018). Hypothalamic–pituitary and growth disorders in survivors of childhood cancer: an Endocrine Society clinical practice guideline. *J Clin Endocrinol Metab* **103**, 2761–84.

Strongman H, et al. (2019). Medium and long-term risks of specific cardiovascular diseases in survivors of 20 adult cancers: a population-based cohort study using multiple linked UK electronic health records databases. *Lancet* **394**, 1041–54.

Swerdlow AJ, et al. (2019). Risk of meningioma in European patients treated with growth hormone in childhood: results from the SAGhE Cohort. *J Clin Endocrinol Metab* **104**, 658–64.

Immune checkpoint inhibitor endocrinopathy

- Immune-mediated endocrinopathies as a consequence of treatment with CPIs include thyroiditis, hypophysitis, insulin-dependent diabetes mellitus (IDDM), and adrenalitis (see also Table 12.5).
- The incidence of endocrine dysfunction increases significantly with combination therapies.

Table 12.5 Endocrine effects of immune checkpoint inhibitors

Drug class	Tumour types	Endocrine effects (incidence)
CTLA-4 inhibitors (ipilimumab)	Melanoma	Hypothyroidism (3.8%) Hypophysitis (3.2%) Hyperthyroidism (1.7%)
Combined CTLA-4 and PD-1 inhibitors (e.g. ipilimumab and nivolumab)	Melanoma	Hypothyroidism (13.2%) Hypophysitis (6.4%) Hyperthyroidism (8%)
PD-1 inhibitors (nivolumab, pembrolizumab)	Melanoma, non-small cell lung cancer, RCC, Hodgkin's lymphoma, head and neck squamous cell carcinoma	Hypothyroidism (7.0%) Hyperthyroidism (3.2%) IDDM (0.9%) Hypophysitis (0.4%) Adrenalitis (rare)
PD-L1 (programme death ligand 1) inhibitors (atezolizumab, avelumab, durvalumab)	Non-small cell lung cancer	Hypothyroidism (3.9%) Hyperthyroidism (0.6%) Hypophysitis (0.1%) IDDM (rarely)

Thyroiditis

- The commonest CPI endocrinopathy. Generally presents as asymptomatic thyrotoxicosis, followed by subclinical or overt hypothyroidism. TPO positivity is present in 33–67%.
- TRAb should be checked if Graves' is suspected, but this is uncommon.
- There have also been rare reports of Graves' ophthalmopathy.
- Management of thyroiditis is the same as usual care to thyroiditis management (see ➔ Thyroiditis, p. 76).

Hypophysitis

- Can present with acute hypoadrenalism, headaches, and rarely mass effect, and typically results in permanent hypopituitarism (see ➔ Hypopituitarism, pp. 138–9). Patients are often asymptomatic but may present with life-threatening illness and should be treated as a medical emergency as per adrenal crisis guidelines until diagnostic information is available (see ➔ Box 3.4).

- Unlike other causes of hypopituitarism, CPI-mediated hypophysitis more frequently causes isolated ACTH deficiency.
- SST may be falsely reassuring if performed within 6–12 weeks of an acute episode of hypophysitis.
- Gonadal and thyroid axes can be suppressed in acute illness and should be repeated when clinical condition improves.

Clinical practice points

1. Endocrine dysfunction associated with immune CPIs often asymptomatic, so routine testing is important.
2. If there are life-threatening clinical signs of cortisol deficiency, after measuring a random cortisol and pituitary function (including ACTH), fluid replacement with saline and systemic 100mg hydrocortisone should be given immediately. If cortisol deficiency is confirmed, urgent MRI should be arranged to exclude chiasmal compression.
3. Recovery of ACTH deficiency is very uncommon, but thyroid axis recovery is seen; therefore, repeat testing is important.

Primary adrenal insufficiency

- 1° AI as a result of CPI therapy is rare.
- Patients may present with life-threatening illness and should be treated as a medical emergency as per adrenal crisis guidelines until diagnostic information is available (see ➔ Acute/severe intercurrent illness, p. 147).

Insulin-dependent diabetes

- Rare and predominantly seen with PD-1 inhibitors, but case reports are noted with other CPIs.
- May present as a medical emergency with DKA and should be treated as per usual DKA guidance.

Further reading

Barroso-Sousa R, *et al.* (2018). Incidence of endocrine dysfunction following the use of different immune checkpoint inhibitor regimens: a systematic review and meta-analysis. *JAMA Oncol* **4**, 173–82.

Gridelli C (2016). Thyroid-induced toxicity of check-point inhibitors immunotherapy in the treatment of advanced non-small cell lung cancer. *J Endocrinol Diabetes* **3**, 1–10.

Higham CE, *et al.* (2018). Society for Endocrinology endocrine emergency guidance: Acute management of the endocrine complications of checkpoint inhibitor therapy. *Endocr Connect* **7**, G1–7.

Iyer PC, *et al.* (2018). Immune-related thyroiditis with immune checkpoint inhibitors. *Thyroid* **28**, 1243–51.

Stamatouli AM, *et al.* (2018). Collateral damage: insulin-dependent diabetes induced with checkpoint inhibitors. *Diabetes* **67**, 1471–80.

Wright JJ, *et al.* (2018). Increased reporting of immune checkpoint inhibitor-associated diabetes. *Diabetes Care* **41**, e150–1.

Syndromes of ectopic hormone production

Definition

Secretion of a hormone or other biologically active molecule into the systemic circulation by a neoplasm (benign or malignant) that has arisen from a tissue that does not normally produce that hormone or molecule, resulting in a clinically significant syndrome. See Table 12.6 for common syndromes associated with ectopic hormone production.

Table 12.6 Common syndromes associated with ectopic hormone production

Syndrome	Ectopic hormone	Typical tumour types
Hypercalcaemia of malignancy	PTHrP	Squamous cell lung carcinoma
		Other squamous cell carcinoma (skin, oesophagus, head and neck)
		RCC
		Breast adenocarcinoma
		Adult T-cell lymphoma associated with human T lymphotropic virus type 1 (HTLV-1)
	1,25(OH)2 colecalciferol	Lymphoma
		Sarcoidosis (non-malignant— because of ↑ active vitamin D)
	PTH	Very rare
SIADH	Vasopressin/ADH	Small cell lung carcinoma
		Squamous cell lung carcinoma
		Bronchial carcinoid
		Mesothelioma
		Pancreatic or gut carcinoid
		Adenocarcinoma of the duodenum, pancreas, and prostate
		PCC
		MTC
		Haematopoietic malignancies (lymphoma, leukaemia)
Cushing's syndrome	ACTH (most commonly)	Small cell lung carcinoma
		Thymic carcinoid tumour
		Bronchial carcinoid tumour
		Pancreatic endocrine tumours (including carcinoid tumours)
		Carcinoid tumours of the gut
		PCC
		MTC
		Other lung cancers (adenocarcinoma, squamous cell carcinoma)
	CRH (rarely)	Carcinoid tumour
	Ectopic expression of receptors for GIP; LH	Macronodular adrenal hyperplasia

Syndrome	Ectopic hormone	Typical tumour types
Non-islet cell hypoglycaemia	IGF-2	Mesenchymal tumours Mesothelioma Fibrosarcomas
Oncogenic osteomalacia	FGF23	Sarcomas Haemangiomas Fibromas Prostate adenocarcinoma Osteoblastomas
♂ feminization	hCG	Testicular neoplasms (seminomas, teratomas) Germinomas Choriocarcinomas
Acromegaly	GHRH	Pancreatic islet cell tumours Carcinoid tumours
	GH	Lung, pancreatic islet cell tumours
Hyper-aldosteronism	Renin	Renal (Wilms' tumour, RCC, haemangiopericytoma) Reninoma Lung (small cell lung cancer, adenocarcinoma) Hepatic carcinoma Ovarian carcinoma
Polycythaemia	EPO	Cerebellar haemangioblastoma, uterine fibroids, PCC, ovarian and hepatic cancers

SIADH due to ectopic vasopressin production

Epidemiology

- The commonest tumours associated with SIADH are those with neuroendocrine features, e.g. small cell lung carcinomas and carcinoid tumours.

Pathology

- SIADH may pre-date radiological evidence of malignancy.
- Small cell lung carcinomas have usually metastasized by the time SIADH is present.
- Lung diseases and neurological disorders may cause SIADH due to aberrant hypothalamic vasopressin release, rather than vasopressin release from the tumour per se. In ectopic SIADH, release of vasopressin from the neurohypophysis may be suppressed.
- Worsening hyponatraemia may be an early sign of disease progression.

Diagnostic criteria for SIADH

(See Table 12.7.)

Table 12.7 Diagnostic criteria for SIADH

	Plasma	Urine
Na	↓ (<130mmol/L)	↑ (> 30mmol/L)
Osmolality	↓ (<270mOsm/kg)	↑ (>100mOsm/kg)
Clinical euvolaemia (or mild hypervolaemia)		
Normal renal, adrenal, and thyroid function		

Treatment

- Acute symptomatic hyponatraemia is a medical emergency and should be managed with hypertonic saline, as per current guidance (see ➔ Hyponatraemia, pp. 236–8).
- Patients who have hyponatraemia for >48h are at risk of neurological sequelae with rapid correction.
- Aim for Na rise ≤10mmol/L (≤8mmol/L for severely malnourished and chronic excess alcohol users) in the first 24h and ≤18mmol/L in the first 48h.

Management of underlying tumour

- Surgical, chemo-, or radiotherapeutic treatments to remove or reduce tumour burden are the most effective method to improve hyponatremia.
- If the patient is symptomatic during treatment or oncology treatment is being delayed, the following strategies may be employed.

Fluid restriction
- Rarely successful in patients with SIADH due to ectopic vasopressin production and high urinary osmolality.
- If considered, the degree of fluid restriction necessary depends on the patient's ability to excrete electrolyte-free water—Furst formula (see Table 12.8).

Table 12.8 Furst formula and fluid restriction

Furst formula = (urinary Na + urinary K)/serum Na	
Ratio	Fluid restriction
>1	Unlikely to be effective; consider other treatments
0.5–1	<0.5L
<0.5	<1L

Demeclocycline
- 150–300mg qds may be used to induce nephrogenic DI.
- This may take 5–7 days to have effect.
- Side effects include nausea, skin photosensitivity, and nephrotoxicity.
- Rarely used.

Tolvaptan
- A potent V2 receptor antagonist—7.5–15mg daily.
- Requires monitoring as can lead to rapid rises in Na.
- Hypotonic fluids may occasionally be required in the event of over-rapid correction of serum Na.
- It is commissioned in the UK when patients are delayed in starting chemotherapy due to their hyponatraemia.
- Fluid restriction should always be removed before starting tolvaptan and patients should drink to their thirst.
- LFTs should be checked due to the risk of liver injury with prolonged use.
- Therapy is contraindicated in hypovolaemic hyponatraemia, those without intact thirst mechanisms, anuric patients, and those with concomitant use of strong CYP3a inhibitors.

> **Clinical pearl**
> There is some evidence that oncology patients may be more prone to over-rapid correction of Na with tolvaptan. We recommend a starting dose of 7.5mg tolvaptan in oncology patients, with close monitoring of serum Na.

Further reading

Garrahy A, et al. (2020). Fluid restriction therapy for chronic SIAD; results of a prospective randomized controlled trial. *J Clin Endocrinol Metab* **105**, E4360–9.

Spasovski G, et al. (2014). Clinical practice guideline on diagnosis and treatment of hyponatraemia. *Eur J Endocrinol* **170**, G1–47.

Specialised Commissioning Team (2016). *Tolvaptan for hyponatraemia secondary to the syndrome of inappropriate antidiuretic hormone (SIADH) in patients requiring cancer chemotherapy.* NHS England: 16051/P. ✆ https://www.england.nhs.uk/wp-content/uploads/2016/12/clin-comm-pol-16051P.pdf

Humeral hypercalcaemia of malignancy

Incidence and epidemiology

Hypercalcaemia of malignancy occurs in ~20% of all cancer patients during their clinical course.

Pathophysiology

Hypercalcaemia may be due to the effect of:
- Ectopic hormone secretion (PTHrP, rarely 1,25(OH)$_2$D, rarely PTH).
- Cytokine mediators that activate osteoclastic bone resorption (RANK ligand (RANKL), IL-6 by myeloma cells).
- Bone destruction from metastases.

Table 12.9 Tumours associated with humeral hypercalcaemia

Type	Frequency (%)	Bone metastases	Causal agent	Tumour type
Humoral	80	Minimal	PTHrP	Squamous cell carcinoma, renal, ovarian, endometrial, breast, HTLV-1, lymphoma
Local osteolysis	20	Common Extensive	Cytokines Chemokines PTHrP	Breast, myeloma, lymphoma
1,25(OH)$_2$D	<1	Variable	1,25(OH)$_2$D	Lymphoma
Ectopic PTH	<1	Variable	PTH	Variable

Parathyroid hormone-related peptide

- PTHrP is similar to PTH in the first 13 amino acid sequences and binds to the PTH/PTHrP receptor subtype, causing osteoclast-mediated bone resorption and reduced renal excretion of Ca.
- Investigations show ↑ Ca, ↓ PO$_4$, and ↓ PTH.
- PTHrP secreted by metastatic cells in bone also causes local osteolysis.
- Tumours that metastasize to bone are more prone to produce PTHrP.
- For tumours associated with humeral hypercalcaemia, see Table 12.9.

Management

- As per normal management of hypercalcaemia (see ➡ Other causes of hypercalcaemia, p. 520).
- *Bisphosphonates* are the mainstay of therapy:
  - As well as controlling osteoclastic bone destruction, they may have antitumour effects.
  - In women with early breast cancer, bisphosphonates have been shown to reduce the rate of bone metastases.
  - Zoledronic acid 4mg IV is the bisphosphonate of choice.
  - Side effects include: fever, arthralgia, and rarely osteonecrosis of the jaw or atypical fracture.

- Bisphosphonates are renally excreted, limiting their use in those with renal disease.
- Serum Ca nadir is typically reached after 2–4 days.
- *Denosumab* is a human monoclonal antibody that binds to RANKL and prevents binding to RANK on osteoclast precursors and mature osteoclasts:
  - Inhibition of activation and function of osteoclasts results in reduced bone resorption.
  - It effectively lowers serum Ca levels and has been shown to reduce the incidence of skeletal-related events (pathological fracture, radiation to bone, spinal cord compression, or surgery to bone).
  - It is cleared through the reticuloendothelial system and thus considered safe in those with renal disease (Ca levels must be carefully monitored).
  - Vitamin D status should be checked prior to administration, and adequate Ca intake ensured.
  - Side effects include refractory hypocalcaemia and osteonecrosis of the jaw.
- *GCs* (prednisolone 40mg) are particularly effective in hypercalcaemia mediated by 1,25(OH)2 colecalciferol.
- If the patient is severely symptomatic and not responding to fluids, *calcitonin* can be used (prolonged use leads to tachyphylaxis), or *haemodialysis* can be considered.

Further reading

British National Formulary. *Zoledronic acid.* ℘ https://bnf.nice.org.uk/drug/zoledronic-acid.html#indicationsAndDoses

Faris Shalayel MH, *et al.* (2017). Bisphosphonates: from bone anti-resorptive to anti-cancer drugs. *J Med Oncol Ther* **2**, 20–3. ℘ https://www.alliedacademies.org/articles/bisphosphonates-from-bone-antiresorptive-to-anticancer-drugs-7372.html

Major P, *et al.* (2001). Zoledronic acid is superior to pamidronate in the treatment of hypercalcemia of malignancy: a pooled analysis of two randomized, controlled clinical trials. *J Clin Oncol* **19**, 558–67.

Modi ND, Lentzsch S (2012). Bisphosphonates as antimyeloma drugs. *Leukemia* **26**, 589–94.

O'Carrigan B, *et al.* (2017). Bisphosphonates and other bone agents for breast cancer. *Cochrane Database Syst Rev* **10**, CD003474. ℘ https://www.ncbi.nlm.nih.gov/pmc/articles/PMC6485886/

Stewart AF (2005). Hypercalcemia associated with cancer. *N Engl J Med* **352**, 373–9.

Vakiti A, Mewawalla P (2020). *Malignancy-related hypercalcemia.* StatPearls Publishing, Treasure Island, FL. ℘ http://www.ncbi.nlm.nih.gov/books/NBK482423/

Walsh J, *et al.* (2016). Society for Endocrinology endocrine emergency guidance: Emergency management of acute hypercalcaemia in adult patients. *Endocr Connect* **5**, G9–11.

Cushing's syndrome due to ectopic ACTH secretion

- Ectopic ACTH secretion is responsible for 10–20% of all endogenous Cushing's syndrome.
- The commonest tumour types are those with neuroendocrine features.
- Ectopic CRH production has been described but is rare.
- Small cell lung cancer and carcinoid tumours are the commonest causes of ectopic ACTH.

(For other causes, see Table 12.10.)

Clinical features

- Despite extremely high cortisol levels, patients often do not manifest central weight gain due to the underlying malignant process and associated cachexia.
- Hypertension, hypokalaemia, and metabolic alkalosis are common features (overwhelming of the enzyme 11β-hydroxysteroid dehydrogenase, resulting in exposure of the MC receptor to high circulating GCs).
- Glucose intolerance, susceptibility to infection, thin skin, proximal myopathy, poor wound healing, and steroid-associated mood disturbance are all common features.
- Patients may be pigmented due to melanocyte-stimulating hormone (MSH) arising from high POMC levels.

Investigations

(See Table 12.10; see also ➔ Chapter 2.)

Table 12.10 Investigations for Cushing's syndrome

Investigation	Result
ACTH	Typically higher in ectopic ACTH disease. Partially processed forms commoner
Cortisol	Higher in ectopic ACTH disease
Hypokalaemia (<3.2)	Commoner in ectopic ACTH
CRH test	Absent response in ectopic disease, exaggerated in pituitary disease
IPSS ± CRH	Non-significant central:peripheral gradient

Management

- Treatment of the underlying tumour is the best treatment
- Medical management (see Table 2.9).
- Bilateral adrenalectomy with GC and MC replacement may be necessary.

Macronodular adrenal hyperplasia causing Cushing's syndrome

- Mostly sporadic, but a few familial cases reported (*ARMC5* mutation) (see ➲ Bilateral adrenal hyperplasia, p. 276).
- Ectopic receptors for GIP, LH, vasopressin, serotonin (5-HT), and β-adrenergic agonists have been reported in adrenal tissue.
- Most commonly due to synthesis of ectopic GIP receptors in adrenal tissues.
- GIP secretion associated with meals results in activation of adrenal glands and food-related hypercortisolaemia.

Carcinoid tumours and ectopic hormone production

(See ➲ Syndromes of ectopic hormone production, p. 746.)

Further reading

Bourdeau I, et al. (2004). Gene array analysis of macronodular adrenal hyperplasia confirms clinical heterogeneity and identifies several candidate genes as molecular mediators. *Oncogene* **23**, 1575–85.

Isidori AM, et al. (2006). The ectopic adrenocorticotropin syndrome: clinical features, diagnosis, management, and long-term follow-up. *J Clin Endocrinol Metab* **91**, 371–7.

Isidori AM, et al. (2015). Conventional and nuclear medicine imaging in ectopic Cushing's syndrome: a systematic review. *J Clin Endocrinol Metab* **100**, 3231–44.

Endocrine dysfunction and HIV/AIDS

Adrenal

Subclinical changes can be detected, including elevated basal cortisol concentrations and lower DHEA concentrations.

Adrenal insufficiency

Uncommon (<4% of patients with AIDS). In patients with clinical signs suggestive of hypoadrenalism (hyponatraemia and hypovolaemia), 30% incidence of inadequate response to Synacthen®.

Causes

- Infection. Histologically common. Adrenal function usually maintained (10% of residual adrenal tissue is adequate for normal function).
- CMV (adrenalitis found postmortem in 40–90% of patients with advanced disease).
- *Mycobacterium avium intracellulare* (MAI) complex, TB.
- *Cryptococcus*.
- Neoplasm: lymphoma, Kaposi's sarcoma.
- Haemorrhage.
- Drug-induced:
  - Rifampicin and PIs (e.g. ritonavir) induce ↑ hepatic metabolism of corticosteroids. In subjects with already compromised adrenal reserve, this may precipitate an Addisonian crisis.
  - Ketoconazole inhibits cortisol synthesis.
  - Megestrol acetate possesses GC activity and may cause 2° AI. Abrupt cessation after long-term treatment may precipitate an adrenal crisis.

Secondary adrenal insufficiency

- Drugs (megestrol acetate).
- Hypopituitarism 2° to toxoplasmosis, *Cryptococcus*, and CMV.
- Idiopathic anterior pituitary necrosis.
- Mild hypercortisolaemia common in all stages of HIV infection, without clinical manifestation of Cushing's syndrome.

Possible causes

- Chronic stress.
- Proinflammatory cytokines.
- Binding protein dysfunction.
- GC resistance.
- Concomitant use of ritonavir and inhaled fluticasone.

Gonads

Males

- SHBG concentrations are often elevated; this can lead to normal total testosterone concentrations, but low free testosterone concentrations.
- Testosterone deficiency common in ♂ patients with AIDS (6% of patients with asymptomatic HIV infection, compared with 50% of patients with AIDS).
- Hypogonadism is associated with wasting, ↓ muscle mass, fatigue, loss of libido, and impotence. Hypogonadism may be 1° or 2°; up to 75% of patients with hypogonadism have low or inappropriately normal gonadotrophins. Testosterone replacement will maintain body weight and lean body weight.

Causes

Primary hypogonadism

- *Testicular destruction/infiltration.* Due to infection (CMV most commonly, MAI, toxoplasmosis, TB) or neoplasm (lymphoma, Kaposi's sarcoma, germ cell tumours).
- *Drug-induced.* Ketoconazole (inhibits steroidogenesis, causing lowered testosterone levels), megestrol acetate, other GCs.

Secondary hypogonadism

- Due to malnutrition, severe acute illness, destructive disorders of the pituitary/hypothalamus (CMV, toxoplasmosis, lymphoma); medications such as megestrol acetate (GC-like action causes HH).

Females

- Hypogonadism in ♀, as evidenced by oligo-/amenorrhoea; less common than in ♂ unless advanced disease. Fertility rates not affected until advanced disease.
- Hypoandrogenism (testosterone, DHEA) common in ♀ with wasting syndrome.

Electrolyte disturbance due to endocrine perturbation in HIV/AIDS

Hyponatraemia

- Very common in advanced disease. Due to SIADH in 50%; AI also a common cause.

Calcium disorders

- Hypocalcaemia. Common (18% of patients with AIDS). Main cause is vitamin D deficiency. Other causes include: severe illness; hypomagnesaemia; altered PTH secretion/metabolism; malabsorption of Ca and vitamin D due to GI tract opportunistic infection; medications (foscarnet—complexes with Ca; pentamidine—induces renal Mg wasting and 2° PTH deficiency).
- Hypercalcaemia. Rare. May relate to lymphoma or granulomatous disease.

Osteoporosis

- Osteoporosis ↑ in HIV, which stabilizes on HAART.

Thyroid

- Overt thyroid dysfunction is uncommon. Commonest thyroid dysfunction is sick euthyroid syndrome (NTI). ↑ TBG often observed (significance unknown). Graves' disease has been reported after initiation of HAART in the later phase of immune reconstitution.
- Subclinical hypothyroidism may occur during HAART.
- Infections.
- Rare; usually postmortem diagnoses. Thyroid function usually euthyroid or sick euthyroid.
- *Pneumocystis carinii (*may also cause thyroiditis).
- Mycobacteria.
- *Cryptococcus neoformans.*
- Aspergillosis.

- Neoplasm. Rare. Usually euthyroid or sick euthyroid; may be hypothyroid due to infiltrative destruction.
- Kaposi's sarcoma.
- Lymphoma.

Pituitary

- Anterior hypopituitarism. Very rare.
- Posterior pituitary dysfunction, causing DI. Common.
- Infection. Toxoplasmosis, TB.
- Neoplasm. Cerebral lymphoma.

Wasting syndrome

Definition

- The involuntary loss of >10% of baseline body weight, in combination with diarrhoea, weakness, or fever. Wasting is an AIDS-defining condition.

Causes

- Unknown but, in part, reflects ↓ calorie intake due to anorexia associated with 2° infection and malabsoprtion 2° to small intestinal infections (usually protozoal) and to partial villus atrophy and crypt hyperplasia. Underlying ↑ resting energy expenditure associated with HIV infection per se. Hypogonadism common in ♂ with wasting syndrome.

Treatment

- HAART. Associated with overall weight gain, though lean body mass may remain unchanged.
- Nutritionally based strategies. Adequate caloric intake to meet metabolic demands. Efficacy limited, as refeeding generally increases fat body mass, with little/less effect on lean body mass.
- Appetite stimulants. Megestrol acetate increases caloric intake and weight, compared to placebo, though most weight gain due to ↑ fat mass. Dronabinol stimulates appetite, but weight gain is minimal.
- Exercise. Although exercise can increase total and lean body mass in patients with AIDS, its role in patients with wasting syndrome is not known.
- Androgen therapy. In hypogonadal ♂ patients with wasting syndrome, testosterone increases overall weight and, in particular, lean body mass. Both IM and transdermal testosterone effective. Testosterone therapy not indicated in eugonadal ♂ with wasting.
- GH therapy. Patients with wasting syndrome generally have GH resistance, as suggested by high serum GH and low IGF-1 levels. The most likely cause for this is undernutrition. High-dose GH has shown improvements in lean body mass and protein balance in patients with acquired GH deficiency or severe catabolic states. Side effects (peripheral oedema, arthralgias, myalgias) common due to high doses required. GH may improve fat redistribution that occurs with refeeding.
- Cytokine modulators. Although many inflammatory cytokines are ↑ during acute illness and sepsis, their specific role in wasting syndrome is not known. Thalidomide, a potent inhibitor of TNF, can increase body weight and reduce protein catabolism, but it has a very high rate of serious side effects and is contraindicated in ♀ of childbearing age due to phocomelia (limb malformation).

Lipodystrophy

- Loss of SC fat, particularly in the face, peripheries, and buttocks—in some cases, with concomitant SC fat deposition, particularly in the abdominal area, neck, dorsocervical area ('buffalo hump'). Visceral fat deposition also occurs.
- Associated dyslipidaemia with hypertriglyceridaemia, low HDL-C, insulin resistance, glucose intolerance, and (less commonly) frank DM. ↑ cardiovascular mortality from MI.
- 25% of patients with HIV who are on treatment have metabolic syndrome.
- Associated with HIV-1 PIs, used as part of HAART; 40% of patients treated with PIs will develop lipodystrophy by 1 year. HIV PI-naive patients have similar body composition and fat distribution to non-HIV-infected men. Indinavir may be less potent in inducing lipodystrophy than ritonavir and saquinavir.
- Abnormal body composition and hypertriglyceridaemia may be part of the refeeding phenomenon consequent upon improved well-being and loss of anorexia per se.
- Nucleoside reverse transcriptase inhibitors may be associated with fat loss and accumulation also, but this may be a separate phenomenon to that seen with PIs.

Management

- Observation in mild cases.
- Very low-fat diets and exercise (particularly resistance exercise).
- Withdrawal or switching of PIs in some circumstances may be warranted.
- Anabolic agents (testosterone, GH) not effective.
- Liposuction from areas of fat accumulation; fat pad insertions for areas of lipoatrophy also used. Semi-permanent fillers for facial lipoatrophy.
- Standard lipid-lowering agents for hypertriglyceridaemia (e.g. gemfibrozil).
- HMG CoA (3-hydroxy-3-methylglutaryl coenzyme A) reductase inhibitors metabolized by P4503A4 (which is inhibited by PIs), so the risk of myopathy may be ↑.
- Role for thiazolidinediones unclear.

Opiates and their endocrine effects

- Opiates use (and abuse) has ↑ significantly since early 2000 and endocrine effects vary, depending on the the dose and length of treatment.
- Opiates act via different receptors (mainly μ, δ, κ), which are also expressed on endocrine glands.
- The most commonly seen endocrine disruption is hypogonadism, particularly in ♂, but amenorrhoea occurs in 50% of ♀. However, other systems can be disrupted (see Table 12.11) and frank AI has been reported (although the incidence of endocrine dysfunction not firmly established).
- Opiates cause osteoporosis by inhibiting osteoblasts and by opiate-induced hypogonadism.
- Intrathecal opiates may cause hypogonadism.
- Testosterone or oestradiol therapy can be void.

Table 12.11 Outline of the effects of acute and chronic opiates on the human endocrine system

Hormone	Acute	Chronic
GH	↑	?
PRL	↑	↑
TSH	↑	?/=
ACTH	↓	↓/=
LH	↓↓	↓↓
FSH	=	=
Oestradiol	↓↓	↓
Testosterone	↓↓	↓↓
AVP	↑/↓	↑/↓
Oxytocin	↓	↓/=

↑, stimulation; ↓, inhibition; ↑/↓, conflicting; =, no change; ?, not studied.

Source: data from Vuong C et al (2010) "The effects of opioids and opioid analogs on animal and human endocrine systems" *Endocr. Rev.* 31(1):98–132.

Further reading

Elliott JA, et al. (2012). Non-analgesic opioids: opioids and the endocrine system. *Curr Pharm Des* **12**, 6070–8.

Katz N, Mazer NA (2009). The impact of opioids on the endocrine system. *Clin J Pain* **25**, 170–5.

Merza Z (2010). Opioids and the endocrine system. *Horm Metab Res* **42**, 621–6.

Vuong C, et al. (2010). The effects of opioids and opioid analogs on animal and human endocrine systems. *Endocr Rev* **31**, 98–132.

Liver disease and endocrinology

Sex hormones—males

(See Table 12.12.)

- Hypogonadism occurs in 70–80% of ♂ with chronic liver disease. There is a combination of 1° testicular failure and failure of hypothalamo–pituitary regulation.
- Alcohol acts independently to produce hypogonadism. There is a combination of 1° testicular failure and failure of hypothalamo–pituitary regulation.
- The effects of elevated oestrogens result in ↑ loss of the ♂ escutcheon, loss of body hair, redistribution of body fat, palmar erythema, spider naevi, and gynaecomastia.
- The ↑ conversion of testosterone and androstenedione to oestrone is attributed, at least in part, to portosystemic shunting. In addition, the large increase in SHBG concentration will increase the oestrogen:testosterone ratio, as testosterone has a higher affinity for SHBG.
- Spironolactone may result in iatrogenic feminization by inhibiting testosterone action.
- There is no evidence that exogenous administration of androgens reverses hypogonadism in chronic liver disease.

Sex hormones—females

(See Table 12.13.)

- Alcoholism increases the frequency of menstrual disturbances and spontaneous abortion but does not affect fertility.
- Liver dysfunction of whatever aetiology is associated with early menopause.
- Alcohol, rather than liver disease, is the prime cause of hypogonadism. Non-alcoholic liver disease is only associated with hypogonadism in advanced liver failure when it is accompanied by encephalopathy and impaired GnRH secretion.
- Plasma testosterone and oestrone concentrations are usually normal; androstenedione concentration is ↑, and DHEA and DHEAS levels are reduced.

Thyroid

- The liver synthesizes albumin, T_4-binding prealbumin (TBPA), and TBG, all of which bind thyroid hormones covalently and reversibly.
- TFTs must be interpreted with caution in patients with liver disease. In acute liver disease, e.g. acute viral hepatitis, TBG levels are↑, which increases the measured total circulating T_4 and T_3 levels. In biliary cirrhosis and chronic active hepatitis, TBG may be ↑. In other chronic liver disease and in hepatomas, TBG is also ↑. In severe cases of acute liver disease, TBG may be low due to reduced synthesis. The liver deiodinates T_4 to T_3, and this is impaired in liver disease. T_4 is preferentially converted to rT_3, and there is an increase in the $rT_3:T_3$ ratio.
- In liver cirrhosis, TBG, T_4, and T_3 are low.
- Table 12.5 summarizes the changes in TFTs with liver disease. Free T_4 and T_3 assays are essential for accurate interpretation of thyroid status in liver disease.

Table 12.12 Sex hormone changes in liver disease

Hormone	Level
Testosterone	↓↓
SHBG	↑
Oestrone	↑
Oestradiol	↑/normal
LH	Inappropriately low/normal
FSH	Inappropriately low/normal
PRL	↑/normal
IGF-1	↓
IGFBP3	↓

Table 12.13 Thyroid function changes in liver disease

Hormone	Acute hepatitis	CAH/PBC	Cirrhosis
T_4	↑	↑	↓
FT_4	↑↑	↑	↑
T_3	↓	↑	↓
FT_3	↓	↓	↓
rT_3	↑	↑	↑↑
TSH	↑	↑	↑↑
TBG	↑	↑	↓

CAH, chronic active hepatitis; PBC, primary biliary cirrhosis.

Adrenal hormones

- Patients who abuse alcohol may develop a clinical phenotype of Cushing's syndrome, with moon facies, centripetal obesity, striae, and muscle wasting, and may have ↑ plasma cortisol concentrations. This is termed pseudo-Cushing's syndrome.
- Reversible (on abstention) adrenocorticoid hyperresponsiveness occurs in alcoholics. In liver disease, cortisol metabolism may be impaired, leading to elevated plasma cortisol levels, loss of diurnal cortisol variation, and failure to suppress with dexamethasone.

Further reading

Malik R, Hodgson H (2002). The relationship between the thyroid gland and the liver. *QJM* **95**, 559–69.

Renal disease and endocrinology

Calcitriol

There is impaired renal conversion of 25-hydroxyvitamin D_3 to $1,25(OH)_2D_3$ in end-stage renal failure (ESRF), leading to metabolic bone disease (see Table 6.6).

Parathyroid hormone and renal osteodystrophy

Serum PTH secretion is stimulated by low serum Ca in ESRF. This is due to:

- $\downarrow\downarrow$ renal PO_4 clearance (resulting in $\uparrow$ Ca/PO_4 mineral ion product, precipitation of vascular calcification, with consequent hypocalcaemia triggering PTH release). Vascular calcification is a major contributor to vascular death in ESRF. High PO_4 per se may increase PTH secretion directly, but evidence of the mechanism for this is lacking.

Impaired renal calcitriol secretion

- As renal function declines, elevated PTH and $\downarrow$ calcitriol can be detected, with Cr clearance of 50mL/min. This rise in PTH is initially sufficient to maintain serum Ca in the normal range.
- In ESRF, patients are markedly hyperphosphataemic and hypocalcaemic. The degree of hyperparathyroidism progresses inversely with the fall in renal function. Tertiary hyperparathyroidism occurs when PTH secretion becomes autonomous, and hypercalcaemia will persist even after renal transplantation.
- Hyperparathyroid bone disease and osteomalacia are the main mechanisms behind the development of high turnover bone disease in renal osteodystrophy. Hypogonadism is also common in both ♂ and ♀ with ESRF. Adynamic bone disease also contributes, probably due to direct toxic effects from urea and other nitrogenous compounds upon bone cells. Renal osteodystrophy causes bone pain and fractures.

Treatment of renal osteodystrophy

- Maintenance of normal PO_4 levels with PO_4 binders (such as calcium carbonate) and treatment of osteomalacia. The $\uparrow$ use of calcium carbonate has been suggested as the cause of the $\uparrow$ incidence of adynamic renal osteodystrophy, but intensive vitamin D therapy and peritoneal dialysis are probably also contributory.
- Alfacalcidol or calcitriol (which do not require renal 1α-hydroxylation) are effective in treating osteomalacia.
- Calcitriol at a dose of 1–2 micrograms/day is used for established renal osteodystrophy. Lower doses of calcitriol (0.25–0.5 micrograms/day) are used in early ESRF to prevent the development of renal osteodystrophy.
- Parathyroidectomy is advocated in bone disease uncontrolled by vitamin D therapy or the development of tertiary hyperparathyroidism.
- Calcimemetics, e.g. cinacalcet, acts directly at the CASR to lower PTH secretion. This markedly improves 2° hyperparathyroidism, Ca and PO_4 levels, and renal osteodystrophy, and is the 1st-line treatment option when parathyroidectomy is high risk or PTH is especially high. Improvement in mortality due to $\downarrow$ vascular calcification has not yet been demonstrated.

Prolactin

Hyperprolactinaemia is common in ESRF but is usually mild, i.e. <1000mU/L. The cause is both ↑ secretion and ↓ renal clearance.

Gonadal function

- Hypogonadism—clinical and biochemical—is common in ESRF.
- In ♂, there is impaired pulsatile release of LH, although basal LH levels are usually elevated due to impaired renal clearance. Serum FSH is usually normal or mildly elevated.
- In ♀, levels of oestradiol, progesterone, and FSH are reported to be within the normal range in the early follicular phase but fail to show the usual cyclical changes. Menstrual disturbance is common. Amenorrhoea, polymenorrhoea, and menorrhagia can also occur on dialysis. Infertility is the rule and conception on dialysis is the exception.
- Sexual dysfunction is common in both sexes but has been better studied in ♂; 60% of ♂ have some degree of impotence, and examination yields 80% to have testicular atrophy and 14% to have gynaecomastia.
- Treatment of hypogonadism in ESRF is suboptimal. Testosterone therapy is not associated with any clinical benefit in ♂.

Growth hormone and growth retardation

- Basal GH levels are normal, but there is impaired secretion following an adequate hypoglycaemic stimulus in 40–70% of patients with ESRF.
- There is impaired growth in children, particularly during periods of greatest growth velocity, and puberty is delayed. This combination leads to short stature. The improved growth velocity after renal transplantation is often too little too late in order to attain a normal stature.
- Recombinant human GH (rhGH) has been shown to be an effective treatment for growth retardation in children with stable CRF and ESRF, as well as after renal transplantation.

Thyroid

The 'sick euthyroid' finding is common in CRF (see ➜ Sick euthyroid syndrome, pp. 878–80).

Adrenal

- The adrenal axis is not impaired clinically by CRF.
- There is evidence of blunted cortisol response to hypoglycaemia, but this is not relevant clinically.
- Urine cortisol is inaccurate in assessing cortisol excess in renal failure.
- Patients with amyloidosis are at risk of hypoadrenalism due to adrenal amyloid infiltration.

Endocrinology in the critically ill

(See Table 12.14.)

ACTH and cortisol

CRH, ACTH, and cortisol increase rapidly during all forms of acute illness.
Low albumin and CBG cause free cortisol to be substantially higher.
This physiological adaptation results in:

- Provision of substrates for major organ energy expenditure (via catabolism).
- Haemodynamic advantages (enhanced sensitivity to angiotensin II, ↑ vasopressor and inotropic response to catecholamines).
- Prevention of an excessive immune response.

Inflammatory cytokines result in ↑ cortisol metabolism and reduced receptors, i.e. peripheral cortisol resistance.

After moderate to severe injuries, plasma cortisol starts to fall after a day or two but only reach normal levels after a week.

Cortisol is elevated for at least 2 weeks in patients with severe burns.

Prolonged critical illness results in low CRH and ACTH, with 'normal' or slightly raised cortisol, perhaps driven by an alternative pathway involving endothelin.

Cortisol deficiency should be suspected in an acutely ill patient with a plasma cortisol of <690nmol/L or an increment of <250nmol/L on a 250-microgram SST (some assay-dependent variation in limits).

Drugs used in intensive care may contribute to AI by:

- Reducing cortisol metabolism, e.g. etomidate (frequently used in induction of anaesthesia) and ketoconazole.
- Promoting cortisol metabolism, e.g. phenytoin, carbamazepine, and rifampicin.

Metabolism

- Hyperglycaemia is common in critical illness (even in non-diabetic subjects) due to ↑ cortisol, catecholamines, GH, and glucagon.
- These hormones and inflammatory cytokines also contribute to insulin resistance.
- IV insulin, titrated to maintain normoglycaemia (glucose <10mmol/l) and to avoid hypoglycaemia.

TSH and thyroid hormones

- TSH levels usually remain stable in acute injury. Total T_4 and T_3 tend to fall but may remain within the normal range.
- Enhanced thyroid hormone metabolism by ↑ activity of liver deiodinase type 3 (peripheral hormone deactivator).
- With prolonged illness, total T_4 tends to fall below the normal range. FT_4 remains in the normal range.
- Total and free T_3 levels fall after injury and may remain suppressed for 2–3 weeks after a severe injury. The rT_3 level rises.
- In prolonged critical illness, the thyroid function conforms to 'sick euthyroid syndrome' (see ➔ Sick euthyroid syndrome, pp. 878–80).

Gonadotrophins and gonadal steroids

In prolonged illness, HH occurs.

Table 12.14 Endocrine and other changes seen in the ill

Acute illness	
ACTH/CRH	↑↑↑
Albumin/CBG	↓
Free cortisol	↑↑
Catabolism	↑↑
Immune response	↓
Inflammatory response	↑↑
Cortisol resistance	↑
Glucose	↑
Insulin resistance	↑↑
TSH	↑
FT_4 and FT_3	↑ ↓
IGF-1, IGFBPs, GH-binding proteins	↓
Prolonged critical illness	
ACTH/CRH	↓↓
Free cortisol	↑
TSH, total T_4	↓
rT_3	↑
LH/FSH/testosterone/oestradiol	↓
GH	↓
Response to GHRH	↓

Growth hormone

- In critical illness, the GH axis is profoundly affected, with initially raised GH secretion, but low IGF-1, IGFBPs, and GH-binding proteins related to peripheral GH resistance.
- Prolonged critical illness of >5–7 days results in low GH and a blunted response to GHRH.
- Recombinant GH was proposed as a beneficial agent for critical illness; however, evidence is lacking and there are reports of a detrimental effect.

Hormone replacement and critical illness

There is no evidence that, other than insulin, hormonal supplementation in the critically ill improves outcome. However, high-dose hydrocortisone is recommended for >3 days in septic shock that is not responsive to fluid and vasopressors, and IV methylprednisolone considered in moderate to severe respiratory distress syndrome, as well as replacement in those found deficient.

Further reading

Annane D, et al. (2017). Guidelines for the diagnosis and management of critical illness-related corticosteroid insufficiency in critically ill patients: Society of Critical Care Medicine and European Society of Intensive Care Medicine. *Intensive Care Med* **43**, 1751–63.

Elleger B, et al. (2005). Endocrine interventions in the ICU. *Eur J Intern Med* **16**, 71–82.

Isidori AM, et al. (2006). The ectopic adrenocorticotropin syndrome: clinical features, diagnosis, management, and long-term follow-up. *J Clin Endocrinol Metab* **91**, 371–7.

Silva-Perez LJ, et al. (2017). Management of critically ill patients with diabetes. *World J Diabetes* **8**, 86–9.

Téblick A, et al. (2019). Anterior pituitary function in critical illness. **8**, R131–43.

Syndromes of hormone resistance

Definition

Reduced responsiveness of target organs to a particular hormone, usually 2° to a disorder of the receptor or distal signalling pathways. This leads to alterations in feedback loops and elevated circulating hormone levels.

Thyroid hormone resistance

(See ⊃ Resistance to thyroid hormones, pp. 58–9.)

Androgen resistance

(See ⊃ Androgen receptor insensitivity syndrome, p. 602.)

Glucocorticoid resistance

- AD and AR forms have been described.
- The resistance can be generalized or tissue-specific, partial or complete, and transient or permanent.
- Several mutations of the human GC receptor gene have been described.
- Diminished sensitivity to GC leads to reduced glucocorticoid feedback on CRH and ACTH, leading to ↑ CRH, ACTH, and cortisol concentrations.
- The clinical features are not due to excess GC, as there is reduced peripheral tissue sensitivity. However, elevated ACTH leads to ↑ secretion of MC (e.g. deoxycorticosterone) and androgens (DHEA and DHEAS). This may lead to hypertension and hypokalaemic alkalosis, hirsutism, acne, oligomenorrhoea in ♀, and sexual precocity in ♂.
- GC resistance may be differentiated from Cushing's syndrome as, despite evidence of ↑ urinary cortisol, abnormal suppression with dexamethasone, and ↑ responsiveness to CRH, the diurnal rhythm of cortisol secretion persists, there are no clinical features of Cushing's syndrome, BMD is normal or ↑, and there is a normal response to insulin-induced hypoglycaemia.
- Low-dose dexamethasone treatment (1–3mg/day) may efficiently suppress ACTH and androgen production.

ACTH resistance

- Rare AR disorders where the adrenal cortex fails to respond to ACTH in the presence of an otherwise normal gland (MC secretion is preserved under angiotensin II control). Very rarely can be due to autoantibodies blocking the ACTH receptor.
- The presenting clinical features include hypoglycaemia, which is often neonatal, neonatal jaundice, ↑ skin pigmentation, and frequent infections.
- Occasionally, ACTH resistance is a component of the triple A syndrome of alacrima (absence of tears), achalasia of the cardia, and ACTH resistance plus neurological disorders.

Biochemical features

- Undetectable or low 9 a.m. cortisol, with grossly elevated ACTH (often >1000ng/mL) and normal renin, aldosterone, and electrolytes, and impaired response to SST.

Treatment
- Steroid replacement.

Mineralocorticoid resistance

(See ➲ Mineralocorticoid deficiency, p. 287.)

Also known as type 1 pseudohypoaldosteronism, this is a rare inherited disorder which usually presents in children with vomiting and anorexia soon after birth, failure to thrive, salt loss, and dehydration. Both AD and AR forms have been described.

Biochemical features
- ↓ serum Na.
- ↑ serum K (hyperkalaemic acidosis).
- ↑↑ urinary Na (despite hyponatraemia).
- ↑ plasma and urinary aldosterone.
- ↑ plasma renin activity.

Diagnosis
- Requires proof of unresponsiveness to MCs (no effect of fludrocortisone on urinary Na).

Treatment

Na supplementation and carbenoxolone have been used successfully. With time, treatment can often be weaned, and salt wasting is unusual following childhood.

Further reading

Charmandari E, *et al*. (2008). Generalized glucocorticoid resistance: clinical aspects, molecular mechanisms, and implications of a rare genetic disorder. *J Clin Endocrinol Metab* **93**, 1563–72.

Kahn LG, *et al*. (2020). Endocrine-disrupting chemicals: implications for human health. *Lancet Diabetes Endocrinol* **8**, 703–18.

Kassotis CD, *et al*. (2020). Endocrine-disrupting chemicals: economic, regulatory, and policy implications. *Lancet Diabetes Endocrinol* **8**, 719-30.

Differential diagnosis of possible manifestations of endocrine disorders

Sweating

- Menopause/gonadal failure.*
- Thyrotoxicosis.*
- Intoxication.*
- Drug/alcohol withdrawal.*
- PCC.
- Acromegaly.
- Carcinoid syndrome.
- Hypoglycaemia.
- DM.
- Parkinsonism.
- Autonomic neuropathy (gustatory sweating).
- RCC.
- Chronic/subacute infection (e.g. TB, endocarditis).
- Haematological malignancy (e.g. lymphoma).
- Anxiety.
- Idiopathic.
- Drugs, e.g. fluoxetine, TCAs, aspirin, NSAIDs, tamoxifen, omeprazole, cocaine, heroin withdrawal, ciprofloxacin, aciclovir, sertraline, esomeprazole.
- Fabry's disease (most commonly causes anhidrosis).

(* Commonest causes.)

Investigation

- History.
- Clinical examination.
- TFTs, serum gonadotrophin levels, blood glucose level.
- Specific investigations, according to clinical suspicion, FBC, ESR, glucose.

Management

- Treat the underlying cause where possible.
- Antiperspirants.
- Topical aluminium chloride ± ethanol.
- Antimuscarinics: propantheline, topical glycopyrronium bromide (or unlicensed oral preparations), oxybutynin (unlicensed).
- Clonidine (unlicensed)—taken at night as can be sedative.
- Iontophoresis.
- Botulinum toxin A injections into affected areas (inhibits the release of acetylcholine at the synaptic junction of local nerves).
- Local excision of axillary sweat glands.
- Sympathetic denervation:
  - Video-assisted endoscopic thoracic sympathectomy: excision or radioablation.
  - Sympathectomy (chain disconnection between T2 ganglion and stellate ganglion).

Palpitations (often associated with sweating)
- Thyrotoxicosis.
- Hypoglycaemia (insulinoma).
- PCC.
- Anxiety states.
- Cardiac arrhythmia.
- Caffeine excess.
- Alcohol/drug withdrawal.

General malaise and tiredness
- Addison's disease.
- Hypo- or hyperthyroidism.
- Hypogonadism.
- Hypopituitarism/GHD.
- Osteomalacia.
- DM.
- Cushing's syndrome.
- Anaemia.
- Drugs (prescription and recreational):
  - Antihistamines, antidepressants, antihypertensives (β-blockers, methyldopa, clonidine), neuroleptics, corticosteroids.
- COVID-19/long COVID.
- Malignancy.
- CFS (may be associated with reduced cortisol output, both basally and in response to a variety of challenges).
- Chronic illness (cardiac, respiratory, hepatic).
- Chronic pain.
- Fibromyalgia.
- Depression.
- Sleep disorders (obstructive sleep apnoea).
- Infection.
- Musculoskeletal/neurological disease (myasthenia gravis).
- Toxins.
- Idiopathic.

Investigation of fatigue
- Careful history-taking:
  - Sleep history and pattern.
  - Duration, onset, recovery, and type of fatigue.
  - Person's usual activity level and level of exercise/exertion.
  - Shift work?
  - Associated symptoms, e.g. focal neurological signs, lymph node enlargement, weight loss, recurrent tonsillitis.
- Clinical examination.
- Serum electrolytes.
- FBC ± serum ferritin, B12, folate level if FBC abnormal.
- Inflammatory markers (ESR, CRP).
- LFTs.
- Random glucose
- Serum Ca and PO_4 levels.
- TFTs.

- CK.
- Urinalysis.
- Assessment of coeliac disease.
- Early morning cortisol or SST only if clinical symptoms suggestive.

Management
- Sleep management.
- Limit rest periods.
- Increase cognitive and physical activity.
- Relaxation techniques.
- Shift sleep pattern with daytime light ± bright light
- Melatonin is sometimes helpful (unlicensed).

Clinical practice point: chronic fatigue syndrome
- Fatigue >6 months, new/recent onset, persistent and unexplained, associated with reduced activity levels and at least one of:
  - Poor sleep.
  - Multisite muscle/joint pain.
  - Painful lymph node (not enlarged).
  - General malaise.

Red flags
- Lymph node enlargement.
- Focal neurological signs.
- Features of connective tissue disorder/inflammatory arthropathy.
- Cardiorespiratory features.
- Significant weight loss.

Flushing
- Gonadal failure (with flushing and sweats).
- Drugs (vasodilators, e.g. calcium channel blockers).
- Chlorpropamide.
- Nicotinic acid.
- Antioestrogens.
- LHRH agonists.
- SSRIs.
- Carcinoid (dry flushing—no sweats).
- Mastocytosis.
- MTC.
- Anaphylaxis.
- Pancreatic cell carcinoma.
- PCC (more often pallor).
- Fever.
- Alcohol.
- Autonomic dysfunction.
- Some foods:
  - Fish.
  - Tyramine-containing food (cheese).
  - Nitrites (cured meat).
  - Monosodium glutamate.
  - Spicy food.

- Gustatory flushing.
- Benign cutaneous flushing.
- Idiopathic.

Initial evaluation of patients with flushing
- Careful history.
- Physical examination (ideally during a flush, although not often possible):
  - Examine skin carefully.
  - Pulse rate.
  - BP.
  - Thyroid examination.
  - Respiratory examination (wheeze).
  - Careful abdominal examination.
  - Urine dipstix.

Biochemistry
- Gonadotrophin levels.
- 2× 24h urinary 5-HIAA measurements.
- Serum chromogranin A.
- 2× 24h urinary catecholamine measurements.
- Plasma metanephrines (if high level of suspicion).
- Serum tryptase level (if suspecting mastocytosis).
- Calcitonin level (if suspecting MTC).
- Plasma VIP (if suspecting pancreatic carcinoma).
- Immunoglobulin (Ig) levels (raised IgE may suggest allergies).
- Specific investigations, according to suspected diagnosis.

Management of flushing
- Treat the underlying cause.
- Nadolol (non-selective β-blocker) effective in some cases of benign cutaneous flushing.
- SSAs can be used to treat flushing associated with carcinoid syndrome.
- Antihistamines may be effective in some histamine-secreting carcinoid tumours.

Further reading

Cleare A (2003). The neuroendocrinology of chronic fatigue syndrome. *Endocr Rev* **24**, 236–52.

Cornuz J, et al. (2006). Fatigue: a practical approach to diagnosis in primary care. *CMAJ* **174**, 765–7.

Eisenach J, et al. (2005). Hyperhidrosis: evolving therapies for a well established phenomenon. *Mayo Clin Proc* **80**, 657–66.

Huguet I (2017). Management of endocrine disease: Flushing—current concepts. *Eur J Endocrinol* **177**, R219.

Izikson L, et al. (2006). The flushing patient: differential diagnosis, workup and treatment. *J Am Acad Derm* **55**, 193–208.

National Institute for Health and Care Excellence (2007). *Chronic fatigue syndrome/myalgic encephalomyelitis (or encephalopathy): diagnosis and management*. Clinical guideline [CG53]. ℛ https://www.nice.org.uk/guidance/cg53

Paisley AN, Buckler HM (2010). Investigating secondary hyperhidrosis. *BMJ* **341**, c4475.

Stress and the endocrine system

Definition

Stress may be considered as a state of threatened, or perceived as threatened, homeostasis. The principal effectors of the stress response are CRH, GCs, catecholamines, AVP, and POMC-derived peptides (especially α-MSH) and β-endorphins.

Endocrine effects of stress

The endocrine response to stress is mediated by CNS and peripheral components. The CNS components mediating the endocrine response to stress are located in the hypothalamus and brainstem and consist of neurones releasing CRH and AVP, and the noradrenergic cell groups in the medulla/pons. Peripheral components of the endocrine stress response include the sympathetic–adrenal medulla system, the parasympathetic system, and the HPA axis.

Hypothalamic–pituitary axis
- ↑ amplitude of synchronized pulsatile release of CRH and AVP (potent synergistic factor of CRH) into the hypophyseal portal system.
- ↑ stimulated ACTH production.
- ↑ adrenal GC and androgen secretion.
- GCs also play a role in termination of the normal stress response by −ve feedback at the pituitary, hypothalamus, and extrahypothalamic regions.

Growth hormone axis
- GCs suppress GH production and inhibit the effects of IGF-1 (thus, children with anxiety disorders may have short stature).
- CRH increases somatostatin production, inhibiting GH production.
- GH response to IV glucagon is blunted.

Thyroid axis
- GCs reduce the production of TSH and limit the conversion of T_4 to the more active T_3 by reducing deiodinase activity.
- Somatostatin suppresses both TRH and TSH release.

  (See ➲ Sick euthyroid syndrome, pp. 878–80.)

Reproductive axis
- CRH reduces GnRH secretion.
- GCs suppress GnRH neurones and pituitary gonadotrophs, and render the gonads resistant to gonadotrophins.
- GCs also render peripheral tissues resistant to oestradiol.
- Chronic stress leads to amenorrhoea in ♀, and low LH and testosterone in ♂.
- Oestrogens increase CRH expression via an oestrogen response element in the promoter region of the *CRH* gene. This may account for the sex-related differences in the stress response and HPA axis activity.
- CRH is produced by the ovary, endometrium, and placenta during the latter half of pregnancy, leading to physiological hypercortisolism.

Metabolism
- GCs, via their direct effect and via reduced GH and sex hormone activity, result in muscle and bone catabolism and fat anabolism.
- Chronic activation of the stress system is associated with ↑ visceral adiposity, ↓ lean body mass, and suppressed osteoblastic activity (which may ultimately lead to osteoporosis).
- GCs induce insulin resistance and other features of the metabolic syndrome.

Other effects
- Immune: activation of the HPA axis inhibits the immune/inflammatory response; most components of the immune response are inhibited by GCs (>20% of genes expressed in human leucocytes are regulated by GCs), increasing susceptibility to infections.

Further reading

Charmandari E, et al. (2005). Endocrinology of the stress response. *Annu Rev Physiol* **67**, 259–84.

Endocrinology of exercise

Exercise and the hypothalamic–pituitary axis

Exercise presents a significant challenge to physiological homeostasis. The endocrine system is integral to the body's ability to adapt to exercise, allowing the mobilization of metabolic fuels and also assisting in key cardio-respiratory responses.

- A 'stress' response is a significant part of this, with both CRH and ADH stimulating the release of ACTH and hence cortisol. This response promotes gluconeogenesis and helps to limit exercise-induced inflammation. Chronically trained athletes demonstrate background hypercortisolaemia, although an attenuated cortisol rise in response to exercise is also seen.
- GH is released in response to acute exercise and remains ↑ until around 2h afterwards, although the mechanisms underlying this are not clear. The response is proportional to both the intensity and the duration of the exercise. In the longer term, both 24h GH secretion and IGF-1 levels correlate well with physical activity and VO$_{2max}$.
- So fluid homeostasis can be maintained, ADH is released in response to exercise in response to osmotic stimuli. However, non-osmotic stimuli can also affect ADH release, and this may contribute to the development of exercise-associated hyponatraemia.
- PRL is secreted in response to an exercise bout, although regular exercise does not seem to affect PRL levels long term. The role of PRL in exercise is not clear, but it may impact on immune function.
- Both PRL and cortisol suppress GnRH secretion, and hence LH/FSH secretion, which may explain why exercise can suppress gonadal function. Potential effects of this are discussed in ➲ The female athlete triad (p. 777).
- TSH is rapidly stimulated in response to acute exercise, but longer-term effects are not clear. Exercise training can inhibit peripheral thyroid hormone metabolism, leading to ↑ levels of rT$_3$ and ↑ levels of T$_3$.

Exercise and bone health

- Physical activity has been shown to ↑ bone mass, especially at load-bearing sites. ~26% of total adult bone mass is gained in 2 years around the time of peak bone gain (12.5 years in girls and 14.1 years in boys), meaning that physical activity may be particularly important around this time.
- Bone strength may be a more important measure than bone mass. Small, but significant, exercise-related increase in bone strength have also been seen in the lower extremities in children.
- In older adults, bone mass is improved with weight-bearing exercise, compared with controls, in general due to the attenuation of normal bone loss, rather than an increase in bone mass, in the intervention group.
- Rates of stress fracture in athletes have been reduced with Ca and vitamin D supplementation, although the evidence is not yet strong enough for supplementation to be recommended routinely. Dosing is also not clear.

The female athlete triad

This has been recognized since the 1990s and is defined as the interplay between:
- Energy deficit (with or without an eating disorder).
- Amenorrhoea.
- Osteoporosis.

HA can develop in the context of stress, weight loss, and exercise. An energy deficit (between intake and expenditure) appears to be essential for weight loss and exercise-related forms, with leptin also playing a key role. Problems with bone health may result from a combination of poor intake of Ca and vitamin D and disruption of gonadal function.

▶ It is vital to ask about energy intake, weight, and menstrual function in young ♀ athletes. A detailed history is key to diagnosis of amenorrhoea, and investigation should rule out alternative causes.

Successful management often takes a multidisciplinary approach, including both dietetic and psychological input. Strategies include:
- Exercise reduction and dietary modification to eliminate the energy deficit and to ensure adequate nutrient intake are important. Weight gain may be required.
- For bone health, ensuring an adequate intake of Ca and vitamin D is important. Whether supplemental doses are required (and if so, what they should be) is not clear. There is no clear evidence for OCP use in this context, although it is widespread.
- Bone densitometry is likely to be helpful both to assess bone health and to evaluate the effectiveness of interventions.
- The OCP is not recommended for amenorrhoea, but consideration of transdermal oestradiol with cyclical progesterone if amenorrhoea persists, despite addressing the fundamental cause, is appropriate.

Relative energy deficiency in sport

- The International Olympic Committee issued a consensus statement that defined RED-S as impaired physiological functioning caused by relative energy deficiency and includes, but is not limited to, impairments of metabolic rate, menstrual function, bone health, immunity, protein synthesis, and cardiovascular health. It also has consequences on psychological well-being and cognitive performance. The aetiological factor is low energy availability (LEA).
- RED-S expands the ♀ athlete triad to include men and other populations, e.g. dancers, the military.
- Endocrine consequences include disruption of the HPA–gonadal axis, alterations in thyroid function, reduced leptin, GH resistance, and ↑ cortisol. In men, loss of LH pulsatility leads to a reduction in testosterone.
- It appears that the endocrine and inflammatory status regains homeostasis after stopping the activity, but studies are related to short-term energy deficit and recovery and there are little data on long-term outcomes and recovery if RED-S is persistent.

Performance-enhancing drugs (PEDs)

PEDs are pharmacologic agents that athletes and non-athletes (e.g. weight-lifters) use to enhance performance. It is referred to as doping when used in competitive sport, but the majority of cases are recreational. Often multiple combinations of PEDs are used and other high-risk behaviours and addiction are commoner in these groups. Drugs are easily available on the Internet without the need for a prescription.

Some of the most popular PEDs are:

- Androgenic anabolic steroids (AAS):
  - AAS are androgenic ($\male$ sexual characteristics) and anabolic (increasing muscle strength and mass), and therefore, anabolic steroids aim to have less androgenic consequences.
  - Adverse effects include cardiovascular (dyslipidaemia and cardiomyopathy), haematologic (raised Hct), psychiatric (mood disorders), neuropsychological (more susceptible to rage, antisocial and violent behaviour), and dependence (through body image and neuroendocrine and hedonic pathways).
  - Commonest hypogonadal effects include infertility, gynaecomastia, sexual dysfunction, hair loss, acne, and testicular atrophy.
  - Unproven techniques adopted to minimize hypogonadism include addition of intermittent SERMs (e.g. clomifene, tamoxifen, raloxifene), antiandrogens (anastrozole, exemestane, letrozole), and hCG.
  - Recovery of the HPA axis takes 12 months in most cases (but can be longer or never recover).
- Opiates. Often used in combination to continue training despite muscle and joint pain.
- EPO. This improves performance by improving O_2 delivery to muscle. The main side effects are ↑ risk of thrombosis and hypertension, ↑ risk of cardiovascular events and stroke, and ↑ risk of death.
- GH. This results in improved muscle mass and reduced fat mass, although there is limited evidence of a performance benefit. Adverse effects are similar to those seen in acromegaly.
- Insulin. This can have beneficial anabolic effects, although side effects, such as hypoglycaemia and weight gain, may make it less attractive.
- Diuretics. These are used to alter weight categories in performance, enhance muscle definition, and dilute urine to reduce the concentration of other PEDs in the urine.
- Gene doping. A theoretical threat of using nucleic sequences or genetically modified cells to enhance performance. There are no known cases of gene doping as of yet. Potential adverse safety are immune reactions to vectors, unregulated gene expression, ↑ cancer risk, and transmission of the new genetic material to offspring.

Further reading

Gordon CM, et al. (2017). Functional hypothalamic amenorrhea: an Endocrine Society Clinical practice guideline. *J Clin Endocrinol Metab* **102**, 1413–39.

Karavolos S, et al. (2015). Male central hypogonadism secondary to expgenous androgens: a review of the drugs and protocols highlighted by the online community of users or prevention and/or mitigation of adverse effects. *Clin Endocrinol (Oxf)* **82**, 624–32.

Mastorakos G, et al. (2005). Exercise and the stress system. *Hormones (Athens)* **4**, 73–89.

McGrath JC, Cowan D (2008). Drugs in sport. *Br J Pharmacol* **154**, 493–5.

Mountjoy M, et al. (2018). International Olympic Committee (IOC) consensus statement on relative energy deficiency in sport (RED-S): 2018 update. *Int J Sport Nutr Exerc Metab* **28**, 316–31.

Pope HG, et al. (2014). Adverse health consequences of performance enhancing drugs: an Endocrine Society scientific statement. *Endocr Rev* **35**, 341–75.

Complementary and alternative therapy and endocrinology

Introduction

Many patients use natural products alongside, or instead of, conventional therapy. Products and information are available from many sources, but in particular the Internet.

- Patients need to be asked specifically about usage.
- Hospital pharmacists can be extremely helpful in sourcing information about natural products, including interactions with conventional medicines.
- Quality control of natural products is usually poor, with content ranging anywhere from 0% of stated level to several fold higher.
- Safety data are often absent or inadequate. Some preparations may also contain pharmacologically active compounds which can interact with other treatments or worsen comorbidities (e.g. alternative and complementary therapies for menopausal symptoms have been shown to contain oestrogenic properties which would be a concern for women with hormone-dependent diseases such as breast cancer).
- Discussion of any natural products listed here is not intended in any way to imply efficacy or safety of these products or to recommend their usage, but rather to illustrate the compounds being promoted for these conditions by alternative information sources.

Alternative therapy used in patients with diabetes mellitus

A major concern with natural products used by patients with DM is that of interaction with conventional medicines, placing the patient at risk of hypoglycaemia.

Hypoglycaemic agents

These work by ↑ insulin secretion from the pancreas or due to direct insulin-like action at the insulin receptor.

- Banaba (*Lagerstroemia speciosa*)—crepe myrtle. Banaba extracts contain corosolic acid and ellagitannins, which may have direct insulin-like effects at insulin receptors.
- Bitter melon (*Momordica charantia*). Contains a polypeptide with insulin-like effects. Used as juice, powder, extracts, and fried food. Often part of Asian and Indian foods.
- Fenugreek (*Trigonella foenum-gracum*). Used as powder or seeds, or as part of dietary supplement. May enhance insulin release and may also decrease carbohydrate absorption due to laxative effect. May also inhibit platelets and thus increase bleeding diathesis.
- Gymnema (*Gymnema sylvestre*), 'gurmar' in Hindi ('sugar-destroying'). Extract 'GS4' also used. May increase endogenous insulin secretion (↑ C-peptide levels noted in users). In some preliminary studies, gymnema improved HbA1c and ↓ insulin or oral hypoglycaemic agent (OHA) requirements.
- Berberine (from *Coptis chinensis*). AMP kinase activator and promotes glucose transporter type 4 (GLUT4) translocation to the cell membrane. Some studies suggest an HbA1c-lowering effect.

Insulin sensitizers

- Cassia cinnamon (*Cinnamomum aromaticum*)—also known as Chinese cinnamon (*Cinnamomum verum* is the usual cinnamon used in the UK, although cassia cinnamon may be contained in ground cinnamon mixes). May increase insulin sensitivity and lower fasting blood glucose levels. Appears safe and well tolerated.
- Chromium. Chromium deficiency is associated with IGT, hyperglycaemia, and ↓ insulin sensitivity. Chromium forms part of a 'glucose tolerance factor' complex, and therefore, supplements are sometimes labelled 'chromium GTF'. In patients with DM and chromium deficiency, addition of chromium improves glycaemic control. However, the role of chromium in patients without deficiency is not clear. The American Diabetes Association (ADA) only recommends chromium usage in patients with documented chromium deficiency. Excessive chromium may cause renal impairment.
- Vanadium. Thought to stimulate hepatic glycogenolysis; inhibit gluconeogenesis, lipolysis, and intestinal glucose transport; and increase skeletal muscle glucose uptake, utilization, and glycogenolysis. High-dose vanadium (taken as vanadyl sulphate) may improve insulin sensitivity and glycaemic control in patients with T2DM, with large doses of elemental vanadium required for these effects—however, doses >1.8mg/day vanadium may cause renal impairment.
- Ginseng (both *Panax ginseng* and American ginseng (*Panax quinquefolius*)). Contain ginsenoisides which may improve insulin sensitivity. Efficacy and safety not established.
- Prickly pear cactus (*Opuntia ficus-indica*), also called opuntia or 'nopals' (referring to the cooked leaves of the cactus). Prominent in Mexican folk medicine as a treatment for DM. *Opuntia streptacantha* stems may improve glycaemic control, either by acting as an insulin sensitizer or by slowing carbohydrate absorption; however, this is not observed with other prickly pear cactus species.
- Reservatrol. Extracted from grapes and red wine. Activates sirtuin 1 (with an indirect effect on substrates, including peroxisome proliferator-activated receptor (PPAR) γ and AMP kinase).
- Cannabinoids activate AMP kinase and PPARγ. Only anecdotal data on glucose lowering available; formal trials ongoing.

Carbohydrate absorption inhibitors

- Soluble fibre. Increases viscosity of intestinal contents, thus slowing gastric emptying time and carbohydrate absorption, resulting in lower postprandial blood glucose levels.
- The following products have some evidence of reducing postprandial blood glucose levels and may also improve TC and LDL-C levels in patients. They may also interfere with absorption of drugs and therefore should not be taken at the same time as conventional medicines:
  - Blond psyllium seed (*Plantago ovata*).
  - Guar gum (*Cyamopsis tetragonoloba*).
  - Oat bran (*Avena sativa*).
  - Soy (*Glycine max*)—contains both soluble and insoluble fibre and may improve insulin resistance, fasting BM, lipid profile, and HbA1c in T2DM.
- Insoluble fibre. Glucomannan (*Amorphophallus konjac*)—can delay glucose absorption.

Other products used by patients with diabetes mellitus
- α-lipoic acid. Antioxidant. May improve insulin resistance. May help symptoms of diabetic neuropathy.
- Stevia (*Stevia rebaudiana*). May enhance insulin secretion. May be toxic.
- Huangqi (*Radix astragali*). Used to treat hypoglycaemia unawareness. May increase neural activation in central glucose-sensing regions in response to hypoglycaemia.

Alternative therapy used in menopause

Phytoestrogens

The main types are isoflavones (most potent and most widespread), lignans, and coumestans.
- Sources:
  - Isoflavones: legumes (soy, chickpea, garbanzo beans, red clover, lentils, beans). Main active isoflavones are genistein and daidzein.
  - Lignans: flaxseed, lentils, whole grains, beans, many fruits and vegetables.
  - Coumestans: red clover, sunflower seeds, sprouts.
  - Other phytoestrogens: chasteberry (*Vitex agnus-castus*).
- Not structurally similar to oestrogen or to SERMs, but contain a phenolic ring that allows binding to oestrogen receptor (ER)-α and β. Effects of binding depend upon ambient oestrogen levels, the relative ratio, the concentration of ER-α and ER-β, and tissue type and location. Relatively much less potent than endogenous oestrogen (by 100- to 10,000-fold).
- Phytoestrogens *in vitro* stimulate proliferation of normal human breast tissue and oestrogen-sensitive breast tumour cells. Theoretically, phytoestrogens may stimulate ER +ve breast cancer and other oestrogen-sensitive tumours. Phytoestrogens may also antagonize the effects of tamoxifen or other SERMs. Phytoestrogens have not been shown to stimulate endometrial growth; however, they are not usually taken with progestagenic compounds. It is not known whether the other serious side effects of conventional oestrogens (e.g. DVT, PE, IHD, stroke) occur with phytoestrogen use. Many sources of phytoestrogens (e.g. coumestans) interfere with warfarin.
- Soy protein (20–60mg/day, containing 34–76mg isoflavones) modestly decreases the frequency and severity of vasomotor symptoms in a proportion of menopausal women.
- Synthetic isoflavones (ipriflavone) do not have antivasomotor activity.
- Phytoestrogens from red clover have not shown consistent improvement in vasomotor symptoms. Other sources of phytoestrogens have not shown improvement in menopausal symptoms.
- Compounds with oestrogenic activity should not be used in women who should not take oestrogen (e.g. in women with breast cancer).

(For use in osteoporosis, see ➜ Alternative therapy used by patients with osteoporosis, pp. 783–4.)

Other compounds with oestrogenic activity
- Kudzu (*Pueraria lobata*).
- Alfalfa (*Medicago sativa*).
- Hops (*Humulus lupulus*).
- Liquorice (*Glycyrrhiza glabra*).
- Panax ginseng (ginseng)—*in vitro* evidence of stimulation of breast cancer cells.

Other substances used
- Black cohosh (*Actaea racemosa*, formerly *Cimicifuga racemosa*)—not to be confused with blue cohosh and white cohosh which are entirely separate plants. Widely used in menopause. Although often advertised as such, black cohosh does not bind to ERs or have oestrogen effects and there is little evidence for efficacy for hot flushes.
- Dong quai (*Angelica sinensis*)—not clear if oestrogenic. *In vitro* evidence of promotion of breast cancer cells.

Alternative therapy used by patients with osteoporosis

Calcium
- Hundreds of preparations available.
- Several types of Ca salts available (including citrate, carbonate, lactate, gluconate, PO_4, etc. between different compounds, with little evidence of superiority of absorption, other than calcium citrate useful in patients with low gastric acidity (e.g. on concomitant PPIs or H_2 antagonists).

Magnesium
- Necessary for release of PTH.
- In itself, not effective in treating osteoporosis, unless patients are deficient in Mg.

Fluoride
- Increases bone density, but not strength—bones less elastic, more brittle—with resultant ↑ fracture rate.

Trace elements
- For example, manganese, zinc, boron, and copper.
- While many trace elements are important for multiple enzyme systems, including those in bone, most patients are not deficient, and thus supplements have negligible +ve effects upon osteoporosis. Moreover, many minerals in high doses cause serious side effects (e.g. manganese doses >11mg/day can cause extrapyramidal side effects).

Vitamin D
- Multiple preparations available, mainly as ergocalciferol or colecalciferol (vitamin D metabolites require prescription).

Isoflavones

(For more detail about the mechanism of action of phytoestrogens, see
→ Alternative therapy used in menopause, pp. 782–3.)

- Soy protein in doses >80mg/day may improve BMD, but no studies of
soy have shown improvement in fracture rate. Possible adverse effects
upon oestrogen-sensitive tissues such as ER +ve breast cancer.
- Ipriflavone—semisynthetic isoflavone, produced from daidzein. No
oestrogenic effects. No evidence of improved fracture outcome. Some
studies of ipriflavone with Ca have reported improved BMD, although
other studies have not shown an improvement. Ipriflavone can cause
serious lymphopenia (<1 × 10⁹ mL/L) which may take up to a year to
recover.

Tea

- Tea consists of green tea (unfermented), oolong tea (partially
fermented), and black tea (completely fermented).
- All teas contain fluoride and have high isoflavonoid content, in addition
to caffeine.
- Coffee (with a high caffeine content) has been associated with ↑ hip
fracture risk. However, tea drinking of all types has been associated
with higher BMD, although no fracture outcome has been reported.

DHEA

(See → Miscellaneous alternative therapy, p. 785.)

Wild yam

Wild yam contains diosgenin which is used commercially as a source for
DHEA synthesis; however, this does not occur in humans.

Other compounds used by patients for osteoporosis

- Flaxseed (α-linolenic acid and lignans).
- Gelatin.
- Dong quai.
- Panax ginseng.
- Alfalfa.
- Liquorice.

  There is no evidence of a +ve effect upon bone of these compounds.

Miscellaneous alternative therapy

Iodine and the thyroid

- Sources: kelp, shellfish-derived products.
- Effects: iodine-induced goitre or hypothyroidism, particularly in patients
with underlying thyroid disease (may have a Wolff–Chaikoff effect in
patients with Graves' disease, causing inhibition of iodide organification,
and thus thyroid hormone production).
- Iodine-induced hyperthyroidism in areas of endemic goitre and iodine
deficiency.
- Selenium and/or Brazil nuts (*Bertholletia excelsa*) rich in selenium: used
in mild to moderate GO.

DHEA—'elixir of youth'

- Reported to slow or improve changes associated with ageing, including general well-being, cognitive function, sexual function, energy levels, body composition, and muscle strength, and to aid weight loss and treat the metabolic syndrome.
- Mechanism of action: DHEA is secreted by the adrenal glands and interconverted to DHEAS. Both DHEAS and DHEA are converted to androgens and oestrogens that then act directly at their receptors.
- DHEA and DHEAS may play a role in replacement of adrenal androgens in patients with AI, resulting in improved well-being, particularly with respect to sexual function.
- Not proven in controlled trials to improve health in other patients without AI.
- Risks of androgenic effects in women when taken at high doses (100–200mg/DHEA daily). Theoretical risk of promoting hormone-sensitive cancers such as prostate and breast cancers. DHEA may also interfere with antioestrogen effects of anastrozole and other aromatase inhibitors.

Endocrine-disrupting chemicals

- Since the early 1960, a growing body of studies have identified effects of various exogenous chemicals on endocrine processes and functions, known as endocrine-disruptive chemicals (EDCs). EDCs can be classified based on their origin: industrial, agricultural, residential, pharmaceutical, and heavy metals.
- Many affect neurodevelopment, child behaviour, weight, and ♂ and ♀ reproductive health.
- Examples:
  - Perfluoroalkyl substances, bisphenols, phthalates, organophosphate pesticides.
  - Ethinyl oestradiol, dexamethasone, levonorgestrel, rosiglitazone, testosterone, lead, cadmium, mercury, arsenic.
- Most EDCs tend to be highly lipophilic; they accumulate in adipose tissue, extending their half-life.
- EDCs can potentially target every endocrine axis; however, the HPT, hypothalamic–pituitary–gonadal, and HPA axes are the main targets.
- EDCs have been linked to adult and child obesity, IGT, and GDM, reduced birthweight, prematurity, and reduced anogenital distance in boys, breast and prostate cancers, reduced semen quality, PCOS and endometriosis, cognitive deficit and attention-deficit disorder in children following prenatal exposure, and possible intergenerational transfer.

Further reading

Kahn LG, et al. (2020). Endocrine-disrupting chemicals: implications for human health. *Lancet Diabetes Endocrinol* **8**, 703–8.

Lauretta R, et al. (2019). Endocrine disrupting chemicals: effects on endocrine glands. *Front Endocrinol* **10**, 178.

Natural Medicines. [Comprehensive database, requires subscription]. ℘ http://www.naturaldatabase.com

Genetic testing in endocrinology

Márta Korbonits and *Paul Newey*

Genetic basis of endocrine disease

- The majority of clinical genetic testing focuses on DNA sequence analysis of genes responsible for monogenic endocrine disorders (see Table 13.1).
- Additional genetic tests are aimed at detecting large chromosomal abnormalities (e.g. aneuploidy or copy number variants (CNVs)).
- Emerging clinical applications include detection of somatic mutations in endocrine cancers to guide therapy (e.g. somatic *RET* mutations in thyroid cancers) and evaluation of genetic variants with potential pharmacogenomic effects.

Monogenic endocrine disease

Monogenic disorders are inherited in one of six patterns:
- AD (e.g. MEN1 due to *MEN1* mutation; MEN2 due to *RET* mutations).
- AR (e.g. CAH due to *CYP21A2* mutations).
- X-linked dominant (e.g. X-linked hypophosphataemic rickets due to *PHEX* mutations).
- XLR (e.g. Kallmann syndrome due to *ANOS* mutations).
- Y-linked (e.g. azoospermia/oligospermia due to loss of *USPY* gene).
- Mitochondrial (e.g. Kearns–Sayre syndrome).

In addition to these modes of inheritance, germline mosaicism, resulting from a post-zygotic mutation in parental germ cells, may result in apparent autosomal patterns of inheritance (i.e. multiple affected offspring from un-affected parents).

- In certain monogenic disorders, parent-of-origin effects may be observed due to genomic imprinting (e.g. phaeochromocytoma/ paraganglioma (PPGL) occurrence due to paternally inherited *SDHD* and *SDHAF2* mutations).
- In a proportion of individuals with monogenic disorders, the mutation is not inherited but rather develops *de novo* (i.e. occurs for the 1st time in the individual).
- Incomplete penetrance can be observed in several AD diseases, which therefore may mask familial disease, making the establishment of a genetic disease more difficult.

Genetic abnormalities resulting in monogenic disease

Several types of genetic abnormality may give rise to monogenic disease, including:
- SNVs: substitution of one nucleotide with another, resulting in missense amino acid substitutions, nonsense mutations (i.e. premature stop codon) or disruption to splice sites.
- Small insertions or deletions ('indels'): result in either in-frame or out-of-frame (i.e. frameshift) mutations.
- Large structural defects/CNVs: include whole or partial gene deletions or duplications.

Frameshift, nonsense, and splice site mutations, as well as whole or partial gene deletions, typically result in loss of gene function.

Disease penetrance and genetic heterogeneity
- Penetrance refers to the likelihood that an individual carrying a disease-causing variant will manifest the respective disorder. High penetrance disorders include MEN1, in which >95% of pathogenic variant carriers develop manifestations by age 50 years. Intermediate penetrance disorders include PPGL due to *SDHB* and *SDHD* mutations, in which 20% and 40% of pathogenic variant carriers develop disease by age 60 years, respectively. Low penetrance disorders include PPGL due to *SDHA* mutations (i.e. estimated to be 1–4%).
- Genetic heterogeneity refers to the situation in which similar clinical phenotypes may result from different genetic abnormalities. For example, mutations in >15 different genes are associated with hereditary PPGL.
- In some instances, variants in the same gene may cause different phenotypes (e.g. gain-of-function germline *RET* variants associated with MEN2, loss-of-function *RET* variants associated with Hirschsprung's disease).

Chromosomal disorders
- Large-scale abnormalities affecting all or part of one or more chromosomes account for several endocrine genetic disorders.
- These include conditions associated with an abnormal number of chromosomes (i.e. aneuploidy) such as Klinefelter syndrome (47,XXY) and Turner syndrome (45,X).
- Alternatively, there may be gains or losses of chromosomal material (e.g. 22q11.2 deletion syndrome, or Prader–Willi syndrome due to losses of genetic material on chromosome 15).
- The majority of chromosomal disorders are not inherited but occur *de novo*, although in some instances, inheritance from a parent may occur (e.g. 15% of those with 22q11.2 deletion syndrome).

Genetic tests

(See Table 13.1.)

Requesting a genetic test: general considerations
- The decision to undertake genetic testing requires careful consideration and should take into account the potential clinical utility of the test, as well as any harms that may arise.
- It is essential that the person requesting testing has sufficient knowledge to provide the individual undergoing testing with appropriate information (see ⟴ Genetic tests, pp. 796–8). When there is uncertainty about the suitability of testing or the testing approach to adopt, there should be involvement of the clinical genetics team.

Table 13.1 Examples of genetic tests employed in endocrinology

Disorder/ phenotype	Gene(s)	Mode of inheritance	Variant type(s)	Testing platform
MEN syndromes				
MEN1	*MEN1*	AD	SNV, indel, gene del	Single/panel MLPA/aCGH
MEN2A/B	*RET*	AD	SNV	Single/panel
MEN4	*CDKN1B*	AD	SNV, indel, gene del?	Single/panel MLPA/aCGH
HPT-JT	*CDC73*	AD	SNV, indel, gene del	Single/panel MLPA/aCGH
VHL	*VHL*	AD	SNV, indel, gene del	Single/panel MLPA/aCGH
NF-1	*NF1*	AD	SNV, indel, gene del	Single/panel MLPA/aCGH
McCune–Albright syndrome	*GNAS*	S. Mos	SNV	Single/panel
Carney complex	*PRKAR1A*	AD	SNV, indel, gene del	Single/panel MLPA/aCGH
DICER1 syndrome	*DICER1*	AD	SNV, indel, gene del	Single/panel MLPA/aCGH
Hypothalamic/pituitary disorders				
FIPA	*AIP*	AD	SNV, indel, gene del	Single/panel MLPA
X-linked acrogigantism	*GPR101*	AD/S. Mos	Duplication	MLPA, duplex PCR
Combined pituitary hormone deficiency	*PROP1, HESX1, LHX3, LHX4, OTX2, POUF1F1, SOX2* + others	AD/AR/ XLD	SNV, indel	Panel ± CNV detection
HH with/ without anosmia	*ANOS1, FGFR1, PROKR2, CHD7, FGF8, PROK2* + others	AD/AR/ XLR	SNV, indel	Panel
Adrenal disorders				
Autoimmune polyglandular syndrome	*AIRE*	AR (AD)	SNV, indel	Single/panel

Table 13.1 (Contd.)

Disorder/ phenotype	Gene(s)	Mode of inheritance	Variant type(s)	Testing platform
CAH	CYP21A2, CYP11B1 CYP17A1	AR	SNV, indel	Single/panel
X-linked adrenoleuko-dystrophy	ABCD1	XLD	SNV, indel	Single/CNV analysis
FGD	MC2R, NNT, MRAP, STAR, TXNRD2 + others	AR	SNV, indel	Single/panel
Hereditary phaeochromo-cytoma/paraganglioma	SDHB, SDHC, SDHD, SDHAF2, MAX, RET, VHL, NF1, TMEM127 + others	AD	SNV, indel, gene del	Single/panel (MLPA/CNV analysis)
Familial hyperaldo-steronism	CYP11B1/ 2, KCNJ5, CACNA1D, CACNA1H	AD	SNV, gene fusion	Single/panel LR-PCR
Calcium-related disorders				
Familial isolated hypopara-thyroidism (FIH)	GCM2, PTH	AD/AR	SNV, indel, gene del	Single/panel
Autosomal dominant hypocalcaemia (ADH)	CASR, GNA11	AD	SNV	Single/panel
22q11.2 deletion syndrome (di George)	3Mb deletion on chromosome 22 (including TBX1 gene)	DN/AD	–	aCGH/FISH/MLPA
Pseudohypo-parathyroidism type 1a/pseudopseudo-hypopara-thyroidism	GNAS	AD	SNV, indel, gene del	Single
Hereditary hyperpara-thyroidism	MEN1, CASR, CDC73, CDKN1B, GCM2	AD	SNV, indel, gene del	Single/panel
FHH	CASR, GNA11, AP2S1	AD	SNV, indel, gene del	Single/panel
Thyroid disorders				
Congenital hypothyroidism	TSHR, PAX8, DUOX2, SLC5A5, TSHB, THRA + others	AR/AD	SNV, indel	Single/panel

(Continued)

Table 13.1 (*Contd.*)

Disorder/phenotype	Gene(s)	Mode of inheritance	Variant type(s)	Testing platform
Thyroid hormone resistance	*THRB, THRA*	AD/(AR)	SNV, indel	Single/panel
Disorders of glucose homeostasis				
Neonatal and infancy-onset diabetes	*ABCC8, KCNJ11, GCK, INS, PDX1* + others	AD/AR/DN	SNV, indel	Single/panel
Autosomal dominant familial mild hyperglycaemia/diabetes (MODY)	*HNF4A, GCK, HNF1A, HNF1B* + others	AD	SNV, indel	Single/panel
Congenital hyperinsulinism	*ABCC8, KCNJ11, GCK* + others	AD/AR	SNV, indel	Single/panel
Disorders of sex development/sex chromosomes				
46,XY disorder of sex development/ambiguous genitalia	*SRY, AR, NR5A1, HSD17B3, MAMLD1, SRD5A2, MAP3K1, NROB1, DHH* + others	NI (AD/AR)	SNV, indel, gene del, CNV	aCGH/FISH/panel
Turner syndrome	Aneuploidy 45,X (loss or partial deletion of X chromosome)	–	NI	Karyotype/aCGH
Klinefelter syndrome	Aneuploidy 47,XXY	NA	–	Karyotype/aCGH
Prader–Willi syndrome	Paternal deletion, maternal uniparental disomy, or translocations involving part of chromosome 15	NA	–	Methylation-specific MLPA/aCGH/FISH

aCGH, array comparative genomic hybridization; AD, autosomal dominant; AR, autosomal recessive; CNV, copy number variant; del, deletion; DN, *de novo*; FISH, fluorescence *in situ* hybridization; indel, insertion or deletion; LR-PCR, long-range polymerase chain reaction; MODY, maturity onset diabetes of the young; MLPA, multiplex-ligation dependent probe amplification; NI, not inherited; S. Mos, somatic mosaicism; SNV, single-nucleotide variant; XLD, X-linked dominant.

'Single' refers to respective single gene test. 'Panel' refers to relevant disease-targeted gene panel.

Adapted from: Newey PJ. Genetic Testing in Endocrinology; current concepts and contemporary challenges. *Clin Endocrinol* (2019); 91; 587–607.

Potential utility of genetic testing

Genetic testing may be useful in several settings, including:

- Establishing a clinical diagnosis, thereby facilitating appropriate patient management and/or treatment. For example, making a genetic diagnosis may:
  - Guide clinical and treatment decision-making (e.g. determine the potential timing of prophylactic thyroidectomy in MEN2 patients harbouring high-risk *RET* mutations).
  - Enable surveillance for manifestations of the disorder that may not be clinically apparent (e.g. tumour surveillance in MEN1).
  - Provide prognostic information for the patient and family (e.g. ↑ risk of malignancy in PPGL due to *SDHB* mutations).
- Facilitating predictive testing of asymptomatic/symptomatic relatives, thereby identifying additional family members who may be at risk of disease (see ⮌ Predictive genetic testing, p. 794).
- Allowing pre-pregnancy genetic counselling/preimplantation genetic diagnosis (PGD) (see ⮌ Preimplantation and prenatal genetic testing, pp. 794–5).

Potential harms of genetic testing may include the possible −ve psychological impact of being diagnosed with a genetic disorder, feelings of guilt over transmission to family members, and any stigmatization or −ve discrimination that might arise.

Consent for genetic testing

- For consent to be valid, the person giving consent should be provided with appropriate information to make an informed decision. This information should be tailored to the individual and take into account the clinical situation (e.g. diagnostic vs predictive setting) and the type of test being performed (e.g. single gene test vs high-content testing).
- The clinician requesting testing should have the relevant knowledge to provide this information and/or make available access to appropriate genetic counselling.
- A 'Record of Discussion' may be used to record the topics covered at the time of consent. Topics that may be discussed include:
  - The potential for test results to inform future, as well as current, health problems.
  - The potential for the test result to have implications for other family members.
  - The potential to identify genetic variants whose significance is not yet known (i.e. variants of uncertain significance).
  - If appropriate, the potential for incidental findings (i.e. genetic changes unrelated to the reason for the test) (see ⮌ Incidental findings, p. 798).
  - Local practices for both DNA and data storage.
  - The potential need for data sharing to aid variant interpretation.
- A common concern of those undergoing testing is the potential impact of genetic testing on obtaining health-related insurance. In the UK, British insurers and the government have a voluntary agreement, such that insurers cannot request the result of a *predictive* genetic test to determine cover, with the exception of Huntington's disease (for policies in excess of £500,000). This code does not cover *diagnostic* testing.

- Where genetic testing is for research purposes, consent should be taken in accordance to project-specific ethical approvals.

Predictive genetic testing
- Predictive genetic testing of asymptomatic individuals at ↑ risk of genetic disease (e.g. 1st-degree relatives of a patient with a known pathogenic variant in a monogenic disease gene) can identify those harbouring the mutation, allowing early introduction of surveillance and/or treatment.
- Predictive testing may also identify family members who do not harbour the family-specific variant and these individuals can be reassured about their future risk of disease and avoid further tests.
- Predictive testing is most widely employed in the endocrine setting for penetrant monogenic tumour syndromes in which identification of 'at-risk' individuals facilitates tumour screening and/or early treatment (e.g. MEN1, MEN2, VHL).
- Predictive testing should be undertaken by the clinical genetics team, with appropriate genetic counselling.
- Predictive testing of young children (with parental consent) should usually only be performed if the disorder has potential clinical consequences in early life (e.g. early-onset tumours in MEN1 or MEN2). For disorders with adult-onset clinical features, predictive genetic testing should be delayed until an age whereby the individual can decide whether they wish to undergo testing.

Preimplantation and prenatal genetic testing
- Preconception genetic counselling is an important component of clinical care for prospective and/or existing parents at risk of transmitting genetic disorders to their future offspring.
- PGD may be offered in some settings in which parents are at risk of transmitting severe monogenic disorders to future offspring, and has been used in the setting of several endocrine disorders (e.g. MEN1, MEN2, CAH).
- PGD is performed in the context of IVF. It involves removal of a small number of cells from the early blastocyst to allow DNA analysis to detect the presence or absence of the specific genetic abnormality. This allows identification of potentially unaffected blastocysts that can subsequently be implanted in the mother's uterus.
- In contrast to PGD, prenatal genetic testing evaluates the genetic status of the fetus once pregnancy is established and can be used to detect a number of genetic abnormalities (e.g. aneuploidy and other chromosomal disorders, single-gene defects).
- Prenatal testing is usually performed when the pregnancy is at ↑ risk of hereditary disease or where antenatal screening has identified features consistent with a potential genetic diagnosis.
- Prenatal genetic testing involves acquisition of fetal DNA for evaluation. Invasive methods include chorionic villous sampling or amniocentesis, each of which incurs a small risk of miscarriage. Non-invasive prenatal genetic diagnosis (NIPD) or testing (NIPT) methods use cell-free circulating fetal DNA obtained from the maternal circulation, which may be detectable from 5 to 6 weeks' gestation.

Further reading

Brezina PR, Kutteh WH (2015). Clinical applications of preimplantation genetic testing. *BMJ* **350**, g7611.

Committee on Bioethics, Committee on Genetics, and American College Of Medical Genetics and Genomics Social, Ethical, Legal Issues Committee (2013). Ethical and policy issues in genetic testing and screening of children. *Pediatrics* **131**, 620–62.

Newey PJ (2019). Clinical genetic testing in endocrinology: current concepts and contemporary challenges. *Clin Endocrinol (Oxf)* **91**, 587–607.

Royal College of Physicians, Royal College of Pathologists, British Society for Genetic Medicine (2019). *Consent and confidentiality in genomic medicine: guidance on the use of genetic and genomic information in the clinic*, 3rd edition. ℛ https://www.rcpath.org/uploads/assets/d3956d4a-319e-47ca-8ece8a122949e701/Consent-and-confidentiality-in-genomic-medicine-July-2019.pdf

Genetic tests

Although the clinician does not require a detailed knowledge of the different genetic testing platforms, it is important that they have an awareness of the types of test available and their potential uses.

Tests to detect chromosomal abnormalities

- Karyotyping: detects abnormalities of chromosome number (e.g. aneuploidy) or structure (e.g. CNVs, inversions, translocations), but with limited genomic resolution (e.g. 3–10Mb).
- Array comparative genomic hybridization (aCGH): increasingly used as 1st-line investigation for detection of structural genetic abnormalities (improved resolution, compared with karyotyping).
- Fluorescence *in situ* hybridization (FISH): can identify abnormalities located to specific chromosomal regions (e.g. translocations).
- MLPA: used to detect whole/partial gene deletions (e.g. for *MEN1*, *VHL*).
- Whole-genome SNP array and droplet digital polymerase chain reaction (ddPCR) employed to detect CNVs.

DNA sequencing

- The diagnosis of the majority of monogenic endocrine disorders relies on high-fidelity DNA sequencing.
- Advances in DNA sequencing technology have resulted in a shift in testing with an ↑ use of 'next-generation sequencing' (NGS) that provides a cost-effective and time-efficient approach to high-content genetic testing.
- NGS relies on 'massive parallel sequencing' which facilitates simultaneous acquisition of DNA sequence data from millions of small DNA fragments. However, it is highly dependent on bioinformatic tools for data acquisition, processing, and analysis.
- Current DNA sequencing tests include: single-gene tests, disease-targeted gene panels, whole-exome sequencing (WES) and whole-genome sequencing (WGS).

Single-gene tests/Sanger sequencing

- Sanger sequencing represents the 'gold standard' for DNA sequencing but is labour-intensive, compared to NGS methods.
- Suitable when the genetic aetiology of the disorder is limited to a single or a very small number of genes.
- Sanger sequencing retains an important role in the predictive testing setting when DNA sequence analysis is limited to the detection of a specific pathogenic variant. It may also be used in some settings to confirm genetic abnormalities detected by NGS methods.

Disease-targeted gene panels

- A widely employed NGS method that provides a cost-effective approach to simultaneous sequence analysis of multiple genes.
- Most suitable for monogenic conditions with marked genetic heterogeneity (e.g. PPGL, Kallmann syndrome) in which sequence analysis of multiple genes is recommended.

- As the content of the panel increases (i.e. number of genes sequenced), so does the potential for uncertain test results (i.e. identification of 'variants of uncertain significance' (VUS)).

Whole exome sequencing whole genome sequencing

- WES is an NGS method that undertakes DNA sequence analysis of all ~30,000 protein-coding genes (~1% of the genome). A modified approach is the clinical exome platform that limits DNA sequence analysis to 4000–7000 genes implicated in human disease.
- WES is suitable for testing of monogenic disorders with unknown genetic aetiology and has been highly successful in disease gene discovery.
- In contrast to WES, WGS represents the most comprehensive DNA sequencing platform, providing sequence analysis of all coding and non-coding regions.
- Both WES and WGS rely on automated bioinformatic pipelines for sequence analysis and variant interpretation.

Variant interpretation

- Establishing whether a given DNA sequence variant is pathogenic (i.e. representing a disease-causing 'mutation') or benign is frequently complex.
- For penetrant monogenic disorders, DNA sequence variants are evaluated based upon the ACMG guidelines, together with other national guidelines (e.g. UK Practice Guidelines for Variant Classification).
- The process of variant interpretation considers multiple gene- and variant-level factors (e.g. population frequency of variant, predicted functional effect on encoded protein, co-segregation of the variant with clinical features in a kindred).
- Following analysis, DNA sequence variants are categorized into one of three broad groups:
  - Benign/likely benign.
  - VUS.
  - Pathogenic/likely pathogenic.
- However, variant interpretation is imprecise and potentially prone to error. Therefore, it is important to interpret the genetic test result alongside the overall clinical assessment, i.e. a combined clinical genetic diagnosis. Where uncertainty exists, multidisciplinary working between the clinician, clinical genetic teams, and laboratory scientists is encouraged.

VUS variants

- Where a definitive classification of a specific variant is not possible, the term VUS is used. This situation arises when there is insufficient and/or conflicting evidence to allow a more definitive classification.
- The frequency of VUS variants has ↑ substantially with the introduction of high-content NGS-based testing methods (e.g. disease-targeted gene panels, WES, WGS).

- In some instances, it may be possible to gain additional information to up- or downgrade VUS variants (e.g. demonstration of segregation of variant with the clinical phenotype in additional family members; establishing whether the variant has occurred de novo; undertaking additional bioinformatic or functional studies).
- There is a debate as to how VUS variants are reported and whether all VUS should be fed back to the requesting clinician and/or patient.
- Responsible data sharing at a national/international level may facilitate improved interpretation.
- Periodic re-evaluation of VUS variants is recommended.

Incidental findings

- Incidental findings refer to pathogenic variants identified during testing which are associated with disorders other than those for which the test was undertaken.
- Previous studies have reported that 1–4% of the general population may have a potentially pathogenic variant in one of 59 'actionable' monogenic disease genes (as defined by the ACMG), including several associated with endocrine tumour syndromes (e.g. *MEN1*, *RET*, *SDHx*, *VHL*), although the challenges of variant interpretation may reduce the reliability of such findings.
- The potential for incidental findings is most relevant to high-content testing platforms (e.g. WES, WGS) and it remains controversial as to whether all WES/WGS data sets should be evaluated for incidental findings.
- However, if there is a possibility of detecting incidental findings during genetic testing, this should be discussed during the consent process.

Further reading

Biesecker LG, et al. (2018). Distinguishing variant pathogenicity from genetic diagnosis: how to know whether a variant causes a condition. *JAMA* **320**, 1929–30.

Ellard S, et al. *ACGS best practice guidelines for variant classification in rare disease 2020.* ℰ https://www.acgs.uk.com

Lek M, *et al.* (2016). Analysis of protein-coding genetic variation in 60,706 humans. *Nature* **536**, 285–91.

Newey PJ, et al. (2017). Utility of population-level DNA sequence data in the diagnosis of hereditary endocrine disease. *J Endocr Soc* **1**, 1507–26.

Newey PJ (2019). Clinical genetic testing in endocrinology: current concepts and contemporary challenges. *Clin Endocrinol* **91**, 587–607.

Richards S, *et al.* (2015). Standards and guidelines for the interpretation of sequence variants: a joint consensus recommendation of the American College of Medical Genetics and Genomics and the Association for Molecular Pathology. *Genet Med* **17**, 405–42.

Whiffin N, *et al.* (2017). Using high-resolution variant frequencies to empower clinical genome interpretation. *Genet Med* **19**, 1151–8.

Pituitary adenomas

Pituitary adenomas have recently been suggested to be renamed as pituitary neuroendocrine tumours (PitNETs), although this attracted some controversies. While the vast majority are sporadic cases with various somatic alterations in their genetic and epigenetic characteristics, some are caused by germline or embryonic genetic abnormalities. The diseases and genes which are currently known to be associated with inherited or congenital pituitary tumourigenesis are listed in Box 13.1.

Box 13.1 Diseases and genes known to be involved with inherited or congenital pituitary tumourigenesis

- MEN1 or MEN1-like syndrome:
  - *MEN1* coding for menin protein (in MEN1).
  - *CDKN1B* coding for p27 protein (in MEN4).
  - *MAX* encodes Max protein (in ?MEN5).
  - *CDKN2B* coding for p15, *CDKN2C* coding for p18, and *CDKN1A* coding for p21.
- FIPA:
  - Aryl hydrocarbon receptor interacting protein (*AIP*).
  - Duplication of *GPR101*, usually in the context of microduplication at Xq26.3; can also be mosaic.
- Carney complex:
  - *PRKAR1A* coding for the regulatory subunit of PKA.
  - *PRKACB* coding for the catalytic subunit of PKA.
- McCune–Albright syndrome—mosaic condition:
  - *GNAS* gene coding for Gsα subunit protein.
- DICER1-related syndrome causing infant pituitary blastoma:
  - *DICER1* gene.
- PPGL associated with pituitary adenoma:
  - *SDH1x*—*SDHA*, *SDHB*, *SDHD*, *SDHC*, and *SDHA2F* genes coding for subunits of the enzyme SDH.
  - *MAX*—large deletion.

Multiple endocrine neoplasia types 1 and 4

(See also Table 14.7.)
- The *MEN1* gene is located on 11q13 and codes for the 610 amino-acid menin protein.[1,2]
- Patients are heterozygous for the disease-causing mutation, and disease penetrance for Ca abnormalities is over 95% by the age of 50 years.[3]
- *MEN1* behaves as a tumour suppressor gene:
  - Three-quarters of the mutations lead to a truncated protein and the majority of MEN1 syndrome-related tumour tissues show LOH at the *MEN1* locus.
- Menin has extensive interactions with other proteins involved in cell proliferation, cell cycle, and transcriptional regulation, but it is currently unclear how lack of the menin protein leads to tumourigenesis in the pituitary or other endocrine organs.
- There are over 1300 mutations identified, with a few hotspot mutations being responsible for 20% of the cases, with no genotype–phenotype correlation.
- PitNETs manifest in about 30–40% of the cases,[4] and pituitary adenoma can be the 1st manifestation of the disease in 15% of the cases.
- The frequency of the adenoma types is prolactinoma > somatotropinoma > corticotropinoma > non-functioning adenoma, in cases where the adenoma is identified due to symptoms, and not via screening.
- Plurihormonal adenomas are commoner in MEN1 syndrome-associated PitNETs, compared to somatic cases.[5]
- Prospective screening, however, identified a high proportion of small, clinically non-functioning pituitary adenomas.[6]
- Clinically manifesting MEN1-related pituitary adenomas are larger and more difficult to treat than sporadic pituitary adenomas.
- Somatic mutations of the *MEN1* gene have been commonly described in sporadic NETs and parathyroid tumours, but very rarely in sporadic pituitary adenomas.

Benefits of testing

- *MEN1* testing can help to establish the clinical diagnosis in the index patient and can lead to search and early identification of other manifestations.
- In addition, it can identify other family members with the mutation, who can enter a clinical screening programme in a timely manner, and at the same time can rule out other family members who therefore do not need any further medical attention in this respect.
- Indications for *MEN1* gene testing are listed in Table 13.2.
- Phenocopies are regularly encountered and need to be carefully considered.

Alternative mutations

- MEN-4—mutations in *CDKN1B* coding for the cyclin-dependent kinase inhibitor (CDKI) p27, coded by *CDKN1B*, are found in 1.5% of patients with MEN1-like phenotype, but with no detectable *MEN1* mutations.
- Mutations in other genes encoding CDKIs (*CDKN2B* [p15], *CDKN2C* [p18], and *CDKN1A* [p21]) can be rarely found, accounting for about 2% of *MEN1* mutation −ve patients.[7,8]

References

1. Chandrasekharappa SC, et al. (1997). Positional cloning of the gene for multiple endocrine neoplasia-type 1. *Science* **276**, 404–7.
2. Lemmens I, et al. (1997). Identification of the multiple endocrine neoplasia type 1 (*MEN1*) gene. The European Consortium on MEN1. *Hum Mol Genet* **6**, 1177–83.
3. Thakker RV, et al. Clinical practice guidelines for multiple endocrine neoplasia type 1 (MEN1). *J Clin Endocrinol Metab* **97**, 2990–3011.
4. Turner JJ, et al. (2010). Diagnostic challenges due to phenocopies: lessons from multiple endocrine neoplasia type 1 (MEN1). *Hum Mutat* **31**, E1089–101.
5. Trouillas J, et al. (2008). Pituitary tumors and hyperplasia in multiple endocrine neoplasia type 1 syndrome (MEN1): a case-control study in a series of 77 patients versus 2509 non-MEN1 patients. *Am J Surg Pathol* **32**, 534–43.
6. de Laat JM, et al. (2015). Long-term natural course of pituitary tumors in patients with MEN1: results from the DutchMEN1 study group (DMSG). *J Clin Endocrinol Metab* **100**, 3288–96.
7. Pellegata NS, et al. (2006). Germ-line mutations in p27Kip1 cause a multiple endocrine neoplasia syndrome in rats and humans. *Proc Natl Acad Sci U S A* **103**, 15558–63.
8. Agarwal SK, et al. (2009). Rare germline mutations in cyclin-dependent kinase inhibitor genes in multiple endocrine neoplasia type 1 and related states. *J Clin Endocrinol Metab* **94**, 1826–34.
9. Korbonits M, et al. (2012). Familial pituitary adenomas: who should be tested for *AIP* mutations? *Clin Endocrinol (Oxf)* **77**, 351–6.
10. Trivellin G, et al. (2014). Gigantism and acromegaly due to Xq26 microduplications and *GPR101* mutation. *N Engl J Med* **371**, 2363–74.
11. Horvath A, Stratakis CA (2008). Clinical and molecular genetics of acromegaly: MEN1, Carney complex, McCune–Albright syndrome, familial acromegaly and genetic defects in sporadic tumors. *Rev Endocr Metab Disord* **9**, 1–11.
12. Forlino A, et al. (2014). *PRKACB* and Carney complex. *N Engl J Med* **370**, 1065–7.
13. O'Toole SM, et al. (2015). 15 years of paraganglioma: The association of pituitary adenomas and phaeochromocytomas or paragangliomas. *Endocr Relat Cancer* **22**, T105–22.
14. de Kock L, et al. (2014). Pituitary blastoma: a pathognomonic feature of germ-line *DICER1* mutations. *Acta Neuropathol* **128**, 111–22.

Table 13.2 Indications for gene testing

Gene	Indication for gene testing	Reference
MEN1	Patient with two or more MEN1-related manifestations	3
	Patient with one MEN1-related manifestation and a 1st-degree family member with MEN1	
	Patient with suspicious MEN1 (with parathyroid adenomas occurring before the age of 35 years; or multigland parathyroid disease, gastrinoma, or multiple pNETs at any age)	
	Patient with atypical MEN1—one classical and one non-classical manifestation (adrenal cortical tumour, carcinoid, facial angiofibroma, collagenoma, thyroid tumours, lipomatous tumour, and meningioma)	
	1st-degree relative of a MEN1 mutation carrier	
AIP	Patient with FIPA	9
	Patient with childhood-onset pituitary adenoma (primarily GH- and/or PRL-secreting) and no MEN1 and Carney complex-related family history	
	Young-onset (<30 years) macroadenoma patient (primarily GH- and/or PRL-secreting) and no MEN1 and Carney complex-related family history	
	1st-degree relative of an AIP mutation carrier	
GPR101 duplication	Patient with extreme growth starting before the age of 5 years and high IGF-1. Patient may have a pituitary adenoma, hyperplasia, or an apparently normal-sized pituitary gland on MRI	10
PRKAR1A	Patient with Carney complex	11
	Patient with a Carney complex-related manifestation and a 1st-degree family member with Carney complex	
	1st-degree relative of a PRKAR1A mutation carrier	
PRKACA duplication	Patient with Carney complex and −ve PRKAR1A sequencing and MLPA tests	12
SDHx and MAX	Patient with pituitary adenoma and PCC or PGL	13
DICER1	Infant (<2 years of age) with large pituitary tumour, usually ACTH-secreting. Personal or family history of manifestations of the DICER1 syndrome such as pleuropulmonary blastoma, cystic nephroma, young-onset multinodular goitre, sex cord tumours, etc.	14

Familial isolated pituitary adenoma

- FIPA is a genetically heterogeneous disease with an AD inheritance pattern, with incomplete penetrance in some of the conditions.
- Patients belonging to the FIPA group can be divided into three subgroups, based on their genotypes according to our current knowledge.
- The phenotypes of these three groups are considerably different.

AIP mutation-associated FIPA

- In 10–20% of FIPA families, a heterozygous germline mutation of the *AIP* gene can be detected.[1,2,3]
- Families with *AIP* mutations typically have at least one member with a GH-secreting tumour, and disease onset is significantly younger (mean age 20–24 years) in these patients, compared to *AIP* mutation −ve FIPA or sporadic pituitary adenoma groups.
- The disease most often manifests in adolescence, but childhood and young adult cases are also common.
- Patients usually have large aggressive adenomas.
  - Somatotroph adenomas often show a sparsely granulated pattern and poor response to SSA treatment.
  - The commonest pituitary adenomas are somatotroph, mammosomatotroph, and PRL-secreting tumours, followed by clinically non-functioning and rarely thyrotroph adenomas.
- The disease can also manifest in patients without apparent family history and their phenotype is not different from the familial cases (simplex cases). About 20% of childhood-onset, apparently sporadic hormone-secreting adenomas are caused by *AIP* mutations.

AIP is located at 11q13 and codes for a 330-amino acid protein. *AIP* is a tumour suppressor gene and LOH has been identified in many *AIP* mutation-related pituitary adenoma tissues. While a number of proteins have been identified to interact with AIP, the exact tumourigenic mechanism is not known. Over 100 different mutations have been described, the majority leading to a truncated protein, with a few genetic hotspots, the commonest being a stop mutation affecting amino acid 304 (p.R304*). This particular mutation has been identified in a large number of young-onset acromegaly patients, including one born in the eighteenth century, supporting the data that this is due to a founder effect about 100 generations ago.[4] No somatic mutations have been identified in somatotroph adenomas to date.

AIP testing indications are shown in Table 13.2. Awareness of *AIP* mutations in affected patients might help to predict the course of the disease[3] and could assist decisions on treatment options. As the only clinical manifestation of FIPA is a pituitary adenoma, the presence of pituitary incidentalomas (a common finding in up to 20% of the general population) could make clinical screening more difficult.

X-linked acrogigantism

A subset of patients with very young-onset gigantism harbour duplication of the G protein-coupled receptor gene *GPR101*, usually as part of a microduplication at Xq26.3.[5,6] This disease has a high and possibly full penetrance. Most cases develop the 1st signs by the age of 1 year and are diagnosed before the age of 5 years. Patients are characterized by extreme growth velocity and final height, unless treated. The majority of the patients are ♀ and harbour a *de novo* germline microduplication, while sporadic ♂ have mosaicism.[6,7,8] A few familial cases have also been described with mother-to-son transmission.[5,9] Patients have GH-secreting pituitary hyperplasia (sometimes with normal pituitary MRI) or adenoma, usually with PRL hypersecretion. Treatment is challenging as response to cabergoline and 1st-generation SSAs are incomplete, while pegvisomant in appropriate doses can normalize IGF-1. Surgery is usually only successful if all the pituitary tissue is removed, and radiotherapy has been successfully applied in some of the cases.[6,9]

FIPA with unknown genetic cause

In the 3rd and by far the largest group of FIPA families, no disease-causing mutation have been identified to date.[3] These patients have an age of onset considerably older than the other two FIPA groups, apparently not dissimilar to sporadic patients. Penetrance is low, less than in *AIP* mutation +ve cases. The clinical phenotype is also more variable. About half the families are homogenous (i.e. all family members have the same type of pituitary adenoma) where GH- or PRL-secreting adenomas predominate, with less non-functioning adenoma and exceptional ACTH-secreting adenoma families. Heterogeneous families can have different types of adenomas, although TSHomas are exceptionally rare. Suggestion for germline mutations in other genes has been suggested in some usually sporadic cases, but these have not been currently confirmed yet in various populations.[10,11]

References

1. Vieimaa O, *et al.* (2006). Pituitary adenoma predisposition caused by germline mutations in the *AIP* gene. *Science* **312**, 1228–30.
2. Daly AF, *et al.* (2010). Clinical characteristics and therapeutic responses in patients with germ-line *AIP* mutations and pituitary adenomas: an international collaborative study. *J Clin Endocrinol Metab* **95**, E373–83.
3. Marques P, *et al.*; FIPA Consortium (2020). Significant benefits of *AIP* testing and clinical screening in familial isolated and young-onset pituitary tumors. *J Clin Endocrinol Metab* **105**, e2247–60.
4. Chahal HS, *et al.* (2011). *AIP* mutation in pituitary adenomas in the 18th century and today. *N Engl J Med* **364**, 43–50.
5. Trivellin G, *et al.* (2014). Gigantism and acromegaly due to Xq26 microduplications and *GPR101* mutation. *N Engl J Med* **371**, 2363–74.
6. Iacovazzo D, *et al.* (2016). Germline or somatic *GPR101* duplication leads to X-linked acrogigantism: a clinico-pathological and genetic study. *Acta Neuropathol Commun* **4**, 56.
7. Daly AF, *et al.* (2016). Somatic mosaicism underlies X-linked acrogigantism syndrome in sporadic male subjects. *Endocr Relat Cancer* **23**, 221–33.
8. Rodd C, *et al.* (2016). Somatic *GPR101* duplication causing X-linked acrogigantism (XLAG)-diagnosis and management. *J Clin Endocrinol Metab* **101**, 1927–30.
9. Beckers A, *et al.* (2015). X-linked acrogigantism syndrome: clinical profile and therapeutic responses. *Endocr Relat Cancer* **22**, 353–67.
10. Hernandez-Ramirez LC, *et al.* (2017). Loss-of-function mutations in the *CABLES1* gene are a novel cause of Cushing's disease. *Endocr Relat Cancer* **24**, 379–92.
11. Zhang Q, *et al.* (2017). Germline mutations in *CDH23*, encoding cadherin-related 23, are associated with both familial and sporadic pituitary adenomas. *Am J Hum Genet* **100**, 817–23.

Carney complex

Carney complex is characterized by spotty skin pigmentation, cutaneous, mucosal, and atrial myxomas, and various endocrine overactivities, as well as other tumours (see also ➲ Chapter 14) (for a detailed review, see Horvath and Stratakis[1]). Diagnosis is made on clinical grounds. Disease penetrance is over 95% by the age of 50 years. Over 70% of all the cases and 80% of the cases involving adrenal Cushing's syndrome are caused by a heterozygous germline mutation in the *PRKAR1A* gene coding for the regulatory subunit of PKA.[2] *PRKAR1A* is located at 17q22-24 and consists of 384 amino acid residues, and is a typical tumour suppressor gene with LOH detected in many human tumour samples. Until now, over 110 mutations have been described, with the majority coding for a truncated protein, and nonsense-mediated decay of the mutant mRNA has been observed. ~10% of cases harbour large gene deletions. There is genotype–phenotype correlation, with large deletions causing more severe disease.[3] A single case has been described with ↑ copy number of the β catalytic subunit (*PRKACB*) of PKA.[4] In some of the *PRKAR1A* mutation −ve families, linkage studies point to the 2p16 locus. PKA is part of the cAMP pathway, which is activated by GHRH in somatotrophs, and other components of this pathway can also cause somatotroph adenomas (G protein α subunit, *GNAS*). Sequence variants in the *PDE11A* gene may have modifying effects on disease manifestations.

The pituitary gland is frequently (70%) affected in Carney complex, manifesting either as somatotroph and lactotroph hyperplasia, with abnormal IGF-1 and PRL levels and GH level dynamics, while true somatotroph or lactotroph adenomas occur only in a small (10%) proportion of the cases. Two cases have been described with corticotroph adenoma.[5,6]

Indications for genetic testing are listed in Table 13.2. It is suggested that family members are tested before the age of 6 months. Carrier family members benefit from early clinical screening, while family members free of the family-specific mutation do not need further follow-up.

References

1. Horvath A, Stratakis CA (2008). Clinical and molecular genetics of acromegaly: MEN1, Carney complex, McCune–Albright syndrome, familial acromegaly and genetic defects in sporadic tumors. *Rev Endocr Metab Disord* **9**, 1–11.
2. Kirschner LS, *et al.* (2000). Mutations of the gene encoding the protein kinase A type I-alpha regulatory subunit in patients with the Carney complex. *Nat Genet* **26**, 89–92.
3. Salpea P, *et al.* (2014). Deletions of the *PRKAR1A* locus at 17q24.2-q24.3 in Carney complex: genotype–phenotype correlations and implications for genetic testing. *J Clin Endocrinol Metab* **99**, E183–8.
4. Lodish MB, *et al.* (2015). Germline *PRKACA* amplification causes variable phenotypes that may depend on the extent of the genomic defect: molecular mechanisms and clinical presentations. *Eur J Endocrinol* **172**, 803–11.
5. Hernandez-Ramirez LC, *et al.* (2017). Corticotropinoma as a component of Carney complex. *J Endocr Soc* **1**, 918–25.
6. Kiefer FW, *et al.* (2017). *PRKAR1A* mutation causing pituitary-dependent Cushing disease in a patient with Carney complex. *Eur J Endocrinol* **177**, K7–12.

McCune–Albright syndrome

McCune–Albright syndrome is not a familial disease. It is caused by an embryonic genetic alteration which results in a mosaic condition (see also ➜ McCune-Albright syndrome, pp. 654–5). It is not transmitted to the offspring of affected subjects. The manifestations can be variable, depending on what stage of development the mutation occurred in and therefore how many organs and sites are affected. The diagnosis of McCune–Albright syndrome is established on clinical grounds, with patients having at least two features of the triad of polyostotic fibrous dysplasia, café-au-lait skin pigmentation, and autonomous endocrine hyperfunction, including precocious puberty, thyrotoxicosis, pituitary gigantism, and Cushing's syndrome. Pituitary disease in McCune–Albright syndrome occurs in 21% of the cases, of which around half manifest as GH- and PRL-producing cell hyperplasia while the other half have adenomas. The average age of onset is 24 years and acromegaly is almost always associated with skull base fibrous dysplasia. These patients are challenging to treat as a surgical approach is difficult; total hypophysectomy is usually needed, and response to radiotherapy and SSAs is poor, while GH antagonist treatment is promising.[1,2]

The disease is caused by an activating mutation in the stimulatory G protein α subunit coded by the *GNAS* gene located on 20q13. Gsα is a ubiquitously expressed 1037-amino acid protein; 15–40% of sporadic somatotroph adenomas carry a somatic *GNAS* mutation. Gsα activates adenylyl cyclase and leads to excess cAMP generation. Mutations in McCune–Albright syndrome usually affect arginine 201 (but usually not residue 227; somatic mutations in sporadic somatotroph adenomas can affect both residues 201 and 227). McCune–Albright syndrome is a clinical diagnosis and genetic testing is not routinely performed, although (90%) +ve from affected tissues. A sensitive method with ddPCR from leucocyte or cell free DNA testing can detect the mutation in the majority of patients.[3]

References

1. Akintoye SO, et al. (2006). Pegvisomant for the treatment of gsp-mediated growth hormone excess in patients with McCune–Albright syndrome. *J Clin Endocrinol Metab* **91**, 2960–6.
2. Salenave S, et al. (2014). Acromegaly and McCune–Albright syndrome. *J Clin Endocrinol Metab* **99**, 1955–69.
3. Romanet P, et al. (2019). Using digital droplet polymerase chain reaction to detect the mosaic *GNAS* mutations in whole blood DNA or circulating cell-free DNA in fibrous dysplasia and McCune–Albright syndrome. *J Pediatr* **205**, 281–5 e284.

SDHx mutation-related pituitary adenoma

The coexistence of pituitary adenoma and PGL or PCC is rare, but it has been described in a number of patients with mutations in *SDHx* genes, most commonly *SDHD* or *SDHB*, and in patients with large *MAX* gene deletions,[1,2] while pituitary adenoma and PCC can rarely be a feature of MEN1 syndrome.[1,3] The *SDHx* and *MAX*-related PitNETs are usually hormone-secreting (PRL and GH) macroadenomas with a relatively aggressive behaviour. A metastatic pituitary carcinoma has also been described.[4] An interesting histological feature of vacuolized cells has been observed in *SDHx* gene-related cases.

References

1. Dénes J, et al. (2015). Heterogeneous genetic background of the association of pheochromocytoma/paraganglioma and pituitary adenoma: results from a large patient cohort. *J Clin Endocrinol Metab* **100**, E531–41.
2. Daly AF, et al. (2018). Pheochromocytomas and pituitary adenomas in three patients with *MAX* exon deletions. *Endocr Relat Cancer* **25**, L37–42.
3. Xekouki P, et al. (2012). Succinate dehydrogenase (SDH) D subunit (SDHD) inactivation in a growth-hormone-producing pituitary tumor: a new association for SDH? *J Clin Endocrinol Metab* **97**, E357–66.
4. Tufton N, et al. (2017). Pituitary carcinoma in a patient with an *SDHB* mutation. *Endocr Pathol* **28**, 320–5.

DICER1 syndrome

Heterozygous germline mutations in *DICER1* are associated with ↑ risk for pleuropulmonary blastoma, cystic nephroma, nasal chondromesenchymal hamartoma, ovarian Sertoli–Leydig cell tumours, botryoid embryonal rhabdomyosarcoma of the uterine cervix, ciliary body medulloepithelioma, pineoblastoma, mesenchymal hamartoma,[1] nodular thyroid hyperplasia or thyroid carcinoma, and pituitary blastoma. These tumours could present in isolation or as a syndromic disease. Pituitary blastoma, originally described in 2008 as a separate entity and pathognomic to DICER1 syndrome,[2] is a low-penetrance (<1%), potentially lethal early childhood (7–24 months old) ACTH-secreting tumour of the pituitary gland. The tissue has an embryonic appearance and previous cases had 40% lethality.[3, 4]

References

1. Apellaniz-Ruiz M, et al. (2019). Mesenchymal hamartoma of the liver and DICER1 syndrome. *N Engl J Med* **380**, 1834–42.
2. Scheithauer BW, et al. (2008). Pituitary blastoma. *Acta Neuropathol* **116**, 657–66.
3. de Kock L, et al. (2014). Pituitary blastoma: a pathognomonic feature of germ-line *DICE5R1* mutations. *Acta Neuropathol* **128**, 111–22.
4. Liu APY, et al. (2021). Clinical outcomes and complications of pituitary blastoma. *J Clin Endocrinol and Metab* **106**, 351–63.

Practical and nursing aspects of endocrine conditions

Anne Marland and *Mike Tadman*

Introduction

Endocrinology nursing is an ever-evolving specialty. This chapter aims to provide expert, innovative practice-based nursing information, underpinned by evidence/research, and complements other chapters of this handbook. It is a comprehensive guide for all nurses working within endocrinology.

Endocrine nursing focuses on a patient-centred approach, thus enhancing the quality and level of care, and recognizes nurses as having a role as a pivotal and equal member within the MDT. Recent developments include the development of autonomous advance nurse practice, which includes prescribing, history taking, physical assessment, and development of nurse-led clinics (NLC). The competency framework for adult endocrine nursing is an excellent recommended educational resource to underpin development within the role and to offer clinical guidance (Kieffer et al 2015)[1].

Reference

1. Kieffer V, *et al.* (2015) Competency framework for adult endocrine nursing: 2nd edition. Society for Endocrinology. *Endocr Connect* **4**, W1–W17.

Thyroid

The endocrine nurse plays an important role in the management of hyperthyroidism and antithyroid drug therapy (ATDT). This includes offering a clear, reassuring explanation of treatment options and commonly used medications, individualized and adapted to the needs of the patient. Websites and written information should be provided in order to reinforce verbal explanation.

Explanation of common treatment options include: carbimazole, PTU, propranolol, radioiodine treatment options, and thyroidectomy (see ➔ Chapter 1).

The nurse should advise and reassure on key points of thyroid disorders, for example: medications prescribed (ensure patient is not asthmatic—contraindicatory to propranolol) and other allergies documented. Explanation of side effects and key points to look out for that require reporting include:

- Sore throat.
- Fever.
- Bruising.
- Mouth ulcers (agranulocytosis).
- Analgesia for pain associated with neck swelling (paracetamol).
- Awareness of eye swelling (ophthalmopathy):
  - (Graves' disease) and for the patient to report promptly in order to facilitate a referral to ophthalmology.
- Pregnancy: should be avoided when using ATDT. If the patient becomes pregnant, then swift referral to the endocrine/obstetrics team.

Thyroid surgery

Endocrine nurses play an important role in the safe preparation of a patient for surgery. This includes encouraging self-administration of medication and educating the patient on safe preparation for surgery. Links should be provided to websites (e.g. British Thyroid Foundation, Thyroid Eye Disease Charitable Trust), and other suitable information provided for the individualized requirements of each patient. This can be a very stressful time for a patient and a strong rapport with the endocrine team will aid in recovery.

Post-operatively, the endocrine nurse will probably see the patient a few weeks after surgery. Key point is to check the wound site, and once completely healed, advise on the use of Bio-Oil® which, when massaged over the well-healed site, will minimize scarring. Concordance with medication again is vital and to be encouraged, and psychological support again is necessary.

Further reading

British Thyroid Association. ℜ https://www.british-thyroid-association.org/
Society for Endocrinology. ℜ https://www.endocrinology.org/
Thyroid Eye Disease Charitable Trust. ℜ http://tedct.org.uk/

Pituitary function

The nurse is key in facilitating investigation, performing tests, and providing education. Psychological support is vital in the diagnostic period when there are many uncertainties for patients. The diagnostic path may be lengthy and follow-up may be lifelong, and it is imperative the nurse is knowledgeable and empowering in order to enable safe preparation and interpretation of the results of investigations. Well-informed, emotionally supported patients often have improved outcomes.

Dynamic tests

Dynamic function tests are carried out as per protocol of each endocrine centre. Many tests are complex and the nurse must be knowledgeable in all aspects of testing, including: safe patient preparation; facilitation of the test; and interpretation of the results. If a nurse is more junior, they must be supported by a senior member of the clinical team. It is recommended, if possible, that clear written information is provided to the patient pretest in order to reduce anxiety and to provide clear instruction on omission of medication and nil by mouth—this is to ensure the test is carried out correctly and safely.

Complex dynamic tests with special considerations

- Informed consent should be obtained for all tests where a pharmacological agent is injected IV or SC.
- Be aware of tests where other medications may interfere with the interpretation of the test results, e.g. oral oestrogens and inhaled/topical steroids for SST (also contraindications with asthma).
- Saline infusion test: suitable antihypertensives presaline infusion test (recent K >3; BP stable); if low K, commence on K supplements.
- ITT (age/normal ECG/concise medical history/cortisol level): test performed by senior healthcare practitioners/two staff members available at all time/rescue equipment available).

Specialist nurse management

Acromegaly
The nurse is involved in the diagnostic testing for acromegaly and discussing treatment options, and plays an active role in the facilitation of dose adjustments, which include dose reduction/increase and dose extension. The main points of consideration are the psychological effects of excessive GH production and the physical issues. Substantial psychological changes are usually present at the time of presentation and a careful plan of care should be implemented. Many patients suffer from an altered body image and experience cognitive dysfunction. Many experience bodily pain, physical dysfunction, and headaches. The patient may go through complex changes in pathways of care and requires support at each point of intervention, e.g. medical therapy, surgery, radiotherapy.

- SSAs are given IM or deep IM, and the nurse may be involved in the administration in hospital settings. The nurse must be educated in safe administration, and information is now widely available (websites on, for example, octreotide/lanreotide). Home care can also be accessed for the patient through collaboration and primary care. The nurse will need to liaise with GP practices regarding training and prescriptions.

- GH receptor antagonists (pegvisomant): very often self-administered by the patient. Careful training should be provided and home care services can be used (as above).
- Education around travel and safe storage of medicines should be provided to the patient, along with practical tips on safe self-administration. There are patient support services available from the Pituitary Foundation and also directly from pharmaceutical companies that manufacture the medications.
- Injection site problems are well documented with all formulations; this includes lipodystrophy, sterile abscess, skin irritation, local discomfort, and lipoatrophy. Patients require reassurance and it is well documented that well-educated patients with balanced expectations have improved outcomes.

Cushing's disease
(See ➲ Definition of Cushing's disease, p. 178.)

Cushing's disease is a serious condition associated with significant morbidity and impacts on patients' QoL. Mortality in patients with Cushing's disease is more than twice than in patients with non-functioning adenomas, implying excess cortisol overexposure contributes to ↑ mortality risk. The nurse's role is vital in all aspects of patient management, especially patient education and psychological support. The nurse is pivotal in facilitating a multidisciplinary approach/referral in the management of comorbidities.

- Common comorbidities and nursing considerations are: sleep dysfunction, weight management, nutrition, and psychological issues.
- The nurse's role includes psychological support through the pathway of treatment for Cushing's disease; this may or will include:
  - Medical therapy: education on medicine used and explanation of possible side effects; psychological support; the aim is for concordance with medication.
  - Surgical treatment (adenomectomy/pituitary surgery): pre- and post-operative preparation, in line with local protocol. Psychological support offered to patient (see ➲ Pituitary surgery, pp. 820–1).
  - Adrenalectomy: offers immediate resolution of hypercortisolism; however, it is essential the patient receives steroid education and understands sick day rules, as now adrenal-insufficient and at risk of adrenal crisis (see ➲ Acute/severe recurrent illness, p. 147). Recommend patient obtains MedicAlert® jewellery and carries a steroid card.
  - Radiation treatment: given in cases of persistent disease to control hypercortisolism. The patient requires psychological support and information to enable safe preparation pretherapy. Psychological support can be accessed through engagement with clinical psychology services. There is also a wealth of support provided by support groups.
  - Patients require long-term follow-up with nurses and all disciplines, and many again require long-term psychological support, as the effects of hypercortisolism are well documented. Many patients have great difficulty in living with a normal level of steroid replacement and remain very anxious. The nurse is integral in building an empowering relationship, creating trust and reinforcement of the clinical pathway.

Further reading

Society for Endocrinology. *Advice for patients who take replacement steroids (hydrocortisone, prednisolone, dexamethasone or plenadren) for pituitary/adrenal insufficiency.* ℛ https://pituitary.org.uk/media/602862/SfE-COVID-advice-statement-28-Apr.pdf

Growth hormone deficiency in adults

The endocrine nurse has an important role in GH diagnosis/initiation, and monitoring and knowledge around the complexities of the diagnosis are imperative.

Criteria for GH treatment in adults are clearly set by NICE (2003) in the UK.

Associated adverse features of GHD in adults are shown in Box 14.1. They may be present in variable degrees in any individual.

> **Box 14.1 Adverse features of growth hormone deficiency in adults**
> • Reduced QoL.
> • Reduced energy levels.
> • Altered body composition:
>   • Reduced lean mass.
>   • ↑ fat mass, especially in the trunk.
> • Osteopenia/osteoporosis.
> • Dry skin (reduced sweating).
> • Reduced muscle strength and exercise capacity.
> • Lipid abnormalities (especially elevated LDL-C).
> • Insulin resistance.
> • ↑ levels of fibrinogen and plasminogen activator inhibitor.
> • Reduced extracellular fluid (ECF) volume.
> • ↑ thickness of intima media of blood vessels.
> • Impaired cardiac function.

Patients who should be under clinical supervision for developing GHD are shown in Box 14.2.

> **Box 14.2 Patients who should be under medical supervision**
> • Patients with known or suspected hypothalamic or pituitary disease.
> • Patients who have received cranial irradiation.
> • Patients with a deficiency of one or more of the other pituitary hormones.
> • Patients who have undergone hypophysectomy.
> • Adults who received GH in childhood for GHD.

Isolated GHD is the commonest pituitary hormone deficiency and can result from congenital or acquired causes, although the majority of cases are idiopathic with no identifiable aetiology (see ℘ https://www.nice.org.uk/guidance/ta64).

Diagnosis and provocative tests: who to test and when

Nurse considerations

- *Single dynamic test required:* patients with severe GHD in adulthood are defined as patients with known hypothalamic–pituitary abnormality and at least one known deficiency of another pituitary hormone, excluding PRL. These patients should undergo a single dynamic diagnostic test in order to diagnose the presence of GHD.
- *Two confirmatory diagnostic tests required:* in patients with childhood-onset isolated GHD (no evidence of hypothalamic–pituitary abnormality or cranial irradiation), two diagnostic tests should be recommended, except for those having low IGF-1 (a marker of GH response) concentrations (SD score <−2), who may be considered for one test.

Tests for diagnosis of GH deficiency

- The ITT is regarded as the 'gold standard' test for adults. The protocol should be followed as per individual unit guidelines.
- A general definition of severe GHD in adults is a peak concentration of <9mU/L (3ng/mL) in response to insulin-induced hypoglycaemia.
- When the ITT is contraindicated in patients over 60 years and those with a cardiac history, brain injury, or previous craniotomy/risk of seizure, other tests—glucagon, GH-releasing hormone + arginine—can be used.

When to test

- Diagnostic test after stabilized treatment of other pituitary deficiencies (at least 3 months).
- Diagnostic test at least 1 month after pituitary surgery.
- Transition at approximately age 18 when the epiphyses have fused/final height achieved (see ➋ Chapter 8).

Transition from child to adult nurse considerations

Transition from paediatric to adult care is an important time to re-evaluate GH status. Once final height is achieved, GH secretion should be retested as a significant percentage of patients with GHD in childhood subsequently have normal GH secretion in adulthood. In those patients with confirmed GHD, continuation of GH treatment through the late adolescent years into early adulthood is recommenced in order to complete somatic development. When height velocity has ↓ to <1.5–2.0cm/year, GH should be discontinued for 6–8 weeks.

From the nurse's perspective, it is always necessary to explain fully to the patient that continuing with GH is important. This is also important for children diagnosed with GHD at an older age, even when already into the transition period, as the patient's expectation is that it is essential for growth velocity alone. This is where a multidisciplinary approach is essential and a transition clinic should be in place. Patients require a full explanation of the continued effects of GH on lipids and body composition, the physiological effects in order to achieve peak bone mass, and the QoL effects and possible reduction in energy and mood. Psychological support is essential at this time to patient and family to assist in a smooth pathway into adult services.

Dose and administration in adult GHD nurse considerations

- Treatment is self-administered by a daily SC injection. Generally, the initial dose is 0.2–0.3mg (0.6–0.9IU) daily (typically 0.27mg, or 0.8IU, daily). The starting dose may differ and the nurse should follow the clinical/prescribed care pathway for their clinical setting.
- For the first 2–3 months, dosage adjustments are made after monthly assessments of serum levels of IGF-1 and in response to the presence of adverse effects, until a maintenance dose is achieved. The currently used median maintenance dose is 0.4mg (1.2IU) daily.
- GH requirements may decrease with age, mirroring the physiological production of GH.
- GH is a SC injection that is self-administered by the patient in the evening in order to mimic normal physiological pulse of GH. Various brands are available and local commissioning protocol/shared care should be followed in each individual case. The nurse is responsible for education of a safe injection technique and for monitoring of injection sites and providing relevant equipment. The nurse is vital in offering psychological support to aid in concordance with medication.

Adverse effects
- Fluid retention (peripheral oedema) is the most commonly reported 'side effect' of GH replacement therapy. Fluid retention, with occasional mild ankle oedema, is a normal part of GH action. This tends to decrease as therapy continues but may occasionally require dose reduction.
- Hyperglycaemia and hypoglycaemia have been reported. GH therapy has also been shown to reduce insulin sensitivity in these patients by antagonizing the action of insulin—this could increase the risk of DM.
- Headache. Persistent headaches require investigation, with fundoscopy for papilloedema recommended if severe or recurrent headache, visual problems, or nausea and vomiting occur. If papilloedema is confirmed, consider benign intracranial hypertension (rare cases reported). This is usually recognized shortly after commencement of therapy. Usually a temporary cessation of treatment resolves the symptoms. A severe and persistent headache should be reported immediately to the endocrinology department.
- Arthralgia (joint pain), myalgia (muscle pain), carpal tunnel syndrome, and paraesthesiae can occur. These effects, if they occur, are usually mild and self-limiting. A reduction in the GH dose may be required while they persist.
- Hypothyroidism can occur, and regular biochemical monitoring of thyroid function is essential and adjustments to medication prudent.
- Reactions at injection site—these are unusual and may also be due to unnecessary use of a spirit-based skin cleanser, which is not recommended.
- Antibody formation can be detected but is rarely of physiological relevance.
- Other side effects may include mild hypertension, visual problems, and nausea and vomiting.

- All of these possible side effects will have been discussed with the patient by the endocrine team before treatment is started and an information leaflet provided.
- There is no evidence to suggest that GH therapy will increase the risk of abnormal or neoplastic growth, either a new growth or a resurgence of an old tumour.

Contraindications
- GH treatment is contraindicated in people with any evidence of tumour activity, those with proliferative diabetic retinopathy, critically ill patients (e.g. after complications following open heart or abdominal surgery, multiple trauma, acute respiratory failure or similar conditions), and also patients with known hypersensitivity to GH or to any of the excipients.
- In patients with tumours, antitumour therapy must be completed before starting GH therapy.
- In pregnancy and lactation.

Common drug interactions
- Corticosteroids: the growth-promoting effect of somatropin may be inhibited by corticosteroids.
- Oestrogens: ↑ doses of GH may be needed when given with oestrogens (when used as oral replacement therapy).

Monitoring

A recognized technique for monitoring the dose of GH is to take regular measurements of IGF-1. IGF-1 levels should increase during therapy. IGF-1 levels should normally be maintained within the normal range during therapy. The aim is to find the dose of GH which moves IGF-1 levels into the normal range, ideally into mid/upper of the reference range.
- The patient will require 4- to 8-weekly IGF-1 blood tests until the optimum maintenance dose is reached.
- Adjustment of the dose where appropriate, and discussion with the patient of any adverse effects experienced.
- Re-evaluation of compliance/concordance and retraining with injection device if required. Monitoring of patient self-administration and observation of injection sites.

Regular clinical and biochemistry assessment should occur 1- to 2-monthly initially:
- Height, weight, and BMI.
- BP.
- HbA1c.
- Lipid profile.
- Serum IGF-1.
- Body composition measurement (Tanita bioimpedance).
- Waist:hip ratio.
- Assessment of QoL (AGHDA).
- Monitoring patient's overall health and well-being.
- Long-term monitoring.
- Pituitary imaging (MRI scan, as appropriate).
- DXA scan 3-yearly.

Steroid education of the patient with adrenal insufficiency

The endocrine nurse is vital in providing education to patients and families in order to optimize replacement therapy and minimize complications of over/under-replacement. It is crucial that patients are empowered with the knowledge of how to manage intercurrent illness and reduce the risk of an adrenal crisis. Nurses also have a role in the education of other healthcare professionals and are a useful resource to our colleagues in other areas, e.g. oncology where treatment causes endocrinopathies/AI.

Steroid teaching evenings can be implemented by endocrine units and evaluated to ensure a strong approach to steroid education.

(See Figs. 3.4 and 3.5 for the new NHS steroid card and sick day rules, respectively.)

Prolonged fasting—Ramadan

During the month of Ramadan, Muslims abstain from eating/drinking/taking oral medication from predawn to sunset. This can put patients at risk. Therefore, it is important that patients are well educated on the management of AI and are aware of alternatives to regular hydrocortisone while fasting. A longer-acting formula, e.g. Plenadren® 20mg or prednisolone 4–5mg at dawn pre-fast, is a recommendation. Practical guidance is outlined by Hussain et al. (2020).[1]

Shift working/air travel

Patients with AI who work shifts or have a change in sleep pattern, i.e. due to air travel, will disturb their cortisol circadian rhythm. The role of the nurse involves education of the patient and facilitating a clinical pathway to follow. Steroid replacement should follow the wake–sleep pattern, i.e. the 1st dose on waking and the last dose no later than before 4–5h of sleep. A short-acting formulation is preferable, as a long-acting formula may result in risk of glucose intolerance and impaired quality of sleep. For example, an emergency worker called in the night must supplement their wake time with an extra dose of hydrocortisone, e.g. 10mg, on being called out and another 5mg if out for 5h or more. This is crucial in preventing an adrenal crisis.

References

1. Hussain S, et al. (2020). Fasting with adrenal insufficiency: practical guidance for healthcare professionals managing patients on steroids during Ramadan. *Clin Endocrinol (Oxf)* **93**, 87–96.

Visual field deficits

Endocrine patients can commonly present with, or develop, visual field deficits. The visual field examination determines the extent of compression to the optic nerve. For driving guidelines, see Box 14.3.

> **Box 14.3 Minimum standards for field of vision—all drivers**
>
> - The minimum field of vision for Group 1 driving is defined in the legislation:
>   - A field of at least 120° on the horizontal measured using a target equivalent to the white Goldmann IIl4e settings.
>   - The extension should be at least 50° left and right. In addition, there should be no significant defect in the binocular field that encroaches within 20° of the fixation above or below the horizontal meridian.
> - This means that homonymous or bitemporal defects that come close to fixation, whether hemianopic or quadrantanopic, are not usually acceptable for driving.
> - If the DVLA needs a visual field assessment for determining fitness to drive, it:
>   - Requires the method to be a binocular Esterman field test.
>   - May request monocular full-field charts in specific conditions.
>   - Exceptionally may consider a Goldmann perimetry assessment carried out to strict criteria.
>
> The Secretary of State's Honorary Medical Advisory Panel for Visual Disorders and Driving advises that, for an Esterman binocular chart to be considered reliable for licensing, the false +ve score must be no more than 20%. When assessing monocular charts and Goldmann perimetry, fixation accuracy will also be considered.

Patients require education and advice in regard to driving and will often require psychological support to manage this situation (℞ https://www.gov.uk/visual-field-defects-and-driving).

Pituitary surgery

Preoperative

The nurse plays an important role in preparing the patient preoperatively and being a link between disciplines within the MDT. There are various surgical approaches and knowledge of each approach is pertinent to the nurse in caring for the patient (the usual approach is transsphenoidal). Very often, it is the nurse who can provide a clear concise explanation post-MDT meeting and it is encouraged that the nurse is present with the patient during the MDT meeting. Psychological support should be offered, and through building a rapport with the patient, this enables a safe preoperative preparation. Each unit should follow their relevant protocol which will include: ECG, visual fields, blood analysis, observations, allergies recorded, and comprehensive history taking, with current hormone dysfunction noted.

Post-operative—example of NLC pathway

The endocrine nurse is usually involved at day 8 post-op when the patient will attend the endocrine unit. The usual pathway is a further review at 6 weeks post-operatively and then an outpatient review at 4 months.

Key points: 8 days post-operatively
- Visual field test: compare to preop and report promptly to medical colleagues if any change.
- Blood analysis as per unit guidelines. Recommended:
  - FBC, U&E, morning cortisol, pituitary profile, plasma osmolality, paired with urine for osmolality.
- Patients should attend at 8.30 a.m., having omitted their previous evening dose and morning dose of hydrocortisone if well.
- Hydrocortisone must not be omitted if the patient is unwell, in the case of craniotomy, or in Cushing's patients (see ➜ Special situations, p. 822).
- Awareness of symptoms of DI: polyuria, polydipsia, excessive thirst, hypotensive, pyrexia.
- CSF leak: presents with clear, odourless rhinorrhoea. Salty, metallic, bitter taste in mouth.
- Infection (risk of meningitis): headache, pyrexia, photophobia, vomiting, lethargy.
- Educate patient on self-care at home and avoiding lifting, blowing the nose, coughing, and picking the nose (transsphenoidal approach).
- Psychological support and discussion/advice on return to work, etc.

Blood results and actions
- If FT3 and FT4 low, commence levothyroxine.
- If cortisol >350mmol/L, stop hydrocortisone.
- If cortisol <350mml/L, continue hydrocortisone, with standard sick day rules (see ➜ Steroid education, p. 818).

Key points: 6 weeks post-operatively
- Blood analysis as per unit guidelines. Recommended:
  - FBC, U&E, lipid profile, pituitary profile, SST, plasma osmolality, and copeptin, paired with urine for osmolality. Visual fields are only carried out if fields at the 8-day review were not normal or the patient describes a new visual field defect.
- Once all results are available, the patient's case and histology should be reviewed within an MDT meeting and the patient informed of the outcome. Pituitary MDT.

Four-month clinic review
- The patient is reviewed in the endocrinology clinic at 4 months post-surgery. At this stage, their case will have been reviewed in the pituitary MDT and a plan made regarding ongoing treatment.
- The 4-month review is particularly important for optimizing the patient's pituitary profile, e.g.:
  - If the patient fails their SST at the 6-week review, this may be repeated at the 4-month review.
  - If the patient has been commenced on levothyroxine post-operatively, this could be withheld for 1 week prior to the 4-week review and blood tests repeated in clinic.
  - Testosterone replacement may be discussed if appropriate.
  - At the 4-month review, a decision is made as to whether the patient will be discharged back to the referring clinician (if appropriate) or remain under the endocrinology team.

Special situations

Craniotomy

- The majority of patients have pituitary surgery performed via the transsphenoidal route. This is associated with excellent outcomes and shorter hospital admissions.
- A minority of patients may need to have pituitary surgery via craniotomy, e.g. if the tumour is difficult to access or they are having redo surgery. This is a more significant surgical procedure, and patients will typically remain in hospital for longer.
- *Craniotomy patients must not have their hydrocortisone stress dose reduced.* They should remain on hydrocortisone 20/10/10mg until their 8-day review, and *should not* omit their hydrocortisone on the evening prior to, and morning of, their review.
- Following assessment at the 8-day review, the patient may reduce the hydrocortisone dose to 10/5/5mg if well. All craniotomy patients will remain on hydrocortisone until their 6-week review.

Cushing's disease (example of NLC pathway)

Preoperative care

- Patients with Cushing's disease are at ↑ risk of developing thrombosis. For this reason, they should be on prophylactic dalteparin. This should be stopped 2 days prior to pituitary surgery. If the patient is on metyrapone, this also should be stopped 2 days prior to pituitary surgery.

Post-operative care

- Early morning cortisol levels should be checked on days 2 and 3 after surgery. A cortisol level of <50nmol/L implies cure and such patients should be commenced on hydrocortisone 20/10/10mg.
- Cortisol results and the clinical status of the patient should be assessed on a daily basis post-operatively, as the hydrocortisone replacement may need individualizing and it may be inappropriate to await repeat results on day 3 prior to hydrocortisone commencement. Days 2/3 9 a.m. cortisol <100mmol/L is still indicative of significant resection/cure of a corticotroph adenoma. If post-operative cortisol levels remain high, this will need discussion with the neurosurgical team, as further surgery/total hypophysectomy may be considered at an early stage.

Post-discharge care

- Patients with Cushing's disease should remain on prophylactic dalteparin for 4 weeks after their operation, as the ↑ risk of clotting seems to be maintained for some time.
- Patients with Cushing's disease and DM on insulin may experience reduced insulin requirements after successful surgery. A careful medication review is therefore essential prior to discharge.
- Hydrocortisone should be gradually weaned, with the aim of the patient being on 10/5/5mg by the time of the 6-week review. If they pass the SST, they should then proceed to overnight dexamethasone suppression test (ODST) to ensure cure.

Diabetes insipidus

- DI is one of the commonest complications of pituitary surgery. The onset of symptoms is usually abrupt, within 12–24h of surgery. In many cases, the condition will be transient, but a minority of patients will be permanently affected and this is more likely if the stalk was disrupted during surgery.
- It can also occur due to infiltrative/inflammatory conditions (see ➔ Diabetes insipidus, pp. 230–4).
- DI is diagnosed on the basis of polyuria (typically >3L/24h), dilute urine (osmolality <300mOsm/kg), and high plasma osmolality (>295mOsm/kg). If access to fluid is unrestricted and the patient's thirst response is intact, plasma Na may remain within the normal range. For patients on fluid restriction, hypernatraemia may be observed.
- If a patient becomes polyuric post-operatively (>200mL/h for 3 consecutive hours), appropriate management is:
  - Urgent U&E, copeptin, plasma and urine osmolality.
  - Relax fluid restriction: patient can drink to thirst.
  - If biochemistry suggestive of DI, administer 1 microgram of desmopressin.
  - Strict fluid balance.
- If a patient become polyuric again once parenteral desmopressin wears off, they may require regular desmopressin. If symptoms occur following discharge, the patient should be admitted to their nearest hospital for urgent assessment as above.
- Patients will need regular blood tests and monitoring while desmopressin doses are being titrated, and either need to remain in hospital or have a clear plan for regular outpatient blood tests, as they are at risk of hyponatraemia.
- If a patient is discharged on desmopressin, they should be advised to delay a dose at least once a week until aquaresis is achieved, to minimize the risk of hyponatraemia, pending their next blood test.
- Patients established on desmopressin prior to surgery require an individualized decision about whether a trial off treatment may be appropriately post-operatively.
- Poorly managed DI can be life-threatening, with fluid overload leading to hyponatraemia or lack of access to fluid and withheld desmopressin (e.g. during hospital admission) associated with recent in-hospital deaths.
- Patients must be informed that they should always ensure endocrine review when admitted to hospital in order to avoid inadvertent discontinuation of desmopressin.
- In patients without an adequate thirst axis (e.g. hypothalamic damage), close nursing/medical supervision with daily weights and patient education is even more crucial.

Male fertility

Fertility in males and initiating treatment

A nurse with advanced skills in this rare area is well placed to aid in the facilitation of treatment of fertility in ♂.

Fertility treatment is conducted in patients with HH due to pituitary dysfunction. HH is failure of the testes to produce adequate amounts of testosterone, spermatozoa, or both due to underlying pituitary disease.

Testosterone therapy may inhibit spermatogenesis (if this was not already affected). Men with HH would normally require therapy with gonadotrophins if fertility is desired.

Responsibilities (example of a possible pathway)

Consultant

- Only an endocrine consultant can refer a patient to have fertility treatment. The medication used is prescribed off licence by the endocrine consultant.
- The endocrine consultant is responsible for checking that the patient meets the criteria to start fertility treatment (HH due to pituitary dysfunction, partner fertility has been investigated, and physical exploration if required).
- Then refer the patient to the endocrine specialist nurse (ESN) to organize the pathway of care.
- The consultant is responsible for prescribing.

Two medications are normally prescribed

- Cautions: severe anaphylactic reaction, prostate cancer, breast cancer. Polycythaemia.

Menopur® (menotrophin)

Usual dose 75U or 150U, three times a week: Mondays, Wednesdays, and Fridays. This medication comes in a multidose vial that the patient will inject as advised.

- Possible side effects:
  - *Common or very common:* GI discomfort; headache; nausea.
  - *Uncommon:* breast abnormalities; diarrhoea; dizziness; fatigue; hot flush; vomiting.
  - *Rare or very rare:* skin reactions.

Ovitrelle®

- 250 micrograms prefilled syringe (choriogonadotropin alfa), normally the patient will take one dose twice a week: Tuesdays and Thursdays. Some patients take their medication on different times, e.g. once a week or once every 10 days, as the doctor advises.
- Possible side effects:
  - *Common or very common:* abdominal pain; fatigue; headache; nausea; vomiting.
  - *Uncommon:* breast pain; depression; diarrhoea; irritability; restlessness.
  - *Rare or very rare:* rash; shock; thromboembolism.

Endocrine specialist nurse considerations and responsibilities
- It is the ESN's responsibility to explain the medication and administration to the patient.
- The medication is to be self-administered by the patient only.
- The ESN will monitor the patient for side effects and liaise with the consultant.
- Liaise with the patient to have blood analysis and ask the doctor to review the results and to provide follow-up and a plan of care.
- Bloods tests and sperm count to be reviewed by a consultant; however, explained by the ESN and psychological support offered as some patients find sperm collection an emotional challenge.

Before start of treatment
- Testosterone, FBC, LFTs, PSA, and sperm count.
- If the patient is on regular testosterone therapy, they will need to stop before they start fertility treatment. Short-acting medications, e.g. gels, need to be stopped 24h before the test. For long-acting medications, e.g. Nebido®, the patient will need to wait until the medication is no longer active before starting fertility treatment.
- If testosterone is high, repeat blood tests weekly until bloods is on target; ideally testosterone needs to be in the low third of the normal range.

After starting treatment
- Blood tests for testosterone and FBC are required 1–2 weeks after the medication is started.
- Regular blood tests for testosterone, FBC, LFTs, U&E, PSA, and sperm counts may be required 3-monthly. Patients are advised to have a sperm count before their endocrine clinic appointment and that they bring the results with them to the appointment, if possible.
- Patients are responsible for organizing the sperm count with their GP, if possible.

Completing treatment
- Usually funding in the UK will cover 12 months of treatment; after this period, treatment will need to be assessed by the consultant to evaluate progress.
- If pregnancy is achieved, treatment will be stopped in the 1st trimester of pregnancy.
- It is highly recommended to inform the patient about sperm banking options in the fertility clinic; this service requires direct contact by the patient privately.
- Patients and their partners undergoing fertility treatment require psychological support.

Testosterone replacement

It is becoming more usual for a suitably qualified nurse to facilitate testosterone replacement. However, certain levels of competency must be achieved to facilitate an often complex pathway. Patients may suffer with complex psychological issues around sexuality/self-image and require psychological support alongside the clinical pathway.

Low testosterone (hypogonadism) is associated with a number of symptoms and signs. Symptoms include sexual dysfunction, loss of energy, fatigue, depression, decrease in cognitive ability, and irritability. Low testosterone can also have −ve effects on bone mass, which results in a significant risk of osteoporosis in hypogonadal men. Progressive reduction in muscle mass and red blood cell mass may also be a symptom of low testosterone in men. In general, clinical manifestations of hypogonadism depend on the age at onset and the severity and duration of the deficiency. Patients can experience one or many of these symptoms and signs.

The causes for low testosterone may be either 1°, i.e. gonadal failure, or 2° to hypothalamic or pituitary disease. 1° hypogonadism is seen in Klinefelter's syndrome, which is a common condition occurring in 1:700 ♂ births, or following radiotherapy, chemotherapy, infection, or surgery to the testicles. 2° causes are normally related to pituitary dysfunction (tumour, irradiation, surgery, inflammation, and infiltrative process).

Testosterone therapy may inhibit spermatogenesis (if this was not already affected). Men with HH would normally require therapy with gonadotrophins if fertility is desired (see ➔ Male fertility, pp. 824–5).

Various replacement medications are available (see ➔ Androgen replacement therapy pp. 418–20).

The nurse is pivotal in providing strategic support to the patient through education and facilitating treatment pathway options with the patient. The aim is to enable concordance with medication, develop coping strategies, and facilitate the reverse of many of the effects of low testosterone, i.e. low mood, low libido, ↓ sexual function, low muscle mass/strength, osteoporosis, and lack of facial/body hair.

IM Nebido® injection (testosterone undecanoate 1000mg/4mL) is a replacement that the nurse will commonly administer in the clinical setting and the following clinical operating considerations are recommended.

Responsibilities (example of NLC pathway)

- The requesting clinician or advanced nurse practitioner (ANP)/qualified prescriber must check that the patient meets the criteria for injection/treatment. It is the responsibility of this individual to review the results and action any follow-up requirements.
- It is the requesting clinician's/ANP's responsibility to explain to the patient the possible side effects of receiving Nebido® (see Table 14.3).
- The nurse is responsible for ensuring that the Nebido® injection is given correctly, following the protocol.
- The nurse is responsible for ensuring that pretest bloods have been reviewed if required (see Table 14.1).
- The nurse is responsible for checking the patient's bloods are within range prior to giving the injection (see Table 14.2).
- The requesting clinician/ANP and nurse will decide when the patient should be transferred back to the GP for ongoing treatment. Very often this is facilitated through a shared care agreement.

Cautions
- Risk of severe anaphylactic reaction, dyspnoea, and difficulty breathing if the medication is administered too quickly.
- Risks associated with complications arising from an IM injection.
- As with all oily solutions, Nebido® must be injected strictly IM and very slowly. Pulmonary microembolism of oily solutions can, in rare cases, lead to signs and symptoms such as cough, dyspnoea, malaise, hyperhidrosis, chest pain, dizziness, paraesthesiae, or syncope. These reactions may occur during or immediately after the injection and are reversible. Treatment is usually supportive, e.g. by administration of supplemental O_2 (🔗 https://www.medicines.org.uk/emc/files/pil.3873.pdf).

Commencing a patient on Nebido®
- Patients who are starting Nebido® for the 1st time must have stopped all other testosterone medications before starting Nebido®.
- If the patient has not had any previous testosterone therapy, then Nebido® may be started straight away as long as the blood results are within the correct parameters (see Table 14.2).
- Inform the patient of the possible side effects (see Table 14.3).

Procedure for Nebido® injection
Prior to giving Nebido® injection
- Check testosterone and FBC levels. Testosterone is recommended to be in the lower third of the normal range (8.7–15.0nmol/L). The Hct is recommended to be within the normal range or under 0.54L/L. Ensure the patient meets the criteria for carrying out the test; check medication and allergy status, and document. Ensure informed consent.
- The patient should be in a comfortable position for the injection on a bed. The bed should be completely flat and the patient's hands should be kept under their head. You should also remind the patient to remain still during the injection.

Where to administer the intramuscular injection
- The preferred site for the IM injection is the gluteus medius muscle, located in the upper outer quadrant of the buttock.
- Care must be taken to prevent the needle from hitting the superior gluteal artery and the sciatic nerve.
- Nebido® should not be split into portions and it should never be administered into the upper arm or the thigh.
- As with all oil-based solutions, Nebido® must be injected strictly IM and very slowly.
- It is recommended to inject Nebido® over ~2min.
- After selecting the injection site, cleanse the area with an alcohol wipe.
- If there is little muscle mass, you may need to pinch up 2–3 edges of the gluteal muscle to provide more volume and tissue to insert the needle.
- Insert the needle into the skin at a 90° angle to ensure it is deeply embedded in the muscle.
- Grasp the barrel of the syringe firmly with one hand. Using the other hand, pull the plunger back to aspirate for blood.
- If blood appears, do not proceed with the injection. Take the needle out of the patient immediately, and replace it with a new needle.

- Carefully repeat the steps for injection.
- If no blood is aspirated, hold the needle position to avoid any movement.
- Apply the injection very slowly by depressing the plunger carefully and at a constant rate until all the medication is delivered (ideally over 2min).
- If possible, use your free hand to probe manually or check for depot formation.
- Withdraw the needle and cover the injection site with a plaster.
- The patient should be observed during and immediately after each injection of Nebido® in order to allow for early recognition of possible signs and symptoms that may indicate pulmonary oil microembolism (POME) and suspected anaphylaxis.

Table 14.1 Nebido® regimen (sample pathway)

Time	Monitoring required	By whom	Looking for
Pretreatment	9 a.m. Testosterone, SHBG, oestradiol, FSH, LH, PSA, prolactin, FBC, lipids (TC, HDL-C, TGs) U&E, LFTs	GP or 2° care	Confirm diagnosis Contraindications to treatment Baseline Hct and PSA
1st injection	Testosterone, FBC before first injection	GP or 2° care	Rise in Hct, testosterone
2nd injection (6 weeks after 1st injection)	FBC and PSA before 2nd injection	GP or 2° care	Rise in Hct, testosterone
3rd injection (12 weeks after 2nd injection)	Testosterone + FBC and PSA before 3rd injection	GP or 2° care	Rise in Hct, testosterone
6–12 monthly review	Testosterone, FBC, PSA	GP or 2° care	Rise in Hct, testosterone, PSA

Table 14.2 Blood results—reference range

Testosterone	Lower third of normal range	<14 If it is ≥14, do not give Nebido®; discuss with requesting clinician
Hct	If <5.4, can give Nebido®	If ≥5.4, speak with referring clinician; patient may require venesection
Hb	130–150 If >180, escalate to doctor	Normally when Hb is high, so is Hct.
PSA	Check this has been done once a year	

Table 14.3 Side effects of Nebido®

Common side effects (may effect up to 1 in 10 patients	Solution
The commonest side effects are acne and pain where the injection is given	Alternating the injection site from left to right side helps to reduce the pain
Abnormally high levels of red blood cells	Inform the patient Venesection
Weight gain	
Hot flushes	
Acne	
Enlarged prostate and associated problems	Inform the patient this is monitored by measuring PSA every 6 months
Various reactions to where the injection was given (e.g. pain, bruising, or irritation)	Alternate the injection site
Uncommon side effects (may affect up to 1 in 100 patients)	**Solution**
Allergic reaction	Staff are trained in managing this if it occurs
↑ appetite, changes in blood test results, e.g. ↑ blood sugars or fats)	'Clinician is monitoring your bloods closely and will inform you of any changes'
Depression, emotional disorder, insomnia, restlessness, aggression, or irritability	Important patients are honest with how they are feeling when they are assessed Psychological support
Headache, migraine, or tremor	
Cardiovascular disorder, high BP, or dizziness	
Bronchitis, sinusitis, cough, shortness of breath, snoring, or voice problems	
Diarrhoea or nausea	
Changes in LFT results	
Hair loss or various skin reactions (e.g. itching, reddening, or dry skin)	
Joint pain, pain in limbs, muscle problems (e.g. spasm, pain, or stiffness), or ↑ creatine phosphokinase (CPK) in blood	
Urinary tract disorders (e.g. ↓ flow of urine, urinary retention, urge to pass urine at night)	

(Continued)

Table 14.3 *(Contd.)*

Common side effects (may effect up to 1 in 10 patients	Solution
Prostatic disorders (e.g. prostatic intraepithelial neoplasia, or hardening or inflammation of the prostate), changes in sexual appetite, painful testicles, painful, hardened, or enlarged breasts, or ↑ levels of ♂ and ♀ hormones	
Tiredness, general feeling of weakness, excessive sweating, or night sweats	
Rare side effects (may affect up to 1 in 1000 patients)	
The oily liquid Nebido® may reach the lungs (pulmonary microembolism of oily solutions) which can, in rare cases, lead to signs and symptoms such as cough, shortness of breath, feeling generally unwell, excessive sweating, chest pain, dizziness, 'pins and needles', or fainting. These reactions may occur during or immediately after the injection and are reversible	
Suspected anaphylactic reactions after Nebido® injection have been reported	
Treatment with high doses of testosterone preparations commonly stops or reduces sperm production, although this returns to normal after treatment ceases. Testosterone replacement therapy of poorly functioning testicles (hypogonadism) can, in rare cases, cause persistent, painful erections (priapism). High-dose or long-term administration of testosterone occasionally increases the occurrence of water retention and oedema (swelling due to fluid retention)	

Gender dysphoria

Patients seeking gender reassignment have complex requirements and require specialist care. The NHS has outlined a pathway of care for gender dysphoria and the endocrine nurse can play a crucial and pivotal part in streamlining a patient pathway and working to develop a service. This patient group have multifactorial needs and the nurse is well placed to support in offering strategic pathways of care, including offering psychological support, medication monitoring, and facilitating blood tests. Some endocrine centres are now commissioned to provide a pathway for such patients who are otherwise untreated or self-purchasing hormone therapies. Patients often wait >2 years to be seen in the initial gender identity clinic that confirms the diagnosis of gender dysphoria and subsequently recommends hormone therapy.

A proposed pathway is recommended of initial triage which follows well-defined criteria. The 1st appointment is consultant-led and then planned following the pathway shown in Box 14.4.

Box 14.4 Proposed pathway

This list is not exhaustive and should be in line with the individual endocrine service requirements.

- Initial nurse triage according to well-defined criteria/protocol, including blood tests.
- 1st consultant appointment and establish medication.
- 3-month consultant review (as may need medication change) plus blood tests.
- 6-month nurse appointment—blood tests plus prescription reissue.
- 9-month nurse appointment—blood tests plus prescription reissue.
- 12-month consultant follow-up.
- 18-month nurse follow-up.
- 24-month consultant follow-up.
- 30-month nurse follow-up.
- 36-month consultant follow-up.
- During the year, anticipate non-face-to-face appointments which will be to deal with queries and give blood test results. (~4).
- Once the patient is stable, then transfer to 1° care, with support available from 2° care if required (shared care).

Neuroendocrine tumours

Nursing care of patients with neuroendocrine tumours

Caring for individuals with NETs is complex and challenging.

- Wide range of diagnoses, including different tumour types, grades, and stages.
- Lack of clear evidence on how to best manage these can lead to uncertainty for patients and their families.
- Complex range of symptoms requiring a wide range of knowledge and skills, and input from many different disciplines and specialties.
- Patients may live with advanced disease for many years; rollercoaster ride of multiple treatments, symptoms, and psychological and social burden of living with a life-limiting illness.

Key issues in nursing NET patients

Gastrointestinal symptoms in NETs

- Major cause of morbidity for many patients with NETs.
- Cause isolation and embarrassment, as well as contribute to other symptoms such as fatigue and weight loss.
- Typically, patients with GEP NETS will have multiple GI symptoms, e.g. abdominal pain, bowel cramps, greasy/oily stools, excessive flatulence, diarrhoea, urgency, lack of appetite, early satiety, and weight loss.
- Accurate assessment and early treatment can significantly improve QoL.
- Often multiple causes. Use of a gastroenterology team and dietetic service experienced in NETs can be invaluable.

(See Table 14.4.)

Table 14.4 Common causes of abdominal symptoms in gastroenteropancreatic NETs

Functional hormonal symptoms (carcinoid, Verner–Morrison, ZES)	Diarrhoea, abdominal cramps, weight loss
Mass effect of tumour	Abdominal pain, obstruction, poor appetite, overflow diarrhoea, weight loss, nausea
Mesenteric fibrosis, and mesenteric angina	Cramping abdominal pain, obstruction, erratic bowel habit—diarrhoea/constipation, early satiety, weight loss
Treatments	Insufficiency symptoms

Management of NET-related diarrhoea

- Common causes of diarrhoea in GEP NETs:
  - Surgery: small intestinal surgery, pancreatic resection, cholecystectomy, duodenectomy.
  - Disease: mesenteric mass, gastrinoma, VIPoma.
  - Medication: both cancer treatments and other medications need to be considered, e.g. SSAs, chemotherapy, targeted therapies such as everolimus, antidepressants, diabetic medications, etc.
  - Syndromes: carcinoid syndrome, ZES, Verner–Morrison syndrome.

NB. ↑ risk in many GEP NET patients of pancreatic exocrine insufficiency, bile acid malabsorpion, and small intestinal bacterial overgrowth.

Assessment of GEP NET-related diarrhoea
- Detailed assessment essential.
- Nature of stool, consistency, colour, frequency, amount, time of day, exacerbating/relieving factors, time in relation to eating. Is stool greasy? Does it float? Is it easy to flush away?
- When did it commence? Was it post-surgery? Was it pre-diagnosis?
- Type of NETs: pNET, small intestinal; is it functional or non-functional?
- Treatments: previous surgery, drug therapy.
- Accompanying symptoms: bloating, abdominal pain, flatulence, weight loss, nausea, vomiting.
- Consider risks of bile acid malabsorption (BAM) and small intestinal bacterial overgrowth.

Management and nursing care
- Manage cause.
  - Carcinoid syndrome: use of SSAs about 70% effective in reducing diarrhoea by >50%. Use of loperamide and opioids. Telotristat has been shown to be effective in patients with diarrhoea refractory to SSAs (currently not licensed in the UK).
  - If BAM suspected, then arrange SeHCAT scan. Use of bile acid sequestrants if confirmed.
  - Small intestinal bacterial overgrowth (SIBO): gastroenterology input, use of antibiotics as per local protocol. Tends to follow chronic fluctuation of symptoms, then need for retreatment.
  - Use of SSAs, antidiarrhoeal agents, pancreatic enzyme replacement therapy (PERT), and PPIs as required.
- For most patients, GI symptoms are ongoing in nature and management strategies aim to improve QoL where possible.
- Patients are often embarrassed and can be isolated.
- Nurses have a key role in assessing patients' symptoms and guiding referral to appropriate teams such as gastroenterology and dietetics.

Ongoing support
- Assisting dose adjustment of PERT and antidiarrhoeal medications.
- Assessing any changes in symptoms and impact on QoL. Referring to appropriate team if exacerbating symptoms.
- Supporting adjusting to living with symptoms.
- Enabling patients to maintain privacy and dignity.
- Advice on fluid intake, dietary changes, medication, hygiene, incontinence aids, wallet cards to assist access to toilet facilities, and also psychological support.

End-of-life care in NETs

- Prognostication is challenging in many low-grade NET patients. Many patients with advanced disease can live for many years with multiple treatments.
- Highly symptomatic patients with high disease burden who do not respond well to initial treatments will have worse prognosis overall.

- Can be difficult to clearly predict when entering more end-of-life trajectory.
  - Clinicians and nurses should engage with discussions about prognosis early on, even when fraught with uncertainty. Can then re-engage with this as treatment options start to run out or performance status diminishes significantly.
  - Patients and family can struggle with the reality that after many years of responding to treatments, they may be entering end-of-life phase.

Aims of care
- Focus on QoL and management of symptoms as per normal principles of palliative care.
- For functional patients, managing the syndrome can be challenging, e.g. insulinoma or small intestinal NET with carcinoid syndrome.

Specific challenges
- Refractory carcinoid syndrome:
  - Continue SSAs to try to reduce the risk of profound diarrhoea. May need to increase frequency. Add in breakthrough short-acting octreotide if effectiveness of long-acting is reduced.
  - Long-acting injections can be painful in cachectic, frail patients. If needed, replace with short-acting octreotide in syringe driver.
  - Trial of antidiarrhoeal agents. Higher-dose loperamide can be trialled (off licence). May not be effective.
  - Good nursing care. Focus on scrupulous skin care, hygiene, and comfort. Open communication and honesty about challenges of managing refractory diarrhoea.

Mesenteric desmoplasia and small bowel insufficiency
- Patients with non-operable mesenteric tumours causing bowel obstructive symptoms may face many challenges in end-of-life care.
- Multiple symptoms: severe cramping abdominal pain, anorexia, cachexia, malnutrition, and diarrhoea. Can be resistant to normal measures.
- Bypass surgery may not remove pain due to bowel ischaemia. High-output stoma can be challenging.
- Will need specialized input from palliative care team. May need high levels of opioid analgesia, nil by mouth, and intensive nursing support.

Role development

Nurse-led clinics

- Work at an advanced level and practise autonomously, as well as within an MDT, and are self-directed.
- Work clinically to optimize health and well-being, demonstrate autonomous decision-making related to comprehensive history taking and physical assessment of patients.
- Work at an advanced level, drawing on a diverse range of knowledge in complex decision-making to determine evidence-based therapeutic interventions, which includes prescribing medication.
- Plan, prioritize, and manage complete episodes of care, working in partnership with others, delegating and referring as appropriate to optimize health outcomes and resource use, and providing direct support to patients and clients. Act as a key worker where appropriate.
- Use professional judgement in managing complex and unpredictable care events.
- Appropriately define boundaries in practice.
- Promote a high standard of advanced specialist nursing by initiating and coordinating assessment, planning, delivery, and evaluation of holistic needs of patients/families through evidence-based practice, following agreed policies, protocols, and guidelines.
- Maintain adequate patient documentation to the Nursing and Midwifery Council (NMC) requirements for all patients seen and advice given in any practice setting, and contribute to clinical activity/data collection as required.

Advanced nurse practice

Royal College of Nursing (RCN) Accreditation of MSc Advanced Practice Programmes

This is the only nationally recognized quality marker for Advanced Nurse Practitioner Programmes in the UK and provides uniformity of standard and quality.

Advanced clinical practice is delivered by experienced, registered health and care practitioners. It is a level of practice characterised by a high degree of autonomy and complex decision making. This is underpinned by a master's level award or equivalent that encompasses the four pillars of clinical practice, leadership and management, education and research, with demonstration of core capabilities and area specific clinical competence (HEE, 2017[1]).

Nurses can also apply for the Society for Endocrinology Masters double module in Endocrine Nursing (⅏ https://www.endocrinology.org/careers/training-and-resources/courses/masters-level-module-in-endocrine-nursing/).

Reference

1. Health Education England. Multi-professional framework for advanced clinical practice in England. 2017. ⅏ https://www.hee.nhs.uk/our-work/advanced-clinical-practice/multi-professional-framework

Diabetes

Gaya Thanabalasingham, Alistair Lumb, Helen
Murphy, Peter Scanlon, Jodie Buckingham,
Solomon Tesfaye, Ana Pokrajac, Pratik Choudhary,
Patrick Divilly, Ketan Dhatariya, Ramzi Ajjan,
Rachel Besser, and Katharine Owen

Classification and diagnosis of diabetes

Background

Diabetes mellitus is a metabolic disorder characterized by chronic hyperglycaemia due to defects in insulin secretion and/or insulin action. In 2019, 3.92 million people in the UK have a diagnosis of diabetes (6% of the UK population) and a further almost 1 million are estimated to have diabetes which is not yet diagnosed. Worldwide, 463 million adults are living with diabetes, and this number is predicted to exceed 578 million by 2030.

Diagnosis

Diabetes is a biochemical diagnosis based on fasting and postprandial (2h) glucose levels during a 75g OGTT and, since 2010, also using HbA1c.

Table 15.1 shows the plasma glucose thresholds associated with different stages of dysglycaemia; these range from normal glucose tolerance through IGT, impaired fasting glycaemia (IFG), and on to frank diabetes. An HbA1c ≥48mmol/mol or 6.5% fulfils the diagnostic criterion for diabetes.

A diagnosis of diabetes is confirmed in any person with typical hyperglycaemic symptoms (e.g. polyuria, polydipsia, weight loss), with a random or postprandial blood glucose ≥11.1mmol/L or fasting plasma glucose ≥7mmol/L. In asymptomatic patients or those with intercurrent illness, a 2nd abnormal result is necessary to establish a definitive diagnosis of diabetes.

Table 15.1 Glucose thresholds for diagnosis of diabetes mellitus and other stages of dysglycaemia

Venous plasma glucose (mmol/L)		
Normal	Fasting	<6.1
	and 2h glucose during OGTT	<7.8
Diabetes	Fasting	≥7.0
	or 2h glucose during OGTT	≥11.1
IGT	Fasting	<7.0
	and 2h glucose during OGTT	≥7.8 and <11.1
IFG	Fasting	≥6.1 and <7.0
HbA1c		
Normal	≤42mmol/mol or ≤6%*	
IGT	43–47mmol/mol or 6*–6.4%	
Diabetes	≥48mmol/mol or ≥6.5%	

* The ADA definition uses a cut-off of 5.7%.

Classification

During the 1980s, the WHO published the first widely accepted classification of diabetes. Diabetes was classified as insulin-dependent diabetes (IDDM) or T1DM, and non-insulin-dependent diabetes (NIDDM) or T2DM. In 1997, the terms IDDM and NIDDM were discarded, with the updated classification system focusing on the specific underlying aetiology of diabetes. These aetiological groups are listed in Box 15.1.

Box 15.1 Aetiological classification of diabetes mellitus

1. *T1DM* (5–10% of cases): β-cell destruction.
* Includes autoimmune and idiopathic forms.
2. *T2DM* (90% of cases): defective insulin secretion, usually with defective insulin action.
3. *Other specific types:*
* Genetic defects of β-cell function:
  * Maturity-onset diabetes of the young (MODY).
  * Mitochondrial DNA mutations.
  * Neonatal diabetes.
* Genetic defects of insulin action:
  * Lipodystrophies.
  * Insulin receptor mutations (includes type A insulin resistance, leprechaunism, Rabson–Mendenhall syndrome).
  * Rare downstream insulin-signalling defects.
  * Monogenic obesity/hyperphagia (e.g. leptin deficiency).
* Diseases of the exocrine pancreas:
  * Pancreatitis, trauma, pancreatectomy, neoplasia, pancreatic destruction (including CF and haemochromatosis), others.
* Endocrinopathies:
  * Cushing's syndrome, acromegaly, PCC, glucagonoma, hyperthyroidism, APS 1 and 2, others.
* Drug- or chemical-induced:
  * GCs, thyroid hormone, diazoxide, β-adrenergic agonists, thiazides, γ-interferon, antiretroviral treatment (HIV).
* Infections:
  * Congenital rubella, CMV, others.
* Uncommon forms of immune-mediated diabetes:
  * 'Stiff man' syndrome (T1DM, rigidity of muscles, painful spasms), anti-insulin receptor antibodies, others.
* Other genetic syndromes associated with diabetes:
  * Down syndrome, Klinefelter syndrome, Turner syndrome, Wolfram syndrome, Friedreich's ataxia, Huntington's chorea, ciliopathies, myotonic dystrophy, others.
4. *GDM.*

Adapted from ADA/WHO classification.

The vast majority of patients with diabetes have either T1DM (2° to autoimmune-mediated β-cell destruction and absolute insulin deficiency) or T2DM (due to insulin resistance and defects of insulin secretion). Table 15.2 outlines the key differences.

Although the remaining aetiological subtypes account for <10% of all diabetes cases, it is important to consider these rarer causes of diabetes, which comprise the entire differential diagnosis, in order to facilitate personalized management of these patients. Rarer forms, such as MODY, largely arise in young adults. These individuals are often assumed to have T1DM or T2DM and frequently experience long delays before the correct diagnosis is reached. Fig. 15.1 illustrates a suggested diagnostic algorithm for young adults.

Table 15.2 Differences between type 1 and type 2 diabetes

	T1DM	T2DM
Peak age of onset (years)	12	60
UK prevalence	0.25%	5–7% (10% of those >65 years of age)
Initial presentation	Polyuria, polydipsia, weight loss, ketoacidosis	Hyperglycaemic symptoms, often with complications of diabetes
Aetiology	Autoimmune β-cell destruction	Combination of insulin resistance, β-cell destruction, and β-cell dysfunction
Presence of β-cell antibodies	>90%	No
Insulin deficient	Yes	Can develop after many years
DKA	Common	Rare
Obesity	Uncommon	Common (use ethnic cut-offs)
Insulin resistance	Uncommon	Common
Treatment	Insulin from outset	Weight loss ± non-insulin hypoglycaemic agents ± insulin

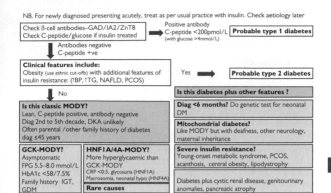

Fig. 15.1 Aetiological diagnosis in diabetes.

Genetics

Although T2DM is much more commonly seen to run in families than T1DM, T1DM is also highly heritable.

Type 1 diabetes

The overall lifetime risk of developing T1DM in a Caucasian population is currently 0.4%. This risk increases to:
- 1–2% if the mother has T1DM.
- 3–6% if the father has T1DM.
- 5–6% if a sibling has T1DM.
- Monozygotic twins have ~50% concordance rate by age 40 years.

Human leucocyte antigen (HLA) genes of the MHC account for half of the heritability of T1DM. The HLA class II DR and DQ loci (respectively encoded by genes *DRB* and *DQB*) carry almost all of T1DM susceptibility from this region; >90% of patients with T1DM have at least one copy of *DRB*301-*DQB*201 or *DRB*401-*DQA*301-*DQB*302.

Other susceptibility loci include variants in the gene encoding insulin (*INS*) which confers a 2-fold ↑ risk. More recent GWAS have ↑ the total number of loci associated with T1DM to >70; however, these loci have a much lower effect size than the *HLA* or *INS* genes.

These genetic studies have confirmed that the pathogenesis of T1DM involves disordered immune regulation.

Type 2 diabetes

The importance of genetic background in the aetiology of T2DM is well established from family and twin studies (concordance between monozygotic twins is 60–100%). Heritability of T2DM is estimated at ~25%.
- >100 genetic susceptibility variants for T2DM have been detected, largely through GWAS.
- *TCF7L2* (encoding transcription factor 7-like 2 protein) on chromosome 10q has the largest effect on T2DM risk described to date, with a per-allele OR of ~1.4.
- Together, the genetic loci found so far only explain a small proportion (~10%) of the overall heritable risk for T2DM.
- Ongoing research is focused on identifying rare genetic variants which might account for the missing heritability in T2DM.
- Potential areas of clinical translation include risk prediction, prevention, pharmacogenetics, and development of novel therapeutics.

Maturity-onset diabetes of the young

MODY, the commonest cause of monogenic β-cell dysfunction, is estimated to be the underlying cause in 0.5–1% of all patients with diabetes. A typical 'MODY patient' has a young age of onset (<45 years, frequently <25 years), an autosomal dominant (AD) family history of diabetes, absence of autoimmune markers, absence of insulin resistance, and remains C-peptide +ve even if insulin-treated. Mutations in a number of different genes have been associated with the MODY phenotype; however, in clinical practice, the vast majority of MODY cases are due to heterozygous mutations in genes encoding the enzyme glucokinase (GCK) and the nuclear transcription factors hepatocyte nuclear factor 1α (HNF1A), hepatocyte nuclear factor 4α (HNF4A), and hepatocyte nuclear factor 1β (HNF1B).

HNF1A-MODY *(previous name MODY3)*

- Accounts for 30–70% of MODY cases.
- Associated with a progressive defect of insulin secretion and treatment requirement.
- Vascular complications are seen at a similar rate to other forms of diabetes.
- Low renal glucose threshold and low CRP (<0.5mg/L).
- An RCT has shown that people with HNF1A-MODY are exquisitely sensitive to sulfonylureas (SUs). Low doses (e.g. gliclazide 20–40mg od) are recommended as 1st-line pharmacological therapy, often maintaining excellent glycaemic control for years.
- In those misdiagnosed as T1DM at onset of diabetes, insulin can frequently be stopped when an SU is commenced (although this is less successful with a longer duration of diabetes).
- Second-line treatments are metformin or DPP-IV.
- The existing low renal glucose threshold means SGLT inhibitor treatment may be less effective than in T2DM, or cause dehydration.

HNF4A-MODY *(previous name MODY1)*

- Accounts for 5–10% of MODY cases.
- Clinical presentation similar to HNF1A-MODY (except normal renal glucose threshold and normal CRP).
- Also sensitive to SUs.
- Affected offspring have hyperinsulinaemia *in utero*, leading to macrosomia and neonatal hypoglycaemia.

GCK-MODY *(previous name MODY2)*

- Accounts for 30–70% of MODY cases.
- Results in a raised glucose threshold for glucose-stimulated insulin secretion, but importantly insulin secretion remains regulated.
- Lifelong, mild, stable fasting hyperglycaemia (FPG 5.5–8mmol/L and HbA1c <7.5%) Low increment of glucose rise following a carbohydrate challenge.
- Hyperglycaemia due to GCK-MODY can be diagnosed at any age. Patients are often asymptomatic, with hyperglycaemia found during screening, e.g. GDM, medicals, hospital admissions.
- A large observational study has shown that diabetes-related microvascular complications are not observed.
- Patients do not require any treatment, except possibly during pregnancy (see ➔ Management of MODY in pregnancy, p. 846).
- 2° care follow-up is not usually required.

HNF1B-MODY *(previous name MODY5)*

- Also known as renal cysts and diabetes (RCAD) syndrome.
- 5–10% of cases of MODY; half are caused by whole gene deletions.
- This is a syndrome of developmental abnormalities featuring renal cysts, genital tract malformations, pancreatic atrophy and exocrine insufficiency, hyperuricaemia, raised LFTs, hypomagnesaemia, and neurodevelopmental or behavioural disorders.
- Affected individuals may present to renal physicians first; renal cysts can be diagnosed during antenatal US.
- Not sensitive to SUs. There is no evidence base to determine treatment, so oral agents may be used as in T2DM, but insulin treatment is usually required within a few years of diagnosis.

Rarer causes of MODY

Mutations in the genes encoding the β-cell K_{ATP} channel *ABCC8* and *KCNJ11*, or in the insulin gene (*INS*) can cause MODY, each accounting for up to 1% of cases. They are a commoner cause of neonatal diabetes (see ➔ Neonatal diabetes, below) for discussion of diagnosis and treatment).

Management of MODY in pregnancy

Although MODY is an uncommon cause of GDM, women with MODY often present for the 1st time with dysglycaemia in pregnancy. Most will be misdiagnosed as GDM and managed according to routine guidelines. There should be a high index of suspicion to screen for MODY in women without the usual risk factors for GDM, or lean women who present early in pregnancy. Those with persistent isolated fasting hyperglycaemia may have GCK-MODY.

For those known to have MODY prior to pregnancy, specific advice on management can be sought from the MODY UK diagnostic centre (ℜ http://www.diabetesgenes.org).

It is now possible in the UK at least to test for the presence of the MODY mutation in the fetus using the free fetal DNA in the mother's blood. This can guide pregnancy management in GCK-MODY and HNF4A-MODY where the fetal mutation status is crucial to the outcome.

For those with HNF1A/HNF4A-MODY already well controlled on low-dose SU agents prior to pregnancy, there is a good argument for using glibenclamide preconception (safe in T2DM) and in the 1st and 2nd trimesters, so long as good control is maintained. Glibenclamide may cross the placenta and increase the risk of macrosomia, so it is recommended to convert to insulin for the final trimester.

In HNF4A-MODY, an affected fetus can develop hyperinsulinaemia, macrosomia, and neonatal hypoglycaemia. Seek specialist advice on fetal monitoring and involve the paediatricians.

In GCK-MODY, an unaffected fetus may develop macrosomia with exposure to the mother's raised blood glucose (an affected fetus has normal growth). Treatment (with insulin) is only recommended if macrosomia is developing; however, evidence shows it is not very effective in normalizing blood glucose and women may feel unwell if large insulin doses lower their glucose level below their usual baseline, due to counter-regulatory hormone release. Early delivery at 37–38 weeks may be required. Blood glucose monitoring is not required until the 3rd trimester.

Neonatal diabetes (diabetes diagnosed up 6 months of age)

- Affects ~1 in 100,000–150,000 live births.
- Diabetes diagnosed before 6 months is likely to be one of the monogenic subtypes of neonatal diabetes, rather than T1DM. *Refer those diagnosed before 6 months for genetic investigation, even if many years later and attending adult clinics.* A genetic diagnosis is found in over 80% of cases and diagnosis could change management at any age.
- Neonatal diabetes may be transmitted by AD or AR inheritance and may lead to either isolated diabetes or diabetes as part of a complex syndrome.

- Where neonatal diabetes is the 1st presentation of a rare syndrome, identifying the cause may guide future clinic management or inform prognosis.
- Transient neonatal diabetes mellitus (TNDM): diabetes usually remits within 3 months—chromosome 6q24 imprinting abnormalities (70% cases), mutations in the K_{ATP} channel genes (20% cases).
- Permanent neonatal diabetes mellitus (PNDM): mutations in the *KCNJ11* and *ABCC8* genes, respectively encoding the Kir6.2 and SUR1 subunits of the β-cell K_{ATP} channel (50% cases); insulin gene (*INS*) mutations (10–15% cases).
- Patients with *KCNJ11* and *ABCC8* mutations can be effectively treated with high-dose SUs and insulin stopped.
- Those presenting with *KCNJ11* and *ABCC8* mutations in adult life respond to lower dose of SU.
- ~20% cases with K_{ATP} channel gene mutations have additional neurological features (DEND syndrome—developmental delay, epilepsy, and neonatal diabetes).
- *INS* mutations should be treated with insulin sensitizers or insulin; agents that stimulate insulin secretion may accelerate β-cell loss through endoplasmic reticulum stress.

Mitochondrial diabetes

Mitochondrial diabetes has a similar prevalence to the rarer forms of MODY and is another important diagnosis not to miss.
- Caused by mutations in mitochondrial DNA (commonest is an A-to-G point mutation at position 3243 in the transfer RNA (tRNA) leucine gene).
- Maternal inheritance.
- Commonly associated with sensorineural deafness (MIDD: maternally inherited diabetes and deafness).
- Clinical features include myopathy, cardiomyopathy, macular retinal dystrophy (which may be detected at retinal screening), CNS disease, and renal disease.
- Clinical phenotype can be variable within the same family, due to heteroplasmy (variable distribution of abnormal mitochondria).
- Clinical management should include cardiology assessment (interval echocardiography), audiology, and clinical genetics advice. This is best delivered in specialist centres—in the UK, these are based in London, Oxford, and Newcastle. Outside these centres, seek expert advice.

Genetic causes of severe insulin resistance

Genetic severe insulin resistance is a little rarer than MODY. It is associated with high cardiovascular risk.
- Characterized by young onset of severe insulin resistance, e.g. acanthosis nigricans, dyslipidaemia, hypertension, hepatic steatosis, PCOS. This constellation of features, particularly in non-obese patients, should raise suspicion of a genetic cause. Treatment can be challenging. Exercise and insulin sensitizers are 1st line, then high-dose insulin. Concentrated insulins, e.g. Toujeo® and Tresiba® U200, may be helpful, or the older Humulin® R U-500 if available.

- *Lipodystrophies.* Abnormal fat distribution leads to insulin resistance due to lack of 'metabolically safe' storage sites, e.g. loss of fat from limbs and ↑ central and ectopic fat. The classic Dunnigan familial partial lipodystrophy is caused by mutations in *LMNA*. Mutations in *PPARG* present with a similar phenotype. The lipodystrophies are more readily diagnosed in ♀ patients—look for absent fat on legs and prominent veins. Consider in patients with a Cushing's disease phenotype but who do not have hypercortisolaemia.
- *Insulin receptor mutations.* Present with a range of severities but, in addition to severe insulin resistance, can present initially with fasting hypoglycaemia and growth defects and hyperandrogenism in women. A classic presentation in the diabetes clinic would be young-onset PCOS and acanthosis in a lean woman.

Assessing newly diagnosed diabetes

There are two issues to address in a patient with a new diagnosis of diabetes: firstly, what the immediate management is (inpatient vs outpatient, appropriate treatment); and secondly, what the underlying aetiology is. Assigning aetiology is usually most challenging in those diagnosed in the 2nd to 4th decades of life where there is overlap of clinical features between both T1DM and T2DM and the rarer forms of diabetes. Reassessment over the months to years after diagnosis can be helpful. If in any doubt over whether this is T1DM, be safe and commence insulin.

Fig. 15.1 illustrates an algorithm for the investigation of young adults.
- *History:* acute or insidious onset, precipitating cause, family history of diabetes, ethnic origin, presence of other autoimmune diseases, features of insulin resistance, other medical history.
- *Examination:* BMI, fat distribution, acanthosis nigricans, vitiligo.
- *Investigations:* presence of ketones, HbA1c; renal, liver, and thyroid function; lipid profile.

Diagnostic tools

No test is absolute, but the following can be useful to confirm a clinical diagnosis or support treatment decisions.

β-cell antibodies

T1DM is associated with raised levels of the islet antibodies glutamic acid decarboxylase (GAD), tyrosine phosphatase (IA-2), and zinc transporter 8 (ZnT8) antibodies at diagnosis. The presence of two or more antibodies, or one +ve antibody with a supportive clinical picture, confirms the diagnosis of T1DM.

Conversely, absence of antibodies at diagnosis in those labelled as T1DM should prompt consideration of a different aetiology.

While antibody testing is helpful, particularly in those presenting under the age of 50, low titres of a single antibody can be difficult to interpret and the old islet cell antibodies (ICA) test should not be used due to poor sensitivity and specificity.

C-peptide

C-peptide is secreted in equimolar quantities with insulin and is a marker of endogenous insulin. C-peptide level varies, depending on insulin sensitivity, and should always be measured with a paired glucose. Generally a random plasma C-peptide of <200pmol/L (0.2nmol/L or 0.6ng/mL) with blood glucose >4mmol/L represents insulin deficiency consistent with T1DM. Ambient glucose level is crucial for interpreting C-peptide, and it is also renally cleared, so is higher in renal impairment.

Genetic testing

Diagnostic testing is available for the MODY subtypes, neonatal diabetes, mitochondrial mutations (particularly the common A3243G variant), and lipodystrophies (*LMNA/PPARG*).

Although testing can be expensive, a clinical diagnosis is not a substitute for a definitive genetic test, especially where treatment decisions, such as stopping insulin, might depend on the outcome. Most countries, including the UK, sequence a panel of 20–30 genes known to cause monogenic diabetes.

Involve clinical genetics services to help with family screening. In the UK, the Genetic Diabetes Nurses network can provide help and expertise (℠ https://www.diabetesgenes.org/training/genetic-diabetes-nurses/).

MODY probability calculator

This online tool (also available as an App) uses a number of clinical features (but not antibodies or C-peptide) to generate a probability of MODY compared to T1DM or T2DM (℠ https://www.diabetesgenes.org/exeter-diabetes-app/ModyCalculator).

Genetic risk score

Genetic risk scores (GRS) for complex diseases are calculated by genotyping a number of risk variants (usually single nucleotide changes detected in GWAS) and attributing a weighted score for each variant detected in the patient. This score is then compared to a gold standard group with the condition. Although largely research tools, the existence of variants which tag high-risk HLA in T1DM means that a T1GRS is a helpful adjunct to assessment of patients, although not a conclusive test in isolation. It can be requested alongside MODY testing in the UK.

Causes of diagnostic confusion

- *Latent autoimmune diabetes of adulthood (LADA).* This presents like T2DM but is a form of T1DM with insidious onset, defined by the presence of any β-cell antibody. Treat like T2DM, but progression to insulin is usually more rapid. Do not call classic T1DM in older people 'LADA'.
- *Ketosis-prone diabetes (KPD).* This presents with DKA or ketosis, but insulin requirements decline over weeks/months and insulin can often be withdrawn. Diabetes may remit for a period of time. Antibodies are −ve. Classically described in those of African origin, but actually seen in all ethnicities. Patients should be advised that they may develop ketosis again during illness and be given ketone-monitoring equipment.
- *'Grey cases'.* An increasing number of adults aged 20–50, particularly in non-white ethnic groups, do not easily fit into a diagnostic category. Some will be started on insulin based on hyperglycaemia ± ketosis at diagnosis. Others will be assumed to have T2DM based on BMI or ethnicity and thus miss out on education or technology offered in T1DM. Be open to reassessing the aetiology using the diagnostic tools discussed in ➔ Diagnostic tools, pp. 840–2.

Monitoring serial C-peptide levels can identify those becoming insulin-deficient, while adding non-insulin agents in people without strong evidence of T1DM can simplify treatment.

Further reading

American Diabetes Association (2021). Diagnosis and classification of diabetes mellitus. *Diabetes Care* **44** (Suppl 1), S15–33.

De Franco E, *et al.* (2015). The effect of early, comprehensive genomic testing on clinical care in neonatal diabetes: an international cohort study. *Lancet* **386**, 957–63.

Diabetes Genes. [The website run by the UK testing centre for monogenic diabetes in Exeter has a wide range of patient and professional resources and also provides advice on testing and clinical management of monogenic diabetes]. ℘ https://www.diabetesgenes.org/

Misra S (2017). Pancreatic autoantibodies: who to test and how to interpret the results. *Practical Diabetes* **34**, 221–23. https://doi.org/10.1002/pdi.2123

Murphy R, *et al.* (2007). Clinical features, diagnosis and management of maternally inherited diabetes and deafness (MIDD) associated with the 3243A>G mitochondrial point mutation. *Diabet Med* **25**, 383–99.

Owen KR (2016). Treating young adults with type 2 diabetes or monogenic diabetes. *Best Pract Res Clin Endocrinol Metab* **30**, 455–67.

Semple RK, *et al.* (2011). Genetic syndromes of severe insulin resistance. *Endocr Rev* **32**, 498–514.

Expert management of type 1 diabetes

Background

This condition is characterized by absolute insulin deficiency 2° to T-cell-mediated autoimmune destruction of the insulin-producing β-cells. Most patients have antibodies to components of the pancreatic β-cell including GAD, IA-2 and ZnT8 (see ➔ Assessing newly diagnosed diabetes, pp. 850–2). These antibodies can be detected for a few years prior to diagnosis and frequently decline from the time of diagnosis. They can be absent in long-standing disease and are not thought to be pathogenic themselves. Age at presentation is bimodal, with a peak around puberty and another peak between 20 and 30 years of age. Incidence rates in those under 5 years have been rising sharply.

Patients who develop T1DM later in life frequently have a more insidious presentation and there may be diagnostic confusion with T2DM (sometimes termed LADA; see ➔ Assessing newly diagnosed diabetes, pp. 850–2). T1DM has a complex genetic background, with over 60 genetic loci associated with susceptibility and HLA DR4-DQ8 and DR3-DQ2 present in 90% of children with T1DM. However, only 13% of patients have a 1st-degree relative with the condition.

Soon after diagnosis, patients commonly go through the 'honeymoon period' when insulin requirements reduce dramatically and patients can even come off insulin for a short duration. This phase can last from a few weeks to a few years (longer with increasing age), but it is important to monitor blood glucose and ketones carefully and reinstate insulin treatment as soon as blood glucose starts to rise. At the time of diagnosis, patients usually have between 10% and 20% of β-cell function left, which can sustain the patient through this phase.

Management

All patients with T1DM should be treated with physiological insulin replacement.

An initial education package will include:

- An explanation of what diabetes is and what it means.
- Action of insulin.
- Aims of treatment (see Table 15.3).
- Self-monitoring of glucose (see ➔ Glucose monitoring, p. 860).
- Injection technique, including site rotation.
- Advice about hypoglycaemia detection and treatment.
- Dietary advice with information on carbohydrate counting.
- Information about annual screening (review) for complications of diabetes, including referral to their local eye screening service.
- Advice regarding DVLA, insurance companies, and Diabetes UK.
- Advice regarding pregnancy (for women of childbearing age).
- Advice about dealing with illness (sick day rules) (see ➔ Sick day rules, p. 866).

Table 15.3 Suggested aims of treatment

Premeal blood glucose	4.5–7.5mmol/L
Post-meal blood glucose (at 2h)	8–10mmol/L
HbA1c	42–58mmol/mol (6.0–7.5%) WITHOUT Recurrent or debilitating hypoglycaemia
Time in target (3.9–10mmol/L)	>70%
Time below target <3.9mmol/L	<4%
BP	<130/80mmHg
BMI	20–25kg/m² ideally
Glucose monitoring	Between 4 and 10 times/day. Ideally a minimum of before each meal (to help judge the dose of insulin required) and pre-bed

Types of insulin

Understanding the action profiles of different insulins is key to understanding when to take them and which insulin may be contributing to high or low glucose readings at any given time.

- Physiological insulin replacement depends on dividing the insulin into basal (background) and bolus (mealtime/quick-acting) insulin. In most patients, aim for a 50/50 split between basal and bolus insulin.
- Background insulin is affected by weight, stress, exercise, alcohol.
- Quick-acting insulin is adjusted, according to carbohydrate intake and exercise, and is also used to correct high readings.
- Biosimilar insulins: Biological copies of analogue insulins made by other companies which may offer cost advantages, e.g. Abasaglar®, Semglee® (both insulin glargine), Lispro Sanofi® (insulin Lispro).
- Inhaled insulin: This was originally available, but withdrawn in 2010 due to concerns over lung side-effects. There is now a commercial preparation (Alfrezza®) marketed in the USA.
- Currently available insulins are listed in Table 15.4.

Insulin regimens

(See Fig. 15.2.)

Basal bolus regimen

- Once- or twice-daily basal insulin is given to balance hepatic glucose output. This should be titrated so that ideally if the patient is fasting, the glucose levels remain constant. The amount of background insulin may need to be reduced in response to exercise or alcohol, or ↑, e.g. in illness as required.
- Bolus insulin should be taken 10–15min premeal to cover carbohydrate intake and/or to correct raised glucose levels.
- This regimen, combined with structured patient education that trains patients to adjust the doses in response to food, exercise, and illness, provides patients with flexibility to be able to lead a more normal life.

Table 15.4 Summary of types of insulin available

Type of insulin	Examples	Peak activity (h)	Duration of action (h)
Bolus (quick-acting) insulin			
Rapid-acting analogues	FiAsp® (faster insulin aspart)	1	3–3.5
	*Humalog® (insulin lispro)	1–1.5	3.5–5
	Lyumjev® (faster insulin Humalog)	1	3–5
	NovoRapid® (insulin aspart)	1–1.5	3.5–5
	Apidra® (insulin glulisine)	1–1.5	3.5–5
Soluble	Actrapid®	1.5–2.5	4–8
	Humulin S®	1.5–2.5	4–8
	Insuman Rapid®	1.5–2.5	4–8
Basal (background) insulin			
Isophane (NPH)	Insulatard®	4–6	10–16
	Humulin I®	4–6	10–16
	Insuman Basal®	4–7	11–20
Long-acting analogues	Levemir® (insulin detemir)	Peakless	12–16
	Lantus® (insulin glargine)	Peakless	18–24
	Toujeo® (insulin glargine—U300)	Peakless	24–28
	*Tresiba® (insulin degludec)	Peakless	42
Mixed insulin			
Isophane with soluble insulin	Humulin M3®	Dual peaks at 2 and 6h	10–16
	Insuman Comb 15®	Dual peaks at 2 and 6h	10–16
	Insuman Comb 25®	Dual peaks at 2 and 6h	10–16
	Insuman Comb 50®		
Biphasic analogue insulin	Humalog Mix 25®	Dual peaks at 2 and 6h	10–16
	Novomix 30®	Dual peaks at 2 and 6h	10–16
Animal insulin	Display similar characteristics to the human insulin above		
	Hypurin® Porcine neutral	1.5–2.5	4–8
	Hypurin® Porcine isophane	4–6	10–16
	Hypurin® Porcine 30/70 mix		

* Available in standard U100 and U200 strength

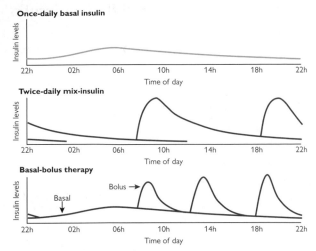

Fig. 15.2 Profiles of common insulin regimens.

Twice-daily fixed mixtures

These are rarely used as 1st line in T1DM in modern practice.

• Pre-prepared mixtures of soluble and isophane insulin, most commonly in the ratio of 30% soluble:70% isophane may be used in some cases. These have the advantage of only two injections a day but offer less flexibility in terms of ability to respond to changes in food, exercise, or illness.

• These may be used in patients who are unable to inject more often or live a very fixed lifestyle and are more commonly used in those with T2DM.

Structured education and flexible insulin therapy

- NICE recommends this should be offered to all patients with T1DM, ideally within a year of diagnosis.
- Patients receive training to adjust insulin doses on the basis of their current blood glucose levels, expected carbohydrate intake, activity, and other variables.
- There are several similar programmes available (DAFNE, BERTIE, EXPERT, etc.) which are based around the following key principles:
  - Separation of meal (quick-acting) and background (basal) insulin.
  - Adjustment of mealtime insulin, based on carbohydrate intake.
  - Correction of doses, based on the correction factor, to return blood glucose back to target.

Insulin:carbohydrate ratio

This is the amount of insulin required for a fixed amount of carbohydrate (usually 10g). A total of 10g carbohydrate is also referred to as a 'CP', or a carbohydrate portion in DAFNE. This can also sometimes be expressed as the number of grams of carbohydrate required to balance 1 unit of insulin (e.g. 8g/unit). A common starting point for a normal-weight adult would be 1unit/10g carbs.

Rule of 400

A simple rule to calculate the insulin:carbohydrate ratio is to divide 400 by the total daily dose (TDD).

For example, for a TDD of 40units, the insulin:carbohydrate ratio will be $400/40 = 10g/unit$. For a TDD of 80units, the insulin:carbohydrate ratio will be $400/80 = 5g/unit$.

This can be tested by checking blood glucose levels 2h post-meal. If these are above target (usually set for <10mmol/L), then this can be ↑.

Insulin sensitivity (correction factor)

This is the degree to which 1 unit of insulin will drop the blood glucose. A common starting point for an adult is 1 unit to drop the glucose by 3 mmol/L.

Rule of 120

$$120/TDD = \text{correction factor in mmol/L}.$$

For example, for a TDD of 40units, correction factor = $120/40 = 3.0$.

Principles of dose adjustments

Patients are advised to measure blood glucose a minimum of four times before breakfast and before bed. Reflect on blood glucose readings at regular intervals to look for patterns over the previous 5–7 days. The only exception to waiting for a pattern is when overnight or fasting hypoglycaemia occurs, when patients should reduce their night-time background insulin by 10–20% the following night.

Some simple rules of adjustment are:
- Make one change at a time.
- Use carbohydrate-free days to adjust the daytime basal.
- Adjust the bedtime basal insulin, based on the fasting glucose.

- If a correction dose is required at the same time every day, consider changing the insulin:carbohydrate ratio or basal insulin active at that time.
- Reduce evening basal insulin after alcohol or exercise by 20–50%.
- Do not correct post-hypo highs.
- If high post-meal readings, increase the insulin:carbohydrate ratio.
- Reduce bedtime basal insulin in response to recurrent unexplained nocturnal hypoglycaemia.

Dawn phenomenon

Most people have a surge in insulin requirements 3–4h before waking up. This is mainly due to ↑ amplitude and frequency of GH pulses but also coincides with a natural rise in cortisol levels. In about 30% of people, this causes >30% increase in insulin requirements. In patients on NPH insulin, this coincides with a reduction in activity of the insulin, leading to fasting hyperglycaemia. Increases in bedtime NPH lead to overnight hypoglycaemia. This effect is less pronounced with analogue basal insulins, which do not wane in function in the early hours. To check for this, we advise patients to check at 3 a.m. and then in the morning, or to use continuous glucose monitoring traces to see if there is a consistent rise between 3 a.m. and waking. If there is, commonly people will need to use an insulin pump that can be programmed to increase insulin delivery at that time to bring glucose readings into target range.

Somogyi effect

Some people confuse the dawn phenomenon with the Somogyi effect. First suggested in 1938, this hypothesized that high fasting glucose readings may be due to a rebound, caused by release of counter-regulatory hormones after overnight hypoglycaemia. However, multiple more recent studies using continuous glucose monitoring have failed to demonstrate that this is a significant cause of fasting hyperglycaemia and this idea is now largely discredited.

Glucose monitoring

Capillary glucose monitoring

Most people with T1DM are recommended to perform a minimum of four capillary glucose measurements per day (before each meal and before bed).

There is a clear correlation between the number of blood glucose measurements performed and the HbA1c achieved, and NICE recommends patients with T1DM to perform 4–10 measurements/day.

Interstitial glucose monitoring

This is either 'flash' glucose monitoring where a sensor is swiped to get the glucose reading, or 'continuous' (CGM) where the glucose value is sent to a connected device with a continuous readout. These systems use a tiny needle that sits just under the skin and measures glucose in the subcutaneous interstitial fluid. This can lag 5–15 minutes behind capillary or venous blood.

Flash glucose monitoring

The FreeStyle Libre is the 1st (and only at time of publication) example of flash monitoring. The user swipes with the reader or mobile phone to obtain the glucose value, along with information about the direction and rate of change of glucose and a trace showing the last 8h of glucose. This form of monitoring is used by over 50% of people with T1DM in the UK. Audit data show improvements in glucose control as well as reductions in diabetes related distress and hospital admissions. The latest version of the system has alarms that alert the patient if glucose is too high or too low.

Continuous glucose monitoring

CGM systems may connect to an insulin pump, a mobile phone App, or a smart watch. These systems have alarms that can be programmed to alert the user of prespecified high or low readings, as well as predicted high or low readings, allowing the user to take appropriate action to avoid them. Clinical trial data have shown improved HbA1c and significant reductions in hypoglycaemia and improvements in QoL with these systems.

Setting alarms

When starting, make sure not to set the alarms to too tight a range, or patients may develop alarm fatigue.

Suggested settings include:
- 'High alert' 14–18mmol/L, depending on the average glucose levels.
- 'Low alert' 3.5–4.5mmol/L, depending on the degree of hypoglycaemia awareness.

Flash glucose monitoring and CGM also display arrows showing the direction and rate of change of glucose (see Table 15.5).

Retrospective CGM

Sometimes CGM can be used for 1–2 weeks to collect 'blinded' data that can be used to then identify changes that may be required to therapy. There are some bespoke systems that can be used for this purpose.

Table 15.5 Arrows and rate of change on CGM

	Rate of change	How long to change by 1mmol/L	How much will it change in 30min
↑	>0.11mmol/L/min	Average 7min	3–4mmol/L
↗	Between 0.11 and 0.06mmol/L/min	Average 15min	2–3mmol/L
→	<0.06mmol/min	>20min	<2mmol/L
↘	Between 0.11 and 0.06mmol/L/min	Average 15min	2–3mmol/L
↓	>0.11mmol/L/min	Average 7min	3–4mmol/L

Arrows denote the direction and rate of change.

Insulin pump therapy: continuous subcutaneous insulin infusion (CSII)

This involves continuous infusion of quick-acting insulin (usually rapid-acting analogue insulin), using a small pager-sized pump through an SC cannula. The cannula is replaced by the patient every 2–3 days. There are also tube-less or patch pumps which have no tubing and stick directly to the skin. There is no need for long-acting basal insulin, as the pump is programmed to deliver a continuous infusion of fast-acting insulin that can be adjusted as required in response to ambient blood glucose during exercise, illness, or other events. When the patient needs a bolus to cover meals or to correct a high glucose value, this can be done easily and unobtrusively by pressing a button on the pump or on a remote control. Most modern pumps have in-built bolus calculators that use pre-programmed values for insulin:carbohydrate ratios, insulin sensitivity, and blood glucose targets to calculate insulin doses. These calculators can take into account any insulin previously delivered to avoid 'stacking' of insulin and help avoid hypogly-caemia. They can also store information on blood glucose readings entered into the pump and insulin delivered for download and review. This is discussed in more detail in the next section.

NICE criteria for insulin pump therapy (technical appraisal TA151)

Insulin pump therapy is recommended as a treatment option for adults and children 12 years and older with T1DM provided:
- Attempts to achieve target HbA1c with multiple-dose injection (MDI) result in disabling hypoglycaemia, OR
- HbA1c remains above 69mmol/mol or 8.5%, despite a high level of care.

CSII is also recommended for children younger than 12 years with T1DM, provided MDI therapy is considered impractical or inappropriate.

Basal rates

A pump delivers basal insulin by infusing rapid-acting insulin continuously. Basal rates can be adjusted to suit the lifestyle of the patient and to negate the impact of the dawn phenomenon.
- Temporary basal rates: the basal rate can be temporarily ↑ or ↓ between 1% and 100%.
  - ↑ basal rate to cover for stress or illness.
  - ↓ basal rate to cover for exercise.

Altered wave boluses

(See Table 15.6.)
   Pumps offer the ability to deliver the bolus over different time periods to cover for different types of food.
- Square wave bolus: this delivers the bolus over a given period of time and is useful if someone plans to eat gradually (e.g. buffet or snacking).

Table 15.6 Types of bolus dose deliverable by pump

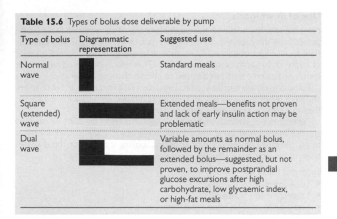

Type of bolus	Diagrammatic representation	Suggested use
Normal wave		Standard meals
Square (extended) wave		Extended meals—benefits not proven and lack of early insulin action may be problematic
Dual wave		Variable amounts as normal bolus, followed by the remainder as an extended bolus—suggested, but not proven, to improve postprandial glucose excursions after high carbohydrate, low glycaemic index, or high-fat meals

Dealing with pump failure

Non-delivery of insulin from a pump is a major risk, and there have been a few deaths with ketoacidosis due to this. This can be due to pump failure or if infusion sets are not changed every 3 days. Patients should keep a supply of SC insulin for use in the event of pump failure.

Sensor-augmented pump therapy

These are systems where CGM links in with an insulin pump. Some systems can stop delivery of insulin when blood glucose drops, or is predicted to drop, below a preset threshold. In sensor-augmented pumps, insulin delivery is reduced or halted when blood glucose drops at a fast rate or drops below a certain threshold. These features are particularly beneficial in patients with impaired awareness of hypoglycaemia or severe hypoglycaemia.

Automated insulin delivery (AID) systems

Hybrid closed loop (HCL)

Commercially available HCL pumps use an algorithm to continuously adjust basal insulin delivery through the pump, based on glucose data obtained from CGM around a selected glucose target. They are called 'hybrid' because the patient still has to 'announce' meals and usually this means they have to carb count. Patients must enter their bolus insulin into the pump as before. HCL pumps have been shown to improve time in range to over 70%, with minimal hypoglycaemia. There are some systems in development that use both insulin and glucagon (dual-hormone closed loops).

DIY closed loops ('open APS')

Expert patient groups have built 'DIY' closed loop systems that use open-source algorithms that connect data from commercial continuous glucose monitors and insulin pumps. These systems are unregulated and untested, but widely peer-supported through an online community. Diabetes UK position on DIY closed looping is that patients should still receive support and care from their diabetes team; however, patients need to be aware of the risks with open APS.

Use of downloads

Most modern home blood glucose meters and all currently available insulin pumps have the capability to download data to a computer. These data can then be used to obtain statistics such as mean glucose, SD, and number of hypo- or hyperglycaemic excursions. They can also be used to look for trends or patterns that can be used to inform changes to therapy.

Pump downloads can be used to evaluate TDD, frequency of set changes, and number of boluses/day and, when combined with data from a meter, they can provide very useful data on patterns.

Patients can download their pumps, insulin pumps, or CGM or capillary glucose meters and send the information electronically to their diabetes team, allowing remote consultations and making it easier for the diabetes team to provide dose adjustment advice.

Suggested use of downloads

- Look for mean tests/day.
- Look for mean boluses/day.
- Look for mean TDD and basal/bolus split.
- Pattern management:
  - Look at different time periods (overnight/post-breakfast/post-lunch, and post-evening meal), and try to identify patterns.
  - Look for low blood glucose readings, and use the download to identify possible causes (high insulin:carbohydrate ratio, correction bolus, basal rate too high).
  - Look for very high blood glucose and for possible causes (missed bolus, inadequate insulin:carbohydrate ratio, overtreatment).

Sick day rules

(See Fig. 15.3.)

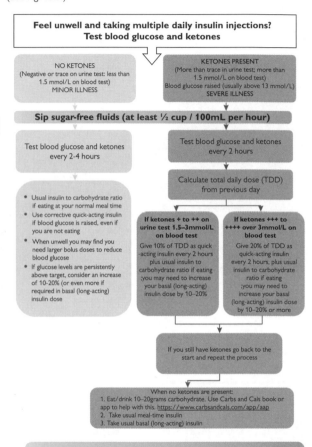

**Feel unwell and taking multiple daily insulin injections?
Test blood glucose and ketones**

NO KETONES
(Negative or trace on urine test: less than
1.5 mmol/L on blood test)
MINOR ILLNESS

KETONES PRESENT
(More than trace in urine test; more than
1.5 mmol/L on blood test)
Blood glucose raised (usually above 13 mmol/L)
SEVERE ILLNESS

Sip sugar-free fluids (at least ½ cup / 100mL per hour)

Test blood glucose and ketones
every 2-4 hours

Test blood glucose and ketones
every 2 hours

Calculate total daily dose (TDD)
from previous day

- Usual insulin to carbohydrate ratio
  if eating at your normal meal time
- Use corrective quick-acting insulin
  if blood glucose is raised, even if
  you are not eating
- When unwell you may find you
  need larger bolus doses to reduce
  blood glucose
- If glucose levels are persistently
  above target, consider an increase
  of 10-20% (or even more if
  required in basal (long-acting)
  insulin dose

If ketones + to ++ on
urine test 1.5–3mmol/L
on blood test
Give 10% of TDD as quick-
acting insulin every 2 hours
plus usual insulin to
carbohydrate ratio if eating
;you may need to increase
your basal (long-acting)
insulin dose by 10–20%

If ketones +++ to
++++ over 3mmol/L on
blood test
Give 20% of TDD as
quick-acting insulin
every 2 hours, plus usual
insulin to carbohydrate
ratio if eating
;you may need to
increase your basal
(long-acting) insulin dose
by 10–20% or more

If you still have ketones go back to the
start and repeat the process

When no ketones are present:
1. Eat/drink 10–20grams carbohydrate. Use Carbs and Cals book or
app to help with this. https://www.carbsandcals.com/app/aap
2. Take usual meal-time insulin
3. Take usual basal (long-acting) insulin

If ketones are still present after 4–6 hours and /or you continue to vomit, are unable to keep
fluids down, or unable to control your blood glucose or ketones, you must go to hospital as an
emergency. You must not stop your basal (long-acting) insulin.

Fig. 15.3 Sick day rules.

Hypoglycaemia

Defining hypoglycaemia

- 3.9mmol/L: 'alert value'—action should be taken.
- 3.0mmol/L: serious hypoglycaemia, associated with cognitive impairment and potential for harm.
- Severe hypoglycaemia: this is defined as an episode associated with cognitive impairment that requires assistance from another person, or that requires hospitalization or parenteral glucose administration or treatment with glucagon.

Normal response to hypoglycaemia

In response to hypoglycaemia, patients experience symptoms that are categorized into autonomic, neuroglycopenic, and general (see Table 15.7). They also generate a counter-regulatory hormonal response that includes glucagon (lost in T1DM after 5 years), adrenaline, and then cortisol and GH.

Table 15.7 Typical symptoms of hypoglycaemia

Autonomic	Neuroglycopenic	General
Sweating	Confusion	Headache
Palpitations	Drowsiness	Nausea
Shaking	Odd behaviour	
Hunger	Speech difficulty	
	Incoordination	

Impaired awareness of hypoglycaemia

Recurrent hypoglycaemia can reduce the hormonal and symptomatic responses to subsequent hypoglycaemia, and over time, after exposure to multiple episodes, patients can lose the ability to recognize hypoglycaemia. Often other people will recognize hypoglycaemia before the patient does. This is termed impaired awareness of hypoglycaemia and is associated with a 3- to 5-fold greater risk of severe hypoglycaemia. Up to 40% of those with long-standing T1DM may have impaired awareness of hypoglycaemia. A simple score to assess awareness of hypoglycaemia is called the GOLD score (see Fig. 15.4).

Gold Questionnaire

'Do you know when your hypos are commencing?'

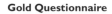

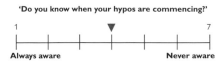

A score of 4 or greater suggests impaired awareness

Fig. 15.4 GOLD score.

Advanced therapies

Immune modulation

Immunotherapy for T1DM is not yet the standard treatment seen in other autoimmune conditions, but many clinical trials are ongoing. The aim of immunotherapy in newly diagnosed T1DM is to maintain some C-peptide which is associated with improved HbA1c and ↓ hypoglycaemia. Prevention trials are also available for antibody +ve 1st-degree relatives of those with T1DM and in babies at high genetic risk. Clinical trials can be accessed in the UK through the Type 1 Diabetes UK Immunotherapy Consortium (℅ https://www.type1diabetesresearch.org.uk/) and internationally through Type 1 Diabetes TrialNet (℅ https://www.trialnet.org/).

Islet cell transplantation

Following the 1st reports of insulin independence following islet cell transplantation in 2000, this has become an established procedure for patients with T1DM fulfilling any one of the following criteria:
• Recurrent disabling hypoglycaemia despite optimal medical therapy.
• Already on immunosuppression for a renal transplant.
• Hypoglycaemia unawareness.

Patients must have T1DM, be aged 18–65 years, and have insulin requirements <0.7U/kg, with body weight <85kg and BMI <28kg/m². Cr clearance must be >60mL/min.

Islets are separated from the donor pancreas and infused intraportally into the liver. The patient requires immunosuppression. Outcomes include improved glucose control, protection against hypoglycaemia, and slowing down in deterioration of nephropathy. Latest data show 70% of patients are insulin-independent at 1 year, dropping to 50% at 4 years.

Pancreas transplantation

Pancreas transplantation is most commonly performed simultaneously with renal transplantation in patients with T1DM and renal failure. Occasionally, it may be performed alone for similar indications as islet cell transplantation in those whom islet cell transplantation is considered inappropriate. This procedure has a 4% operative mortality, with 10–15% risk of relaparotomy. At 1 year, 95% are insulin-independent, with between 65% and 70% insulin-independent at 5 years. The outcomes are better for simultaneous pancreas–kidney (SPK) transplantation than pancreas transplantation alone (PTA) or pancreas after kidney (PAK) transplantation. These procedures should be carried out at centres with expertise in transplantation and diabetes management following multidisciplinary assessment.

For details on islet and pancreas transplantation in the UK, see ℅ https://bts.org.uk/wp-content/uploads/2019/09/FINAL-Pancreas-guidelines-FINAL-version-following-consultation.-Sept-2019.pdf

Further reading

American Diabetes Association (2005). Defining and reporting hypoglycemia in diabetes: a report from the American Diabetes Association Workgroup on Hypoglycemia. *Diabetes Care* **28**, 1245–9.

Hovorka R, et al. (2010). Manual closed-loop insulin delivery in children and adolescents with type 1 diabetes: a phase 2 randomised crossover trial. *Lancet* **375**, 743–51.

Juvenile Diabetes Research Foundation Continuous Glucose Monitoring Study Group (2008). Continuous glucose monitoring and intensive treatment of type 1 diabetes. *N Engl J Med* **359**, 1464–76.

National Institute for Health and Care Excellence (2004). *Diagnosis and management of type 1 diabetes in children, young people and adults.* ℘ http://guidance.nice.org.uk/CG15/Guidance//Adults

National Insitute for Health and Care Excellence (2008). *Continuous subcutaneous insulin infusion for the treatment of diabetes mellitus.* ℘ https://www.nice.org.uk/guidance/ta151

[No authors listed] (1995). Effect of intensive therapy on the development and progression of diabetic nephropathy in the Diabetes Control and Complications Trial. The Diabetes Control and Complications (DCCT) Research Group. *Kidney Int* **47**, 1703–20.

[No authors listed] (1997). Hypoglycemia in the Diabetes Control and Complications Trial. The Diabetes Control and Complications Trial Research Group. *Diabetes* **46**, 271–86.

Pickup J, et al. (2002). Glycaemic control with continuous subcutaneous insulin infusion compared with intensive insulin injections in patients with type 1 diabetes: meta-analysis of randomised controlled trials. *BMJ* **324**, 705.

Shapiro AM, et al. (2006). International trial of the Edmonton protocol for islet transplantation. *N Engl J Med* **355**, 1318–30.

Walker GS, et al. (2018). Structured education using Dose Adjustment for Normal Eating (DAFNE) reduces long-term HbA1c and HbA1c variability. *Diabet Med* **35**, 745–9.

Expert management of type 2 diabetes

Background

T2DM is a major UK public health issue. In 2019, there are over 4 million people living with T2DM in the UK. This includes ~1 million people who have not yet been formally diagnosed. The UK prevalence of T2DM has doubled to 6–7% over the last two decades, in parallel with increasing rates of obesity. T2DM was traditionally diagnosed in older individuals but can present at any age, including in childhood and adolescence. The prevalence of T2DM in ethnic minority communities is 3–5 times higher than in the white British population.

T2DM is characterized by insulin resistance and reduced insulin secretion (see Table 15.2). It is commonly associated with obesity, reduced physical activity, dyslipidaemia, and hypertension. At the time of diagnosis, 30% of individuals have diabetes-related complications. Atherosclerotic CVD is the leading cause of death in those with T2DM. The aims of treatment are to reduce complications and to maintain QoL. This requires a patient-centred approach to effectively manage dysglycaemia and other cardiovascular risk factors.

Management: key recommendations

- Lifestyle management (including advice on dietary quality, calorie restriction, weight management, and ↑ levels of physical activity).
- Offer access to a structured diabetes education programme (that meets the Department of Health and Diabetes UK Patient Education Working Group criteria) at the time of diagnosis, with annual review and reinforcement to improve overall understanding and self-management of T2DM.
- Assess and optimize cardiovascular risk: BP, smoking cessation advice, and dyslipidaemia.
- Set and agree an individualized HbA1c target with the patient, and provide a level of care to achieve and maintain that target.

Glucose targets

HbA1c is the 1° measure of overall glycaemic control in T2DM. HbA1c is a less reliable marker of glycaemic control in end-stage renal failure, pregnancy, and those with haemoglobinopathies. Early intensive management of blood glucose levels in T2DM has long-term benefits in terms of reductions in all diabetes-related complications, including CVD. HbA1c targets should be individualized and take into account patient comorbidities, including frailty and overall life expectancy. A reasonable HbA1c target for most non-pregnant adults with sufficient life expectancy to benefit from reduced microvascular complications (~10 years) is 53mmol/mol (7%) to 58mmol/mol (7.5%). Those managed by diet and lifestyle and/or metformin monotherapy should achieve a target HbA1c level ≤48mmol/mol (6.5%).

Self-monitoring of blood glucose levels is not routinely offered, unless taking medications which have an ↑ risk of hypoglycaemia (such as insulin) or the person is pregnant or planning to become pregnant.

Glucose-lowering medications: current guidelines

Metformin is the recommended initial glucose-lowering medication for most patients with T2DM. If the individualized HbA1c target is not reached with metformin alone, then a 2nd-line glucose-lowering agent should be added. Factors to consider when choosing which agent should be used include drug efficacy, costs, side effect profile, patient preference, and comorbidities. Current NICE guidelines (published in 2015) recommend the addition of a DPP-IV inhibitor, an SU, or pioglitazone as 2nd-line therapies. In contrast, the ADA/European Association for the Study of Diabetes (EASD) consensus statement (published in 2018) recommend that medications with proven benefits in CVD, heart failure, and renal protection should be prioritized for at-risk patients. This is based on recently published cardiovascular outcome trials (CVOTs) which have demonstrated that specific SGLT2 inhibitors and GLP-1 receptor agonists substantially improve cardiovascular outcomes, heart failure, and progression of renal disease.

Glucose-lowering medications

(See Table 15.8 for summary.)

Metformin

Metformin remains the preferred 1st-line medication for most people with T2DM. The United Kingdom Prospective Diabetes Study (UKPDS) showed that metformin reduced all-cause mortality and MI in patients with T2DM. Metformin lowers blood glucose levels by reducing hepatic gluconeogenesis and increasing muscle glucose uptake/metabolism.

Side effects, contraindications, and special precautions

Metformin is usually well tolerated, weight neutral, and unlikely to cause hypoglycaemia. GI side effects occur commonly but are usually transient. If the starting dose is low (e.g. 500mg od), most people develop tolerance and are able to take higher doses. A trial of slow-release metformin should be offered to those in whom GI side effects prevent continued use. Metformin should not be used in those with renal impairment (eGFR <30mL/min/1.73m²). Lactic acidosis can rarely occur, usually in the context of acute kidney injury. Therefore, patients should be advised to temporarily stop metformin during acute severe illness, dehydration, and vomiting, and for 48h after an iodinated contrast imaging scan.

Sulfonylureas

SUs include gliclazide, glipizide, glimepiride, and glibenclamide. SUs are effective and inexpensive glucose-lowering medications. They bind to and close the ATP-sensitive K channel in pancreatic β-cells, leading to membrane depolarization, Ca influx, and subsequent insulin release.

Side effects, contraindications, and special precautions

The main side effects are hypoglycaemia and weight gain. Hypoglycaemia is likely under-reported, with recent data suggesting that up to 50% of patients taking SUs experience at least one hypoglycaemic episode every year. The longer-acting older agents, such as glibenclamide, have a higher risk of hypoglycaemia and should be avoided if possible. Cautious use of SUs in the elderly and those with chronic kidney disease (CKD) is sensible. In the UKPDS, the mean weight gain seen after 10 years of therapy was 2.3kg. These medications should not be prescribed in patients with porphyria.

SGLT2 inhibitors

SGLT2 inhibitors include empagliflozin, canagliflozin, dapagliflozin, and ertugliflozin. These medications enhance urinary excretion of glucose. They inhibit glucose reabsorption by SGLT2 in the proximal renal tubules. These medications have high efficacy to lower blood glucose levels in those with normal renal function; currently, these agents are approved for use when eGFR is >45mL/min/1.73m². These agents lead to weight loss and lower BP, and do not increase the risk of hypoglycaemia when used alone or in combination with metformin. Furthermore, recent CVOTs have demonstrated that empagliflozin, canagliflozin, and dapagliflozin improve cardiovascular outcomes in patients with established, or at high risk of, CVD. These CVOTs also reported +ve 2° outcomes; empagliflozin, canagliflozin, and dapagliflozin reduced the risk of hospitalization for heart failure and slowed the progression of diabetic nephropathy.

Table 15.8 Glucose-lowering medications

Class (example)	HbA1c reduction	Weight effect	Adverse effects	Cardiovascular benefit	Renal benefit
Biguanide (metformin)	0.8–1.0% 9–12mmol/mol	Neutral	GI	Yes	N/A
SU	0.8–2.0% 9–22mmol/mol	↑	Hypoglycaemia	N/A	N/A
SGLT2 inhibitor	0.4–0.8% 5–9mmol/mol	↓	Genitourinary infections	Yes	Yes
GLP-1 receptor agonist	0.5–1.8% 6–20mmol/mol	↓	GI	Yes	Yes
Thiazolidinedione (pioglitazone)	0.6–1.5% 7–17mmol/mol	↑	Oedema Bone fractures (rare) Bladder cancer (rare)	Yes	N/A
DPP-IV inhibitor	0.40% 5mmol/mol	Neutral	Pancreatitis (rare)	No	No

Side effects, contraindications, and specific precautions
Common side effects of SGLT2 inhibitors include genitourinary infections (e.g. vaginitis in women, balanitis in men), dehydration, and orthostatic hypotension. The use of SGLT2 inhibitors can rarely cause ketoacidosis which can occur in the absence of marked hyperglycaemia, i.e. euglycaemic DKA. Eugycaemic DKA can be a diagnostic challenge, leading to delays in recognition and initiation of treatment. Therefore, it is important to counsel patients about the risk of this potentially life-threatening condition and to stop this medication when acutely unwell. Canagliflozin has been associated with an ↑ risk of lower limb amputation and fractures. There have been very rare reports of necrotizing fasciitis of the perineum (Fournier's gangrene) with SGLT2 inhibitor use.

GLP-1 receptor agonists
The incretin hormone GLP-1 is released from the GI tract after a meal and stimulates glucose-dependent insulin secretion. Additional actions of GLP-1 include inhibition of glucagon secretion, slowing of gastric emptying, and central effects on the brain, leading to satiety and reduced appetite. These glucose-lowering agents are therefore particularly attractive due to the low rates of hypoglycaemia and potential weight loss of up to 6kg over 6 months. GLP-1 receptor agonists are delivered by SC injection. Structural differences among the GLP-1 receptor agonists affect the duration of action and may contribute to the differences in efficacy, side effect profile, and cardiovascular effects. Exenatide is administered twice daily, liraglutide and lixisenatide once daily, and dulaglutide, exenatide extended-release, and semaglutide once weekly. Recent CVOTs have demonstrated that liraglutide, dulaglutide, and semaglutide reduce the risk of major cardiovascular adverse events in patients with established, or at high risk of, CVD.

Oral semaglutide has recently been licensed.

Side effects, contraindications, and specific precautions
GI side effects, such as nausea, vomiting, and diarrhoea, are common, but usually transient. GLP-1 receptor agonists do not appear to increase the risk of pancreatitis or pancreatitic cancer, as suggested by early studies. The SUSTAIN 6 trial reported ↑ risk of retinopathy complications with semaglutide, especially in those with baseline retinopathy whose glycaemic control had rapidly improved.

Thiazolidinediones

TZDs are insulin-sensitizing agents which activate PPAR-γ. Pioglitazone is currently the only available TZD in the UK; rosiglitazone was withdrawn in 2011 after reports of ↑ cardiovascular mortality. Pioglitazone has been shown to reduce cardiovascular events, increase HDL-C, and reduce hepatic steatohepatitis.

Side effects, contraindications, and specific precautions
Patients should be warned about the possibility of significant weight gain and oedema with TZDs. Pioglitazone should not be used in people with evidence of heart failure or those with previous or active bladder cancer. There is ↑ risk of bone fractures and so cautious use is advised in those with known osteoporosis or who have risk factors for osteoporosis.

Dipeptidyl peptidase IV inhibitors

DPP-IV inhibitors include sitagliptin, vildagliptin, saxagliptin, alogliptin, and linagliptin. These agents potentiate the action of incretin hormones, including GLP-1, by inhibiting their enzymatic breakdown. These agents are generally well tolerated, with a very low risk of hypoglycaemia, and are weight-neutral. They have modest glucose-lowering effects. Recent CVOTs demonstrated cardiovascular safety, but no cardiovascular benefits for these agents.

Side effects, contraindications, and specific precautions

The SAVOR-TIMI 53 trial reported an ↑ risk of hospitalization for heart failure with saxagliptin. This was not seen in the CVOTs evaluating alogliptin and sitagliptin. ↑ rates of pancreatitis have been reported with DPP-IV inhibitors.

Less commonly used glucose-lowering agents

There are other glucose-lowering agents such as α-glucosidase inhibitors (e.g. acarbose) and prandial insulin secretagogues (e.g. rapeglinide, nateglinide); these medications are not commonly used in the UK. Acarbose reduces postprandial glucose peaks by inhibiting the digestive enzyme α-glucosidase which breaks down carbohydrates into their monosaccharide components. The passage of undigested carbohydrates into the large intestine results in bacterial breakdown and the development of unpleasant GI side effects. Repaglinide and nateglinide stimulate insulin secretion with a short duration of action. These medications are taken just before eating a meal. The short duration of action is associated with low rates of hypoglycaemia. They should not be used in people with renal and hepatic impairment.

Insulin therapy

The majority of people with T2DM will require insulin injections at some point in their lives. Various insulin formulations are available, which differ in terms of onset and duration of action and the risk of hypoglycaemia (see Table 15.7).

Insulin is highly efficacious and can be used to achieve almost any glycaemic target if not limited by hypoglycaemia. The main disadvantages of insulin, compared with other glucose-lowering therapies, are hypoglycaemia, weight gain, and the need for glucose monitoring. Successful use of insulin therapy is highly dependent on appropriate patient selection, provision of adequate patient training and support, and frequent review and dose titration to safe glucose targets.

Most guidelines recommend the addition of basal insulin to the existing therapeutic regimen when other glucose-lowering therapies are unable to achieve or maintain sufficient glycaemic control. Basal insulin refers to longer-acting insulin that aims to cover the individual's basal metabolic requirement. Options for basal insulin include once- or twice-daily isophane (NPH) insulin or long-acting analogue insulin. Analogue insulins are more expensive, compared to NPH insulins, with relatively modest benefits in clinically relevant risks of hypoglycaemia and glycaemic efficacy in people with T2DM. Many patients initiated on basal insulin will require further intensification to a basal-bolus regimen or a twice-daily premixed insulin regimen. Risk factors for not achieving adequate glycaemic control with basal insulin alone include higher pretreatment HbA1c, higher BMI, and longer duration of diabetes.

Remission of type 2 diabetes

Recent studies have challenged the long-held belief that T2DM is a permanent and chronically progressive condition. Significant weight loss can normalize blood glucose levels and lead to remission of T2DM. Remission rates are highest in people with a short duration of T2DM, before the development of irreversible damage to the pancreatic β-cells. Very low-calorie diets and bariatric surgery are currently the most effective methods to achieve diabetes remission. Almost 50% of participants on a very low-calorie diet (~800kcal/day for 3–5 months) in the Diabetes Remission Clinical Trial (DiRECT) attained diabetes remission after 1 year. Importantly, this trial demonstrated that diabetes remission is a practical target in 1° care. Even higher diabetes remission rates are seen after bariatric surgery. (For a full discussion of bariatric surgery, see ➔ Bariatric surgery, pp. 1018–1022.) An individual who has achieved diabetes remission, regardless of the method used, will need ongoing support to prevent weight gain and thereby minimize the risk of relapse of T2DM. It is unknown what effect diabetes remission has on the development or progression of diabetes-related complications, and so it is important that these individuals are recalled for annual review, including retinal screening.

Further reading

Davies MJ, et al. (2018). Management of hyperglycaemia in type 2 diabetes. A consensus report by the American Diabetes Association (ADA) and the European Association for the Study of Diabetes (EASD). *Diabetologia* **61**, 2461–98.

Holman RR, et al. (2008). 10-year follow-up of intensive glucose control in type 2 diabetes. *N Engl J Med* **359**, 1577–89.

Home P (2019). Cardiovascular outcome trials of glucose-lowering medications: an update. *Diabetologia* **62**, 357–69.

National Institute for Health and Care Excellence (2015, updated 2019). *Type 2 diabetes in adults: management.* ℘ https://www.nice.org.uk/guidance/ng28

Taylor R (2019). Calorie restriction for the long-term remission of type 2 diabetes. *Clin Med* **19**, 37–42.

Living with diabetes

Driving

Diabetes can influence the ability to drive safely because of hypoglycaemia or complications such as a reduction in visual acuity or fields. It has been found to carry a similar risk of accidents to epilepsy, and restrictions are placed on some drivers with diabetes. This can be a difficult subject for people with diabetes, but the DVLA in the UK sets legal requirements which must be met. If the DVLA is not informed appropriately, a driving licence and insurance may be invalid. Different standards apply for Northern Ireland and are administered by the Driver and Vehicle Agency (DVA; ℘ https://www.nidirect.gov.uk/contacts/driver-vehicle-agency-dva-northern-ireland).

Box 15.2 summarizes good practice for driving with diabetes.

Medical standards for assessing fitness to drive

The guidance outlined here was produced by the DVLA Drivers Medical Unit in 2016 and last updated in March 2020. Full details are available on the DVLA website (℘ https://www.gov.uk/guidance/diabetes-mellitus-assessing-fitness-to-drive#diabetes-mellitus). It is important to check for the latest information, as the standards are reviewed every 6 months. Different standards apply for licensing to drive group 1 vehicles (including cars and motorcycles) and group 2 vehicles (including large lorries and buses).

▶ *Hypoglycaemia*

Group 1

Hypoglycaemia is a significant risk factor for accidents while driving. In order to obtain a group 1 licence, a person with insulin-treated diabetes must meet all of the following criteria:
- Must have adequate awareness of hypoglycaemia (defined as the ability to bring their vehicle to a safe, controlled stop). This should not rely on alarms from glucose monitoring devices.
- No more than one episode of severe hypoglycaemia (defined as an episode requiring the assistance of another person) while awake in the preceding 12 months and the most recent episode occurred >3 months ago.
- Practises appropriate glucose monitoring.
- Not regarded as a likely risk to the public while driving.
- Under regular review.

Group 2

People with diabetes can apply for a group 2 licence as long as they meet the qualifying conditions. For those on insulin, they must also undergo an independent medical examination and sign a commitment to follow medical advice. The procedure for application is detailed on the DVLA website.

For a group 2 licence, the following criteria must be met:
- Must have full awareness of hypoglycaemia.
- No episode of severe hypoglycaemia in the preceding 12 months.
- Monitors capillary glucose at least twice daily on days when not driving and at times relevant to driving (see Box 15.2).
- Interstitial glucose monitoring is not accepted for a group 2 licence.
- Demonstrates an understanding of the risks of hypoglycaemia.
- There are no other disqualifying complications of diabetes.

Holding a group 1 licence (cars and motorcycles)

Those not treated with insulin

As long as there are no problems with hypoglycaemia and there are no other contraindications to driving (e.g. from neuropathy/visual problems), the DVLA does not need to be informed. Drivers on any treatment, other than diet alone, need to be under regular medical review. Drivers using treatments with a risk of hypoglycaemia (including SUs and glinides) need to undertake appropriate blood glucose monitoring at times appropriate to driving and should be prescribed monitoring equipment.

Those treated with insulin

Must inform the DVLA of their diabetes. As long as there are no problems with hypoglycaemia, short-term (1–3 years) licences are issued under the following conditions:
- Must perform appropriate blood glucose monitoring.
- Must not be regarded as a likely source of danger to the public while driving.
- Must meet standards for visual acuity and visual field.

> **Box 15.2 Good practice for driving with diabetes**
> - Test blood glucose before driving, even short distances, and every 2h during longer journeys if there is any possibility of hypoglycaemia. The 1st test during a journey should be no more than 2h after the pre-driving blood test.
> - If blood glucose is <4.0mmol, carbohydrate (CHO) should be taken and driving delayed for at least 45min to allow any cognitive deficit to recover.
> - If glucose is <5mmol/L before driving, extra CHO should be strongly considered.
> - Keep a source of rapid-acting CHO (e.g. glucose tablets) easily available in the vehicle to treat symptoms of hypoglycaemia arising while driving.
> - Do not continue to drive once symptoms of hypoglycaemia develop.
> - Move out of the driver's seat to treat hypoglycaemia.

Temporary insulin treatment

The DVLA does not need to be informed initially as long as under medical supervision and not considered to be at risk of disabling hypoglycaemia. The DVLA must be informed if:
- Disabling hypoglycaemia develops.
- Treatment continues for longer than 3 months (3 months post-partum in the case of GDM).

Holding a group 2 licence (large lorries and buses)

Those managed using agents carrying a risk of hypoglycaemia (including insulin)

For this group, the DVLA must be informed and the above criteria must be met. For those on insulin, they must also undergo an independent medical examination and sign a commitment to follow advice. The procedure for application is detailed on the DVLA website.

Those using other treatment with no other contraindications

If on diet alone, the DVLA does not need to be informed. For other treatment, drivers must be under regular medical review and test glucose regularly. The DVLA must be informed but will usually issue a licence.

Interstitial glucose monitoring

Group 1 drivers

Flash glucose monitoring and real-time continuous glucose monitoring systems may be used for glucose monitoring. Fingerprick glucose monitoring should also be available and should be used to confirm the interstitial glucose readings when:

- Glucose is 4.0mmol/L or below.
- Symptoms of hypoglycaemia are being experienced.
- The glucose reading is not consistent with current symptoms (e.g. symptoms of hypoglycaemia, but the glucose reading does not reflect this).

Individuals with complete hypoglycaemia unawareness cannot use CGM alarms to warn of impending hypoglycaemia. Should a driver become reliant on these alarms to advise them that they are hypoglycaemic, they must stop driving and notify the DVLA.

Sport and exercise and diabetes

The suggested amount of exercise is the same for those with diabetes as for the general population (see Box 15.3). The health benefits, such as alterations in BP and lipids, may be particularly helpful in diabetes. However, metabolic changes during exercise can make the management of diabetes difficult. When encouraging people with diabetes to exercise, it is important to take account of any complications. For example, weight-bearing exercise is unlikely to be appropriate for an individual with significant peripheral neuropathy. Cardiovascular risk should also be assessed, and formal assessment arranged if appropriate.

For advice on sport and diabetes, see ℘ https://extod.org/.

Type 1 diabetes

Lower-intensity (aerobic) exercise

In those without diabetes, insulin levels decrease during exercise of lower intensity and longer duration. The difficulty of achieving this with exogenous insulin therapy means that the commonest problem in diabetes is hypoglycaemia. Fear of hypoglycaemia is recognized as the most important factor limiting people with T1DM for adopting a more active lifestyle. Post-exercise hypoglycaemia is a real concern, particularly in young men sleeping alone.

Higher-intensity (anaerobic) and resistance exercise

In contrast, high-intensity exercise and resistance exercise (particularly involving the upper body) can cause significant ↑ glucose through ↑ catecholamines. This is often unexpected and can cause confusion and frustration.

General advice

- Avoid hypoglycaemia before exercise.
- Test blood glucose before, during, and after exercise where possible.
- Aim to keep blood glucose between 7 and 10mmol/L before and during exercise.
- If below 7mmol/L before exercise, have 15–20g CHO.
- Ensure a supply of fast-acting CHO is freely available.
- Ensure safety—make sure those around are aware and can treat hypoglycaemia. If alone, ensure somebody knows where you are supposed to be and the expected time of return.

Strategies for dealing with hypoglycaemia

- Avoid bolus insulin injection near exercising muscle (e.g. legs if running/cycling).
- Adequate dietary energy consumption is important. This will vary with factors such as body weight and duration and intensity of exercise.
- If exercise is within 2h of a meal, bolus insulin dose with that meal should be ↓ by 50%.
- Extra rapid-acting CHO can be taken during exercise; 0.5–1g/kg body weight/h may be needed, although absorption of >60g/h can be problematic. Ideally taken from around 15–20min into exercise and gradually in small amounts thereafter.
- A post-exercise snack may be needed, with 50% of the usual insulin bolus. Insulin requirements with an evening meal post-exercise may also be reduced by 50%.

- A decrease in basal insulin injection of 10–20% may be required on the night after exercise to avoid nocturnal hypoglycaemia.
- CSII therapy can be very useful for exercise. Basal rate should be ↓ to 20–50% of normal around 60–90min before exercise and then returned to normal at the end.
- A 10s high-intensity sprint can help to stop glucose falling, but this should not be used as a treatment for hypoglycaemia.
- Insulin pumps can be removed for exercise, although there is a significant risk of hyperglycaemia ± ketosis. A hybrid approach where 20–50% of basal insulin is given by injection and the rest via the pump can support prolonged pump removal.
- Post-exercise CSII basal rate should be ↓ by 20% from bedtime for 4–6h.

> **Box 15.3 Physical activity recommendations for health**
> - At least 150min each week of moderate-intensity physical activity in blocks of at least 10min (e.g. 30min on at least 5 days each week), 75min of vigorous activity each week, or a combination of the two.
> - At least two sessions of muscle strengthening activity each week. These should not be on consecutive days.

Strategies for dealing with hyperglycaemia
- Ensure adequate hydration, and avoid excess CHO replacement.
- 50% of the usual calculated correction bolus can help to reduce glucose after exercise.
- If the glucose rise with an activity is predictable, a small dose of insulin before activity may be helpful. Start with 0.5–1U.
- A low-intensity warm-down can also be used.

Type 2 diabetes

Both aerobic and resistance exercise are beneficial in T2DM. There is also benefit in reducing the risk of 'prediabetic' states (IFG and IGT) developing into diabetes.

The main benefits are:
- Improvement in glycaemic control.
- Insulin sensitivity increases acutely with a single bout of exercise and chronically with sustained exercise, leading to ↓ insulin requirements.
- Cardiovascular risk factors improve.
- Help with weight control, both through altered energy balance and a reduction in insulin requirements.
- Improvements in general well-being and functional capacity.

Alcohol and diabetes

People with diabetes can continue to drink alcohol without problems as long as they do so sensibly. Excess alcohol should be avoided (see Box 15.4). It is best to avoid or limit sweet alcoholic drinks, such as sweet wines and alcopops, and mixers should be of the 'sugar-free' or 'diet' varieties.

▶ Alcohol increases the risk of hypoglycaemia, with larger amounts increasing the risk. The risk can persist for up to 16h.

- Avoid drinking alcohol on an empty stomach—starchy snacks may be helpful if drinking throughout an evening.
- Alcoholic drinks contain carbohydrate but should not be used to replace meals or snacks.
- After consuming larger amounts of alcohol, ensure that some CHO is eaten before going to bed (especially if treated with insulin). Healthy snacks are better, but chips or pizza, for example, are an alternative. Breakfast should be eaten the following morning.
- Alcohol intoxication may reduce hypoglycaemic symptoms. Remember a hypo could be confused with drunkenness if alcohol is on the breath.

Box 15.4 Diabetes UK recommended alcohol limits

- In line with government advice, it is recommended to drink no more than 14U per week.
- This limit is the same for men and for women.
- For more information about units, visit ✆ https://www.drinkaware.co.uk

---

Recreational drug use and diabetes

In questionnaire surveys:
- 5–25% of those aged 12–20 and 29% of those aged 16–30 have experienced recreational drug use during their lifetime.
- >50% of young people with DKA admitted into a tertiary centre over a 10-month period admitted to drug use, although only 20% volunteered this on initial questioning.

The index of suspicion for drug use needs to be high, as drug use is significantly associated with risk of death from acute diabetes-related events (OR 5.7). In those where there is significant suspicion, urinary drug screening should be considered. Box 15.5 lists some of the adverse effects reported with recreational drugs in diabetes.

Mechanisms by which recreational drugs affect diabetes are variable:
- Effects on judgement and decision-making. For example:
  - Missed insulin doses, resulting in hyperglycaemia/DKA.
  - Alterations in food intake, resulting in hyper- or hypoglycaemia.
  - Reduced ability to recognize hyper- or hypoglycaemia and to treat appropriately due to impaired perception.
- Catecholamine toxicity.
- ↑ lipolysis.
- Altered renal handling of ketones and bicarbonate.

Advice about being as safe as possible when using recreational drugs should be made available to people with diabetes. This may include:
- Being as well informed as possible about potential effects.
- Choosing as safe an environment as possible.
- Never experimenting the 1st time alone.
- Carrying something identifying you as having diabetes.
- Ensuring at least one person present knows you have diabetes and ideally knows how to handle any emergency and remains capable of providing assistance.

Box 15.5 Observed consequences of common recreational drugs

- MDMA (ecstasy): DKA and hyponatraemia.
- Ketamine: DKA (acidosis out of proportion to ketosis), rhabdomyolysis.
- Heroin: hyperglycaemic hyperosmolar state (HHS) following heroin OD; lethal levels of methadone in a patient who died of DKA.
- Cocaine: HHS and DKA (one study has shown cocaine use to be a strong independent risk factor for recurrent DKA).
- Cannabis: direct effects minimal, although may lower blood glucose in large amounts.

Travel and diabetes

People with diabetes need to plan ahead prior to travelling on holiday or for business (see Box 15.6). If possible, take more medication (especially insulin) than should be required in case there is a problem. When obtaining insulin abroad, it is important to remember that not every country uses U100 (i.e. 100U/mL) insulin which is the standard in the UK. Some countries use U40 or U80.

Crossing time zones can be complex. The day is longer travelling east to west, and extra insulin doses may be required. Travelling west to east, the day is shorter, so doses of basal insulin may overlap and require reduction. Insulin requirements may alter when on holiday due to ↑ temperature (↓), unaccustomed exercise (↓), and a change in diet (↑ or ↓). FRÍO® packs (℘ https://friouk.com/) are useful for keeping insulin cold for hours when a fridge is not available.

> **Box 15.6 Travelling by plane with diabetes**
> - Contact the airport and airline well in advance.
> - Have a letter from the healthcare team, explaining the need to carry medication, delivery devices (including needles), and monitoring equipment in hand luggage.
> - Ensure insulin does not travel in the hold—low temperatures may cause degradation, and there will be problems if luggage is lost.
> - Carry CHO-containing food for the journey.
> - Inform airlines in advance of use of CSII/CGM technology—airlines differ on rules for device use on board (most people with diabetes technology travel without incident).
> - May need to disconnect pump or handsets during take-off and landing.
> - Should not go through X-ray machines or full body scanners wearing insulin pump/CGM—ask for 'pat-down' search.
> - There is a medical device information card produced in conjunction with the Civil Aviation Authority and Airport Operators Association (download from ℘ https://www.caa.co.uk/home/).

Ramadan and diabetes

Fasting during Ramadan, the holy month of Islam, is a duty for all healthy adult Muslims. Although illness allows exemption from fasting, most Muslims with diabetes do not consider themselves unwell and choose to fast. Many Muslims also fast for 1–2 days each week throughout the year. Fasting includes omission of all oral intake, including liquids and medications, between sunrise and sunset. Blood glucose monitoring is allowed.

Fasting is broken at sunset with the Iftaar meal, which is a social occasion spent with family and friends. This can involve people with diabetes managing a large carbohydrate intake. Suhoor is a smaller meal taken just before sunrise, and the start of the day's fast.

Fasting is not meant to create excessive hardship, and advice should be sought from healthcare professionals as to the risks. Healthcare providers must advise honestly, but be sensitive to an individual's spiritual views, with advice sought from religious leaders where appropriate. Missed fasts due to chronic illness can be compensated for by paying a charitable donation known as fidya.

The main risks during Ramadan are:
- Hypoglycaemia.
- Hyperglycaemia.
- DKA.
- Dehydration and thrombosis.

A pre-Ramadan medical assessment is helpful where advice can be given about management of diabetes and fasting (see Box 15.7) and a risk stratification performed.

Low/moderate risk of harm from fasting includes those with HbA1c <8%/64mmol/mol, who are hypo aware, treated with agents that do not cause hypoglycaemia, and aged <75 years. Previous experience of fasting without problems is helpful.

In T1DM, willingness to self-monitor regularly, the ability to adjust insulin, and a good understanding of when to break the fast all lower the risk of problems.

Those with a recent diagnosis of T1DM, pregnancy, HbA1c >8%, frequent hypoglycaemia, hypo unawareness, use of SGLT2 inhibitor therapy, a history of DKA in the last year, and CKD and other complications of diabetes should be advised that fasting would be high risk. Children with diabetes should not fast. Fasting should also be avoided on days where intense physical activity or prolonged driving is required.

Management strategies can be suggested for those who do elect to fast. Ramadan-focused structured education may be helpful.

Box 15.7 Managing diabetes during Ramadan

- Blood glucose should be monitored more frequently.
- Try to avoid dose changes or new therapies immediately before Ramadan.
- Most non-insulin therapies can be continued without dose change; however, consider stopping or reducing SUs.
- Insulin doses may need to be ↓, e.g. reducing basal by 20%.
- Match rapid-acting insulin doses to the size of the Iftaar and Suhoor meals.
- Type of insulin may need to be changed. Premixed insulin is less easy to manage during fasting.
- Consume low glycaemic index food before the fast. Fruit, vegetables, and salad should be included.
- Limit high glycaemic index and fatty foods when breaking the fast.
- Avoid dehydration—increase fluid intake during non-fasting hours.
- Break the fast in the event of hypoglycaemia (blood glucose <3.9mmol/L) and significant hyperglycaemia (blood glucose >16.7mmol/L).
- Avoid fasting on 'sick days'.

Language matters: life, language, and diabetes

Arguably, of all the common chronic diseases, diabetes has the most pervasive impact on day-to-day life. People with diabetes, particularly those on insulin, have to think about the effect on blood glucose of everything they eat or drink and manage the consequences of activity, stress, illness, hormones, and multiple other influences. People with obesity and T2DM also face the frequent judgement that they have brought diabetes on themselves through poor lifestyle choices. Having diabetes is really difficult.

Imagine now, that instead of being supportive and empathetic of the challenges, a healthcare professional talks about 'poor control' or 'non-compliance' and the person with diabetes comes to clinic worried about being 'told off'.

The language used by healthcare professionals can have a profound impact on how people living with diabetes, and those who care for them, experience their condition and feel about living with it day-to-day. At its best, good use of language—verbal, written, and non-verbal (body language)—which is more inclusive and values-based, can lower anxiety, build confidence, educate, and help to improve self-care. Conversely, poor communication can be stigmatizing, hurtful, and undermining of self-care and have a detrimental effect on clinical outcomes.

Resources and position statements on Language Matters can be found at ℘ https://www.languagemattersdiabetes.com/. The documents suggest practical examples of positive, empowering language that will encourage positive interactions with people living with diabetes.

Further reading

Living with diabetes
Diabetes UK. [The website has useful information about all topics on diabetes and life]. ℘ http://www.diabetes.org.uk

Sport
Lumb AN, Gallen IW (2009). Diabetes management for intense exercise. *Curr Opin Endocrinol Diabetes Obes* **16**, 150–5.
ExCarbs. ℘ https://excarbs.sansum.org/ [aimed at patients].
EXTOD (Exercise for Type 1 Diabetes). [Aimed at healthcare professionals currently, although patient advice will follow]. ℘ https://extod.org/
Runsweet. [Aimed at patients]. ℘ http://www.runsweet.com/

Drugs and diabetes
Lee P, et al. (2009). Managing young people with type 1 diabetes in a 'rave' new world: metabolic complications of substance abuse in type 1 diabetes. *Diabet Med* **26**, 328–33.

Ramadan
Ibrahim M, et al. (2020). Recommendations for management of diabetes during Ramadan: update 2020, applying the principles of the ADA/EASD consensus. *BMJ Open Diab Res Care* **8**, e001248.
Hussain S, et al. (2020). Type 1 diabetes and fasting in Ramadan: time to rethink classification of risk? *Lancet Diabetes Endocrinol* **8**, 656–8.
Al-Arouj M, et al. (2010). Recommendations for management of diabetes during Ramadan. *Diabetes Care* **33**, 1895–902.

Language and diabetes
Language Matters Diabetes. ℘ https://www.languagemattersdiabetes.com/
NHS England (2018). *Language matters. Language and diabetes.* [UK working group position statement]. ℘ https://www.england.nhs.uk/wp-content/uploads/2018/06/language-matters.pdf

Hospital inpatient diabetes management and diabetes-related emergencies

Data from the National Diabetes Inpatient Audit suggest that the number of hospital inpatients with diabetes ranges from ~10% to over 30%. This does not mean that up to 1 in 3 inpatients are in hospital *because* of their diabetes but that they happen to have diabetes, in addition to whatever other condition has necessitated their admission. Whatever the reason for admission, people with diabetes often have longer lengths of hospital stay, and the presence of diabetes remains an important comorbidity that must be dealt with by staff who are competent and confident in its management.

Over the last few years, the Joint British Diabetes Societies Inpatient Care Group has published several national guidelines on the management of several aspects of inpatient diabetes care. These guidelines are being regularly reviewed and updated, with guidance on new subjects also being published regularly.

The following guidelines are largely derived from those, and full versions can be found on the Internet (⅌ https://abcd.care/joint-british-diabetes-societies-jbds-inpatient-care-group).

The aim of these guidelines is to improve standards of diabetes care within hospitals. Support for people with diabetes admitted to hospital commonly now includes diabetes inpatient nurse teams.

Diabetes-related hyperglycaemic emergencies

Diabetic ketoacidosis

The diagnosis of DKA is dependent on the combined presence of three biochemical abnormalities:

- Ketonaemia ≥3mmol/L or significant ketonuria (>2+).
- Blood glucose >11mmol/L or known diabetes.
- Bicarbonate (HCO_3^-) <15mmol/L and/or venous pH <7.3.

The presence of any of the following should prompt consideration of admission to a level 2/high dependency unit (HDU) environment:

- Blood ketones >6mmol/L, HCO_3^- level <5mmol/L, pH <7.1.
- Hypokalaemia (<3.5mmol/L).
- Abnormal Glasgow Coma Scale (GCS) or AVPU score.
- O_2 saturation <92% on air.
- Systolic BP <90mmHg, pulse >100 or <60bpm.
- Anion gap >16 [anion gap = $(Na^+ + K^+) - (Cl^- + HCO_3^-)$].

Management of DKA

The resolution of DKA depends upon the suppression of ketonaemia, and measurement of blood ketones now represents best practice in monitoring the response to treatment. Bedside ketone monitors should be used to measure plasma ketone concentrations (in particular, 3β-hydroxybutyrate) because this is a direct marker of disease severity.

Where available, the specialist diabetes team should ideally be involved as early as is practical after admission.

Monitoring should be by using venous blood gases (the differences in arterial and venous pH, HCO_3^-, and K^+ are not great enough to alter management). Plasma ketones, venous pH, and HCO_3^- measurements should be used as treatment markers (see Box 15.8).

Use a weight-based, fixed-rate intravenous insulin infusion (FRIII) at 0.1U/kg/h (e.g. 7U/h for a 70kg individual). This enables rapid blood ketone clearance. The fixed rate may be adjusted in insulin-resistant states if the response is not fast enough. The rate of intravenous insulin infusion may be reduced to 0.05unit/kg/h once the glucose drops to <14mmol/L. There is no need for a bolus dose of insulin if the IV insulin infusion (IVII) is set up promptly.

Continue SC basal insulin analogues. They provide background insulin when the IVII is discontinued. Short-acting insulin should be given 30–60min before discontinuing the IVII.

HCO_3^- should not be given because it may worsen intracellular acidosis and may precipitate cerebral oedema, particularly in children.

Box 15.8 Metabolic treatment targets in DKA

- Reduction in blood ketones by 0.5mmol/L/h.
- Increase in venous HCO_3^- by 3.0mmol/L/h.
- Reduction in capillary blood glucose by 3.0mmol/L/h.
- K maintained at 4.5–5.5mmol/L.
  If these rates are not achieved, then the FRIII needs adjusting.

Initial actions (1st hour of treatment)

- Rapid assessment and resuscitation; commence IV fluids.
- Full clinical examination, with assessment of:
  - Respiratory rate; temperature; BP; pulse; O_2 saturation.
  - Assess GCS. Consider NG tube if GCS is <12.
- Initial investigations should include:
  - Bedside capillary ketones and capillary glucose.
  - Venous gases for glucose, U&E, pH, and HCO_3^-. If Cl^- is available, calculate the anion gap.
  - FBC, blood cultures.
  - ECG, CXR, midstream urine (MSU).
- Continuous cardiac monitoring and pulse oximetry.
- LMWH.
- Consider any precipitating causes, and treat appropriately.

Fluid resuscitation

If the systolic BP is <90mmHg, consider causes other than fluid depletion such as heart failure, sepsis, etc. Give 500mL of 0.9% NaCl solution over 10–15min, and repeat if necessary. If there is no improvement in BP, consider the need for circulatory support.

If systolic BP is >90mmHg, use the rate of fluid replacement shown in Table 15.9.

Potassium replacement

Hypo- and hyperkalaemia are common in DKA (see Table 15.10).

Table 15.9 Fluid replacement rates

Fluid	Volume
0.9% NaCl 1L	1000mL over 1st hour
0.9% NaCl 1L with KCl	1000mL 2-hourly × 3
0.9% NaCl 1L with KCl	1000mL 4-hourly × 2
Reassessment of cardiovascular status at 12h is mandatory; further fluid may be required.	

Table 15.10 Potassium replacement for different levels

K level in first 24h (mmol/L)	K replacement in mmol/L of infusion solution
Over 5.5	Nil
3.5–5.5	40mmol/L
Below 3.5	Additional K needed—either through ↑ infusion rate or use of concentrated K infusion (check local guidelines—may require transfer to HDU)

Insulin infusion

- Start a continuous FRIII via an infusion pump; 50U human soluble insulin (Actrapid®, Humulin S®), made up to 50mL with 0.9% NaCl solution.
- Infuse at a fixed rate of 0.1U/kg/h (e.g. 7mL/h if weight is 70kg). The rate of intravenous insulin infusion may be reduced to 0.05unit/kg/h once the glucose drops to <14mmol/L.

Ongoing management of DKA after the first 60min is covered in detail in the national guidelines (⅍ https://abcd.care/sites/abcd.care/files/site_uploads/JBDS_02%20_DKA_Guideline_amended_v2_June_2021.pdf).

This involves continual monitoring and reassessment to ensure that metabolic targets are being achieved (see Box 15.8), stabilization and treatment of precipitating factors, and other medical interventions or monitoring (e.g. NG tube, catheter) are not required.

Practice points

Infusion of large volumes of normal saline may lead to hyperchloraemic metabolic acidosis; however, this is not a cause of significant morbidity or prolongation of inpatient stay.

Convert to SC insulin when biochemically stable (blood ketones <0.3, pH >7.3) and the individual is eating and drinking. If they are not ready to eat or drink, but are biochemically no longer in DKA, then a variable-rate intravenous insulin infusion (VRIII) may be necessary.

Involve the specialist diabetes team at an early stage. The commonest causes of DKA are infections with failure to follow sick day rules and failure of self-management, so assessing the reasons behind admission and re-education to prevent recurrence are vital.

Hyperosmolar hyperglycaemic state

While there is no formal definition of HHS (previous name HONK), the following criteria have been adopted nationally across the UK:

- Hypovolaemia.
- Marked hyperglycaemia (30.0mmol/L or more).
- No significant ketonaemia (<3.0mmol/L) or acidosis (pH >7.3, HCO_3^- >15mmol/L).
- Osmolality usually ≥320mmol/kg.

$$\text{Calculated osmolality} = 2\ Na^+ + glucose + urea$$

NB. A mixed picture of HHS and DKA may occur.

HHS typically occurs in the elderly, but as T2DM is diagnosed in younger adults and teenagers, it is likely that HHS will present at younger ages as well. Unlike DKA, which usually comes on over a matter of hours, HHS comes on over many days, and consequently, the dehydration and metabolic disturbances are more extreme.

Management of HHS

(See ℘ https://abcd.care/sites/abcd.care/files/resources/JBDS_IP_ HHS_Adults.pdf)

Initial assessment

Hyperglycaemia results in osmotic diuresis and renal losses of water in excess of Na and K. Fluid losses are estimated to be between 100 and 220mL/kg. Despite these severe electrolyte losses and total body volume depletion, the typical person with HHS may not look as dehydrated as they are because the hypertonicity leads to preservation of intravascular volume.

The goals of treatment of HHS are to gradually and safely:

- Normalize osmolality.
- Replace fluid and electrolyte losses.
- Normalize blood glucose.
- Treat the underlying cause.
- Prevent arterial or venous thrombosis.
- Prevent other potential complications, e.g. cerebral oedema/central pontine myelinolysis.
- Prevent foot ulceration.

As with DKA, venous blood can be used to assess pH, HCO_3^-, U&E, glucose, etc. in a blood gas analyser.

The presence of any of the following should prompt consideration of admission to a level 2/HDU environment:

- Osmolality >350mOsm/kg, Na >160mmol/L.
- Venous/arterial pH <7.1.
- Hypokalaemia (<3.5mm/L) or hyperkalaemia (>6.0mmol/L).
- GCS score <12 or abnormal AVPU score.
- O_2 saturation <92% on air.
- Systolic BP <90mmHg, pulse >100 or <60bpm.
- Hypothermia.
- Acute or serious comorbidity, e.g. MI, CCF, or CVA.
- Urine output <0.5mL/kg/h or other evidence of acute kidney injury.

Fluid replacement and changes in osmolality

The goal of the initial therapy is expansion of the intra- and extravascular volumes and to restore peripheral perfusion. Replace fluid with 0.9% NaCl. Measurement or calculation of osmolality should be undertaken every hour initially, and the rate of fluid replacement adjusted to ensure a +ve fluid balance sufficient to promote a gradual decline in osmolality. Fluid replacement alone (without insulin) will lower blood glucose which will reduce osmolality, causing a shift of water into the intracellular space. This inevitably results in a rise in serum Na.

The aim of treatment should be to replace ~50% of estimated fluid loss within the first 12h and the remainder in the following 12h, although this will be determined by the initial severity, the degree of renal impairment, and associated comorbidities, which may limit the speed of correction.

A blood glucose target of between 10.0 and 15.0mmol/L is a reasonable goal. Complete normalization of electrolytes and osmolality may take up to 72h.

Role of insulin in HHS

If significant ketonaemia is present (3β-hydroxybutyrate is >1.0mmol/L), this indicates relative hypoinsulinaemia, and insulin should be started at time zero.

If significant ketonaemia is not present (3β-hydroxybutyrate <1.0mmol/L), here is an argument for not starting insulin treatment immediately, because fluid replacement alone will result in a falling blood glucose and reducing this too quickly may lead to lowering the osmolality precipitously. Insulin treatment, prior to adequate fluid replacement, may result in cardiovascular collapse, as water moves out of the intravascular space, with a resulting decline in intravascular volume.

With the administration of IV fluids, a fall in glucose at a rate of up to 5.0mmol/L/h is ideal. Once the blood glucose has ceased to fall following initial fluid resuscitation, reassess fluid intake and renal function. Insulin may be started at this point. The recommended insulin dose is a FRIII given at 0.05U/kg/h (e.g. 4U/h in an 80kg person). However, if insulin was already in place, the infusion rate is ↑ by 1U/h.

Potassium replacement

This is the same as in DKA.

Anticoagulation

Because of the ↑ risk of arterial and venous thromboembolism, people with HHS should receive prophylactic LMWH for the full duration of admission unless contraindicated. Full treatment dose anticoagulation should only be considered in those with suspected thrombosis or acute coronary syndrome.

Other electrolytes

Hypophosphataemia and hypomagnesaemia are common in HHS; however, as with DKA, routine replacement is not recommended.

Foot protection

These individuals are at high risk of pressure ulceration. An initial foot assessment should be undertaken, and heel protectors applied in those with neuropathy, PVD, or lower limb deformity. The feet should be re-examined daily and documented.

Intravenous insulin infusions used in hyperglycaemia

These can be either FRIII or VRIII.

Fixed-rate intravenous insulin infusions

These are used in the initial stages of DKA until ketones are <0.3mmol/L *and* pH >7.3 *and* venous HCO_3^- >18mmol/L, or in those with HHS once their blood glucose has stopped dropping at 5.0mmol/L/h with initial use of 0.9% NaCl. The starting doses are 0.1U/kg/h for DKA, and 0.05U/kg/h for HHS. In DKA the rate of the intravenous insulin infusion may be reduced to 0.05unit/kg/h once the glucose drops to <14mmol/L.

IV crystalloid solution must always be given with an FRIII. In DKA, if blood glucose concentrations are >14.0mmol/L, then this should be 0.9% NaCl; if blood glucose levels are <14.0mmol/L, then 10% glucose solution should be run *alongside* the saline infusion. Saline is for volume resuscitation, and 10% glucose is the substrate for the insulin.

Variable-rate intravenous insulin infusions

The aim of the VRIII is to achieve and maintain normoglycaemia. It should be made up in 50mL syringe with 0.9% NaCl—making a concentration of 1U/mL. See Table 15.11 for an example of how to prescribe a VRIII. More details on the use of a VRIII can be found at ℘ https://abcd.care/sites/abcd.care/files/resources/JBDS_IP_VRIII.pdf

Use of intravenous insulin infusion

- If the patient is already on a long-acting insulin analogue, these should be continued.
- Monitor blood glucose hourly.
- If blood glucose remains >12.0mmol/L for three consecutive readings and is not dropping by 3.0mmol/L/h or more, the rate of insulin infusion should be ↑.
- If blood glucose is <4.0mmol/L, the insulin infusion should be reduced to 0.5U/h and the low blood glucose should be treated, irrespective of whether the patient has symptoms. If the individual has continued on their basal insulin, then their VRII can be switched off, but the regular blood glucose measurements need to continue. Ensure basal insulin has been given before stopping VRII.

Table 15.11 Prescribing a VRIII

Bedside capillary blood glucose (mmol/L)	Initial rate of insulin infusion (unit/h)
<4.0	0.5 (0 if basal insulin has been continued)
4.1–7.0	1
7.1–9.0	2
9.1–11.0	3
11.1–14.0	4
14.1–17.0	5
17.1–20	6
>20	Seek diabetes team or medical advice

Perioperative management of diabetes

Poor perioperative glycaemic control leads to poor outcomes in every surgical specialty. There is detailed guidance available in the Joint British Diabetes Societies guideline on the perioperative management of adult patients with diabetes undergoing surgery or procedures (🖰 https://abcd.care/sites/abcd.care/files/site_uploads/CPOC_Diabetes_Surgery_Guideline_March_2021.pdf).

There are several reasons why patients experience problems:
• Failure to identify people with diabetes.
• Lack of institutional guidelines for management of diabetes.
• Poor knowledge of diabetes among staff delivering care.
• Complex polypharmacy and insulin-prescribing errors.

It is advocated that for elective surgery, HbA1c should be below 69mmol/mol (8.5%) prior to surgery where this is safe to achieve.

For most procedures where only one meal will be missed, hypoglycaemic therapy can be adjusted, as outlined in Table 15.12 (OHAs) and Table 15.13 (insulin). The use of the VRIII (see Table 15.11) should be limited to those who will miss more than one consecutive meal, those who require emergency surgery, and those for whom there was no time to optimize their glycaemic control prior to surgery. The rate of insulin infusion is as described in Table 15.11.

Table 15.12 Guideline for perioperative adjustment of non-insulin medication (short starvation period—no more than ONE missed meal)

Tablet	Day prior to admission	Day of surgery		
		AM surgery	PM surgery	If a VRIII is being used
Acarbose	Take as normal	Omit AM dose if NBM	Give AM dose if eating	Stop until eating and drinking normally
Meglitinide (repaglinide or nateglinide)	Take as normal	Omit AM dose if NBM	Give AM dose if eating	Stop until eating and drinking normally
Metformin (procedure not requiring use of contrast media)*	Take as normal	Take as normal	Take as normal	Stop until eating and drinking normally
SU	Take as normal	Once daily—AM omit	Once daily—AM omit	Stop until eating and drinking normally
		Twice daily—AM omit	Twice daily—omit AM and PM	Stop until eating and drinking normally

Table 15.12 (Contd.)

Tablet	Day prior to admission	Day of surgery		
		AM surgery	PM surgery	If a VRIII is being used
Pioglitazone	Take as normal	Take as normal	Take as normal	Stop until eating and drinking normally
DPP-IV inhibitor	Take as normal	Take as normal	Take as normal	Stop until eating and drinking normally
GLP-1 analogue (daily or weekly, PO or SC)	Take as normal	Take as normal	Take as normal	Take as normal
SGLT2 inhibitors**§	Omit from 24h prior to admission	Omit	Omit	Restart after 7 days and when eating and drinking normally

AM, morning; NBM, nil by mouth; PM, afternoon; PO, oral; SC subcutaneous.

* If contrast medium is to be used and eGFR <50mL/min/1.73m², metformin should be omitted on the day of the procedure and for the following 48h.

** If there is likely to be a period of reduction in oral intake prior to a procedure, e.g. colonoscopy, then the drug needs to be omitted starting on the day of the reduced intake. This may mean omitting the drug the day prior to the procedure, as well as the day of the procedure.

§ If the individual is likely to have a low-carbohydrate diet for several weeks, e.g. prior to bariatric surgery, then the drug must be stopped from commencement of the diet.

Table 15.13 Guideline for perioperative adjustment of insulin (short starvation period—no more than ONE missed meal; in all cases, check blood glucose on admission)

	Insulins	Day prior to admission	Day of surgery	
			AM surgery	PM surgery
Long-acting insulin	Once-daily basal (AM)	No dose change*	Reduce dose by 20% and check blood glucose on admission	Reduce dose by 20% and check blood glucose on admission
	Once-daily basal (lunchtime)	Reduce dose by 20%	Restart insulin at normal when eating and drinking normally	Restart insulin at normal when eating and drinking normally
	Once-daily basal (evening)	Reduce dose by 20%	No dose change*	No dose change*
	Twice-daily basal insulin	No change to AM dose Evening dose will need to be reduced by 20%	Reduce AM dose by 20% and check blood glucose on admission Evening dose remains unchanged	Reduce AM dose by 20% and check blood glucose on admission Evening dose remains unchanged
Self-prepared by patient	Twice daily (two different types of insulin) combined by the patient into one injection	No dose change to AM or evening doses	Give half TDD as intermediate-acting insulin in AM and check blood glucose on admission	Give half TDD as intermediate-acting insulin in AM and check blood glucose on admission
Short-acting insulin	Short-acting insulin with meals (2–4 doses a day)	No dose change	Omit AM and lunchtime doses and check blood glucose on admission	Take usual AM insulin dose. Omit lunchtime dose and check blood glucose on admission

	Day prior to admission	Day of surgery	
Insulins		AM surgery	PM surgery
Premixed insulin prepared by manufacturers			
Twice daily (premixed insulin)	No dose change	Halve the usual AM dose and check blood glucose on admission	Halve the usual AM dose and check blood glucose on admission
Three times per day (premixed insulin)	No dose change	Halve the usual AM dose. Omit the lunchtime dose and check blood glucose on admission	Halve the usual AM dose. Omit the lunchtime dose and check blood glucose on admission

AM, morning; PM, afternoon.

* Some units would advocate a reduction of the usual dose of a long-acting analogue by one-third. This reduction should be considered for any patient who 'grazes' during the day. Warn the patient that their blood glucose control may be erratic for a few days after the procedure.

Emergency management of hypoglycaemia

(See also ➔ Expert management of type 1 diabetes, pp. 854–7.)

Hypoglycaemia is the commonest side effect of insulin and SU treatment. Hypoglycaemia should be excluded in any person with diabetes who is acutely unwell, drowsy, unconscious, unable to cooperate, or presenting with aggressive behaviour or seizures. The hospital environment presents additional obstacles to the maintenance of good glycaemic control and the avoidance of hypoglycaemia.

Management of hypoglycaemia

Algorithm A: adults who are conscious, orientated, and able to swallow

Give 15–20g of quick-acting carbohydrate of the patient's choice:

- 5–7 Dextrosol® tablets (or 4–5 Glucotabs®).
- One bottle (60mL) of Glucojuice®.
- 150mL of non-diet cola (a small can).
- Five Jelly babies or fruit pastilles or ten Jelly beans.
- 3–4 heaped teaspoons of sugar dissolved in water*.
- 150–200mL of pure fruit juice*.

(* Some centres advocate ONLY glucose for the treatment of hypos. Repeat capillary blood glucose measurement 10–15min later. If blood glucose is <4.0mmol/L, repeat step 1 up to three times.)

If blood glucose remains <4.0mmol/L after 45min or three cycles, consider 1mg of glucagon IM (remembering that this may be less effective in patients prescribed SU therapy chronic liver disease or those with frequent recurrent hypoglycaemia) or 10% glucose IV infusion at 100mL/h.

Once blood glucose is above 4.0mmol/L and the patient has recovered, give 20g of long-acting carbohydrate:

- Two biscuits.
- One slice of bread.
- 200–300mL glass of milk (not soya).
- Normal meal if due (must contain carbohydrate).

DO NOT omit insulin injection if due (a dose review may be required).

The long-acting carbohydrate may not be needed in pump users as they can adjust the basal rate after a hypo.

Relative hypoglycaemia

Adults who have poor glycaemic control may start to experience symptoms of hypoglycaemia above 4.0mmol/L. Adults who are experiencing symptoms but have a blood glucose level >4.0mmol/L should consume a small carbohydrate snack only (e.g. one medium banana or a slice of bread). All adults with a blood glucose level <4.0mmol/L, with or without symptoms of hypoglycaemia, should be treated as outlined in ➔ Management of hypoglycaemia, above.

Algorithm B: adults who are conscious but confused, disorientated, unable to cooperate, or aggressive but are able to swallow

- If the patient is unable to follow algorithm A but is able to swallow, give *either* 2 tubes of GlucoGel®/Dextrogel®, squeezed into the mouth between the teeth and gums, *or* (if ineffective) give glucagon 1mg IM.
- Monitor blood glucose levels after 15min. If still <4.0mmol/L, repeat steps 1 and 2 up to three times.
- If blood glucose concentration remains <4.0mmol/L after 45min, give 10% glucose IV infusion at 100mL/h.
- Once blood glucose is above 4.0mmol/L and the patient has recovered, give a long-acting carbohydrate.
- DO NOT omit insulin injection if due (a dose review may be required).

NB. Patients given glucagon require a larger portion of long-acting carbo-hydrate to replenish glycogen stores (double the suggested amount above).

Algorithm C: adults who are unconscious and/or are having seizures and/or are very aggressive OR patients who are nil by mouth

- Assess the patient.
- If the patient has an insulin infusion *in situ*, stop it immediately.
- The following two options are both appropriate:
  - Glucagon 1mg IM (remembering that this may be less effective in patients prescribed SU therapy and may take up to 15min to work).
  - If IV access available, give 75mL of 20% glucose or 150mL of 10% glucose over 12–15min. Repeat capillary blood glucose measurement 10min later. If blood glucose is <4.0mmol/L, repeat.
- Once blood glucose is >4.0mmol/L and the patient has recovered, give a long-acting carbohydrate.
- DO NOT omit insulin injection if due (dose review may be required).
- If the patient was on IV insulin, continue to check blood glucose every 30min until it is above 3.5mmol/L; then restart IV insulin after review of the dose regimen.

Management of stroke patients with diabetes

(See ℅ http://www.diabetologists-abcd.org.uk/JBDS/JBDS_IP_Enteral_
Feeding_Stroke.pdf)

Swallowing difficulties may be temporary or long-lasting following stroke.
Fig. 15.5 shows the management of those with diabetes who need enteral
feeding.

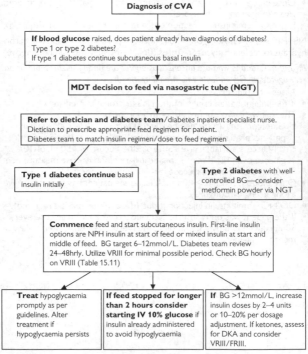

Fig. 15.5 Algorithm for managing diabetes in patients with swallowing difficulties
following a stroke.

The critically ill patient

There is controversy regarding the best way to treat hyperglycaemia in critically ill patients. There have been a number of studies done in this population, although the vast majority have been done on patients in intensive care or cardiac surgical patients. The results have not been consistent, with some studies showing benefit and others showing potential harm. In addition, there is currently little consensus on the best way to treat hyperglycaemia-associated poor outcomes following an episode of acute coronary syndrome; however, studies to assess this are ongoing. If one accepts the premise that high blood glucose levels are associated with harm, then a pragmatic approach is to keep the blood glucose between 6.0 and 10.0mmol/L using whatever means necessary—oral medication, where appropriate, or a VRIII (see Table 15.11). Local guidelines should be followed and guidance sought from diabetes specialist teams.

Further reading

Centre for Peri-operative Care (2011, updated 2021). *Management of adults with diabetes undergoing surgery and elective procedures: improving standards.* ℘ https://abcd.care/sites/abcd.care/files/site_uploads/CPOC_Diabetes_Surgery_Guideline_March_2021.pdf

Furnary AP, et al. (1999). Continuous intravenous insulin infusion reduces the incidence of deep sternal wound infection in diabetic patients after cardiac surgical procedures. *Ann Thorac Surg* **67**, 352–62.

Gandhi GY, et al. (2007). Intensive intraoperative insulin therapy versus conventional glucose management during cardiac surgery: a randomized trial. *Ann Intern Med* **146**, 233–43.

Joint British Diabetes Societies for inpatient care. *Diabetes at the front door.* ℘ https://abcd.care/sites/abcd.care/files/site_uploads/JBDS_Diabetes_Front_Door_amended_FINAL_27032020.pdf

NICE-SUGAR Study Investigators (2009). Intensive versus conventional glucose control in critically ill patients. *N Engl J Med* **360**, 1283–97.

Savage MW, et al. (2011). Joint British Diabetes Societies guideline for the management of diabetic ketoacidosis. *Diabet Med* **28**, 508–15.

Stanisstreet D, et al. (2010). *The hospital management of hypoglycaemia in adults with diabetes mellitus.* ℘ https://abcd.care/sites/abcd.care/files/site_uploads/JBDS_01_Hypo_Guideline_FINAL_23042021_0.pdf

Van den Berghe G, et al. (2001). Intensive insulin therapy in the surgical intensive care unit. *N Engl J Med* **345**, 1359–67.

Diabetes and pregnancy

Background

Diabetes is the commonest medical complication of pregnancy, affecting ~1 in 250 pregnancies. Of the 650,000 women giving birth in England and Wales each year, 2–5% will involve women with diabetes. ~87.5% of pregnancies complicated by diabetes are due to GDM (which may, or may not, resolve after pregnancy), with the remaining 12.5% being due to pre-existing T1DM and T2DM. In T1DM and T2DM, there are risks to both the mother and the fetus, with a congenital anomaly rate of up to 10% or 4–5 times that of the background maternity population in women with unplanned pregnancy and poor glycaemic control (periconception HbA1c >86mmol/mol or 10%). The risks can be reduced, but not entirely eliminated, by optimal periconception glycaemic control (HbA1c <48mmol/mol or 6.5% or lower, if safely achievable without hypoglycaemia) and 5mg folic acid supplementation (see Box 15.9).

Risks

Serious adverse pregnancy outcomes

- Congenital anomaly: cardiac and neural tube defects occur during the first 40 days, stressing the importance of optimizing glycaemic control before conception. The risk of having an infant with a major congenital anomaly is comparable for women with T1DM and T2DM (4–5%) and more than twice that of the background maternity population (1–2%). The contributions of hyperglycaemia and maternal obesity to the pathogenesis of congenital malformations are well recognized. Alterations in O_2 free radicals, myoinositol, arachidonic acid, and zinc metabolism have also been implicated.
- Stillbirth (14 per 1000 births, with ↑ risk if poor glycaemic control and in infants who are large or small for gestational age).
- Neonatal death (10 per 1000 births in mothers with T1DM and T2DM).

Fetal and neonatal complications

- Large for gestational age (birthweight above the 90th percentile) remains the commonest complication of diabetic pregnancy, affecting ~50% of offspring born to mothers with T1DM and 25% of offspring born to mothers with T2DM. Fetal hyperinsulinaemia causes growth of insulin-sensitive tissues, with ↑ abdominal circumference, due to hypertrophy of the fetal pancreatic cells, liver, and heart. As well as causing birth trauma and delivery complications, large-for-gestational age infants have ↑ longer-term risks of insulin resistance, obesity, and T2DM, persisting during childhood and adolescence.
- Preterm delivery (before 37 weeks' gestation) occurs in ~40% of T1DM and 20% of T2DM pregnancies, with resulting complications of neonatal hypoglycaemia, jaundice, and polycythaemia.
- Neonatal intensive care unit admission: ~40% of infants born to mothers with T1DM and 20% of infants of mothers with T2DM require additional neonatal care, most typically for complications of preterm delivery and neonatal hypoglycaemia.

Box 15.9 Preconception management

- Preconception glycaemic control optimized, aiming for HbAlc <48mmol/mol (6.5%) if safely achievable without severe hypoglycaemia.
- High-dose folic acid supplements (5mg/day).
- Review potentially teratogenic medications, including ACEIs and statins.
- Advice on losing weight for all women with BMI >27kg/m².
- Advice on stopping smoking, reducing alcohol intake, and avoiding unpasteurized dairy products.
- Screening for retinopathy and nephropathy.
- Metformin may be used as an adjunct or alternative to insulin. All other OHAs should be discontinued and replaced with insulin. In HNF1A/4A-MODY already well controlled on low-dose SU, glibenclamide can be substituted (see ➔ Management of MODY in pregnancy, p. 846).

Maternal

- ↑ risk of severe hypoglycaemia, particularly during early pregnancy. Historically, the prevalence of severe hypoglycaemia was up to 30–40% in T1DM but is now declining (12% in T1DM pregnancy, 2% in T2DM pregnancy) with widespread use of insulin analogues and ↑ use of insulin pump therapy.
- ↑ risk of pre-eclampsia, which is related to glycaemic control and complicates ~15% of diabetes pregnancies.
- Worsening of diabetic nephropathy and progression of retinopathy: renal and retinal screening is recommended before and during pregnancy, usually at booking and at 28 weeks.
- ↑ risk of DKA. Although rare, affecting <3% of pregnancies, historically, DKA is associated with fetal loss in up to 20% of episodes. Women with suspected DKA should be admitted to level 2 critical care for immediate medical and obstetric care.
- ↑ delivery by Caesarean section (60% in T1DM, 50% in T2DM).
- Thromboembolic disease, while rare, is responsible for a third of all maternal deaths. All women with risk factors (age >35, BMI >30kg/m², proteinuria >5g/day) and/or other comorbidities should receive prophylactic LMWH throughout pregnancy.
- Thyroid dysfunction is three times commoner in T1DM pregnancy and should be assessed during pregnancy and post-partum.

Type 1 and type 2 diabetes

- Most women (>98%) deliver live babies. Congenital anomaly and spontaneous abortion rates are higher when HbA1c is elevated (>6.5%; 48mmol/mol).
- Pregnancy is not recommended in women with HbA1c >86mmol/mol (10%). They should be prescribed safe effective contraception until optimal glucose control has been achieved.

Management during pregnancy

All pregnant women should be managed in a multidisciplinary clinic and reviewed every 1–2 weeks. A checklist for the clinic visit is listed in Box 15.10.

Optimal glycaemic control

Optimal glycaemic control reduces the risk of serious adverse outcomes, including congenital anomaly, stillbirth, and neonatal death. However, even with near-perfect glucose control, there is a small, but significant ↑ risk of cardiac malformations and stillbirth.

A basal bolus regimen is used in conjunction with a healthy balanced diet (typically 20–30g of carbohydrate at breakfast and 40–50g for lunch and dinner) to achieve the tight postprandial glucose targets. Fast-acting insulin analogues are preferred and safe for use in pregnancy. Prandial insulin should be given 15min before eating in early pregnancy (<20 weeks) and at least 30–40min before eating in late pregnancy (>20 weeks).

Levemir® (but not Lantus®) is licensed for use during pregnancy. However, both Lantus® and Levemir® are widely used before and during pregnancy to reduce the risk of maternal hypoglycaemia.

CGM is associated with improved glucose control and reduced risk of large for gestational age, neonatal intensive care admissions, and neonatal hypoglycaemia. The NHS 10-year plan states that by 2020/21, all pregnant women with T1DM will be offered CGM, helping to improve neonatal outcomes.

Insulin pump therapy (CSII) is indicated for women with T1DM who cannot achieve optimal glycaemic control on multiple daily injections without disabling hypoglycaemia.

Insulin therapy

In T1DM, insulin requirements often fall in early pregnancy (from 8 to 14 weeks), and then continue to rise from about 16 until 36 weeks, falling back to pre-pregnancy levels, or even lower, after delivery.

Women with T1DM should be advised about the ↑ risk of severe hypoglycaemia and that hypoglycaemia awareness may decrease, especially during early pregnancy. Advice regarding care with driving (do not drive below 5mmol/L) is essential. Partners should be instructed how and when to administer glucagon.

Monitoring of microvascular complications during pregnancy

Screening for nephropathy and retinopathy is advised at the 1st antenatal appointment and repeated at 28 weeks. Diabetic retinopathy should not be considered a contraindication to rapid optimization of glucose control. If serum Cr is abnormal (120micromol/L or more) or the eGFR is <45mL/min/1.73m^2, referral to a nephrologist is indicated.

Fetal monitoring

- Scanning of the fetus at 10–12 weeks to confirm dates, looking for congenital abnormalities.
- Screening for congenital malformations at 18–20 weeks.
- Fetal growth assessments at 28, 32, and 36 weeks.

Management of delivery and after delivery

- Women should be offered elective birth through induction of labour or by elective Caesarean section typically around 37-38 weeks in T1DM, 38-39 weeks in T2DM and between 39-40 weeks in GDM.

> **Box 15.10 Checklist for type 1/type 2 diabetes in pregnancy during clinic visit**
>
> - Capillary glucose monitoring before and 1h after meals and before bed, i.e. 7–8 tests per day.
>   - Fasting glucose of <5.3mmol/L.
>   - 1h postprandial glucose of <7.8mmol/L.
> - CGM or Libre to optimize maternal glucose control in T1DM pregnancy.
> - HbA1c <48mmol/mol (6.5%) and CGM time in range 3.5–7.8mmol/L (70%).
> - Insulin therapy—basal bolus or insulin pump therapy. Metformin may be continued.
>   - Reinforce risk of hypoglycaemia during 1st trimester (e.g. education on driving, glucagon injection) and DKA (e.g. ketone testing during illness).
> - Monitoring of maternal weight, BP, and urinalysis.
>   - Reinforce dietary advice throughout pregnancy.
>   - Physical activity (at least 30min daily), with advice on monitoring blood glucose and adjusting diet and/or insulin.
>   - Assessment for nephropathy and retinopathy at 1st antenatal visit and at 28 weeks.
> - Screening for thyroid disorders.
> - Fetal monitoring:
>   - Scanning at 18–20 weeks for congenital abnormalities.
>   - Growth scanning at 28, 32, and 36 weeks.
>   - Review 1- to 2-weekly.
> - At 36 weeks' clinic visit, discuss and document:
>   - Mode and timing of delivery.
>   - Blood glucose management and insulin infusion rate for delivery.
>   - Benefits of breastfeeding (mother and baby).
>   - Options for safe, effective post-partum contraception.
> - Induction of labour or elective Caesarean section is usually advised by 38 weeks' gestation.

- During labour, capillary glucose should be monitored on an hourly basis and maintained between 4 and 7mmol/L if safely achievable. For insulin treated women an intrapartum target range of 5 and 8mmol/L may be more applicable to minimise risks of maternal hypoglycaemia.
- IV glucose and insulin infusion is recommended during labour and birth for women if blood glucose is not 4–7mmol/L or 5–8mmol/L.
- Blood glucose testing should be carried out routinely in babies of women with diabetes at 2–4h after birth.
- Women should commence preconception insulin doses or reduce late pregnancy doses by at least 50% as soon as possible after birth.

The potential for hypoglycaemia in mothers who are breastfeeding should be discussed. Extra carbohydrate snacks for the mother are often needed (10–15g CHO per feed), along with further reductions in preconception insulin requirements. One day's worth of breast milk contains about 50g of carbohydrate.

Gestational diabetes

Epidemiology

Pregnancy induces a state of insulin resistance, with ↑ levels of GH, progesterone, placental lactogen, and cortisol all contributing to impaired glucose disposal. Hyperglycaemia during pregnancy occurs in up to 10–13% of women and is associated with ↑ risk of subsequent T2DM in up to 50% of women over the next decade. The risk of subsequent T2DM is significantly reduced by diet and lifestyle and breastfeeding (exclusively for 6 months' duration) and by metformin.

There is a clear association with increasing hyperglycaemia and poorer maternal and fetal outcomes. Intensive treatment of severe hyperglycaemia reduces the risk of serious perinatal morbidity (death, shoulder dystocia, bone fracture, and nerve palsy). Treatment of less severe antenatal glycaemia with diet, metformin, and insulin (required in 10–20% of women) reduces the risk of gestational weight gain, Caesarean delivery, maternal hypertensive disorders, fetal growth acceleration, and neonatal adiposity measures, including large for gestational age, macrosomia, and skinfold thickness.

Diagnostic criteria for GDM are listed in Table 15.14.

High-risk groups

Most women with GDM are detected on routine screening at 24–28 weeks, but certain high-risk groups should be screened earlier. These risk factors include:

• Previous GDM.
• A large baby in their last pregnancy, e.g. >4.5kg.
• Maternal obesity (BMI above 30kg/m²).
• Family history of diabetes (1st-degree relatives).
• Minority ethnic family origin with a high prevalence of diabetes.

Consider a diagnosis of MODY or T1DM in women who have GDM with no classic risk factors (many women with MODY have a history of GDM).

Screening

Screening is recommended at 16 weeks if previous GDM and, if normal, should be repeated at 24–28 weeks in high-risk groups. Box 15.11 details the methods of screening.

Table 15.14 Diagnosis of gestational diabetes, according to the NICE and IADPSG/WHO 2013 diagnostic criteria

	Plasma glucose (mmol/L)	
NICE	Fasting >5.6mmol/L	Postprandial level ≥7.8mmol/L at 2h
IADPSG	≥5.1mmol/L	≥10.1mmol/L at 1h or ≥8.5mmol/L at 2h

The International Association of Diabetes and Pregnancy Study Groups (IADPSG) criteria, based on the Hyperglycaemia and Adverse Pregnancy Outcome (HAPO) study were endorsed by WHO in 2013.

Box 15.11 Methods of screening

- The NICE guidelines recommend screening for GDM only in high-risk groups.
- The 2h 75g OGTT should be used at 24–28 weeks, with earlier testing (16–18 weeks) and/or capillary glucose testing indicated in women with previous GDM.
- FPG, random blood glucose, HbA1c, glucose challenge test, or urinalysis should not be used for assessing risk of GDM.
- Glycosuria of 2+ or 1+ on two or more occasions may indicate undiagnosed GDM. Further testing to exclude GDM should be considered.

Treatment

- Initial treatment is with dietary advice and exercise. Carbohydrates that are unrefined and high in fibre, with a low glycaemic index (below 55) create a slower and lower rise in glucose levels after eating. There is ↑ emphasis on the quality and quantity of carbohydrate at main meals (especially breakfast) and snacks, lean proteins, including oily fish, and a balance of polyunsaturated fats and monounsaturated fats.
- Thirty minutes of daily physical activity is recommended.
- Women with pre-pregnancy BMI ≥27kg/m² should also be advised to restrict calorie intake (to 25kcal/kg/day or less) and avoid excessive gestational weight gain.

Oral hypoglycaemic therapy

Oral hypoglycaemic treatment is recommended if diet and exercise fail to maintain glucose levels in the target range (3.9–7.8mmol/L) and/or the growth scans suggest fetal growth acceleration.

Metformin and/or glibenclamide are not licensed for use in pregnancy. Metformin is commonly used and has beneficial maternal and neonatal outcomes. However, it does cross the placenta, and some have concerns about longer-term metabolic programming effects on the offspring.

Insulin therapy

- Required in 10–20% of GDM pregnancies to maintain fasting blood glucose 3.9–5.3mmol/L and 1h postprandial glucose <7.8mmol/L.
- Used in conjunction with diet and exercise or in addition to metformin.
- Regimen should be tailored to glycaemic profile and patient acceptability: boluses alone, basal alone, mixed or basal bolus.
- Most (but not all) women can stop insulin and/or oral hypoglycaemic treatments immediately after birth.

Post-partum follow-up

- Women with GDM should be offered lifestyle advice (including weight control, diet, and exercise) and an FPG measurement at the 6-week postnatal check and diabetes screening annually thereafter.
- NICE does not recommend a post-partum OGTT, but this is often used in high-risk multiethnic groups at ↑ risk of T2DM.

  (See Box 15.12 for a checklist for GDM during clinic visits.)

Box 15.12 Checklist for gestational diabetes during clinic visit

- Monitoring blood glucose, aim:
  - Fasting blood glucose <5.3mmol/L.
  - 1h postprandial blood glucose <7.8mmol/L (some advocate lower blood glucose targets for obese women, e.g. <5.1 fasting and <7.0 after meals).
- Monitor maternal weight, BP, and urinalysis.
- Monitor fetal size (abdominal circumference).
- Treatment:
  - Diet and lifestyle advice.
  - Metformin if diet and exercise inadequate
  - Insulin—NPH and/or rapid-acting insulin analogues (aspart and lispro).
- Reinforce dietary advice throughout pregnancy.
- Advice on physical activity (at least 30min daily).
- At 36 weeks' clinic visit, discuss and document:
  - Mode and timing of delivery.
  - Blood glucose management plan for delivery.
  - ↑ risk of T2DM and evidence for delaying and prevention (diet and lifestyle, breastfeeding, metformin).
  - Benefits of breastfeeding (mother and baby).
  - Options for safe, effective post-partum contraception.
- Post-partum follow-up—fasting glucose or OGTT 6 weeks post-delivery.

Further reading

Barbour LA, et al. (2018). A cautionary response to SMFM statement: pharmacological treatment of gestational diabetes. Am J Obstet Gynecol **219**, 367.e1-367.e7.

Feig DS, et al. (2017). Continuous glucose monitoring in pregnant women with type 1 diabetes (CONCEPTT): a multicentre international randomised controlled trial. Lancet **390**, 2347–59.

International Association of Diabetes and Pregnancy Study Groups Consensus Panel (2010). International Association of Diabetes and Pregnancy Study Groups recommendations on the diagnosis and classification of hyperglycemia in pregnancy. Diabetes Care **33**, 676–82.

Lowe WL, et al. (2018). Association of gestational diabetes with maternal disorders of glucose metabolism and childhood adiposity. JAMA **320**, 1005–16.

Metzger BE, et al. (2008). Hyperglycemia and adverse pregnancy outcomes. N Engl J Med **358**, 1991–2002.

Murphy HR, et al. (2017). Improved pregnancy outcomes in women with type 1 and type 2 diabetes but substantial clinic-to-clinic variations: a prospective nationwide study. Diabetologia **60**, 1668–77.

National Institute for Health and Care Excellence (2015). Diabetes in pregnancy: management of diabetes and its complications in pregnancy from the pre-conception to the postnatal period. https://www.nice.org.uk/guidance/ng3/resources/diabetes-in-pregnancy-management-from-preconception-to-the-postnatal-period-pdf-51038446021

Ratner RE, et al. (2008). Prevention of diabetes in women with a history of gestational diabetes: effects of metformin and lifestyle interventions. J Clin Endocrinol Metab **93**, 4774–9.

Paediatric and transition diabetes

Diabetes is the 3rd commonest chronic condition in childhood. The National Paediatric Diabetes Audit collates data on outcomes on children and young adults under the care of paediatric teams in England and Wales.

- Prevalence—there are 29,000 children and young people under 19 with diabetes in England and Wales: 95% T1DM, 2.5% T2DM, and 2.5% other types. The others are made up of 2° diabetes, e.g. cystic fibrosis-related diabetes, as well as single-gene abnormalities (monogenic diabetes).

Type 1 diabetes

Epidemiology

- T1DM incidence varies greatly among different populations. Incidence in England and Wales is currently around 25 per 100,000 among 0- to 15-year-old children per year. This is rising at around 4% per year in most developed countries, and even faster in some developing nations.
- Age of onset is typically from 6 months onwards, although younger onset cases have been reported.

Pathogenesis

- Chronic immune-mediated pancreatic β-cell destruction, leading to severe insulin deficiency.
- Majority autoimmune, as indicated by presence of islet autoantibodies (IAAs)—GAD, IA2, ZnT8, ICA.
- Multifactorial aetiology, including genetic susceptibility (>60% risk loci: HLA is biggest contributor with 30–50% risk), environmental factors (including enteroviruses), and effect on immunity.
- Age-dependent expression of autoantibodies (IAA, ZnT8 commoner <10 years vs GAD, IA2 >10 years).
- Typically two peaks of onset—at around ages 5–6 and 12–13 years.
- Antibodies can be present within months of life and can precede T1DM onset by years.

Diagnosis

- Presentation typically with osmotic symptoms: polyuria, polydipsia, nocturia, weight loss, enuresis. Less common symptoms are polyphagia, blurred vision, and behavioural change.
- Young children, including babies and toddlers, may have less easily recognized symptoms—constipation, lethargy, thrush, and poor feeding.
- 20–25% present with DKA in England and Wales—higher in those under 5 (30%).

At 1st presentation, the diagnosis should be made by doing a random capillary blood glucose measurement. If blood glucose >11mmol/L, the child should be referred for hospital assessment on the same day. In hospital, diagnosis of diabetes is confirmed on venous blood glucose ≥11mmol/L accompanying classic symptoms and/or HbA1c ≥48mmol/mol (6.5%).

Management in children is highly specialized and all children should be referred to 2° care centres who have an appropriate MDT with training in diabetes in children.

Type 2 diabetes

Worldwide incidence in children and adolescence varies greatly. In white Europeans, incidence is <1 per 100,000, while in indigenous populations in the USA, it is around 50 per 100,000. The majority of T2DM in children arises in the 15- to 19-year age group. Incidence is increasing worldwide, especially in ethnic minority youth and those from poor socioeconomic backgrounds.

Pathogenesis is a combination of insulin resistance (often with signs of acanthosis nigricans) and relative insulin deficiency, due to the contribution of genetic and lifestyle factors, in particular obesity and a sedentary lifestyle. Family history is common. Early peripheral insulin resistance is compensated by insulin secretion, but when sustained over time, β-cell failure and insulin deficiency follow.

Other types of diabetes

Neonatal, syndromic, and monogenic diabetes are covered in ➜ Classification and diagnosis of diabetes, pp. 840–2 and ➜ Genetics pp. 844–8.

Cystic fibrosis-related diabetes

- Prevalence of diabetes in cystic fibrosis rises with age, with around 20% of adolescents affected and 30–40% of adults.
- In children with cystic fibrosis, weight loss and frequent infections are signs of possible diabetes onset.
- CGM may be the best way of diagnosing subtle changes in glucose tolerance.
- All teenagers with cystic fibrosis should be screened for diabetes as insulin treatment improves lung function.
- Management is with insulin

Management of children with diabetes

In the UK, standards for best practice in caring for children with diabetes have been linked to payment of a '*best practice tariff*—a set amount of funding for each young person cared for (up to their nineteenth birthday). To qualify for this, the following must apply:

- Every child or young person with diabetes will be cared for by a specialist team of healthcare professionals (consisting of a doctor, a nurse, and a dietician as a minimum) who have specific training in paediatric diabetes. The diabetes specialist nurse (DSN) caseload is 70–100 patients.
- For new diagnoses: the case must be discussed with the specialist team within 24h of the diagnosis and seen on the next working day.
- An age-appropriate structured education programme offered at diagnosis and with updates, as needed.
- Four clinic appointments/year with HbA1c check.
- Annual dietician contact.
- At least eight additional contacts per year from members of the specialist team (not all face-to-face) are recommended.
- Annual review with BP and retinopathy/renal screening from age 12.
- Annual psychology assessment and access to psychology services.
- 24h emergency phone advice for families/other health professionals.
- Involvement in the National Paediatric Diabetes Audit and Paediatric Diabetes Network.
- Policy for transition to adult services.
- Policy on managing high HbA1c and infrequent clinic attendance.

Managing type 1 diabetes in children

Insulin

Insulin is started based on body weight, with higher doses in puberty. Insulin regimens are the same as in adults, varying from centre to centre, with very little evidence base for one being superior. In toddlers, basal insulin tends to be given in the morning, moving to the evening in children aged >5 years, or twice daily in some circumstances (e.g. insulin levemir). Prandial insulin doses for food can be anything from 0.5U for 40g of CHO in babies to 3–4U for 10g during puberty.

Continuous subcutaneous insulin infusion pumps

(See ➜ Insulin pump therapy: continuous subcutaneous insulin infusion (CSII), pp. 862–4.)

In the UK, guidelines allow for pumps to be funded in children under the age of 12 in whom multiple insulin injections are considered to be impractical or inappropriate. Children aged over 12 have the same funding rules as adults.

Education

As in adults, this is the mainstay of management to allow parents, and then children to self-manage their own condition.

- *Carbohydrate counting*. This may be taught at any stage but is better if done soon after diagnosis, so that it becomes routine for the family and drives improved glycaemic control.
- *Multiple carers*. One of the main differences between children and adults with diabetes is the need to teach many family members about the condition, including grandparents and childminders.

- *Blood glucose testing.* Before every meal and at other times, to work out whether mealtime doses are correct, as well as at other times for troubleshooting. Many children require 6–8 blood tests per day, more for younger children.
- *SC CGM.* This is available for some patients (e.g. preschool) under NICE criteria. Flash glucose sensing (Libre) is becoming more widespread as long as patients meet the criteria laid out by the National Health Service (NHS) England.
- *Exercise.* Children's exercise levels vary enormously from one day to the next. Therefore, advice about how to cope with blood glucose variability is essential and built into most structured education programmes.
- *Management at school and nursery:*
  - Children spend around a third to half of waking hours at school.
  - Schools need to support intensive management of diabetes.
  - This works best when volunteers at 1° school are taught diabetes management. This includes either supervising or doing blood glucose testing, insulin injections, or pump boluses, and, in some places, use of algorithms to calculate insulin doses for food and blood glucose correction. This involves a lot of education, usually by the DSN.
  - All school staff (1° and 2°) should be aware of the symptoms of hypoglycaemia in a particular child and should know how to treat hypoglycaemia.

Acute complications are mainly treated as in adults (see ❐ Living with diabetes, pp. 878–80; ❐ Hospital inpatient diabetes management and diabetes-related emergencies, p. 891). Specific points relevant to children are described in the following sections.

Hypoglycaemia
- Parents and carers should look out for symptoms, as children may not recognize them reliably until around 10 years old.
- Dose of glucagon for severe lows with fits or unconsciousness: 0.5mg if under 8 years old or who weigh less than 25kg, and 1.0mg if older or who weigh 25kg or more.

Complications and associated conditions

Annual review should include:
- Height, weight, and BP at all ages.
- Microalbuminuria, lipid, and retinopathy screening: annually when >12 years.
- Assess feet to instil good practice.
- Coeliac disease recommended at diagnosis and if symptomatic (many do this as part of annual blood screen).
- Annual TFTs (3–8% co-existent autoimmune hypothyroidism, 0.5–6% hyperthyroidism).
- Addison's disease—no screening, but consider if recurrent hypoglycaemia and lethargy.

Diabetic ketoacidosis

Diagnosis and management in those <18 years should be according to the British Society for Paediatric Endocrinology and Diabetes guidelines (℘ https://www.bsped.org.uk/clinical-resources/guidelines/).

New guidelines (published in April 2020) emphasize adequate restoration of circulatory volume in order to treat shock, while minimizing the risk of cerebral oedema. Careful fluid management, according to strict protocols, needs to be followed to reduce complications of DKA (see ➔ Diabetic ketoacidosis, p. 892).

- Delay in insulin administration until after 1–2h of fluids may reduce the risk of cerebral oedema. FRIII (0.05–0.1unit/kg/h) is used to switch off ketogenesis until resolution of acidosis and SC insulin is started. In patients with established T1DM, the long-acting insulin should be continued and in new patients, consideration should be given to starting a long-acting SC insulin, alongside IV insulin.
- Mortality from DKA can be caused by:
  - Cerebral oedema.
  - Hypokalaemia.
  - Aspiration pneumonia.
  - Inadequate resuscitation.

Puberty and diabetes

- Insulin requirements rise from ~0.7U/kg/day to up to 2.0U/kg/day in early puberty in girls and in late puberty in boys (timed with the growth spurt) due to insulin resistance associated with puberty.
- Puberty and adolescence can make the management of T1DM challenging; most teenagers want to be accepted into a peer group and feeling different in any way makes this hard.
- Therefore, some young people will stop doing blood glucose testing or miss insulin doses, particularly when out with friends.
- Supportive management with short-term goal-setting and counselling is important.
- Young people often need to be seen more frequently, rather than less, during this time.

Eating disorders

Missed insulin injections are often a way of controlling weight. Mild forms are common, especially, but not exclusively, in girls. Should be managed by specialized services, alongside diabetes management.

Transition from paediatric to adult services

During the teenage years, there is a gradual shift in responsibility from parental management of the diabetes to the young people themselves being responsible for their own diabetes self-management. This process is gradual and, like a ball, can be passed between parent and young person, until the latter feels completely able to self-manage. This process may continue into young adulthood and the time course is highly variable. HbA1c levels often deteriorate during adolescence, due to a combination of factors. Research evidence shows that the longer parents remain involved, the better the outcomes in terms of HbA1c and QoL. Therefore, young people should be seen with their parents as long as they wish to, and this should be a family decision. Seeing patients alone initially and increasing the time spent learning how to navigate an outpatient clinic alone can be helpful towards increasing independence and forming a new relationship with their diabetes as they approach a more independent life.

The transition model

- The service should have a transition protocol, which should include agreeing the timing of transfer with the young person, discussed well in advance.
- Transfer should be to a service with a hospital-based young adult clinic with expertise in managing young people with T1DM, rather than to 1° care.
- Some evidence suggests that transition is more successful if there is a joint clinic between the paediatric and adult MDT.
- A dedicated transition service DSN should keep in contact with young people in the community when they default from clinics.
- There is evidence that non-attenders have higher HbA1c levels, and so they do need to be followed up in specialist care.

Educational aspects of transition

It is helpful to run an education programme relevant to the transition age group, with accessible information offered from the early teenage years and for it to take place with parents absent. The paediatric team will usually have spent many years communicating more with the parents than with the children. However, now the young person may need to be helped to understand their diabetes for themselves, often requiring a new process of education and to help them form a new relationship with their diabetes as an emerging adult.

Transition education should include information on
- Alcohol.
- Driving: a doctor is required to sign the provisional driving licence application form. DVLA rules apply.
- Smoking.
- Recreational drugs.
- Sex, contraception, and preconception care.
- Travelling.
- Managing exams.
- Sick day rules—to take account of living alone for the 1st time.
- Higher education:
  - Often 2° specialist care is kept at home for appointments during the holidays, with local GP registration with the university/college student health system. Young people on insulin need a fridge to be provided in their university accommodation and to let people on their corridor know about diabetes. A discussion about how they will manage 'fresher's week', especially with alcohol, and other issues is helpful.

Diabetic eye disease

Epidemiology

Diabetic retinopathy (DR) is a microvascular complication of diabetes which remains the commonest cause of blindness in the working age group globally, even though DR screening and better control of diabetes have contributed significantly to reductions in the rate of blindness in the working age group in the UK. DR is extremely common with long durations of diabetes, which may be some years before the diagnosis of T2DM. Cataracts are also commoner in people with diabetes. A 2012 study of the global prevalence of DR showed a prevalence of 35% for any DR, 7% for proliferative diabetic retinopathy (PDR), 7% for macular oedema, and 10% for sight-threatening diabetic eye disease (STED). Since 1985, people with diabetes have experienced lower rates of progression to PDR and severe visual loss, probably reflecting improvements in diabetes care. Some studies have suggested that non-white ethnic groups have higher prevalences of DR. However, this has been difficult to separate from confounding risk factors such as age, duration of diagnosed diabetes, HbA1c, and BP.

(See Box 15.13 for classification of DR.)

Box 15.13 Classification and features of diabetic retinopathy

- Background retinopathy (graded as R1 by the NHS Diabetic Eye Screening Programme in England):
  - Microaneurysms.
  - Haemorrhages—dot and flame-shaped.
  - Hard exudates.
  - Soft exudates/cotton wool spots.
- Pre-proliferative retinopathy (graded as R2):
  - Multiple blot haemorrhages.
  - Intraretinal microvascular abnormalities (IRMAs).
  - Venous beading.
  - Venous reduplication.
- Proliferative retinopathy (graded as R3):
  - New vessels on the disc (NVD) or within 1 disc diameter (DD) of it.
  - New vessels elsewhere (NVE).
  - Fibrovascular proliferation ± tractional retinal detachment.
  - Pre-retinal or vitreous haemorrhage.
  - Rubeosis iridis (± neovascular glaucoma).
- Maculopathy (graded as M0 if absent, and M1 if present):
  - Exudate within 1 DD of the centre of the fovea.
  - Group of exudates within the macula.
  - Any microaneurysm or haemorrhage within 1 DD of the centre of the fovea only if associated with a best VA of ≤6/12 (if no stereo).
  - Retinal thickening within 1 DD of the centre of the fovea (if stereo available).

Other grades
- R0—no retinopathy.
- O—other non-diabetic lesions seen (e.g. drusen and macular degeneration).
- P—evidence of previous laser therapy/retinal photocoagulation.
- U—unclassifiable, often due to cataracts.

Clinical and histological features of diabetic eye disease

The classification of DR is based on clinical examination or on grading of retinal photographs, but changes in the pathophysiology may explain some of the clinical findings.

One of the 1st histological changes seen is thickening of the basement membrane and loss of pericytes embedded within it, forming acellular capillaries. Breakdown in endothelial cell tight junctions leads to ↑ capillary permeability. Microaneurysms are the hallmark of retinal microvascular disease in diabetes. Microaneurysms may be asymmetrical dilatations of the capillary wall where it is weakened or damaged, following the loss of supporting pericytes and localized increases in hydrostatic pressure. Smooth muscle cell death, capillary weakening and closure, with the occurrence of IRMAs, and impaired autoregulation are all features of DR.

The natural progression, with increasing retinal ischaemia, is from background to pre-proliferative DR to PDR and ultimately to sight-threatening DR. Maculopathy can occur at any of these stages but does occur more frequently with more advanced disease.

Background retinopathy

Capillary microaneurysms are the earliest feature, seen clinically as red 'dots'. Dot haemorrhages also occur, and these can be difficult to distinguish from microaneurysms and are collectively referred to as HMA. Small intraretinal haemorrhages or 'blots' also occur, as can haemorrhage into the nerve fibre layer, which are often more flame-shaped. With capillary leakage, hard exudates, which are lipid deposits, can also be seen.

A *cotton wool spot* is a delay in transmission along the axoplasm of the nerve fibre layer of the retina, caused by ischaemia. It used to be considered a pre-proliferative feature, but because it is not a good indicator of progression to PDR, it is now included in the background R1 category in the NHS Diabetic Eye Screening Programme in England.

Pre-proliferative retinopathy

With increasing ischaemia, the retina shows signs of increasing numbers of blot haemorrhages, which are usually in a deeper layer of the retina than dot or flame-shaped haemorrhages.

IRMAs are tortuous intraretinal vascular segments, varying in calibre. They derive from remodelling of the retinal capillaries and small collateral vessels in areas of microvascular occlusion.

Venous beading is a localized increase in the calibre of the vein, and the severity is dependent on the increase in calibre and the length of the vein involved.

Venous reduplication is dilation of a pre-existing channel or proliferation of a new channel adjacent to, and approximately the same calibre as, the original vein.

The Early Treatment of Diabetic Retinopathy Study (ETDRS) provided evidence that certain features were more indicative of progression to PDR and suggested a '4–2–1' rule:

- 4 quadrants of severe haemorrhages or microaneurysms.
- 2 quadrants of IRMAs.
- 1 quadrant with venous beading.

If you have one of these features, there is a 15% risk of developing PDR within the next year; if two are present, the risk rises to 45%.

Proliferative retinopathy

(See Fig. 15.6.)

New vessels developing in DR are characterized according to whether they develop at or near the optic disc (NVD) or elsewhere in the retina (NVE). They usually develop from the venous circulation and grow forward in the vitreous gel, but they can also develop from the arterial circulation.

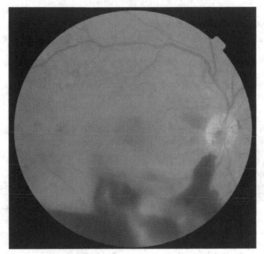

Fig. 15.6 This photograph shows NVD and haemorrhage from these new vessels in front of the inferior temporal arcade.

NVD are defined as any new vessel developing at the optic disc or within 1 DD of the edge of the optic disc.

NVE are defined as any new vessel developing >1 DD away from the edge of the optic disc.

Both give no symptoms but cause the problems of advanced retinopathy, such as haemorrhage, scar tissue formation, traction on the retina, and retinal detachment, which actually results in loss of vision.

The Diabetic Retinopathy Study (DRS) recommended prompt treatment with panretinal photocoagulation in the presence of DRS high-risk characteristics, which reduced the 2-year risk of severe visual loss by 50% or more and were defined by:

- The presence of pre-retinal or vitreous haemorrhage.
- Eyes with NVD equalling or exceeding 1/4 to 1/3 disc area in extent with no haemorrhage.
- NVE equalling >1/2 disc area with haemorrhage (from the NVE).

Untreated, eyes with high-risk characteristics had between 25.6% and 36.9% chance of severe visual loss within 2 years.

Proliferative eyes without high-risk characteristics had the following risks of severe visual loss:

- Untreated—2 years, 7.0%; 4 years, 20.9%.
- Treated—2 years, 3.2%; 4 years, 7.4%.

Because the side effects of modern laser treatment are considerably less than the early lasers, most ophthalmologists treat eyes that develop new vessels of either high- or low-risk categories.

Diabetic macular oedema

Diabetic macular oedema, or maculopathy, may be classified into focal, diffuse, and ischaemic types.

In focal maculopathy, focal leakage tends to occur from microaneurysms, often with a circinate pattern of exudates around the focal leakage.

In the diffuse variety, there is generalized breakdown of the blood–retina barrier and profuse early leakage from the entire capillary bed of the posterior pole, sometimes accompanied by cystoid macular changes.

In ischaemic maculopathy, enlargement of the foveal avascular zone (FAZ) due to capillary closure is found with variable degrees of visual loss.

The ETDRS reported that focal photocoagulation of 'clinically significant' diabetic macular oedema (CSMO) substantially reduced the risk of visual loss.

CSMO is defined as:

- Thickening of the retina at or within 500 microns of the centre of the macula.
- Hard exudates at or within 500 microns of the centre of the fovea, if associated with thickening of the adjacent retina (no residual hard exudates remaining after the disappearance of retinal thickening).
- A zone, or zones, of retinal thickening 1 disc area or larger, any part of which is within 1 DD of the centre of the macula.

More recently, with the advent of VEGF inhibitors, diabetic macular oedema is further classified into whether there is centre-involving or non-centre-involving diabetic macular oedema.

Eye screening

National screening programmes

The development of screening in Europe was first encouraged by the St Vincent Declaration which, in 1989, set a target for the reduction of new blindness by one-third in the following 5 years.

National screening programmes, with consensus grading protocols, were introduced in the UK in 2002–2004. The UK National Screening Committee recommended that those with T1DM and T2DM have their eyes screened at the time of diagnosis and annually thereafter until 2015 when they recommended that, for people with diabetes at low risk of sight loss, the interval between screening tests should change from 1 to 2 years. Those at low risk were defined as those having two consecutive screening results showing no DR. This extension is expected to be introduced in the NHS Diabetic Eye Screening Programme in England during the period 2020–2022. There are differences in the protocols used globally in screening programmes. In England, the method used is two-field mydriatic digital photography, with screening performed by technician screeners or optometrists. Fixed locations and mobile units are both used. Monitoring of programme performance is via Quality Assurance Standards and Key Performance Indicators against which individual screening programmes are assessed.

Ad hoc eye examinations

It is important to remember that patients who are most at risk of developing sight-threatening DR and visual loss are regular non-attenders for screening. The eyes of patients who have not attended for routine screening can be examined using the following method.

Visual acuity

Use a standard Snellen chart for distance and check each eye separately. Let the patient wear their glasses for the test, and if vision is worse than 6/9, also check with a pinhole, as this will correct for any refractive (glasses) error. If it does not correct to 6/9 or better, consider a more careful review; some maculopathy changes cannot be seen easily with a handheld ophthalmoscope, and an ophthalmology review may be needed. Cataracts are a more likely cause, so look carefully at the red reflex.

High blood glucose readings can lead to myopia, and low blood glucose to hypermetropia. In both these circumstances, one would expect the vision to improve with a pinhole.

Eye examination

- Dilate the pupil before looking into the eye.
  - Use tropicamide 1%—dilates the pupil adequately in 15–20min and lasts 2–3h.
  - In those with a dark iris, you may also need phenylephrine (2.5%), added soon after tropicamide, to give adequate views.
  - The main reasons not to dilate are closed angle glaucoma and recent eye surgery, but as such, patients are usually under an eye clinic already; most people are suitable for dilatation.

- Once the pupil is dilated, look at the red reflex to check for lens opacities. Examine the anterior chamber, as although rare, rubeosis iridis is important to pick up. The vitreous is examined before examining the retina. When examining the retina, use the optic disc as a landmark; follow all four arcades of vessels out from it; examine the periphery, and at the end, examine the macula. It is usually much easier for the patient to look directly at the light if a smaller spot size or a target on a green background are chosen for this aspect of the examination.

When to refer

Referral will depend on local preferences but are based on NSC management guidelines, as outlined in Box 15.14.

Box 15.14 Reasons for, and timing of, referral to ophthalmologist

- Immediate referral:
  - Rubeosis iridis/neovascular glaucoma.
  - Vitreous haemorrhage.
  - Advanced retinopathy with retinal detachment.
- Urgent referral (<2 weeks):
  - R3/proliferative retinopathy, as untreated high-risk PDR carries a 40% risk of blindness in <2 years and laser treatment considerably reduces this.
- Routine referral (<13 weeks):
  - R2/pre-proliferative changes.
  - M1/maculopathy.
- Routine non-DR referral:
  - Cataracts.
- Other categories:
  - R0/no retinopathy—annual screening, moving to 2 yearly if two −ve screens.
  - R1/background retinopathy—annual screening and inform diabetes care team.

Medical treatment for diabetic eye disease

Box 15.15 shows the risk factors for worsening retinopathy.

Glycaemic control

The Diabetes Control and Complications Trial (DCCT) and UKPDS confirmed the link between glycaemic control and the onset and progression of diabetic eye disease.

Worsening of DR can occur when glycaemic control improves rapidly, so careful monitoring of DR is needed during this period (e.g. pregnancy). However, the long-term benefits of improved glycaemic control greatly outweigh the risks of early worsening.

Blood pressure control/therapy

The UKPDS also showed that good BP control is vital to reduce the onset and progression of DR.

Lipid control/therapy

Evidence that elevated serum lipids are associated with macular exudates and moderate visual loss and that partial regression of hard exudates may be possible by reducing elevated lipid levels comes from several studies. The FIELD study suggested that the use of fenofibrate in T2DM might reduce the need for laser treatment of DR over a 5-year period. However, caution is needed with this interpretation, as the numbers of events were small.

Lifestyle advice

Stopping smoking may reduce the risk of DR in T1DM. Changes to alcohol consumption or physical activity show no consistent effect.

Box 15.15 Risk factors for developing/worsening of diabetic retinopathy

- Modifiable risk factors for DR:
  - Glucose control.
  - Systemic hypertension.
  - Blood lipids.
  - Smoking in T1DM.
- Non-modifiable risk factors for DR:
  - Duration of diabetes.
  - Age.
  - Genetic predisposition.
  - Ethnicity.
  - Pregnancy.

Surgical treatment for diabetic eye disease

Laser treatment

- The ETDRS protocol for panretinal photocoagulation recommends 1200–1600 argon laser burns of 500-micron spot size, with the treatment performed in two or more episodes, no more than 2 weeks apart, and that no more than 900 burns should be applied in one session.
- Laser therapy is usually performed as two sessions of outpatient treatment on conscious patients. Topical local anaesthetic drops allow a contact lens to be placed on the cornea for application of the laser through the contact lens. Modern multispot laser machines with reduced duration of the burn and the ability to apply predetermined pattern types, which can administer up to 25 spots at a time, have reduced the time taken and the discomfort of panretinal laser treatment. However, more burns need to be applied, with a minimum of 2187 burns in the Manchester Pascal laser study. Because of the reduction in discomfort of the procedure, panretinal photocoagulation can usually be applied with local anaesthetic drops.
- The laser energy is absorbed by the choroid and the pigment epithelium.
- Laser treatment for clinically significant macular oedema reduces visual loss by >50%.
- Laser treatment aims to prevent further visual loss, especially in maculopathy, not to restore vision, and the distinction must be emphasized to all patients requiring treatment. The benefits from laser therapy currently outweigh the risks, which include accidental burns to the fovea if the eye moves during therapy, a reduction in night vision, and, in a small number, interference with visual field severe enough to affect the ability to drive. Most patients, however, retain the minimum field for driving (88% of those who have received bilateral panretinal photocoagulation), although the risk to the driving field is greater for those patients with more ischaemic eyes that require bilateral vitrectomy procedures.

Vitrectomy

The surgical techniques of vitrectomy for advanced DR have improved over the last 30 years, which has been demonstrated by the improved surgical results during this period. Most modern systems employ three small (20–25 gauge) entry 'ports' into the eye, and a cutting/suction device, an intraocular light source, and an infusion cannula are inserted through these trans-scleral incisions.

The reasons why vitrectomy may be required are:
- Non-clearing vitreous haemorrhage.
- A large subhyaloid macular haemorrhage.
- Tractional retinal detachment.
- Combined rhegmatogenous (due to retinal tear)/tractional retinal detachment.
- Progressive severe fibrovascular proliferation.
- Taut posterior hyaloid in diabetic macular oedema.

Alternative surgical treatment—use of intravitreal VEGF inhibitors and intravitreal steroids

Ocular neovascularization (angiogenesis) and ↑ vascular permeability have been associated with VEGF, which does also have a neuroprotective effect.

There are three potential VEGF inhibitors: aflibercept, ranibizumab, and bevacizumab. Ranibizumab is an antibody fragment derived from bevacizumab, which is a full-length humanized monoclonal antibody against human VEGF.

The Diabetic Retinopathy Clinical Research Network reported the results of a multicentre, randomized clinical trial of 854 eyes in 691 participants that evaluated ranibizumab plus prompt or deferred laser or triamcinolone plus prompt laser for diabetic macular oedema. Intravitreal ranibizumab with prompt or deferred laser was more effective through at least 1 year, compared with prompt laser alone, for the treatment of diabetic macular oedema involving the central macula.

In 2013, a NICE appraisal recommended the use of ranibizumab in cases of diabetic macular oedema when the person has a central retinal thickness of 400 microns or more at the start of treatment. In 2015, NICE made a similar recommendation for the use of aflibercept in diabetic macular oedema.

These agents are being increasingly used for treatment of centre-involving diabetic macular oedema where the centre thickness is 400 microns or more. In the 1st year, it is expected that 7–9 anti-VEGF injections would be required, 2–4 in the 2nd year, and 1–3 in the 3rd year. The main risk is endophthalmitis, of which reports of frequency vary between 1 in 1000 and 2.5 in 10,000. Theoretical risks of an increasing frequency of MI or stroke do not appear to have materialized, according to current studies.

These agents are also starting to be used in PDR, but there is still uncertainty over how long they would need to be used for to control the condition.

Of those patients with diabetic macular oedema who do not respond to intravitreal VEGF inhibitors, some will respond to intravitreal dexamethasone implant which has been approved by NICE in those people who have had cataract surgery in that eye in the past.

Cataract extraction

This is a common procedure, with a slightly higher complication rate than in the non-diabetic population. Although diabetes is a risk factor for the development of cataracts, and studies have shown an ↑ risk of ocular complications in people with diabetes after cataract surgery, modern surgical techniques and appropriate preoperative laser treatment have led to an overall good visual outcome in the majority of patients.

Further reading

[No authors listed] (1985). Photocoagulation for diabetic macular edema. Early Treatment Diabetic Retinopathy Study report number 1. Early Treatment Diabetic Retinopathy Study research group. *Arch Ophthalmol* **103**, 1796–806.

[No authors listed] (1987). Indications for photocoagulation treatment of diabetic retinopathy: Diabetic Retinopathy Study Report no. 14. The Diabetic Retinopathy Study Research Group. *Int Ophthalmol Clin* **27**, 239–53.

[No authors listed] (1991). Grading diabetic retinopathy from stereoscopic color fundus photographs--an extension of the modified Airlie House classification. ETDRS report number 10. Early Treatment Diabetic Retinopathy Study Research Group. *Ophthalmology* **98**(5 Suppl), 786–806.

Keech AC, et al. (2007). The FIELD study. *Lancet* **370**, 1687–97.

Klein R, et al. (2008). The twenty-five-year progression of retinopathy in persons with type 1 diabetes. *Ophthalmology* **115**, 1859–68.

National Institute for Health and Care Excellence (2013). *Ranibizumab for the treatment of diabetic macular oedema.* ℅ https://www.nice.org.uk/guidance/ta274/resources/ranibizumab-for-treating-diabetic-macular-oedema-pdf-82600612458181.

National Institute for Health and Care Excellence (2015). *Aflibercept for treating diabetic macular oedema.* Technology appraisal guidance [TA346]. ℅ https://www.nice.org.uk/guidance/ta346/chapter/1-guidance

Sivaprasad S, et al. (2017). Clinical efficacy of intravitreal aflibercept versus panretinal photocoagulation for best corrected visual acuity in patients with proliferative diabetic retinopathy at 52 weeks (CLARITY). *Lancet* **389**, 2193–203.

Wong TY, et al. (2009). Rates of progression in diabetic retinopathy during different time periods: a systematic review and meta-analysis. *Diabetes Care* **32**, 2307–13.

Yau JW, et al. (2012). Global prevalence and major risk factors of diabetic retinopathy. *Diabetes Care* **35**, 556–64.

Diabetic nephropathy and chronic kidney disease

Background

Diabetic nephropathy is now a major cause of end-stage renal disease (ESRD) worldwide, responsible for over 50% of patients on renal replacement therapy (RRT) in many Middle and Far Eastern countries (27% in the UK), with the majority having T2DM. Cardiovascular morbidity and mortality are much greater in patients with diabetes and nephropathy, and many of them will die before reaching ESRD.

Definition

Diabetic nephropathy is defined as a deterioration of kidney function from long-standing diabetes usually in the presence of proteinuria. Chronic kidney disease (CKD) can be diagnosed by either eGFR <60mL/min/1.73m^2 on two occasion within a 3-month period or by albumin:creatinine ratio (ACR) in the urine of >3mg/mmol (NICE clinical guideline [CG182]).

Early stages of CKD are asymptomatic, but as kidney function declines, waste products and fluid accumulate and uraemia develops. Diabetic nephropathy is an independent marker of mortality and morbidity from cardiovascular causes. The risk increases with a decline of eGFR and the amount of protein in the urine, being the highest for those who have all: T2DM, reduced eGFR, and albuminuria (55% above the general population). Classification of CKD is based on cardiovascular risk and serves as a basis for frequency of monitoring (see Table 15.15). Unfortunately, nephropathy screening uptake is the lowest among all complication screening processes in the UK, at 63% according to the National Diabetes Audit (NDA) in 2018.

Not all CKD in patients with diabetes is caused by diabetes. It is important to recognize other causes (autoimmune disease, renal artery sclerosis, obstruction, malignancy, and myeloma) that need to be investigated and treated differently.

Epidemiology

The duration of diabetes is a major risk for the development of nephropathy, making point prevalence studies are hard to interpret. In addition, the incidence appears to be declining, at least in T1DM, so historical prevalence rates may be misleading. In an inception cohort of 277 T1DM patients from Denmark studied from 1979 to 2004, cumulative incidences were 34% and 15% for microalbuminuria and clinical neprhropathy, respectively. For ESRD, rates of 2.2% and 7.8% have recently been reported from Finland after 20 and 30 years' duration, respectively.

Because a true date of onset of T2DM is hard to determine, cumulative incidence data are less reliable. However, the annual incidence of microalbuminuria was around 2% in the UKPDS, which is slightly more than that seen in T1DM, and 3% per annum for clinical nephropathy in those with established microalbuminuria. Rates of ESRD are very dependent upon background ethnicity. In the UKPDS population of mainly white European patients, ESRD occurred in 0.6% after 10 years. Prevalence is equal in men and women. The rates are at least double for those of South Asian background.

Table 15.15 Suggested frequency of CKD monitoring

GFR categories, description, and range (mL/min/1.73m²)			Albuminuria stages, description, and range		
			A1 Normal to mildly ↑ <30mg/g (<3mg/mmol)	A2 Moderately ↑ 30–300mg/g (3–30mg/mmol)	A3 Severely ↑ >300mg/g (>30mg/mmol)
G1	Normal or high	≥90	≤1	1	≥1
G2	Mild	60–89	≤1	1	≥1
G3a	Mild to moderate	45–59	1	1	2
G3b	Moderate to severe	30–44	≤2	2	≥2
G4	Severe	15–29	2	2	3
G5	Kidney failure	<15	4	≥4	≥4
			Frequency of monitoring eGFR (number of times per year)		

CKD, chronic kidney disease; eGFR, estimated GFR; GFR, glomerular filtration rate.

Adapted from Levin A et al (2013) "KDIGO 2012 Clinical Practice Guideline for the Evaluation and Management of Chronic Kidney Disease: Summary of Recommendation Statements" *Kidney International Supplements* 3(1):5–14, © 2013 International Society of Nephrology, with permission from Elsevier.

Making the diagnosis of diabetic renal disease

Timed urine collections are too cumbersome for routine clinical care, so spot samples (preferably 1st morning void specimens) are used, and in order to allow for urine concentration, the albumin content is corrected for Cr, giving an ACR. A +ve dipstick test or an ACR on two or more occasions over 6 months is usually enough to confirm the diagnosis. Remember to exclude potential confounding causes of a +ve test (see Box 15.16).

An increased ACR in a person with T1DM is almost always due to diabetic kidney disease, but up to 15% of T2DM patients with microalbuminuria have atypical appearances on renal biopsy. Presence of retinopathy makes diabetic glomerulosclerosis much more likely. Nephrosclerosis and tubulointerstitial changes are the most commonly seen non-diabetic changes.

Rapidly developing nephrotic-range proteinuria, an accelerated loss of GFR (>5mL/min/year), presence of features of other systemic disease (such as connective tissue disorders or myeloma), or accelerated hypertension should prompt investigation, as these features may suggest alternative, potentially treatable conditions. An increase in serum Cr of >30% after initiation of ACEI therapy suggests possible renal artery stenosis.

Pathology

The earliest pathological feature in T1DM patients is kidney enlargement, mostly due to tubular hypertrophy and hyperplasia in response to glycosuria. These changes are not completely reversible with glycaemic correction, and their link to later nephropathy is uncertain. eGFR is also increased in newly diagnosed patients (termed hyperfiltration), but this usually returns to normal with glycaemic correction.

Within 5 years of T1DM onset, a small, but significant increase in glomerular capillary basement membrane (GBM) thickness is seen due to an accumulation of matrix material, and recent studies have linked this to hyperfiltration. As diabetic nephropathy progresses, GBM width continues to increase and matrix accumulation occurs in the glomerular mesangium (diffuse glomerulosclerosis). In advanced nephropathy, these accumulations can form large acellular (Kimmelstiel–Wilson) nodules (nodular glomerulosclerosis). Ultimately, glomerular capillaries are obliterated by matrix material and they become sclerosed and non-functional. The increase in GBM width leads to increased passage of albumin into the filtrate. At the same time, there is detachment and loss of podocytes on the epithelial side of the GBM, reducing the integrity of the filtration barrier to circulating proteins, thus leading to increasing proteinuria. These changes are also seen in T2DM, although this has been less well studied and pathological appearances are often confounded by coexisting hypertension and ischaemia.

Tubulointerstitial changes are also seen, particularly in advanced nephropathy and T2DM, and are due to a combination of nephron loss secondary to global glomerulosclerosis and direct disease, perhaps secondary to increasing proteinuria. A combination of glomerular capillary loss and tubulointerstitial disease results in a progressive loss of eGFR towards ESRD.

> **Box 15.16 Causes of a false positive test for albuminuria**
> - Vigorous exercise.
> - Urinary tract infection.
> - Presence of blood, e.g. menses.
> - Concentrated urine (less likely using ACR).
>
> *Causes of a false negative test for albuminuria*
> - Dilute urine (less likely using ACR).

Pathogenesis

Hyperglycaemia

Experimental studies suggest that an interaction between metabolic and haemodynamic changes caused by hyperglycaemia are the drivers for nephropathy. Hyperglycaemia results in a glycation of structural proteins (such as collagen), making them less easy to metabolize and altering their function. Rising levels of advanced glycation end-products (AGEs) in blood and tissue have been linked to microvascular and macrovascular complications.

Hyperglycaemia also induces the polyol (sorbitol) and hexosamine pathways and results in activation of protein kinase C which increases flux through glycolysis. In experimental studies, these changes can cause increased oxidative stress, increased thrombosis, and alterations in blood flow which can result in microvascular damage.

In human diabetes, epidemiological studies have shown that both, duration and severity of hyperglycaemia, are strong determinants of nephropathy risk. Moreover, cross-sectional studies have largely supported a role for these mechanisms.

Haemodynamic alterations

A raised eGFR in people with newly diagnosed T1DM (and, to a lesser extent, T2DM) has been shown in experimental studies to be due to dilatation of the afferent glomerular arteriolae. This leads to a rise in glomerular capillary pressure which drives hyperfiltration. The rising pressure results in a mechanical stress in the GBM which, in turn, is thought to stimulate matrix production and thickening via production of profibrotic cytokines, such as transforming growth factor (TGF)-β. Angiotensin II is thought to be a key mediator of these changes. Hyperfiltration is associated with later nephropathy development in T1DM, but the link is no longer significant when corrected for hyperglycaemia. Its role in T2DM is much less certain.

Genetic predisposition and ethnicity

Studies in families with multiple siblings with T1DM have shown concordance for nephropathy development, but it is not possible to completely exclude confounding factors. Over 20 different genetic polymorphisms have been linked to nephropathy; those linked to the *ACE* gene appear to be the strongest. No major gene effect has yet been identified.

Nephropathy rates are much higher in certain ethnic subgroups, notably the Pima and other Native American communities, Pacific Islanders, Australian Aborigines, and non-Ashkenazi Jews. Rates are also higher in those from Afro-Caribbean and Asian populations, compared to white European age- and duration-matched cohorts in the UK. The reasons are unclear, but may be related to greater insulin resistance in the Asian population.

Other factors

Hypertension and obesity frequently coexist with T2DM. They are inde-pendent risk factors for kidney function decline. Other known contributors are: recurrent urinary tract infections, urinary tract obstruction, PVD, and smoking. Prompt treatment of all contributing factors will have a positive effect on kidney function preservation.

Diagnostic approach to kidney disease in diabetes

Early stages of kidney disease are asymptomatic and it is therefore important to actively screen at-risk populations and act on findings. Early intervention slows down the decline of kidney function and prevents progression of CVD.

Forty per cent of people with T2DM have some form of CKD, of whom 18–30% have CKD stages 3–5. As 70% of all medications are cleared by the kidneys, identification of reduced eGFR has important implications to medi-cation dose adjustment. It is predicted that the prevalence of CKD stages 3–5 in Europe will increase by 50% from 2012 to 2025.

Screening

Screening for diabetic nephropathy should be a part of the annual review for all people with diabetes and should involve a blood test for eGFR and a urinary test for the ACR. Depending on findings, the frequency of screening may need to be increased, as shown in Table 15.15. If impaired renal func-tion or albuminuria are detected, it is important to exclude other causes that would require a specific management approach (see Figs. 15.7 and 15.8). Upon detection of kidney disease, it is advised to arrange:

• US of kidneys to exclude an obstruction.
• Autoimmune screening to look for glomerulonephritis in cases of proteinuria.
• Prompt referral to urology for painless haematuria.
• Myeloma screening in the appropriate population, especially if anaemia is detected at the same time.

Kidney function declines with age. With increasing life expectancy, eGFR will often be <60 mL/min/1.73/m², which does not necessarily mean that the person has a significant diabetic nephropathy. A level of albuminuria is a stronger predictor of renal function decline and cardiovascular morbidity and mortality.

Protein intake can cause a significant variation in creatinine levels, and consequently eGFR. Ideally, renal function should be assessed >12h after a protein-rich meal. Due to dietary variations in renal function, diagnosis of kidney disease should be based on two samples 90 days apart.

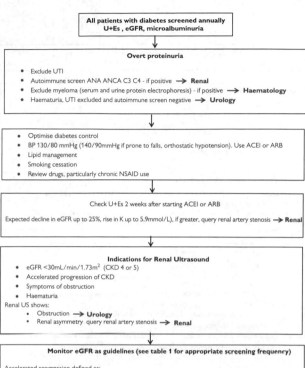

Fig. 15.7 Diabetic renal algorithm.

© Dr Ana Pokrajac 2016, used with courtesy of the author.

eGFR < 45mL/min/1.73m² in a well patient

Does patient have retinopathy/other microvascular complication?
If not, consider non-diabetic kidney disease

Screen for anaemia with FBC

B12, folate, and iron studies

Exclude non-renal causes of anaemia (more likely with higher eGFR)

Iron deficiency in renal disease defined as: % hypochromic red cells >6%, reticulocyte Hb <29pg, transferrin saturation <20%, ferritin <100 micrograms/L

If oral iron ineffective, or remaining anaemic when iron replete ⟶ **Renal for IV iron +/-ESA (erythropoiesis-stimulating agent)**

Monitoring bone profile, Vit D and PTH

If Vit D deficient, treat with Vit D alone and no calcium supplements, doses per Vit D guidelines

If PTH raised but normal phosphate + Vit D, check in 6 months

If PTH rise > 3x upper limit of normal ⟶ **Renal for consideration of hydroxylated vit D**

If phosphate high ⟶ **Renal for dietician and consideration of phosphate binders**

Indications for referral to renal clinic

- eGFR <30 mL/min/1.73m² consistently
- Decline in renal function over 12 months: eGFR decrease of >15 mL/min/1.73m² or decrease of 25% and change in CKD category
- K >5.9 mmol/L on two consecutive samples
- Phosphate >2.0 mmol/L on two consecutive samples
- Anaemia of chronic disease Hb<110, requiring IV iron and/or ESA
- Suspicion of renal artery stenosis

Fig. 15.8 Diabetic renal algorithm: monitoring and onward referral.

Treatment for kidney disease in people with diabetes

Once other specific causes of kidney disease in people with diabetes are excluded, treatment is based on:
- Lifestyle modification to address obesity and smoking
- Glycaemic control
- BP control
- Lipid management
- Uric acid control

When eGFR falls below 45 mL/min/1.72m², it is necessary to include screening and management of CKD complications, anaemia, and bone disease in the care process.

Glycaemic control

Evidence links intensive glucose control to better renal outcomes, expressed as a composite end-point of: renal death, ESRF, eGFR <30 mL/min/1.73m², and macroalbuminuria.

As eGFR declines, glucose control paradoxically improves due to:
- Effect of uraemia on appetite suppression
- Reduced insulin clearance by the kidneys
- Reduced gluconeogenesis

A progression of CKD leads to increased risk of hypoglycaemia accompanied by reduced hypo awareness, so the approach to glucose management has to be reviewed. Hypoglycaemia is often under-reported, not only due to reduced warning signs, but also due to implications for driving. In this particular group of patients with high cardiovascular risk, it is believed that hypoglycaemia triggers either ischaemic events or arrhythmia leading to death. A severe hypoglycaemic episode is associated with 3.5-fold greater mortality.

The Association of British Clinical Diabetologists and Renal Association UK have published guidelines with glycaemic targets specific to the type of diabetes and the stage of CKD (see Table 15.16).[4]

Table 15.16 Glycaemic targets specific to type of diabetes and stage of CKD

Type 1 diabetes	
CKD stages 1 and 2	48–58mmol/mol (6.5–7.5%)
CKD stages 3 and 4	58–62mmol/mol (7.5–7.8%)
CKD stage 5 (on dialysis)	58–68mmol/mol (7.5–8.4%)
Type 2 diabetes	
CKD stages 1 and 2	48–58mmol/mol (6.5–7.5%)
CKD stages 3 and 4 (on non-hypo-inducing agents)	52–58mmol/mol (6.9–7.5%)
CKD stage 3 (on hypo-inducing agents)	53–63mmol/L (7.0–7.9%)
CKD stages 4 (on hypo-inducing agents) and 5 (on dialysis)	58–68mmol/mol (7.5–8.2%)

Many anti-hyperglycaemic drugs are excreted via the kidneys and their dose needs to be reduced with eGFR decline. Hypoglycaemia-inducing drugs like SUs, meglitinides, and insulin need to be dose-adjusted. Table 15.17 provides an overview of dose adjustments for commonly used anti-hyperglycaemic drugs.

There is emerging evidence that SGLT2 inhibitors have renal benefits, independently of their glucose-lowering effect. This renoprotective effect of the class is starting to translate into licence extension for treatment of CKD and reduction of risk of hospitalization with heart failure in people with and without T2DM.

Blood pressure

There are no data supporting a role of antihypertensive therapies (specifically agents which block the renin–angiotensin system (RAS)) in the prevention of nephropathy in normoalbuminuric, normotensive people with either T1DM or T2DM. The benefit of RAS blockade increases with the rise in albuminuria and BP. Targets for BP control in relation to diabetes type and CKD stage are given in Table 15.18.

Lipid management

High rates of CVD and unfavourable lipid profiles seen in people with nephropathy make these attractive treatment targets. In the Heart Protection Study (mainly T2DM patients), there was a reduction in cardiovascular events by around 25%, but few participants had nephropathy. The SHARP trial reported a significant reduction in risk of cardiovascular events of 17% in over 6000 people with pre-dialysis CKD randomized to simvastatin/ezetimibe vs placebo.

There are a number of guidelines for lipid management in diabetes with CKD. A joint publication from the Association of British Clinical Diabetologists and the Renal Association UK suggested the following:
- Lipid-lowering to a target LDL-C of <2mmol/L should be undertaken in all people with diabetes and CKD.
- Treatment with statins is recommended for all people with any type of diabetes and CKD stage 3 and above. For those with milder kidney disease, statin treatment is advised for:
  - *T1DM and:*
    - Any microvascular disease and older than 30 years.
    - 18- to 30-year olds with a microvascular disease and an additional cardiovascular risk factor.
    - Rapidly progressive loss of renal function >5mL/min/year.
  - *T2DM and:*
    - Rapidly progressive loss of renal function >5mL/min/year.
    - Age over 40 years.
    - Persistent micro-/macroalbuminuria.
- Statins are also advised for those on dialysis and previously on statins, but if previously not statin-treated, there is no significant benefit of commencing the treatment. Statin treatment is also indicated for those post-pancreas and/or kidney transplant and for post-transplant diabetes.

Table 15.17 Overview of dose adjustments for commonly used anti-hyperglycaemic drugs

Drug	Class of drug	Renal impairment—CKD stage					
		1 (eGFR >90)	2 (eGFR 60–90)	3a (eGFR 45–59)	3b (eGFR 44–30)	4 (eGFR 29–15)	5 (eGFR <15)
Metformin	**Biguanide**				Reduce dose to 500 mg bd'	eGFR may underestimate in obesity; potential role for 500 mg	
Gliclazide	**SU**				Dose reduction advised	*Off licence*, high risk of hypoglycaemia	
Repaglinide	**Meglitinide**					Dose reduction advised	Dose reduction advised
Sitagliptin	**DPP-IV inhibitor**			<50mL/min: reduce dose to 50mg	Reduce dose to 50mg	Reduce dose to 25mg	Reduce dose to 25mg
Saxagliptin	**DPP-IV inhibitor**			<50mL/min: reduce dose to 2.5mg	Reduce dose to 2.5mg	Reduce dose to 2.5mg	
Linagliptin	**DPP-IV inhibitor**						
Pioglitazone**	**Thiazolidinedione**						
Lixisenatide	**GLP-1 agonist**			Caution if CrCl§ <50mL/min			
Exenatide	**GLP-1 agonist**			Caution if CrCl§ <50mL/min	Conservative dosing		

		Renal impairment—CKD stage		
Exenatide MR	GLP-1 agonist	Stop if CrCl§ <50mL/min		
Liraglutide	GLP-1 agonist		Dose reduction may be needed	Off licence‡
Semaglutide	GLP-1 agonist		Dose reduction may be needed	Off licence‡
Dulaglutide (e.g. Trulicity®)	GLP-1 agonist		Dose reduction may be needed	Off licence‡
Dapagliflozin	SGLT2 inhibitor			¶
Canagliflozin	SGLT2 inhibitor	Reduce dose to 100mg	#¶	
Empagliflozin	SGLT2 inhibitor	Reduce dose to 10mg	†¶	
Insulin		Dose reduction may be needed		Dose reduction should be needed

* Sick day guidance.

** Monitor for fluid retention; contraindicated in heart failure and macular oedema.

§ CrCl, creatinine clearance—as an estimate of glomerular filtration rate, usually calculated using the Cockroft–Gault equation.

‡ Use of liraglutide for eGFR <15mL/min/1.73m^2 is off licence as there is insufficient high-grade evidence; some studies suggest no harm, which is in keeping with its liver metabolism.

\# No significant glucose-lowering effect, but renal function benefit demonstrated in the CREDENCE trial.

† No significant glucose-lowering effect, but used in clinical trials, with no higher incidence of side effects demonstrated in the EMPA-REG trial.

¶ No evidence of harm but due to rapidly changing licence refer to latest SPC.

- High doses of statins can be used for those with the highest cardiovascular risk. There is some evidence to use ezetimibe, in addition to statins, in those who do not attain targets of TC <4 mmol/L and LDL-C <2 mmol/L. There is no role for fibrates in advanced CKD (stage 3b and above), as the risk of side effects exceeds benefits. In people with CKD stage 3a and below, fibrates can be used in addition to statins for residual dyslipidaemia or instead of statins in statin-intolerant people.

Table 15.18 Overview of BP targets for diabetes and CKD

	Stage of kidney function impairment				
	Normal renal function, normo albuminuria	Normal renal function, micro albuminuria	CKD stages 1–3 (non-dialysis)	CKD stages 4–5	CKD stage 5 (dialysis)
T1DM	≤140/80	≤130/80	≤130/80	≤140/90	≤140/90
				≤130/80 for albuminuric	Interdialytic BP
T2DM	≤140/90	≤130/80	≤130/80	≤140/90	≤140/90 interdialytic BP
	≤150/90 for ≥80 years			≤130/80 for albuminuric	

Diet

High dietary protein has been shown to damage the kidneys in experimental diabetes. In T1DM, protein restriction can reduce the rate of loss of eGFR, albuminuria, and mortality in people with established nephropathy. The data are less strong in T2DM. A dietary protein content <0.8 g/kg is suggested, but patients find long-term adherence to be difficult.

As with all patients with CKD, people with diabetes may develop: anaemia, hyperphosphataemia, vitamin D deficiency, and hyperkalaemia; particularly in stage 4 CKD. All of these may require expert dietary and nephrology input and should prompt referral.

When to refer to nephrology

(See Fig. 15.8.)

Current CKD guidance from NICE suggests a referral of all patients with CKD stage 4 or worse (GFR <30 mL/min/1.73m^2) to nephrology. All those with a rate of progression that suggests that they will develop ESRD within 2 years should be referred for preparation for RRT, as there is good evidence that survival is better with careful planning. Those with stable CKD, no significant albuminuria, and well-controlled BP and glycaemia may not need referral.

Complications of CKD, such as anaemia and secondary hyperparathyroidism, or unusual features suggestive of non-diabetic CKD, such as nephrotic-range proteinuria, the presence of signs of non-diabetic systemic disease, or a rapidly declining eGFR, should also prompt a referral.

Survival in those requiring RRT is best for those who receive a renal transplant, although it remains less good than for those with non-diabetic renal disease. A simultaneous pancreas transplantation has not been shown to improve survival, although there are some data suggesting improved QoL in those achieving normoglycaemia.

Further reading

Dasgupta I, et al. (2017). Association of British Clinical Diabetologists (ABCD) and Renal Association clinical guidelines: hypertension management and renin–angiotensin–aldosterone system blockade in patients with diabetes, nephropathy and/or chronic kidney disease. Summary of recommendations. Br J Diabetes **17**, 160–4.

Mark P, et al. (2017). Management of lipids in adults with diabetes mellitus and nephropathy and/or chronic kidney disease: summary of joint guidance from the Association of British Clinical Diabetologists (ABCD) and the Renal Association (RA). Br J Diabetes **17**, 64–72.

National Institute for Health and Care Excellence (2014). Chronic kidney disease in adults: assessment and management. Clinical guideline [CG182]. ℗ https://www.nice.org.uk/guidance/cg182

Neuen B, et al. (2019). SGLT2 inhibitors for the prevention of kidney failure in patients with type 2 diabetes: a systematic review and meta-analysis. Lancet Diabetes Endocrinol **7**, 845–54.

Winocour P (2018). Diabetes and kidney disease: insult added to injury. Br J Diabetes **18**, 78–89.

Zoungas S, et al. (2017). Effects of intensive glucose control on microvascular outcomes in patients with type 2 diabetes: a meta-analysis of individual participant data from randomised controlled trials. Lancet Diabetes Endocrinol **5**, 431–7.

Diabetic neuropathy

Definition

Involvement of cranial, peripheral, and autonomic nerves may be found in patients with diabetes and is termed diabetic neuropathy; this usually suggests a diffuse, predominantly sensory peripheral neuropathy. The effects on nerve function can be both acute or chronic, as well as transient or permanent. The commonest clinical consequences of neuropathy are:

- Altered sensation (both pain and insensitivity to normal sensation).
- Neuropathic ulcers, usually on the feet.
- Erectile dysfunction (with autonomic neuropathy (AN)).
- Charcot arthropathy.

(See Box 15.17 for classification.)

Pathology

DN is one of the microvascular complications of diabetes. Pathologically, distal axonal loss occurs with focal demyelination and attempts at nerve regeneration. The vasa nervorum often shows basement membrane thickening, endothelial cell changes, and some occlusion of its lumen. This results in slowing of nerve conduction velocities or complete loss of nerve function. Both metabolic and vascular changes have been implicated in its aetiology.

Pathogenesis

Hyperglycaemia is probably the major underlying cause of the histological and functional changes, although vascular risk factors, such as hypertension and hyperlipidaemia, may also have a role. Several possible mechanisms have been suggested:

- Overloading of the normal pathways for glucose metabolism, resulting in ↑ use of the polyol pathway which leads to ↓ levels of sorbitol and fructose and ↓ levels of myoinositol and glutathione. This may result in more free radical damage and also lowers nitric oxide levels, thus altering nerve blood flow. Experimental models, using aldose reductase inhibitors which can improve aspects of DN, support this theory.
- Accumulation of AGEs (via non-enzymatic glycation) may contribute.
- In the more acute neuropathies, acute ischaemia of the nerves due to vascular abnormalities has been suggested as the cause. The underlying reason for this is still unclear. Treatment-induced neuropathy of diabetes (TIND; also known as 'insulin neuritis') may occur when there is a rapid fall in glucose with insulin or oral hypoglycaemic therapy.
- Other potential aetiological factors include changes in local growth factor production and oxidative stress.

Further work is needed to clarify the exact role of each of the above mechanisms. In the meantime, studies showing improvements in neuropathy associated with good diabetic control strengthen the argument for the role of hyperglycaemia and offer us a treatment option.

Box 15.17 Classification of diabetic neuropathies

Polyneuropathies

Peripheral sensory motor neuropathy
- Combined large and small fibre neuropathy.
- Predominantly large fibre neuropathy.
- Predominantly small fibre neuropathy.

Autonomic neuropathy
- Cardiovascular:
  - Resting tachycardia.
  - Orthostatic hypotension.
  - Exercise intolerance.
  - Sudden death.
  - Heat intolerance.
  - Foot vein distension and arteriovenous shunting.
  - Oesophageal dysfunction.
- Gastroparesis:
  - Diarrhoea.
  - Constipation.
  - Faecal incontinence.
- GI.
- Bladder hypomotility.
- Erectile dysfunction.
- Retrograde ejaculation.
- Altered sudomotor function:
  - Gustatory sweating.
  - Reduced peripheral sweating.
- ↓ diameter of dark adapted pupil.

Focal neuropathies
- Mononeuropathies.
- Mononeuritis multiplex.
- Proximal motor neuropathy (amyotrophy).
- Thoracoabdominal neuropathy.
- Entrapment neuropathies:
  - Carpal tunnel syndrome.
  - Ulnar neuropathy.

Peripheral sensorimotor neuropathy

(See Box 15.18.)

Although hyperglycaemia can alter nerve function and often gives some sensory symptoms at diagnosis, correcting the hyperglycaemia can often resolve these. Chronic sensorimotor neuropathy (also known as diabetic peripheral neuropathy (DPN) or distal symmetrical polyneuropathy) is the commonest feature of peripheral nerve involvement seen in patients with diabetes. The exact prevalence of DPN varies in most studies because of the different definitions and examination techniques used. For example, sensitive nerve conduction studies can show over 50% of patients have abnormal results. In more normal practice, however, around 30% of patients have either symptomatic neuropathy or abnormalities on examination which are clinically significant. But at least 50% of these patients are asymptomatic. Prevalence increases with increasing duration of diabetes, so although 7–8% of T2DM patients have clinical neuropathy at diagnosis, 50% can be expected to have symptoms or signs 25 years later.

> **Box 15.18 Features of peripheral sensorimotor neuropathy**
>
> - Usually insidious onset with numbness or paraesthesiae, often found on screening, rather than as a presenting problem.
> - Starts in the toes and on the soles of the feet, then spreads up to mid-shin level in a symmetrical fashion. Less often, in more severe cases, it also involves the fingers and hands.
> - Affects all sensory modalities and results in reduced vibration perception thresholds, pinprick, fine touch, and temperature sensations.
> - ↓ vibration sensation and absent ankle reflexes are often the 1st features. A risk factor for ulceration is the inability to feel a 10g monofilament.
> - Less often, the skin is tender/sensitive to touch (allodynia) or frank pain can occur.
> - Painful neuropathy affects up to 20% of a general clinic population. This pain may be sharp, stabbing, electric-shock like, or burning in nature and at times very severe. This is also associated with sleep disturbance, mood disorders, and loss of QoL.
> - There may also be some wasting of the intrinsic muscles of the foot, with clawing of the toes.

Mononeuropathies

Peripheral mononeuropathies and cranial mononeuropathies are not uncommon. These may be spontaneous or may be due to entrapment or external pressure. Of the peripheral mononeuropathies, median nerve involvement and carpal tunnel syndrome may be found in up to 10% of patients and require nerve conduction studies and then surgical decompression. Entrapment of the lateral cutaneous nerve of the thigh is also seen more commonly in those with diabetes, giving pain over the lateral aspect of the thigh. Common peroneal nerve involvement, causing foot drop and tarsal tunnel syndrome, is also recognized but is less common.

Cranial mononeuropathies usually occur suddenly and have a good prognosis. Palsies of cranial nerves III and VI are most commonly seen (but still infrequent). In cranial nerve III palsy, sparing of pupillary responses is usual. Spontaneous recovery is slow over a few months, and no treatment, apart from symptomatic help such as an eye patch, is needed. Unlike entrapment neuropathies where decompression may help, no effective treatment is currently available in most cases of spontaneous mononeuropathy.

Proximal motor neuropathy (diabetic amyotrophy)

This is an uncommon, but disturbing condition to have, mostly affecting men in their fifties with T2DM. It presents with severe pain and paraesthesiae in the upper legs and is felt as a deep aching pain which may be burning in nature and can keep patients awake at night and cause anorexia, resulting in marked cachexia. This, with proximal muscle weakness and wasting of the quadriceps, in particular, can be very debilitating. The lower motor neurones of the lumbar sacral plexus are affected, and improvement is usually spontaneous over 3–4 months. Before making this diagnosis, however, consider other causes such as malignancies and lumbar disc disease. An MRI scan of the lumbar sacral spine is advisable.

Oral antidiabetic agents may play a part in the aetiology of this problem, and conversion to insulin therapy is advised, although anorexia experienced when the pain is severe can make this difficult. Although recovery happens over many months, only 50% recover fully, but no other treatment is currently known to improve on this.

Foot examination

- Mandatory at diagnosis and at least yearly in all asymptomatic patients.
- A gold standard examination would test vibration, fine touch (with a 10g monofilament), and reflexes.
- Using a neurothesiometer or biosthesiometer gives a more quantitative measure of vibration than a 128Hz tuning fork. Inability to feel the vibrating head at >25V in the toes is associated with a significant risk of neuropathic ulceration.
- The 10g monofilament is applied to ten sites across the soles of the two feet. Abnormal sensation is detection of seven or fewer sites.
- In practice, most GP foot screening uses a 10g monofilament and clinical examination to diagnose at-risk feet.

Differential diagnoses of peripheral neuropathy

- Uraemia.
- Vitamin B12 deficiency.
- Infections (e.g. HIV and leprosy).
- Toxins (e.g. alcohol, lead, mercury).
- Drugs (chemotherapeutic agents).
- Malignancy.

Treatment

(See Box 15.19.)

For all patients

Review by a podiatrist and, if indicated, an orthotist to give education on foot care and suitable footwear. If followed by regular podiatry review, this can help to prevent problems developing.

Asymptomatic patients

Apart from good glycaemic control, no drugs are yet available.

Painful diabetic peripheral neuropathy

Pharmacological treatment of painful DPN is not entirely satisfactory, as currently available drugs are often ineffective and complicated by side effects.

- Tricyclic compounds (TCAs) have been used as 1st-line agents for many years, but many patients fail to respond to them and side effects are frequent. Amitriptyline or imipramine 10mg taken at night may be started. Depending on side effects, the dose can be gradually ↑ up to 75mg/day.
- Duloxetine, a selective serotonin–noradrenaline reuptake inhibitor (SNRI), is a 1st-line treatment for painful DPN. It relieves pain by increasing synaptic availability of 5-HT and noradrenaline in the descending pathways that inhibit pain impulses. Duloxetine for painful DPN has been investigated in three identical trials, and pooled data from these show that 60–120mg/day doses are effective in relieving symptoms, starting within a week and lasting the full treatment period of 12 weeks. The main side effect is nausea, but this is often self-limiting. It is advisable to start at 30mg/day, taken with food for a few days.
- The anticonvulsant gabapentin, gradually titrated from 100mg bd to 1800mg/day, is also effective. Doses of up to 3600mg/day can be used.

Box 15.19 Pharmacological treatment of painful DPN

Only two drugs duloxetine and pregabalin have been formally approved by the EMA and FDA for the treatment of painful DPN.

- TCAs:
  - Amitriptyline 25–75mg/day.
  - Imipramine 25–75mg/day.
- SNRIs:
  - Duloxetine 60–120mg/day.
- Anticonvulsants:
  - Gabapentin 300–3600mg/day.
  - Pregabalin 300–600mg/day.
- Opiates:
  - Tramadol 200–400mg/day.
  - Oxycodone 20–80mg/day.
  - Morphine sulfate SR 20–80mg/day.
- Capsaicin cream (0.075%)—applied sparingly 3–4 times per day.
- Capsaicin 8% patch—applied over 30min using protective wear.
- IV lidocaine (for refractory painful neuropathy)—5mg/kg, given IV over 1h, with ECG monitoring.

- Pregabalin has been shown in clinical trials to be effective in the management of painful DPN. Starting dose is 75mg bd, ↑ to a maintenance dose of 150mg bd, with a maximum dose of 600mg/day.
- Other drugs include other anticonvulsants, in particular carbamazepine, opiates, such as tramadol and oxycodone, and, for refractory cases, IV lidocaine. Topical capsaicin, a substance P depleter, is also used; local discomfort at the site of application initially means many patients do not persevere with treatment to see a favourable outcome. For some patients with refractory painful DPN, the 8% capsaicin patch may also be tried in specialist units. A single application over 30min can provide 12 weeks of pain relief, but again there can be severe pain at the site of application. The antioxidant α-lipoic acid was shown to be effective in a small meta-analysis and is widely used in Germany, Eastern Europe, and China.

Despite these treatments, however, many sufferers have suboptimal pain relief. Non-pharmacological treatments, such as acupuncture, transcutaneous electrical nerve stimulation (TENS), and, for severe resistant cases, electrical spinal cord stimulation, may be used. Consensus panels and NICE have evaluated all published clinical trial data and recommended that 1st-line therapies for painful DPN to be a TCA, the SNRI duloxetine, or the anticonvulsants pregabalin or gabapentin, taking into account patient comorbidities and cost.

General treatments

Specific treatments for each form of neuropathy have already been discussed, but there is some evidence for more general therapies.

- Poor diabetic control appears to be associated with worsening neuropathy, and there is level A evidence for improved glycaemic control in preventing/ameliorating DPN in T1DM, while there is level B evidence in T2DM. Thus, good diabetes control is advocated in any patient, especially if neuropathy is present.
- Cardiovascular risk factors, such as hypertension, smoking, obesity, and hyperlipidaemia (especially hypertriglyceridaemia), are risk factors for peripheral neuropathy. Well-designed clinical trials using appropriate end-points are now required to test whether cardiovascular risk reduction improves neuropathy outcomes in T2DM.

Autonomic neuropathy

The commonest effect of AN is erectile dysfunction, which affects 40% of ♂ with diabetes (although this is multifactorial). The widespread use of sildenafil and other similar agents has highlighted this. Some may also have exercise intolerance. Only a small number develop severe GI, cardiac, or bladder dysfunction. Abnormal autonomic function tests can be expected in 20–40% of a general diabetic clinic population. The potential problems during surgery from cardiac involvement should be remembered.

Clinical features

- Erectile dysfunction.
- Postural hypotension—giving dizziness and syncope in up to 12%.
- Resting tachycardia or fixed heart rate/loss of sinus arrhythmia—in up to 20%.
- Gustatory sweating—sweating after tasting food.
- Delayed gastric emptying, nausea/vomiting, abdominal fullness.
- Constipation/diarrhoea.
- Urinary retention/overflow incontinence.
- Anhidrosis—absent sweating on the feet is especially problematic, as it increases the risk of ulceration.
- Abnormal pupillary reflexes.

Assessment

If AN is suspected, check:
- Lying and standing BP (measure systolic BP after 2min standing; normal is <10mmHg drop; >20mmHg is abnormal).
- Pupillary responses to light.

Other less commonly performed tests to consider if the diagnosis is uncertain or in high-risk patients include:
- *Loss of sinus arrhythmia.* Measure inspiratory and expiratory heart rates after 5s of each (<10 bpm difference is abnormal; >15 bpm is normal).
- *Loss of heart rate response to Valsalva manoeuvre.* Look at the ratio of the shortest R–R interval during forced expiration against a closed glottis, compared to the longest R–R interval after it (<1.2 is abnormal).
- *BP response to sustained hand grip.* Diastolic BP prior to the test is compared to diastolic BP after 5min of sustaining a grip equivalent to 30% of maximal grip. A diastolic BP rise >16mmHg is normal; <10mmHg is abnormal. A rolled-up BP cuff to achieve the required hand grip may be used.
- For gastroparesis, a radioisotope test meal can identify delayed gastric emptying. Blood glucose should be <10mmol/L, as hyperglycaemia exacerbates delayed gastric emptying.

Treatment

This is based on the specific symptom and is usually symptomatic only.
   In all patients, improvement in diabetic control is advocated in case any of it is reversible, but this is not usually very helpful or effective.

Postural hypotension

- Stopping drugs that may result in, or exacerbate, postural hypotension, including diuretics, β-blockers, anti-anginal agents, tricyclic agents, etc.
- Advising patients to get up from the sitting or lying position slowly and crossing the legs.
- Increasing Na intake up to 10g (185mmol) per day, and fluid intake to 2.0–2.5L per day (caution in elderly patients with heart failure).
- Raising the head of the bed by 10–20°, as this stimulates the renin–angiotensin–aldosterone system and results in a decrease in nocturnal diuresis.
- Drinking ~500mL of water before or with meals, which stimulates a significant pressor response and improves symptoms of postural hypotension.
- Using custom-fitted elastic stockings extending to the waist.
- Pharmacological treatment with fludrocortisone, starting at 100 micrograms per day, while carefully monitoring for supine hypertension, ankle oedema, and hypokalaemia. K supplementation may be required when higher doses are used, and it is important to monitor U&E.
- In severe cases, the following drugs α1-adrenal receptor agonist midodrine (2.5–10.0mg tds), sympathomimetic ephedrine (25mg tds), and occasionally octreotide and erythropoietin (25–75U/kg three times a week until a Hct level approaching normal is achieved) may be tried.

Erectile dysfunction

Libido is not normally affected and pain is also unusual, so look for hypogonadism and Peyronie's if these features are present. AN is the likely cause, but many drugs, especially thiazides and β-blockers, can also cause it, as can alcohol, tobacco, cannabis, and stress. These should be assessed by direct questioning. Examination should include:

- Genitalia and 2° sexual characteristics.
- Peripheral pulses—as vascular insufficiency may play a part.
- Lower limb reflexes and vibration thresholds—to confirm that neuropathy is present.

Biochemical screening should at least include:

- PRL.
- Testosterone.
- Gonadotrophins (LH/FSH).

Exacerbating factors, such as alcohol and antihypertensive drugs, should be modified. The main therapies are:

- PDE-5 inhibitors, including sildenafil (e.g. Viagra®), tadalafil (e.g. Cialis®), avanafil, and vardenafil. Most are taken 30–60min before intercourse is desired, although a daily dose of tadalafil is also licensed.
- Intraurethral alprostadil.
- Intracavernosal alprostadil.
- Vacuum devices.

None of these are ideal. Sildenafil, although an oral therapy, is effective in only 60% of those with diabetes and is contraindicated in those with severe heart disease and those on nitrates.

A specialist erectile dysfunction clinic is advised for discussion of treatments other than oral PDE-5 inhibitors.

Gastroparesis

Management of diabetic gastroparesis includes:

- Optimization of glycaemic control, as hyperglycaemia can delay gastric emptying. Insulin pump therapy is commonly used.
- Stopping drugs that can delay gastric emptying such as calcium channel blockers, GLP-1 analogues, and anticholinergic agents such as antidepressants, etc.
- Antiemetics (metoclopramide and domperidone).
- Erythromycin which may enhance activity of the gut peptide motilin.
- Gastric electrical stimulation ('pacing') is a treatment option in patients with drug-refractory gastroparesis and can increase the QoL and decrease hospital admissions by alleviating nausea and vomiting.

Severe gastroparesis, causing recurrent vomiting, is associated with dehydration, swings in blood sugar, and weight loss and is therefore an indication for hospital admission. The patient should be adequately hydrated with IV fluids, and blood sugar should be stabilized by IV insulin; antiemetics could be given IV, and if the course of the gastroparesis is prolonged, total parenteral nutrition or feeding through a gastrostomy tube may be required.

Autonomic diarrhoea

The patient may present with diarrhoea which tends to be worse at night, or alternatively some may present with constipation. Both the diarrhoea and constipation respond to conventional treatment, but can be extremely problematic to treat at times.

- Diarrhoea associated with bacterial overgrowth may respond to treatment with a broad-spectrum antibiotic such as doxycycline 100mg bd, erythromycin 250mg qds for 7 days or tetracycline 250mg bd for 7 days.
- Bile acid malabsorption may be treated with colestyramine.
- The antidiarrhoeal synthetic opioids (e.g. loperamide 2mg qds) and codeine phosphate (30mg qds) can improve symptoms by decreasing peristalsis and increasing rectal sphincter tone.
- Refractory diarrhoea may be treated with the α2-adrenergic receptor agonist clonidine and the SSA octreotide. Octreotide suppresses GI motility and inhibits the release of motilin, serotonin, and gastrin but may result in recurrent hypoglycaemia due to impaired counter-regulation.

Neuropathic bladder

- Bladder dysfunction is a rare complication of AN involving the sacral nerves. The patient presents with hesitancy of micturition, ↑ frequency of micturition, and, in serious cases, urinary retention associated with overflow incontinence.
- Patients are prone to urinary tract infections. US scan of the urinary tract, IV urography, and urodynamic studies may be required.
- Treatment manoeuvres include mechanical methods of bladder emptying by applying suprapubic pressure or use of intermittent self-catheterization.
- Anticholinesterase drugs, such as neostigmine or pyridostigmine, may be useful.
- Long-term indwelling catheterization may be required in some, but this unfortunately predisposes the patient to urinary tract infections and long-term antibiotic prophylaxis may be required.

Anhidrosis

Dry feet can cause cracks in the skin and act as a site for infection. Emollient creams may help prevent this.

Gustatory sweating

↑ sweating, usually affecting the face and often brought about by eating (gustatory sweating), can be very embarrassing to patients and difficult to treat.

- Oral anticholinergic agents, including oxybutynin, propantheline, and glycopyrronium bromide, may improve symptoms; however, adverse reactions, including dry mouth, constipation, potential worsening of gastroparesis, and confusion, limit their use.
- Clonidine has been used with some success but is also limited by side effects, including hypotension and dry mouth.
- Systemic side effects have led to the investigation of non-systemic approaches. Topical glycopyrronium bromide, an antimuscarinic quaternary ammonium compound, has been shown to significantly decrease the incidence, severity, and frequency of sweating with eating and is tolerated well.
- Botulinum toxin has been used for gustatory sweating, though, in most literature, it is limited to use in unilateral, surgically related cases.

Further reading

Gibbons CH (2020). Treatment induced neuropathy of diabetes. *Auton Neurosci* **22**, 102668.

National Institute for Health and Care Excellence (2013, updated 2020). *Neuropathic pain: pharmacological management.* NICE guideline [CG173]. ℘ https://www.nice.org.uk/guidance/cg173/evidence/full-guideline-pdf-4840898221.

Pop-Busui R, et al. (2017). Diabetic neuropathy: a position statement by the American Diabetes Association. *Diabetes Care* **40**, 136–54.

Sloan G, et al. (2021). Diabetic peripheral neuropathy: mechanisms and management. *Nature Rev Endocrinol* **17**, 400–20.

The diabetic foot

Diabetic foot problems are a leading cause of morbidity. Box 15.20 illustrates the burden of diabetic foot ulceration in the UK. (See Table 15.19 for clinical features, and Table 15.20 for classification of diabetic foot lesions.)

Risk factors for foot ulcer development

Several factors predispose to ulcer formation, and awareness of these should highlight 'at-risk' patients for education and other preventive strategies. Ulcers can occur anywhere on the foot, but load-bearing areas are the most frequent sites. Risk factors include the following.

Neuropathy

- Sensory neuropathy—observed in up to 80% of patients. It reduces awareness of pain and trauma caused by footwear, foreign bodies, callus, or heat. Examine for reduced sensation with 10g monofilament and reduced vibration perception thresholds.
- AN—leads to anhidrosis, therefore increases the tendency of skin to crack, allowing a portal of entry for infection.
- Motor neuropathy—can result in altered foot muscle tone, wasting of small muscles, raising of the medial longitudinal arch, and clawing of the toes, hence increasing forefoot pressures and predisposing to callus and ulcer formation.

Peripheral vascular disease

PVD and *microvascular circulatory disease* lead to local ischaemia, the potential for ulcer formation and delayed wound healing. Always examine peripheral pulses, and consider Doppler studies or further specialist assessment if there are abnormal pulses or PVD is a concern.

Previous ulceration

Anyone with previous foot disease needs very careful monitoring/follow-up, as they will always be at risk of further foot complications.

Renal replacement therapy

Requiring RRT is an independent risk factor for developing a foot ulcer.

Other factors

Duration of diabetes, increasing age, and presence of other microvascular complications (e.g. nephropathy and retinopathy) are all risk factors for foot ulcer development.

Mechanical, chemical, or thermal trauma/injury

Injury or pressure often initiates a foot ulcer. Therefore, employment, pastimes, and mobility should be considered during foot assessment.

Box 15.20 Epidemiology of foot ulceration in the UK

Prevalence of foot ulceration in diabetes	5–10%
Number of people with diabetes who have foot ulcers	~80,000
Number of people with diabetes undergoing lower limb amputation per year	~8500
Two-year mortality following major amputation	50%
Annual NHS expenditure on diabetes foot-related care	~£650 million

Table 15.19 Clinical features of diabetic feet

Neuropathic feet	Ischaemic feet
Warm	Cold/cool
Dry skin	Atrophic/often hairless
Palpable foot pulses	No palpable foot pulses
No discomfort with ulcer	More often tender/painful
Callus present	Claudication/rest pain
	Skin blanches on elevation and reddens on dependency

Table 15.20 SINBAD classification of diabetic foot lesions

Category	Definition	Score
Site	Forefoot	0
	Mid-foot or hindfoot	1
Ischaemia	Blood flow intact	0
	Absent pulses ± clinical signs of peripheral arterial disease	1
Neuropathy	Sensation intact	0
	Impaired sensation	1
Bacterial infection	None	0
	Clinical signs of infection	1
Area	<1cm²	0
	≥1cm²	1
Depth	Superficial	0
	Tendon or bone	1

Source: data from Ince P et al (2008) "Use of the SINBAD classification system and score in comparing outcome of foot ulcer management on three continents" *Diabetes Care* 31:964–967.

Management of the foot in diabetes

All people with diabetes should have regular screening with regard to their risk of developing a foot complication. This should be at least an annual assessment.

Management of the foot in diabetes requires a multidisciplinary approach with collaboration between diabetologists, DSNs, podiatrists, orthotists, vascular/plastic/orthopaedic surgeons, microbiologists, and the person with diabetes.

Management is aimed at several distinct situations, namely:
- At-risk feet with no current ulceration.
- Treating existing ulcers.
- Treating infection.
- Treating vascular insufficiency.

At-risk feet with no current ulceration

When at-risk feet are identified, patients should be provided with advice and education. This should include:
- General advice on nail care, hygiene, and footwear.
- The importance of daily examination of the feet by the patient or carer and rapidly seeking care if a problem is discovered.
- Avoiding barefoot walking.
- Regular podiatry review where beneficial.
- For those who have had a previous foot problem, consider if bespoke footwear would be beneficial in preventing future ulceration.

Treating existing ulcers

Table 15.20 shows the SINBAD classification for diabetic foot lesions. The higher the combined score, out of a maximum of 6, the more severe the ulcer.

Treatment usually requires
- Regular debridement of callus and dead tissue by an appropriately trained clinician, following an adequate vascular assessment.
- Pressure offloading and reduction of trauma. This is usually achieved via modified insoles or footwear, casting, pneumatic boots, immobilization, or resting. This needs to be tailored to the individual, and involvement of orthotists and podiatrists is essential.
- Regular wound review and dressing with appropriate materials, taking care not to impair circulation or cause further skin damage.
- Optimizing glycaemia.
- Reduction of oedema to aid healing.

Early referral to an MDT for more severe cases is essential.

Treating infection

There should be a high index of suspicion with regard to infection when managing diabetic foot ulcers, as the normal inflammatory response may be reduced. If infection is suspected, prompt action and close monitoring are required as deterioration can be rapid.

Tissue samples should be taken, where possible, for microbiological testing which can be used to guide antibiotic choices as required. If tissue samples are not possible, a swab can be taken. These should be taken before starting antibiotic therapy, if possible, but should not delay the start of therapy.

For all diabetic foot infections where there is a deep or chronic wound, or there is the ability to probe to bone, then osteomyelitis should be suspected. Imaging (e.g. X-ray, MRI) can be useful in confirming a clinical diagnosis.

Antibiotic choices should be guided by local prescribing guidelines, and urgent specialist advice sought for limb-threatening or systemic infection. Rapid surgical input may be required in these situations and patients should be urgently referred to the MDT.

Treating vascular insufficiency

Always consider coexisting vascular disease. Vascular bypass grafting/reconstruction or angioplasty can give excellent results, with a 70–95% limb salvage rate often quoted. The improved blood supply will also help healing of existing ulcers and may negate the need for amputation or allow the area requiring resection to be minimized.

If vascular intervention is unsuccessful or not possible, or all options have been explored, then amputation may be required, preferably as a below-knee procedure to give better mobilization potential post-operatively.

The Charcot foot

Epidemiology

This is a relatively rare complication of diabetes, representing ~10% of the caseload of a specialist diabetic foot clinic. Prevalence in the wider population is much lower.

Pathogenesis

Pathogenesis is unclear. It is suggested that blood flow increases due to sympathetic nerve loss, causing osteoclast activity and bone turnover to increase, so making the bones of the foot more susceptible to damage. It is also thought that repeated microtrauma to the foot through gait, in conjunction with neuropathy, can make a person more susceptible to the condition.

Clinical features

Early presentation of an acute Charcot foot is a red, hot, swollen foot ± a history of trauma ± pain ± deformity. Peripheral pulses are invariably present, and peripheral neuropathy is evident clinically. Differential diagnoses are cellulitis, gout, DVT, or soft tissue injury.

Plain radiographs may be normal initially and later show fractures with osteolysis and joint reorganization, with subluxation of the metatarsophalangeal joints and dislocation of the large joints of the foot. MRI or other imaging techniques may be useful to aid diagnosis.

In the untreated patient, or if there is a late presentation, two classic deformities are seen:

* A 'rocker bottom' deformity due to displacement and subluxation of the tarsus downwards.
* Medial convexity due to displacement of the talonavicular joint or tarsometatarsal dislocation.

Management

Treatment of the condition should be managed under the care of the foot MDT. Where active Charcot foot is suspected, urgent onward referral should be made.

The aim of treatment is to immobilize the foot to prevent or reduce joint destruction and deformity. This is usually achieved by below-knee casts or pneumatic boots for at least 2–3 months, while bone repair/remodelling is going on. In some cases, this may need to continue for 12–18 months. Following resolution of the acute Charcot foot, the patient is likely to require bespoke footwear.

Further reading

Ince P, et al. (2008). Use of the SINBAD classification system and score in comparing outcome of foot ulcer management on three continents. *Diabetes Care* **31**, 964–7.

National Institute for Health and Care Excellence (2015). *Diabetic foot problems: prevention and management*. NICE guideline [NG19]. ℜ https://www.nice.org.uk/guidance/ng19/resources/diabetic-foot-problems-prevention-and-management-pdf-1837279828933.

Macrovascular disease

People with diabetes have a significantly greater risk of macrovascular complications (CHD, cerebrovascular disease, and PVD) than the non-diabetic population. Around three-quarters of people with diabetes will die as a result of macrovascular disease, and a diagnosis of T2DM equates to a cardiovascular risk equivalent of ageing 10–15 years.

Epidemiology

The exact prevalence and incidence of macrovascular disease and its outcomes will vary, depending on the age, gender, and ethnic mix of the patients being assessed. The previous belief that CVD is less common in T1DM has been proven wrong, and in general, vascular complications account for around three-quarters of deaths in both T1DM and T2DM. Although the atheroma seen is histologically the same as in a non-diabetic population, it tends to be more diffuse and progresses more rapidly. It also occurs at an earlier age, and women with diabetes lose the cardiovascular protection seen in the non-diabetic population.

- Overall, PVD occurs in up to 10% of patients, and they have up to 15-fold greater risk of needing a non-traumatic amputation than the non-diabetic population.
- Thromboembolic cerebrovascular events increase in individuals with diabetes, compared to the non-diabetic population.
- The risk of having an MI is also ↑ 2–4 times in individuals with diabetes.

Secondary prevention

- Stop smoking.
- Strict control of BP.
- Lipid-lowering drugs.
- Early control of blood glucose.
- Aspirin: this is *no longer* recommended for 1° cardiovascular protection in subjects with diabetes.

Pathogenesis

The risk factors for atherosclerosis, such as smoking and family history, still apply in the diabetic population. Some factors, however, are commoner in those with diabetes and may also confer a greater risk to the diabetic population. These include:

- *Glycaemic control.* Short-term studies, such as ACCORD, VADT, and ADVANCE, investigating the effects of tight glycaemic control on the development of macrovascular disease have been disappointing. These showed that optimizing glucose control has no value in preventing vascular ischaemic events. However, longer-term studies, such as DCCT-EDIC in T1DM and UKPDS in T2DM, have clearly demonstrated that early glycaemic control is key for the prevention of CVD later in life. However, strict glycaemic control should not occur at the expense of ↑ hypoglycaemia, which can be life-threatening. Interestingly, recent studies show that the type of hypoglycaemic agent used determines the risk of vascular events and cardiovascular mortality.

- *Hypertension*. Commoner in both T1DM and T2DM patients and results in vascular endothelial injury, so predisposing to atheroma formation. The UKPDS suggests BP control is a more important individual risk factor for CVD than glycaemic control. Therefore, there are strict criteria to control BP in patients with diabetes, particularly in the presence of microvascular complications.

- *Hyperlipidaemia*. Common; for example, hyperinsulinaemia in insulin-resistant T2DM patients causes reduced HDL-C, elevated TGs (and VLDL), and smaller denser, and therefore more atherogenic, LDL-C. Results from the FIELD study, investigating the effects of lowering TG levels with fibrate treatment in diabetes, failed to show a beneficial effect on vascular complications, which may have been partially related to study design. On the other hand, use of statins in diabetes has been shown to reduce cardiovascular events in a number of studies, and this is now routine practice for both 1° and 2° cardiovascular protection in diabetes.

- *Obesity*. An independent risk factor, commoner in T2DM patients. Central obesity, in particular, is more atherogenic. However, individuals with T1DM can also become overweight, which increases their risk of diabetes complications and this subpopulation has been referred to as having double diabetes.

- *Insulin resistance* or elevated circulating insulin/proinsulin-like molecule levels are known to increase the risk of atherosclerosis in both diabetic and non-diabetic populations. Endothelial dysfunction is a feature of insulin resistance, explaining the clustering of risk factors in individuals who display a decrease in their insulin sensitivity.

- *Altered coagulability*. Circulating fibrinogen, plasminogen activator inhibitor (PAI)-1, and von Willebrand factor levels are altered in diabetes, whereas platelet activity is enhanced. Antiplatelet agents, mainly aspirin, were previously recommended for 1° cardiovascular protection. However, recent evidence from the largest study to date, the ASCEND trial, addressing the role of aspirin in 1° prevention in diabetes, has shown that the beneficial effects of reducing vascular events by this agent are largely counterbalanced by ↑ risk of bleeding. Therefore, aspirin should not be given routinely for 1° prevention, although it may be considered on a case-by-case basis and after careful assessment of risks and benefits. On the other hand, aspirin continues to be used for 2° cardiovascular protection in diabetes. No specific treatment exists at present to address changes in level/activity of coagulation factors. However, the relatively recent COMPASS trial, using rivaroxaban (factor X inhibitor), has shown a reduction of vascular events in individuals with and without diabetes, but at the expense of ↑ bleeding risk, particularly when the agent is combined with aspirin. Therefore, anticoagulant agents for the prevention of vascular ischaemic events are reserved for specialist use.

The UKPDS has shown the major risk factors for CHD in T2DM patients to be elevated LDL-C, ↓ HDL-C, hypertension, hyperglycaemia, and smoking. Lifestyle changes can address smoking and low HDL-C, while medical therapies can effectively control LDL-C, hypertension, and hyperglycaemia.

(See Box 15.21 for the management of MI in those with diabetes.)

Box 15.21 Management of acute myocardial infarction

Patients with diabetes are more likely to have an MI and more likely to die from it than individuals without diabetes. This is partly due to a greater likelihood of myocardial pump failure in diabetes. Several older studies (ISSI-2, GUSTO, GISSI-2) recruited relatively large numbers of people with diabetes and so provide useful outcome data. More recent studies have shown that agents in the SGLT2 inhibitor class improve cardiac function and reduce hospitalization for heart failure in those at risk of a cardiovascular event.

Around 20–30% of patients admitted to hospital with an MI will have hyperglycaemia, many of whom will not have been previously diagnosed with diabetes.

As in the non-diabetic population, thrombolytic therapy, aspirin, P2Y12 inhibitors, and acute angioplasty have proven benefits. The previous contraindication for thrombolysis in those with PDR has been questioned by many, although this is less of an issue these days as 1° angioplasty is replacing thrombolytic therapy.

Tight glycaemic control (blood glucose 7–10mmol/L using IV glucose and insulin for at least 24h, followed by SC insulin, as used in the DIGAMI study, also has benefits. In DIGAMI, patients with an admission blood glucose >11.0mmol/L who were treated with this regimen had a 7.5% absolute risk reduction in mortality at 1 year and an 11% risk reduction at 3.5 years, compared to the control group (i.e. 33% mortality with treatment vs 44% in controls at 3.5 years). This equates to one life saved for every nine treated with this regimen. The exact reason for this is unclear. The DIGAMI 2 study failed to show a benefit for insulin therapy post-MI, but the various groups had similar glycaemic control, making results interpretation from this trial problematic.

- It is suggested that all patients with a blood glucose >11mmol/L benefit from glucose-lowering therapy, whether previously known to have diabetes or not. Using admission HbA1c to differentiate those with undiagnosed or stress-related hyperglycaemia can be useful but should not result in withholding acute treatment of hyperglycaemia in such patients. It may, however, help to identify those who may be at greater risk of hypoglycaemia and may not therefore be suitable for SC insulin or SUs in the intermediate or long term.
- Using ACEIs early after an MI gives a 0.5% absolute risk reduction of 30-day mortality and a 4–8% risk reduction over 15–50 months in the general population. Analysis of the diabetes subgroup in the GISSI-3 study showed a 30% relative risk reduction in 6-week mortality (8.7% vs 12.4%), compared to a 5% reduction for those without diabetes. In view of the greater proportion of diabetes individuals with poor left ventricular function after an MI, compared to the non-diabetic population, this difference is important.
- The use of SGLT2 inhibitors will further reduce heart failure in individuals with diabetes.
- Despite advancement in therapies, mortality following an MI remains significantly higher in diabetic individuals, compared with the non-diabetic group.

Lipid abnormalities in patients with diabetes

Hyperlipidaemia in a patient with diabetes, at any level of cholesterol, is associated with a greater risk of macrovascular disease than someone without diabetes. Patients with diabetes may have altered activity of insulin-dependent enzymes, such as LPL, which results in delayed systemic clearance of certain lipids. This, combined with altered hepatic production of ApoB-containing lipoproteins, gives a more atherogenic profile.

Usual findings are of ↑ TG-containing lipoproteins, chylomicrons, and VLDL. Although commoner in insulin-resistant T2DM patients, this can also be seen in T1DM patients, particularly in those who are overweight or with above-target HbA1c. Another abnormality is low HDL-C (HDL2 especially), commonly seen in T2DM and individuals with insulin resistance. Other atherogenic changes include a tendency to develop small, dense LDL-C particles and a greater tendency to oxidative damage which renders them even more atherogenic. Lpa levels, which are thought to contribute to the atherothrombotic process, are also often raised.

Other causes of lipid abnormalities should be kept in mind when assessing individuals with diabetes such as FH or FCH (see ➔ Primary hyperlipidaemias, p. 988 91). Screening for 2° causes of hyperlipidaemia, such as hypothyroidism, obstructive liver disease, nephrotic syndrome, and alcohol abuse, should also be performed.

Evidence from trials

The diabetes subgroups from the major lipid-lowering trials (see Table 15.21), such as the 4S study (Scandinavian Simvastatin Survival Study), CARE (Cholesterol and Recurrent Events Trial), LIPID (Long-term Intervention with Pravastatin in Ischaemic Disease), and WOSCOPS (West of Scotland Coronary Prevention Study), show impressive reductions in mortality, reinfarction, and stroke, although the numbers in each were relatively small. In 4S, for example, the simvastatin-treated subgroup of individuals with diabetes had a 23% rate of major coronary events, compared to 45% in diabetes patients assigned to placebo. This compares with 19% and 27%, respectively, in the groups without diabetes. On the basis of this, it is suggested that if 100 people with diabetes who have angina or are post-MI are treated with simvastatin for 6 years, 24 of the 46 expected coronary deaths and non-fatal MIs can be prevented.

Diabetes-specific lipid-lowering trials, such as CARDS (Collaborative Atorvastatin Diabetes Study), showed significant benefit of statin treatment in this population. Atorvastatin seems to be better tolerated than simvastatin and is the safest cholesterol-lowering agent to be used in those with renal impairment.

Table 15.21 Important lipid-lowering studies

Study	4S	WOSCOP	CARE	LIPID
Type of study	2° prevention of CHD	1° prevention of CHD	2° prevention of CHD	2° prevention of CHD
Duration of study (years)	6	5	5	6
Number studied	4444	6595	4159	9014
Mean total cholesterol (mmol/L) (cholesterol at inclusion)	6.8 (5.5–8.0)	7.0 (>6.5)	5.4 (<6.2)	5.6 (4.0–7.0)
Age range (years)	35–70	45–64	21–75	31–75
% men	81	100	86	83
% with diabetes	4.5	1	17	8.6
Treatment	Simvastatin 20–40mg daily	Pravastatin 40mg daily	Pravastatin 40mg daily	Pravastatin 40mg daily
Event reduction	34% and 55% for those without and with diabetes, respectively	31% overall	23% for individuals without diabetes 25% for individuals with diabetes	23% overall

Management

Patients with diabetes are given dietary advice to help control blood glucose, which also contributes to improving the lipid profile. In a patient who is already following a 'healthy diet', however, there is often not much room for improvement.

Other standard advice should also be given:
- Stop smoking—reduces the risk of death by about 50% over a 15-year period.
- Reduce weight if overweight/obese.
- Increase physical activity.

Lipid-lowering therapy

The most recent combined European Society of Cardiology (ESC)-EASD international guidelines advocate aggressive lipid management in individuals with diabetes and suggest dividing patients into three categories:

1. Moderate risk: T1DM <35 years old or T2DM <50 years old with diabetes duration of <10 years and no other risk factors.
2. High risk: patients with diabetes duration of >10 years, usually with an additional risk factor, but no end-organ damage.
3. Very high risk: patients with established CVD, target organ damage, multiple risk factors, or diabetes duration >20 years.

Treatment aims for lipids

- TC <4.0mmol/L.
- LDL-C: moderate risk <2.5mmol/L; high risk <1.8mmol/L; very high risk <1.4mmol/L or at least 50% reduction from baseline.
- HDL-C >1.0mmol/L.
- TGs <2.3mmol/L.

The reduction of LDL-C is usually achieved with use of statins (1st line), with ezetimibe added in case targets are not reached. The relatively novel PCSK9 inhibitors are currently reserved for high-risk resistant cases or for those who are statin-intolerant, and these agents are usually given under specialist supervision. LDL-C targets have been established from T2DM studies and robust outcome trials in T1DM are lacking. However, given the high risk of vascular disease in the latter group, it is not unreasonable to apply the same lipid criteria to individuals with T1DM.

Pharmacological interventions to increase HDL have not been shown to improve clinical outcome. HDL can be raised non-pharmacologically using lifestyle measures (weight loss, exercise, and stopping smoking).

Remember that generally a fit patient with diabetes has a similar risk when compared to an individual without diabetes of the same age and gender who has also had a cardiovascular event (although the RR can vary with age). More strict lipid targets are advocated by many, especially for those who have had coronary revascularization procedures.

In those with mixed hyperlipidaemia, consider a fibrate or a statin licensed for this indication. A fibrate will reduce TGs by 30–40% and LDL-C by <20%, while a statin would reduce TGs slightly less (10–15%) and LDL-C slightly more (25–35%). Fibrates also alter LDL-C to its less atherogenic form. The choice of agent must be tailored to the individual patient. For hypercholesterolaemia alone, a statin is 1st choice, as in individuals without diabetes, and in severely resistant patients, combination therapy with statins and ezetimibe or statin and fibrates may be required. Combination of statin and ezetimibe may reduce LDL-C more effectively than increasing the statin dose alone, although there is no evidence that such combination therapy is translated into better clinical outcome, compared to monotherapy with higher-dose statin.

Hypertension

Epidemiology

Hypertension is twice as common in individuals with diabetes than in those without, and standard ethnic differences in the prevalence of hypertension still hold true. It is known that hypertension worsens the severity and increases the risk of developing both microvascular and macrovascular disease. Using a cut-off of >160/90mmHg, hypertension occurs in:

- 10–30% of patients with T1DM.
- 20–30% of microalbuminuric T1DM patients.
- 80–90% of macroalbuminuric T1DM patients.
- 30–50% of Caucasians with T2DM.

Using the UKPDS suggested target of 140/80mmHg, hypertension is even commoner.

Pathogenesis

- *T1DM patients.* Hypertension is strongly associated with diabetic nephropathy and microalbuminuria, and occurs at an earlier stage than that seen in many other causes of renal disease. It is also more prevalent in those T1DM patients who are overweight.
- *T2DM patients.* Hypertension is associated with insulin resistance and hyperinsulinaemia. Hyperinsulinaemia can directly cause hypertension by ↑ sympathetic nervous system activity, enhanced proximal tubule Na reabsorption, and stimulation of vascular smooth muscle cell proliferation.

Management of hypertension

Treatment aim

NICE guidelines recommend all people with diabetes should have a BP <140/80mmHg or <130/80mmHg in the presence of diabetic complications.

The hypertension study in the UKPDS highlights the benefits for T2DM patients of such a treatment level on mortality, diabetes-related end-points, and microvascular end-points. In this study, a 10/5mmHg difference in BP was associated with a 34% risk reduction in macrovascular end-points, a 37% risk reduction in microvascular end-points, and a 44% risk reduction in stroke. The Hypertension Optimal Treatment (HOT) study supports these targets.

Predisposing conditions

Other conditions causing both hypertension and hyperglycaemia should be considered, e.g. Cushing's syndrome, acromegaly, and PCC.

End-organ damage

Assess for evidence of end-organ damage (eyes, heart, kidneys, and peripheral vascular tree, in particular).

Assessment of cardiac risk factors

Treat associated risk factors for CHD.

Treatment

General

Modify other risk factors such as glycaemic control, smoking, and dyslipidaemia. Then consider:
* Weight reduction if obese.
* Reduced salt intake (<6g/day).
* Reduced alcohol intake (government guidelines <14 units per week).
* Exercise (20–40min of moderate exertion 3–5 times/week).

Pharmacological

Most agents currently available will drop systolic BP by no more than 20mmHg at most. In the UKPDS BP study, one-third of those achieving the current BP targets required three or more drugs. The NICE guidelines for BP treatment advocate an 'A/CD' approach—that is starting with 'A', an ACEI (or an angiotensin II receptor blocker/antagonist if the ACEI is not tolerated), and then adding in either a 'C'/calcium channel blocker or a 'D'/thiazide-type diuretic, with an α-blocker, a β-blocker, or further diuretic therapy then added if this fails to reduce BP adequately.
* In the presence of microalbuminuria or frank proteinuria, an ACEI is 1st line, or an angiotensin II receptor antagonist if not tolerated.
* In African/African-Caribbean patients, ACEIs and β-blockers are less effective than calcium channel blockers and diuretics. A diuretic may be needed to improve the efficacy of the ACEI in these patients.

- Several agents, such as high-dose thiazides and β-blockers, can, in theory, worsen diabetes control and exacerbate dyslipidaemia, so tailor the drugs chosen to each patient. Interestingly, studies with the SGLT2 inhibitor class of hypoglycaemic agents have shown consistent reduction of BP, which is likely to be one mechanism for the beneficial effect of these agents on improving cardiac function. In those with angina, a β-blocker has added benefits.
- In those with PVD, consider vasodilators, e.g. calcium channel blockers.

In summary, to reduce the risk of macrovascular complications in diabetes, we should ensure:
- Early glycaemic control: to achieve HbA1c of 6.5% or less, with avoidance of hypoglycaemia. In individuals with long-standing diabetes and advanced arterial disease, strict glucose control is probably less effective at reducing cardiovascular events.
- Strict BP control: aiming for BP <140/80mmHg or <130/80mmHg for those with micro- or macrovascular complications.
- Treatment of dyslipidaemia, aiming for TC <4.0mmol/L, LDL-C <2.0mmol/L (even as low as <1.4mmol/L in very high-risk individuals), HDL-C >1.0mmol/L, and TG <2.3mmol/L.
- Patient should be encouraged to lose weight through a healthy diet and regular exercise.
- Aspirin therapy has currently no role in 1° cardiovascular protection, although it may be considered in higher risk patients and it continues to be in routine use for 2° prevention.

Further reading

Ajjan RA, Grant PJ (2011). The role of antiplatelets in hypertension and diabetes mellitus. *J Clin Hypertens* **13**, 305–13.

ASCEND Study Collaborative Group; Bowman L, et al. (2018). Effects of aspirin for primary prevention in persons with diabetes mellitus. *N Engl J Med* **379**, 1529–39.

Betteridge DJ (2011). Lipid control in patients with diabetes mellitus. *Nat Rev Cardiol* **8**, 278–90.

Chrysant SG, Chrysant GS (2011). Current status of aggressive blood glucose and blood pressure control in diabetic hypertensive subjects. *Am J Cardiol* **107**, 1856–61.

Cosentino F, et al.; ESC Scientific Document Group (2019). 2019 ESC Guidelines on diabetes, pre-diabetes, and cardiovascular diseases developed in collaboration with the EASD. *Eur Heart J* **41**, 255–323.

Hill D, Fisher M (2010). The effect of intensive glycaemic control on cardiovascular outcomes. *Diabetes Obes Metab* **12**, 641–7.

National Institute for Health and Care Excellence (2016). *Cardiovascular disease: risk assessment and reduction, including lipid modification.* ℘ https://www.nice.org.uk/guidance/cg181

National Institute for Health and Care Excellence (2019). *Type 2 diabetes in adults: management.* ℘ https://www.nice.org.uk/guidance/ng28/chapter/1-Recommendations

Newman JD, et al. (2018). The changing landscape of diabetes therapy for cardiovascular risk reduction: JACC state-of-the-art review. *J Am Coll Cardiol* **72**, 1856–69.

UKPDS Group (1998). Tight blood pressure control and risk of macrovascular and microvascular complications in type 2 diabetes: UKPDS 38. *BMJ* **317**, 703–13.

Lipids and hyperlipidaemia

Fredrik Karpe

Lipids and coronary heart disease

Physiology

The two main circulating lipids, triglycerides (TGs) and cholesterol, are bound with phospholipid and apolipoproteins to make them more water-soluble for transportation throughout the body. The apolipoproteins on the surface of these soluble complexes have functional characteristics and are specific for each lipoprotein:

- *Chylomicrons.* Contain 85% TGs and 4% cholesterol, and can be up to 0.001mm in diameter (light-scattering and presence therefore gives a milky appearance to plasma). Main transport vehicle of fat (50–150g/ day) from the intestine, and assembled and secreted by the mucosa of the small intestine after fat ingestion. Their TG content is broken down in peripheral tissues by lipoprotein lipase (LPL). Initially, they contain apoprotein (Apo) B-48 (ApoB-48) and acquire ApoE and ApoC-II from circulating HDL. Following TG removal in the capillary bed, the chylomicron remnants are removed by specific apoB and apoE receptors in the liver.

- *Very low-density lipoproteins (VLDLs).* Contain 50% TGs, 15% cholesterol, and 18% phospholipid. They are the main carrier of TGs from the liver (~50g/day). VLDLs contain ApoB-100 and apoE. VLDL TGs are also broken down by LPL in peripheral tissue to generate intermediate-density lipoproteins (IDLs) or other remnants (LDL) which are removed by the liver.

- *IDLs.* These VLDL remnants contain mostly cholesterol and phospholipid, and are either removed by the liver or metabolized to form LDLs.

- *Low-density lipoproteins (LDLs).* Contain 45% cholesterol, 10% TGs, and 20% phospholipid. LDL has ApoB-100 on its surface and is the predominant cholesterol transport vehicle in the circulation. The liver has specific LDL receptors (LDLRs) to extract it from the circulation. Half of the body's circulating LDL is removed from the plasma each day, mostly by the liver. Small, dense LDL (5–50% of the LDL pool) is easily oxidized. This is likely to occur while the LDL particle has been retained in the vascular wall. Modified LDL is taken up by macrophages, and an extensive uptake will be the basis of foam cell formation in the atheromatous plaque.

- *High-density lipoproteins (HDLs).* Made in the liver and gut; contain 17% cholesterol, 4% TGs, and 24% phospholipid. HDL transports 20–50% of circulating cholesterol. The main apoprotein is apoAl which attracts free cholesterol from peripheral tissues to form the 1st step of 'reverse cholesterol transport', i.e. transport of cholesterol from peripheral tissues back to the liver. However, it seems this process in not related to HDL-C concentration in blood.

In clinical practice, patients are managed according to levels of cholesterol (total, LDL, HDL) and TGs. Elevated TC or LDL-C with normal TGs is *hypercholesterolaemia*. Isolated elevation of TGs is *hypertriglyceridaemia*, and both together is *combined or mixed hyperlipidaemia*.

There is an exponential relationship between hypercholesterolaemia and CHD. A man with a TC level of 6.5mmol/L has double the risk of CHD in a man with a TC level of 5.2mmol/L, and half the risk of a man with a cholesterol level of 7.8mmol/L. Intervention studies show that reductions in TC and LDL-C reduce coronary and cerebrovascular events, as well as mortality.

HDL-C has an inverse relationship with CHD, i.e. ↑ levels appear protective. However, there is now abundant evidence from HDL raising therapies and genomic studies (Mendelian randomization) that there is no causal relationship between the HDL-C concentration and cardiovascular outcomes. Low HDL-C concentrations may be due to lack of physical exercise, obesity, or perhaps, in particular, to the presence of raised plasma TGs, and it also occurs in smokers. Indeed, low HDL-C is very often seen in the presence of hypertriglyceridaemia. The specific role of low HDL-C is less clear, as the monogenic 'low HDL syndromes' often do not carry an excessive CHD risk.

Although much debated over the past decades, robust evidence now suggests that hypertriglyceridaemia is directly and causally related to CHD. Combined hyperlipidaemia carries a substantially excessive CHD risk and this is often simply explained by the presence of large numbers of atherogenic lipoprotein particles.

A useful way of quantifying the presence of potentially atherogenic lipoprotein concentrations in the plasma is to measure the plasma apoB concentration, which is a marker of lipoprotein particle number.

Pathogenesis

Hyperlipidaemia is nearly always due to a combination of genetic and environmental factors:
- 1° *hyperlipidaemias:* usually largely genetically determined.
- 2° *hyperlipidaemias:* due to a combination of other conditions, drugs, and dietary anomalies, but often with a polygenic background.

Obesity, in particular abdominal fatness, is one of the strongest 2° factors for atherosclerosis and CHD.

Atherosclerosis

In atherosclerosis, subintimal plaques start in medium-sized blood vessel walls when cholesterol in apoB-containing lipoprotein particles accumulates in the subintima. Macrophages take up the particles and form foam cells that, in turn, trigger an inflammatory reaction. This leads to the formation of a cholesterol-rich necrotic core, surrounded by smooth muscle cells and fibrous tissue. These plaques can calcify. If the surface of the plaques ulcerates, thrombosis occurs which can obliterate the lumen of a blood vessel.

The initial endothelial cell damage may be due to:
- Physical trauma, e.g. with hypertension.
- Toxins, e.g. tobacco or alcohol.
- Low-grade inflammation.

CHD/atherosclerosis risk factors

The ♂ gender, increasing age, and a +ve family history are all linked with a greater risk for atherosclerosis. There are also several modifiable risk factors:

- *Cigarette smoking.* >10 cigarettes/day increase the CHD OR by 6.7-fold, while stopping smoking reduces the risk of MI by 50–70% within 5 years.
- *Hypertension.* Increases the CHD OR by 2.7-fold. Each 1mmHg drop in diastolic BP reduces the MI risk by 2–3%. But remember, aspirin reduces MI risk by 33%.
- *Abdominal obesity.* Effects are both direct and indirect through the origins of becoming obese, hypertension, and hyperlipidaemia.
- *DM.* Effects of DM are both direct and indirect through concomitant obesity, hyperlipidaemia, and hyperglycaemia.
- *Hyperlipidaemia.* A 10% fall in TC results in a 25% decrease in CHD risk, and plaque regression with reducing lipids is well documented.

Assessment of CVD risk

Risk assessment tables/calculators for CVD or CHD are widely available, such as the Sheffield tables, the New Zealand tables, the Joint British Societies Coronary Risk Prediction Chart (JBS3), and QRISK. These calculate the likelihood of the patient's absolute risk of CVD over a period of years and/or the individual's relative risk, assuming CVD is not present at this time. The data used for assessment include sex, age, ethnicity (sometimes) blood pressure, presence of left ventricular hypertrophy, smoking, diabetes mellitus, and the measured values of TC, HDL-C, or the ratio of TC:HDL cholesterol. The tables give a prediction which is useful for estimating the future risk for CVD and thus prioritization for lipid lowering treatment. They should not be used for patients in secondary prevention.

Risk assessment tables/calculators can be accessed online, as detailed below.

JBS3

- Available at: ℘ http://www.jbs3risk.com/
- This chart was last updated in 2014 and includes older patients aged >70 years and shows risk thresholds of <10%, 10–20%, and >20% over 10 years (in line with NICE guidance for statin use).

QRISK®3

- Available at: ℘ https://qrisk.org/three/
- This uses data from British subjects and appears to be better at predicting outcome, but is still limited due to the fact that it is developed from the UK Clinical Practice Research Datalink (CPRD) database, so draws its information from GP records in the UK only. QRISK® also takes ethnicity into account and allows UK postcode entry to estimate an impact of deprivation.

UKPDS risk engine

- Available at: https://www.dtu.ox.ac.uk/riskengine/
- The UKPDS Risk Engine provides risk calculation for people with T2DM.

General cautions applied when interpreting calculated risk

CVD risk may be higher than indicated in the charts for:
- Those with a family history of premature CVD ($\male$ <55 years and $\female$ <65 years). This is accounted for in QRISK®, but there is a caution as cases with known or suspected monogenic conditions, such as familial hypercholesterolaemia (FH), are not applicable (likely to grossly underestimate the risk).
- Those with raised TG levels.
- Those with impaired glucose tolerance.
- Women with premature menopause.
- Those approaching the next age category. As the risk increases exponentially with age, the risk will be closer to the higher age range for the last 4 years of each decade.

The estimates of CVD risk from the chart are based on groups of people. In managing an *individual*, the physician also has to use clinical judgement in deciding how intensively to intervene on lifestyle and whether or not to use drug therapies.

Individuals at risk of hyperlipidaemia
- Those with premature CHD (<55 years in $\male$, <65 years in $\female$).
- Those with signs of other atherosclerotic disease (e.g. PVD, ischaemic cerebrovascular disease).
- Those with abdominal obesity.
- Those with DM.
- Those with clinical signs of insulin resistance such as acanthosis nigricans.
- Post-menopausal $\female$ not on HRT.
- Those with a high alcohol intake ($\female$ >14 units/week, $\male$ >21).
- Those with a family history of hyperlipidaemia.
- Those with a family history of early CHD or other atherosclerotic disease.
- Those with known 2° causes of hyperlipidaemia (see ➲ Secondary hyperlipidaemias, pp. 992–3).

Lipid measurements
- Measurements should not be taken during an acute illness or during periods of rapid weight loss, as these artificially lower the results. This is particularly important from 24h after an MI for up to 6 weeks, as during this time, the levels of TC and LDL-C may be falsely reduced.
- Pregnancy or recent weight gain will increase lipid levels. Following rapid weight gain or weight loss, leave at least 1 month before reassessing lipid levels.
- A full lipid profile measures TC, HDL-C, LDL-C, and TGs.
- This needs to be a fasting sample. If non-fasting, only TC and HDL-C measurements are accurate. TGs rise postprandially, and LDL-C is usually calculated using the formula below, so it is inaccurate if not fasting. It is also invalid if TGs are >4.5mmol/L.

$$\text{LDL-C (in mmol/L)} = \text{TC} - \text{HDL-C} - 0.45\,(\text{TGs})$$

- The use of TC alone can be misleading, as isolated HDL-C elevation can increase the value. However, once on a lipid-lowering treatment, in particular a statin, a change in TC normally reflects a change in LDL-C as long as TGs are stable. The TC:HDL-C ratio is used for risk estimation but is less useful for individual therapeutic decisions.
- Variations between assay methods is low for TC, but higher for HDL-C. The analytical method for TGs has a low variation, but within-person, TGs can change substantially and rapidly. A full lipid breakdown should be performed before any decision to intervene with lipid-lowering treatment.

ApoB

ApoB is the carrier protein of LDL and VLDL. As there is one molecule of apoB per lipoprotein particle, measuring apoB level in plasma gives insight to the total number of potentially atherogenic lipoprotein particles. Some studies suggest that apoB is a more accurate CVD risk indicator than LDL-C or non-HDL-C and may therefore serve as a very useful CVD risk indicator. ApoB concentration is largely independent of fasting.

Primary hyperlipidaemias

Background

A 1° hyperlipidaemia is normally defined as a causal monogenic or polygenic trait. Although the clinical features of 1° hyperlipidaemia are often driven by a specific defect, the phenotype is also susceptible to environmental exposures. Some of the 1° hyperlipidaemias are very aggressive and need strict clinical attention. At present, the family history and phenotypic findings in other family members are used as a surrogate for a genetic diagnosis. DNA-based diagnosis is now widely available for familial hypercholesterolaemia (FH) and also used for type III hyperlipidaemia.

Severe isolated hypertriglyceridaemias are classically recessive, and genetic diagnosis can be of help but is not widely available in clinical practice.

Polygenic hypercholesterolaemia

This is the commonest cause of isolated hypercholesterolaemia. A large number of genetic loci contribute. There is a significant impact on the LDL-C concentration in individuals carrying many LDL-raising variants, which can be summarized as a polygenic score. In fact, in a given population, the top percentile of high LDL polygenic score is likely to have an LDL-C concentration not far from what is seen in FH. Patients with a polygenic background to their hypercholesterolaemia do not normally show characteristic xanthelasmata or extensor tendon deposits (xanthomata) as is often seen in FH. If young offspring of people with polygenic hypercholesterolaemia are tested, it would be expected to see normal cholesterol concentrations, which is in contrast to children of those with FH. Instead polygenic hypercholesterolaemias present later in life, typically as an augmented feature of age-dependent rise in plasma cholesterol.

Familial hypercholesterolaemia

FH is an autosomal dominant disorder. The gene frequency is thought to be 1 in 300 in Western Europe and North America. The typical lipoprotein phenotype shows a rise in LDL-C. In FH, >95% of mutations are caused by disruption of the LDLR (on the short arm of chromosome 19), decreasing the number of high-affinity LDLRs by up to 50%, thus reducing LDL clearance and prolonging the circulating time of LDL. More than 1000 different mutations have so far been described. Less commonly, FH is caused by familial defective apoB-100 (3–4%) and proprotein convertase subtilisin/kexin 9 (*PCSK9*) gene mutation (<1%). The nature of the mutation will have different consequences and impact on LDL-C concentration:

- Not producing any LDLRs.
- Failure of LDLRs to move or recirculate to the cell surface.
- Subnormal binding to the LDLR.
- Inability to adequately internalize LDL for degradation.

Patients with untreated FH are at very high risk of premature CHD. (See Box 16.1 for clinical features.)

Box 16.1 Clinical features of FH

- TC >7.8mmol/L (>12.5mmol/L in homozygotes), LDL-C high from birth, normal TGs.
- Clinical stigmata: xanthelasmic deposits around the eyes and on tendons (i.e. fingers, hands, elbow, knee, and Achilles) appearing with age. Tendon xanthoma is more specific for FH than corneal arcus or xanthelasma; 7% of heterozygote FH (aged >19 years) and 75% of homozygotes have tendon xanthomas (but may not be present until age >40 years).
- Achilles tendonitis in childhood.
- Homozygotes can have CHD presenting in childhood and certainly before the age of 30. Such cases must be treated in specialist centres providing apheresis.
- Heterozygotes usually present after 30 years of age.
- FH may occur without clinical stigmata, but with strong family history of early-onset CHD, e.g. <50 years.

Familial combined hyperlipidaemia (FCH)

- FCH is a high-risk syndrome for CHD.
- Population frequency has been estimated to 1 in 200.
- Although original descriptions of the conditions assumed dominant heritance which has lead to search for major disease-causing genes, such gene variants have not been detected. Instead it is now thought that FCH is a truly polygenic trait just as described for polygenic hypercholesteroleamia, but obviously including both LDL-C- and TG-raising alleles.
- It is the commonest type of inherited dyslipidaemia, estimated to cause 10% of cases of premature CHD.
- It has no unique clinical manifestations, and the diagnosis is based on raised lipids (>95th centile for age) and a family history of premature CHD in 1st-degree relatives. In contrast to FH, tendon xanthomata should not be present.
- The lipid phenotype can vary within individuals and family members such that combined hyperlipidaemia, isolated hypercholesterolaemia, and isolated hypertriglyceridaemia can be seen within the same individual at different times and in different family members. Raised plasma ApoB concentrations are very likely.
- It should be treated aggressively and very often needs the combination of several different pharmacological agents.

Familial hypertriglyceridaemia

- Defined as a subentity of FCH, but clearly less common, perhaps with a frequency of 1 in 1000. It is assumed this condition is polygenic and is seen in people with a high polygenic score for TG-raising alleles. TG concentrations are rarely >10mmol/L.
- Suspect this condition where there is moderate hypertriglyceridaemia without any obvious causes (obesity, T2DM, etc.), together with a +ve CHD or a family history of stroke.
- The condition can sometimes be surprisingly responsive to statins.

Severe hypertriglyceridaemias with known genetic background

These conditions normally follow a recessive pattern and therefore are normally not seen as a familial trait. LPL is the only TG lipase responsible for removal of TGs from VLDL and chylomicrons. Therefore, homozygosity for LPL deficiency or mutations in the cofactor for LDL (ApoC-II) invariably leads to severe hypertriglyceridaemia. This is rare and seen with a prevalence of ~1/1,000,000 in the UK, but can be commoner in consanguineous populations or enriched in families with consanguinity. This type of hyperlipidaemia is sometimes called familial chylomicronaemia syndrome (FCS). People with FCS will need to adhere to an extremely low-fat diet, being prone to developing hypertriglyceridaemia-induced pancreatitis.

In the search for additional genetic causes in cohorts of extreme hypertriglyceridaemia, mutations in the protein binding LPL to the endothelium (GP1-HDLBP) and APOA5 have been discovered. The overwhelming clinical concern with extreme hypertriglyceridaemia is pancreatitis. Strict adherence to a low-fat diet is always the core treatment, but a new therapy for FCS is emerging—monoclonal antibodies against ApoCIII (volanesorsen).

Pseudohypertriglyceridaemia should be suspected when very stable hypertriglyceridaemia (typically around 5mmol/L) is seen in someone without any obvious 2° causes (obesity, T2DM, etc.). The condition is X-linked (essentially restricted to ♂) and caused by glycerol kinase (GK) deficiency. Typically, upon inspection of a fasting plasma sample, it is clear (hypertriglyceridaemia in the range of 5mmol/L always shows some opalescence). Test for free glycerol. This is a harmless condition that should be left untreated.

Familial dysbetalipoproteinaemia

- Also known as type III hyperlipidaemia or broad beta disease.
- This is an uncommon disorder affecting 1/10, or less, of people with the *ApoE2/E2* genetic background (which is 1/100 in most populations), and nearly only men. It is associated with early-onset CHD.
- The condition leads to specific elevation of small cholesterol-rich VLDL and chylomicron remnants. Typically, the rise of cholesterol and TGs is equimolar, and very high concentrations can be seen (15mmol/L of TGs and 15mmol/L of plasma cholesterol).
- A characteristic clinical feature is the presence of palmar striae xanthoma; tubero-eruptive xanthomata, found over the tuberosities of the elbows and knees, may also be present.
- An *ApoE2/E2* genetic background is not enough to precipitate the syndrome; an additional factor is needed. This is typically obesity, T2DM, hypothyroidism, β-blocker, or thiazide diuretic medication. The OCP can also elicit type III hyperlipidaemia.
- Diagnosis is confirmed by genetic testing. Due to the recessive nature of the *APOE2* allele and the required additional environmental pressure, family history is rarely revealing.

Elevation of lipoprotein a

Lipoprotein a (Lp(a)) is an LDL-like lipoprotein particle, but it is not cleared via the LDLRs. Less than 5% of the population have raised Lp(a) and the distribution is very skewed. Synthesis appears to be highly genetically driven. Recent evidence suggests this is a highly atherogenic lipoprotein particle.

Raised Lp(a) should be suspected in someone with early presentation of CHD, stroke, or PVD, with moderately elevated cholesterol that is seemingly resistant to statin therapy. At present, the only available pharmacological means by which lowering of Lp(a) can be achieved is with niacin or PCSK9 inhibitors (limited effect). However, there is no formal evidence to show that these agents reduce cardiovascular events in people with raised Lp(a).

Rare familial mixed dyslipidaemias

- These should be considered in any patient with unexplained neurology, organomegaly, or corneal opacities.

Familial lecithin:cholesterol acyltransferase (LCAT) deficiency

- In this recessively inherited disorder, an enzyme necessary for intravascular lipoprotein metabolism is deficient, resulting in elevated cholesterol and TGs. Clinically, corneal lipid deposits result in visual disturbances, and renal deposits in glomerular damage, proteinuria, and often renal failure. Haemolytic anaemia may occur.

Tangier disease (analphalipoproteinaemia or familial alphalipoprotein deficiency)

- In this AR condition, ApoA-I, which is found on HDL, is deficient. HDL-C concentration is very low, as is TC, while TGs are normal or high. Cholesterol accumulation gives enlarged orange-coloured tonsils, hepatosplenomegaly, polyneuropathy, and corneal opacities.

Fish eye disease

- A rare disorder from northern Sweden, with high VLDL levels, low HDL, and a TG-rich LDL. As well as hypertriglyceridaemia, dense corneal opacities occur, giving visual impairment.

Abetalipoproteinaemia

- Results in intestinal fat accumulation due to failure of secreting chylomicrons. Normally detected in infancy with failure to thrive (malabsorption). Cholesterol levels are low, absence of normal LDL and VLDL in plasma, with severe impact on lipid transport in the body, including fat-soluble vitamins. Vitamin E injections may prevent some of the neurological abnormalities observed (ataxia, nystagmus, dysarthria, and motor plus sensory neuropathies), but usually not retinitis pigmentosa and acanthocytes, which also feature.

Hypobetalipoproteinaemia

This AD inherited condition gives a TC level of up to 4mmol/L and can be associated with organomegaly and neurological changes in middle age due to fat deposition and abnormal red cell morphology. The homozygous state is similar to abetalipoproteinaemia.

Hyperalphalipoproteinaemia or HDL hyperlipoproteinaemia

Results in mildly elevated HDL and TC and may be beneficial. If very high HDL is seen together with a type III-like pattern, hepatic lipase deficiency could be suspected. Raised HDL can also occur with exercise, exogenous oestrogen, and phenytoin and phenobarbital use, or from alcohol. Very high consumption of alcohol is one of the few circumstances when high HDL is seen together with raised TGs.

Secondary hyperlipidaemias

Background

Secondary hyperlipidaemias are common, and the predominant precipitating factors are obesity and T2DM or extreme diets. They may feature as elevations of cholesterol or TGs in isolation or in combination. Treatment is primarily based on managing the precipitating disorder before making a further decision on the raised lipids. Not infrequently, >1 cause is apparent in 2° hyperlipidaemias.

Causes

(See summarized in Table 16.1.)

- *Obesity* (see ⊃ Consequences of obesity, p. 1013).
- *DM* (see ⊃ Lipid abnormalities found in patients with diabetes, pp. 974–6).
- *Fatty liver disease.* Almost invariably associated with elevated TGs.
- *Diet.* Excessive consumption of saturated fats, carbohydrate, sugary drinks, and alcohol. Raised TGs by alcohol are normally only seen after excessive consumption. Occasionally, the unusual combination of elevated HDL-C with raised TGs is seen.
- *Hypothyroidism.* Estimated to occur in 4% of those with hyperlipidaemia, and compensated (subclinical) hypothyroidism in a further 10%. Usually resulting in hypercholesterolaemia with a TC level of 7–12mmol/L, dominated by a rise in LDL-C.
- *Chronic renal disease.* ↓ Cr clearance is accompanied by hypertriglyceridaemia and ↓ HDL-C. Proteinuria, in nephrotic syndrome, is associated with hypercholesterolaemia and combined hyperlipidaemia and also raises Lp(a). After kidney transplantation, ciclosporin may increase LDL.
- *Liver disease.* Particularly with cholestasis, resulting in abnormal LDL-C. Primary biliary cirrhosis (PBC) often results in TC >12mmol/L, which is close to treatment resistance. The accumulating cholesterol is contained in a lipoprotein fraction called LpX, which is absent in healthy humans. These are large aggregates of phospholipids and free cholesterol and do not resemble conventional lipoproteins. However, severe hepatocellular damage may also lower LDL-C by decreasing production of its component parts and the enzymes which metabolize it.
- *Cushing's syndrome.* GCs increase VLDL production, thus is linked with hypertriglyceridaemia. Associated weight gain and glucose intolerance can make this effect more pronounced.
- *Lipodystrophies.* A rare group of disorders, the hallmark of which is regional, partial, or generalized fat loss, associated with hyperlipidaemia, especially unusually raised TGs. People with lipodystrophies are extremely sensitive to hypercaloric situations, including dietary fat, which can lead to extreme hypertriglyceridaemia. The condition is associated with insulin resistance, fatty liver disease, and early presentation of T2DM and CVD (see ⊃ Genetic causes of severe insulin resistance, pp. 847–8).

- *Drugs.* Medications commonly implicated are:
  - β-blockers, especially the non-cardioselective ones.
  - Thiazide diuretics.
  - Exogenous oestrogens.
  - Anabolic steroids.
  - GCs.
  - Isotretinoin.
  - Antipsychotic agents
  - PIs (said to cause hyperlipidaemia in 50% after 10 months of treatment).
- *Pregnancy.* Cholesterol rises throughout pregnancy, mostly in the 2nd trimester. TGs also rise, but in the final trimester and mostly in those with underlying genetic abnormalities. Both return to normal by 6 weeks postpartum.

Table 16.1 Secondary causes of dyslipidaemia

Elevated LDL-C	Elevated TGs	Reduced HDL-C
Diet (high saturated fats, high calories)	Diet (weight gain + excess of sugary drinks and alcohol)	Diet (some low-fat diets)
Drugs (GCs, thiazide + loop diuretics, ciclosporin)	Drugs (GCs, β-blockers, oestrogens, isotretinoin)	Drugs (anabolic steroids, tobacco, β-adrenergic blockers)
Hypothyroidism	Hypothyroidism	T2DM
Nephrotic syndrome	T2DM	Insulin resistance syndromes/obesity
Chronic liver disease	Insulin resistance syndromes	CRF
Cholestasis + biliary obstruction	Cushing's syndrome	
Pregnancy	CRF	
	Peritoneal dialysis	
	Pregnancy	

Management of dyslipidaemia

Background

Hyperlipidaemias are common, and a decision to use pharmacological means to lower hyperlipidaemias should depend on estimated cardiovascular risk. For this purpose, useful risk scoring systems (see ➔ Assessment of CVD risk, pp. 984–6) have been developed, but it is important to use these wisely. Importantly, they should not be used for certain 1° and familial conditions with very high cardiovascular risk.

It can be a challenge for the physician to describe benefits of the medication or the necessity of a change in lifestyle to the patient, as treatment rarely comes with an obvious 'reward' and the true effect may only be described as a certain CHD risk reduction noticeable a decade or more ahead.

Overall, the use of statins has an extremely good evidence base, whereas most alternative or complementary options have less solid evidence.

Primary and secondary prevention

It is universally accepted that lowering hypercholesterolaemia using statins in 2° prevention reduces future cardiovascular events and overall mortality. It is estimated that a 10% fall in TC results in a 20% decrease in CHD risk. Regression and remodelling of atheromatous lesions in patients who have had drastic reductions of their lipid risk factors have been demonstrated. Acute coronary syndrome should be treated aggressively, which has shown early benefit with statin treatment.

A decision to reduce cholesterol in 1° prevention relies on the overall cardiovascular risk (see ➔ Assessment of CVD risk, pp. 984–6). The reduction in absolute risk is marginal in patients with few other risk factors and should be evaluated critically. An estimated risk of CHD >2% per annum has unquestionable support for initiation of pharmacological treatment. However, even young patients with 1° and familial conditions should be treated aggressively without applying risk scoring systems.

Specific interventions

Dietary advice

Current recommendations are that fats should constitute <30% of energy consumed and saturated fats must be <30% of the total fat content. To achieve this, vegetable and marine mono- and polyunsaturated fats should be high in the diet, whereas animal and dairy fat should be low. Total dietary cholesterol should ideally not exceed 300mg per day. Foods advocated include fresh fruit and vegetables, which are sources of fibre and antioxidants. A high-fibre content lowers cholesterol. At least 4 months should be given to see if dietary manipulation will work in patients with low to moderate risk and this time frame is also right to demonstrate any significant weight loss. It is unusual to see >15% fall in cholesterol from dietary measures, but certain individuals can respond better.

- *Alcohol*, <14U/week for a ♀ and <21U/week for a ♂, although current UK guidelines are 14U/week (112g) for both ♂ and ♀.
- *Plant sterols and stanols*, 2–3g daily, can reduce blood cholesterol by 10–15%. They are available commercially in enriched margarine spreads, yoghurt, and milky drinks.
- *Weight control*. All overweight patients should be encouraged to lose weight. Weight reduction is closely attuned to dietary advice and physical exercise. A 10kg weight loss in an obese subject can reduce LDL-C by 7% and increases HDL-C by 13%. The effect on raised TGs can be much greater and clinically very useful.
- *Physical activity*. Physical activity, especially aerobic exercise, is recommended. This should be realistic and adapted to the individual's capacity. Although exercise levels in the range of 70% of VO_2max for 30–40min at least 3–5 times per week is extremely useful, it is often unrealistic, and very good effects are seen by walking, etc. Acute exercise will transiently change lipoprotein levels and increase LPL activity. These effects become more permanent with regular training. TG levels fall, HDL-C levels rise, especially the HDL2 subfraction with more vigorous exercise, and the LDL subfraction that is less dense and less atherogenic begin to emerge, perhaps even without seeing a clear drop in total LDL-C. The changes are dose-dependent with ↑ exercise, and a 20% alteration in each variable is achievable after 6 weeks. Particularly good effects are seen in T2DM.
- *Modification of other risk factors*. Other risk factors, such as hypertension, smoking, and DM, must be addressed.

Drug therapy

Numerous agents can be used for both 1° and 2° prevention in patients in whom non-pharmacological approaches have been either unsuccessful or deemed insufficient.

HMG CoA reductase inhibitors (statins)

Statin therapy is unquestionably the number one option for most hypercholesterolaemias due to overwhelming abundance of evidence on efficacy and safety. Table 16.2 shows the comparative potency of common statins.

Indications

Raised LDL, heterozygous + homozygous FH, mixed hyperlipidaemia. Not all these medications are licensed for use in children and should be used with caution in ♀ of childbearing age because of potential teratogenicity. The medication should be stopped for at least 3 months before pregnancy is planned. Women of childbearing age must ensure effective contraception when on these drugs.

Mechanism of action

Inhibition of HMG CoA which is the rate-limiting enzyme in cholesterol synthesis. Reduced hepatocyte cholesterol increases LDLR numbers which leads to ↑ clearance of LDL and VLDL remnants from blood. (See Table 16.2 for comparative lipid-lowering profile, and Table 16.3 for dosage.)

Side effects

Statins are usually very well tolerated. The commonest side effect is muscle ache which, in extremely rare cases, also develops into myositis. Hepatotoxicity is not common but does exist and can be dose-dependent (nearly only seen with simvastatin 80mg or atorvastatin 80mg). LFTs and CK should be measured before they are prescribed and used with caution in those with an excessive alcohol intake. It is recommended that the medications should be discontinued if the liver enzymes aspartate transaminase (AST) and/or alanine transaminase (ALT) show >2- to 3-fold elevation above the upper limit of normal. LFTs should therefore be checked within 3–4 months of treatment and, at most, annually in the long term if the patient is without symptoms. Myositis is rare, but the frequency increases with concomitant medications, e.g. ciclosporin, fibrates, or when renal impairment or untreated hypothyroidism are present. Clinically, there is a picture of swollen tender muscles and CK being >10 times the upper limit of normal. Rhabdomyolysis is even rarer.

Interactions

Several statins are metabolized through CYP3A4. Grapefruit juice should be avoided. Statins can interact with ciclosporin. There is interaction with warfarin for atorvastatin, simvastatin, and rosuvastatin, but it is often not clinically significant and would only lead to small adjustments of the warfarin dose. Erythromycin interacts with all statins. Digoxin interacts with atorvastatin and simvastatin. Rifampicin interacts with fluvastatin and pravastatin. Atorvastatin and rosuvastatin may also interact with the OCP, antacids, and some antifungals.

Management of statin intolerance

Muscle problems after start of statin treatment is common. Although it has been demonstrated that Q10 is reduced in muscle samples after statin treatment, there is no evidence from RCTs that supplementation with Q10 is of any benefit. The two main strategies are to change statin or to reduce the dose. The 1st option normally involves switching from simvastatin or atorvastatin to a low dose of rosuvastatin (5 or 10 mg). The 2nd option involves a very low dose of rosuvastatin (5mg) every 2nd day, or even once a week, or using pravastatin. Non-statin agents are possible but should be used with caution, as the evidence base for cardiovascular benefits is low (e.g. fibrate alone, ezetimibe alone, etc.).

Table 16.2 Comparative lipid-lowering profile of statins

Statin (mg)	% fall in LDL-C	% fall in TGs	% rise in HDL-C
Atorvastatin (40)	38–54	13–32	3–7
Fluvastatin (40)	17–34	8–12	3–6
Pravastatin (40)	18–34	5–13	5–8
Rosuvastatin (20)	50–63	10–28	3–14
Simvastatin (40)	26–48	12–38	8–12

Add-on therapy to statins

Specific cholesterol absorption blocker
- Ezetimibe is the only available compound.
- Indications:
  - Should be used primarily as 2nd-line treatment after a statin when the reduction of LDL-C achieved by the statin is insufficient.
  - LDL-C lowering in patients who are intolerant of statins. Also in the very rare condition of sitosterolaemia where there is ↑ absorption of plant sterols.
- Mechanism of action:
  - Dietary and biliary cholesterol absorption is selectively inhibited. Ezetimibe (10mg) monotherapy produces, on average, an 18% fall in LDL-C and an increase in HDL-C of 1–3%, while TGs are not affected.
- Interactions:
  - None significant.

PCSK9 inhibitors
Currently available drugs are alirocumab and evolocumab. These are humanized monoclonal antibodies against PCSK9 that require repeated injections. Good evidence for cardiovascular prevention as add-on therapy with statins.
- Indications:
  - Add-on therapy to statins to achieve additional lowering of LDL-C.
  - Achievement of effective LDL-C lowering in instances when statins cannot be used.
- Mechanism of action:
  - Binding of the antibody to PCSK9 reduces the plasma concentration of PCSK9. The PCSK9 protein binds to the LDLR and after internalization of the receptor complex, the presence of bound PCSK9 signals destruction of the receptor, whereas absence of bound PCSK9 enables reutilization of the LDLR. Low abundance of PCSK9 therefore increases the presence of LDLRs and enhances elimination of LDL-C from plasma.
  - Normally very potent LDL-lowering effect, which often gives 50% or more LDL lowering than what has been achieved with a statin.
- Side effects:
  - Negligible.
- Interactions:
  - Negligible.

Bile acid sequestrants
- Indications:
  - High LDL, i.e. hypercholesterolaemia. Nowadays rarely used because of low cholesterol-lowering efficacy, cumbersome dosing, and multiple interactions. They are also the only drug licensed for use during pregnancy.
- Mechanism of action:
  - Binds bile acids in the intestine, so reducing enterohepatic circulation and increasing bile acid excretion. This increases hepatocyte cholesterol requirements which increases LDLR production, so reducing circulating LDL levels. Under optimum conditions, LDL-C can be reduced by 20–30%; TGs often rise by 10–17%, and HDL-C increases by 3–5%.
- Side effects:
  - These agents remain in the gut, so constipation, bloating, nausea, and abdominal discomfort are not uncommon. Constipation, found in 35–40% of those on these agents, can be helped with bulking laxatives. Less often, a bleeding tendency due to vitamin K malabsorption can be seen. These agents can also exacerbate hypertriglyceridaemia. To reduce the side effects, start with low doses and build up gradually over the next 3–4 weeks, while maintaining a good fluid intake.
- Interactions:
  - These agents can reduce the absorption of warfarin, digoxin, β-blockers, pravastatin, fluvastatin, and hydrochlorothiazide. Many other agents, such as simvastatin, have not been checked, so to avoid any potential interaction, advise patients to take all other drugs 1–3h *before* or 4–6h *after* the resin.

Bempedoic acid
- Reduces LDL-C by ·15% on top of a statin. This is a new drug and large-scale data providing evidence of cardiovascular prevention have not been released.
- Mechanism of action:
  - The drug is an adenosine triphosphate citrate lyase (ACLY) inhibitor, which interferes with early steps in cholesterol precursor molecule production.
- Side effects:
  - Rise in serum uric acid. The relevance of this is not clear in terms of precipitating gout.
- Interactions:
  - Negligible.

Fibrates
- Indications:
  - Raised plasma TGs or IDL, i.e. mixed hyperlipidaemias which have not responded adequately to diet or other therapies. Fibrates should normally be seen as add-on therapy beyond statins. However, fibrates constitute 1st-line therapy in type III hyperlipidaemia and extreme hypertriglyceridaemia. Fibrates have low efficacy in lowering LDL-C. They reduce TGs by 20–60%, increase HDL by 5–20%, and reduce LDL by 5–25%.

- Mechanism of action:
  - Increases VLDL TG clearance by increasing LPL activity and LDLR-mediated LDL clearance, while increasing HDL synthesis. Most of these effects are achieved by upregulating the synthesis of ApoC-III. The effect on LDL-C may vary in isolated hypertriglyceridaemia, and an increase in LDL-C can be seen in type IV hyperlipidaemia. (See Table 16.3 for dosages.)
- Side effects:
  - Occasionally cause nausea, anorexia, or diarrhoea and precipitate gallstones. They should not be used in patients with severe liver disease (AST/ALT >2–3 times the upper limit of normal) and renal dysfunction (e.g. avoid fenofibrate if eGFR <30mL/min/1.73m², reduce if eGFR 30–59), as they are conjugated in the liver prior to excretion by the kidney. Myopathy, although rare, is the main concern, and the risk of this increases if used with statins.
- Interactions:
  - Use with caution in combination with statins. Can enhance the effects of warfarin and antidiabetic agents, and is contraindicated in those on orlistat.

Nicotinic acid and acipimox

These agents are nowadays rarely used because of lack of evidence on cardiovascular prevention and observed side effects in terms of diabetogenic effects.

- Indications:
  - High LDL, VLDL, IDL, or TGs. Nicotinic acid also increases HDL-C. In practice, however, their use is limited by their side effect profile, especially flushing.
- Mechanism of action:
  - Work by inhibiting lipolysis in adipocytes, so altering fatty acid flux and reducing VLDL synthesis and HDL clearance, or by inhibiting VLDL TG synthesis. Plasma TGs fall by 20–50%, and LDL by 5–25%, while HDL levels rise by 10–50%.
- Side effects:
  - Common, with 30% unable to tolerate these agents. Vasodilatation, giving cutaneous/facial flushing, occurs in most patients but tends to improve after 2–3 weeks of therapy. Pruritus and dry, burning sensation in the skin can be seen. High doses of aspirin were previously given to reduce this effect, but this is now rarely practised due to side effects of high-dose aspirin. Patients should also be instructed to avoid hot drinks and spicy food. Gastritis is also a common side effect, whereas liver side effects are rare. Raises uric acid almost invariably and exacerbation of gout can be seen. Rarely, precipitation of acanthosis nigricans and retinal oedema are also recognized side effects. *Nicotinic acid* can adversely affect glucose control in prediabetes states and in DM. *Acipimox*, a nicotinic acid analogue, seems to be less problematic but is also less potent. In 2013, following the results of the HPS2-THRIVE study, the EMA suspended licences for nicotinic acid preparations on the grounds that they were ineffective and associated with adverse effects. Acipimox remains available.

Omega-3 fatty acids (Omacor®, Maxepa®)
- Indications:
  - Hypertriglyceridaemia.
- Mechanism of action:
  - Inhibit the secretion of VLDL due to ↑ intracellular ApoB-100 destruction. Usually there is a fall in VLDL and LDL, but LDL may rise in the hypertriglyceridaemic individual. Should be seen as add-on therapy to statins. There is mixed evidence for efficacy in cardiovascular prevention, but studies using high and TG-lowering doses (equivalent to 2g bd of 20:5/22:6 enriched formulas) have shown some with some +ve effects on cardiovascular prevention.
- Side effects:
  - Nausea and belching.
- Interactions:
  - None significant.

(For drug choice for specific circumstances, see Box 16.2.)

Further reading

Bhatnagar D, et al. (2008). Hypercholesterolaemia and its management. *BMJ* **337**, a993.

Chapman MJ, et al.; European Atherosclerosis Society Consensus Panel (2011). Triglyceride-rich lipo-proteins and high-density lipoprotein cholesterol in patients at high risk of cardiovascular disease: evidence and guidance for management. *Eur Heart J* **32**, 1345–61.

Hippisley-Cox J, et al. (2017). Development and validation of QRISK3 risk prediction algorithms to estimate future risk of cardiovascular disease: prospective cohort study. *BMJ* **357**, 2099.

National Institute for Health and Care Excellence (2014). *Cardiovascular disease: risk assessment and reduction, including lipid modification.* ℛ https://www.nice.org.uk/guidance/cg181

National Institute for Health and Care Excellence (2008). *Familial hypercholesterolaemia: identification and management.* ℛ https://www.nice.org.uk/guidance/cg71

Newman C, et al. (2018). Statin safety and associated adverse events: a scientific statement from the American Heart Association. *Arterioscler Thromb Vasc Biol* **39**, E38–81.

Newman C, et al. (2020). Lipid management in patients with endocrine disorders: an Endocrine Society clinical practice guideline. *J Endocrinol Clin Metab* **105**, 3613–82.

Piepoli M, et al. (2016). 2016 European Guidelines on cardiovascular disease prevention in clinical practice: The Sixth Joint Task Force of the European Society of Cardiology and Other Societies on Cardiovascular Disease Prevention in Clinical Practice (constituted by representatives of 10 societies and by invited experts). *Eur Heart J* **37**, 2315–81.

Valle DL, et al. *The online access to metabolic and molecular bases of inherited disease. Part 12: Lipids.* ℛ Available at: https://ommbid.mhmedical.com/

Watts GF, Karpe F (2011). Triglycerides and atherogenic dyslipidaemia: extending treatment beyond statins in the high-risk cardiovascular patient. *Heart* **97**, 350–6.

Box 16.2 Which drug to use when?

Elevated LDL-C only
- 1st choice:
  - Statins.
- 2nd choice:
  - Cholesterol absorption blocker.
  - PCSK9 inhibitor.
- Then:
  - Fibrates.
  - Nicotinic acid (not available in Europe).
  - Bile acid sequestrants.

Elevated triglycerides only
- 1st choice:
  - Statins (if TGs are <5mmol/L).
  - Fibrates (if TGs are drastically raised).
- 2nd choice:
  - Omega-3 fatty acids.

All three groups can occasionally be used together if one or two of the above groups are insufficient.

Mixed hyperlipidaemia
- 1st choice:
  - Statin.
- 2nd choice:
  - Statin + fibrate (but needs close monitoring).
  - Statin + fibrate + PCSK9 inhibitor.
  - As with elevated LDL alone, combination therapy may sometimes be useful, with emphasis on avoiding side effects and interactions as above.

The relative doses of lipid-lowering drugs are shown in Table 16.3.

Aims of treatment
- 1° prevention:
  - Reduction of non-HDL-C by 40% or more.
  - Ideally TGs should be <1.7mmol/L.
- 2° prevention—the target should be:
  - TC <4mmol/L.
  - LDL-C <2mmol/L.
  - Ideally TGs should be <1.7mmol/L.
  - ApoB <1g/L.

Table 16.3 Dosage of lipid-lowering drugs

Drug	Dose/day
Statins	
Atorvastatin	10–80mg
Fluvastatin	20–80mg
Pravastatin	10–40mg
Rosuvastatin	10–40mg (5–20mg in patients of Asian origin)
Simvastatin	10–40mg
PCSK9 inhibitors	
Alirocumab	150mg once a fortnight (option for lower dose and higher dose with ↑ dosing interval)
Evolocumab	140mg once a fortnight (option for lower dose and higher dose with ↑ dosing interval)
Fibrates	
Bezafibrate	400–600mg
Ciprofibrate	100mg
Fenofibrate	67–267mg
Gemfibrozil	0.9–1.2g
Anion exchange resins	
Colestyramine	12–36g (in single dose or up to qds)
Colestipol hydrochloride	5g 1–2×/day (max 30g/day)
Colesevelam	1–2g bd
Nicotinic acid group	
Acipimox	500–750mg in divided doses
Nicotinic acid MR	375–2000mg
Nicotinic acid	300mg–6g in divided doses
Nicotinic acid with laropriprant	1000–2000mg
Omega-3 fatty acids	
Omacor®	1–4g/day
Cholesterol absorption blocker	
Ezetimibe	10mg

Obesity

John Wilding

Definition of obesity

Obesity is defined as an excess of body fat sufficient to adversely affect health. The BMI and waist circumference, as a measure of fat distribution, are the most commonly used measures, but a clinical staging system is increasingly used to determine risk and management (see Box 17.1). BMI is an imprecise measure of adiposity and does not account for fat distribution, which may better determine metabolic and cardiovascular risk at lower BMI.

Lower cut-off values for BMI and waist circumference are applicable to non-Caucasian ethnic groups: cut-off points for ↑ risk varies from 22kg/m² to 25kg/m² in different Asian populations, and for high risk from 26kg/m² to 31kg/m².

Central obesity may reflect ↑ visceral (intra-abdominal fat) stores and/or 'ectopic' fat (fat stored in the liver, muscle, pancreas, and epicardium) more directly linked to pathophysiology such as insulin resistance.

Assess overall clinical status, using BMI, waist circumference, and stage (see Box 17.1).

Obesity is associated with ↑ secretion of adipose tissue products, including hormones, cytokines (adipokines), and growth factors, such that it is now regarded as a disease of chronic low-grade systemic inflammation. Many of its adverse sequelae relate to this pathology.

Box 17.1 Edmonton Obesity Staging System (EOSS)

Stage 0
- No apparent obesity-related risk factors, physical symptoms, psychopathology, functional limitations, and/or impairment of well-being.

Stage 1
- Obesity-related subclinical risk factor(s) (borderline hypertension, impaired fasting glucose, elevated liver enzymes, etc.), mild physical symptoms (e.g. dyspnoea on moderate exertion), psychopathology, functional limitations, and/or impairment of well-being.

Stage 2
- Established obesity-related chronic disease(s): hypertension, T2DM, sleep apnoea, OA, reflux disease, PCOS, anxiety disorder; moderate limitations in activities of daily living and/or well-being.

Stage 3
- Established end-organ damage: MI, heart failure, DM complications, incapacitating OA; significant psychopathology, functional limitation(s), and/or impairment of well-being.

Stage 4
- Severe (potentially end-stage) disability/ies from obesity-related chronic diseases, disabling psychopathology, functional limitation(s), and/or impairment of well-being.

Reprinted from Sharma A M and Kushner R F (2009) "A proposed clinical staging system for obesity" *Int. J. Obesity* 33:289–295, with permission from Springer Nature.

Epidemiology of obesity

Overweight and obesity are rapidly increasing globally; the highest rates of obesity (>30%) are seen in the USA, Mexico, and the Middle East. In 2016, nearly 2 billion adults were overweight (BMI >25kg/m²), of whom 650 million were obese. When Asian-specific cut-off points for the definition of obesity are taken into account, the number of adults considered obese globally is over 700 million.

In England, the prevalence has doubled in 25 years; 27.1% of men (aged 16 years and over) and 30% of women were obese in 2017, and 64% of the population are either overweight or obese.

Global estimates of childhood obesity suggest 340 million school-aged children are either overweight or obese, of whom 41 million are obese.

In England, 13% of boys and 11% of girls aged 5–7 years and 25% of boys and 26% of girls aged 13–15 years are obese. The prevalence of obesity varies with age (peak prevalence at 50–70 years) and increases with social deprivation (in adults in England, 21% in the highest income quintile to 34% in the lowest income quintile).

Aetiology of obesity

Overweight and obesity result from a complex interaction between environmental pressures and risks and genetic susceptibility. Heritability of obesity is between 40% and 70%, but the rapid increase in obesity prevalence over the past 30 years argues in favour of predominantly environmental drivers. However, there is increasing interest in the possibility of epigenetic influences on obesity related to maternal obesity, diet, GDM, and even possibly environmental pollutants such as polyfluorinated compounds and polycyclic aromatic hydrocarbons.

Genetic factors

Monogenic obesity

Mutations in genes (usually related to appetite control within the hypothalamus) are associated with obesity of early childhood onset, usually with hyperphagia. However, only about 5% of all severe childhood obesity and 2% of adult obesity are associated with identified genetic causes. Of these, mutations in the melanocortin 4 receptor (*MC4R*) gene are the most frequent and are associated with ↑ linear growth, fat, and lean mass, as well as hyperphagia (moderate) and severe hyperinsulinaemia, but normal puberty and fertility. Prader–Willi syndrome (see ➲ Prader–Willi syndrome, p. 414), due to an imprinting defect on chromosome 15, is found in 1:15,000 live births; it is a common cause of early-onset obesity and is associated with short stature, learning difficulties, and difficult-to-manage hyperphagia.

Other obesity genes

Several hundred genes associated with the development of obesity have been identified through GWAS. The 'fat mass and obesity associated' (*FTO*) gene was originally linked to T2DM; the association was actually found to be due to the higher BMI of diabetic cases, in comparison to non-diabetic controls; common variants in the 1st intron of *FTO* result in a +0.4kg/m² elevation in BMI per risk allele. Similar to the situation with T2DM, possession of 'risk' single nucleotide polymorphisms (SNPs) only accounts for a small increase in susceptibility to obesity or adult BMI. The genetic contribution to BMI can be considered a continuum, with people who are constitutionally lean having the lowest number of susceptibility genes and those who are obese having the most.

Environmental factors

The drivers of obesity can be considered under two main headings—↑ energy (food) intake or ↓ energy expenditure due to physical inactivity—as the major determinants of obesity in genetically susceptible individuals. Societal changes, e.g. ↑ availability of high-caloric density foods and sedentary lifestyle, have been one of the main causes of changes in this balance.

Secondary causes

These are uncommon because, even when linked to weight gain, the disease usually manifests itself from its particular pathophysiology.

- Hypothyroidism: an important cause to exclude in children, but rarely presents simply with weight gain in adults.
- Cushing's disease/syndrome (see ➋ Definition of Cushing's disease, p. 178): rare, but an important cause to exclude in people with obesity presenting with 'overlap' signs and symptoms which can include striae, depression, T2DM, and hypertension.
- Hypothalamic lesions (see ➋ Hypothalamus, p. 246): gonadal failure, visual disturbances, headache, or raised intracranial pressure often predominate as presenting signs, rather than weight gain and hyperphagia.
- PCOS (see ➋ Polycystic ovary syndrome, pp. 340–3): strongly linked to overweight and obesity, but mechanism unclear. Features of hyperandrogenism and oligomenorrhoea may result from obesity itself.
- Iatrogenic: drugs, e.g. antipsychotic medication, glucose-lowering medication (sulfonylureas and insulin), GCs. Also recreational drugs, e.g. cannabis.

Pathophysiology of obesity

Energy balance and body weight are regulated, but the main drive of this allostatic physiology is towards energy acquisition (and thus fat deposition) and defence against weight loss. Although physiology can be 'overridden' by cognitive and behavioural control (e.g. diet, exercise) long term, these mechanisms (within our obesogenic environment) usually prove insufficient in the long term either to protect against or to reverse weight gain.

Long-term signals associated with body fat stores are provided by leptin and insulin. In human obesity, leptin levels are high, rather than low, correlating with fat mass, suggesting either that leptin 'resistance' is present or that leptin is a starvation, rather than an obesity, signal (see Box 17.2 and Table 17.1).

Gut peptide hormones released after food intake provide acute signals of hunger, satiety, and fullness (see Box 17.3). Although originally thought to be short-term signals, the importance of the gut–brain axis as a regulator of body weight in humans has become increasingly apparent from the effects of bariatric surgery. Ghrelin, a hunger hormone, rises before, and probably is involved with, initiation of food intake. Satiety hormones released after food include GLP-1, incretin hormone secreted by ileal L-cells in the distal intestine that stimulates insulin secretion, and peptide YY secreted from the ileum and colon. Oxyntomodulin (also derived from preproglucagon) reduces food intake and increases energy expenditure after systemic administration.

Weight is gained or lost usually in the proportion of 70% fat and 30% lean tissue, implying that ~30MJ (7000kcal) surplus or deficit is needed to gain or lose 1kg in body mass. However, adaptive hormonal and metabolic changes leading to reduced energy expenditure in response to weight loss means that weight loss in response to a fixed energy deficit is less than predicted from this simple model, and eventually reaches a plateau. Maintenance of lost weight is difficult because changes in gut hormones and leptin also drive an increase in hunger.

Box 17.2 Leptin
- Synthesized and secreted by adipose tissue (SC > visceral).
- Encoded by the *LEP* gene (chromosome 7q31.3).
- Hypothalamic receptors, activated through entry via the arcuate nucleus (exposed to peripheral circulation), decrease food intake and increase energy expenditure (by sympathetic activation).
- Stimulated by GCs.
- Human obesity persists despite high circulating levels of leptin (proportional to fat mass), suggesting either resistance to effects or that in human physiology, leptin signals low body fat stores such as in starvation.
- Mutations in *LEP* lead to a rare syndrome of hyperphagia, obesity, hypogonadism, and impaired immunity. Features are reversed by recombinant leptin replacement.
- In conditions of selective decrease in adipose tissue mass (lipodystrophy, HIV or HIV therapy-associated lipoatrophy, severe anorexia nervosa), leptin replacement therapy reverses insulin resistance.
- In response to fasting, leptin levels fall rapidly before, and out of proportion to, changes in fat mass, triggering the neuroendocrine response to acute energy deprivation.
- Trials of leptin augmentation in common obesity do not lead to weight loss or maintenance of weight loss.

Table 17.1 Monogenic obesity

Type	Frequency	Features
Congenital leptin deficiency	Rare	Hyperphagia, hypogonadism
(AR inheritance of *LEP* mutations)		Advanced bone age
		Hyperinsulinaemia
		Immune dysfunction
Heterozygous *LEP* variant	2%	Clinically unaffected
Leptin receptor gene mutations	Rare	Hypogonadotrophic, abnormal GH and TSH secretion
POMC mutation	Rare	ACTH deficiency, red hair, pale skin
MCR4 mutation	Rare	↑ growth
		↑ BMD

Box 17.3 Gut peptide hormones linked to weight regulation

Ghrelin
- The only known 'hunger' hormone.
- Derived from preproghrelin secreted in the stomach, cleaved to the active form acyl ghrelin (28-amino acid peptide) and obestatin.
- Acts on hypothalamic GH secretagogue receptors (GHSR1a) to increase the release of GH from the pituitary.
- Peripherally injected ghrelin increases food intake through the stimulation of ghrelin receptors on hypothalamic neuropeptide Y-expressing neurones and Agouti-related protein-expressing neurones.
- Levels in obesity not consistently elevated, but markedly reduced by bariatric surgery (sleeve gastrectomy and gastric bypass).
- Circulating ghrelin increases preprandially and decreases postprandially, and is thought to regulate premeal hunger and meal initiation.
- GHSR1a is also expressed in other brain areas, linking to the mesolimbic reward neuropathway and to central pathways of energy balance.
- Ghrelin is also involved in modulating reward and motivation in enhancing the hedonic and incentive response to food-related cues.

Glucagon-like peptide-1
- Secreted by L-cells in the distal intestine.
- Stimulates insulin secretion and (in animals) islet cell differentiation and proliferation.
- Inhibits glucagon secretion; inhibits gastric emptying.
- Unlike GIP, levels of GLP-1 are reduced in patients with DM.
- Levels raised preferentially by protein, accounting, in part, for protein's higher satiating effects, compared to other macronutrients.
- GLP-1 analogues (liraglutide) are associated with ~5% weight loss, e.g. liraglutide.
- Liraglutide and semaglutide (see ➲ *GLP-1 receptor agonists*, p. 874), in higher doses than used for DM treatment, produce when used for diabetes treatment sustained weight loss of >10% in people without diabetes.
- Levels markedly elevated after bariatric surgery.

Peptide YY
- A 36-amino acid peptide synthesized and released in L-cells in the distal tract.
- Conversion of PYY1-36 to active PYY3-36 by DPP-IV.
- PYY3-36 shows affinity for hypothalamic neuropeptide Y neurones.
- PYY levels are low in the fasting state, rapidly increase in response to food intake, peak at 1–2h after a meal, and remain elevated for several hours.
- In addition to regulating food intake, PYY3-36 has additional metabolic beneficial effects on energy expenditure and fuel partitioning.

Consequences of obesity

Most metabolic, physiological, and organ systems are affected by obesity and can be considered under the 'four M' headings: mental, metabolic, mechanical, and monetary (see Table 17.2).

- Mortality rates rise steadily at BMI >25kg/m². Obesity and physical inactivity have both independent and dependent effects on all-cause mortality.
- Loss of life expectancy: BMI >35kg/m²—5–7 years at age 45.
- T2DM: elevation in BMI, the dominant risk factor for development of DM. RR in overweight men 2.4, women 12.4; at BMI 30kg/m²: >10; ↑ to 50- to 90-fold at BMI >35.
- Hypertension: RR for overweight men 1.8, women 2.4.
- Dyslipidaemia: moderate relationship with TC, closer relationship with TGs and HDL-C.
- Stroke: RR 1.2 for overweight and 1.5 for obese men and women.
- Asthma: obese twice and overweight 1.4 times more likely to develop asthma.

Table 17.2 Obesity associations and consequences

'Mental'	'Mechanical'	'Metabolic'	'Monetary'
Depression	Sleep apnoea	T2DM	Lower educational attainment
Low self-esteem and stigma	Hypoventilation	Dyslipidaemia	Employment discrimination
Attention-deficit disorder	OA	Hypertension	Lower income
Eating disorder	Chronic pain	IHD	Chronic disability
Cognitive impairment	Gastro-oesophageal reflux	Gout	↑ healthcare costs
	Incontinence	Non-alcoholic fatty liver disease (NAFLD) and non-alcoholic steatohepatitis (NASH)	
	Thrombosis	Cancer	
	Intertrigo		

Management of people with obesity

The use of a structured approach, modified from management of other chronic diseases, consists of *Ask*, *Assess*, *Advise*, *Agree*, and *Assist* (five As).

Ask permission to discuss weight

A non-judgemental approach, using motivational interviewing techniques, that also explores the patient's readiness to change is recommended.

Assess 'root causes' of obesity and obesity-related risk

History

- Weight history from birth onwards (early onset may suggest genetic syndromes).
- Previous treatment/management strategies and their success.
- Current eating habits and triggers for eating/activity levels.
- Family history of obesity and obesity-related disease.
- Symptoms or previous diagnosis of obesity-related diseases, including CVD, DM, psychological issues (eating disorder, depression, low self-esteem), OA, obstructive sleep apnoea, and PCOS.
- Symptoms of reflux.
- Other risk factors such as smoking and alcohol intake.
- Drugs that might exacerbate weight gain.
- Patient's beliefs and expectations.
- Optimal management of other diseases, obesity-related or not.

Examination

- Height, weight, fat distribution.
- General: evidence for syndrome (e.g. small hands and facies in Prader–Willi syndrome), mood.
- Skin: acanthosis nigricans and skin tags (insulin resistance), intertrigo, fat distribution (partial lipodystrophy).
- Cardiovascular: hypertension, heart failure, and other causes for breathlessness.
- Respiratory: airway, obstructive sleep apnoea (somnolence), pulmonary hypertension, cardiopulmonary fitness (consider 6min walk test).
- GI: hepatomegaly, herniae (may influence bariatric surgery).
- Musculoskeletal: mobility.
- Consider other diagnoses: hypothyroidism, Cushing's syndrome, haemochromatosis.

Investigations

- Blood count and iron studies (iron deficiency anaemia from reflux or GI bleeding; polycythaemia from hypoventilation).
- Renal function.
- Liver function (NASH).
- Glucose, HbA1c, and possibly insulin (prediabetes, DM).
- Fasting lipid profile (raised TGs, TC, and LDL-C; lowered HDL-C).
- Vitamin D (often deficient in the obese).
- Thyroid function (hypothyroidism).
- ECG (atrial fibrillation, LVH).
- 24h urine cortisol, overnight dexamethasone suppression test for cortisol (to diagnose Cushing's)

Additional tests
- Liver US if abnormal liver function to confirm NAFLD; liver elastography (FibroScan®) may also be helpful.
- Echocardiography and N-terminal pro B-type natriuretic peptide (NT-proBNP) if heart failure suspected.
- Pharmacological stress testing if IHD suspected (subject may be unable to undertake exercise test).
- Endoscopy if anaemia—gastroscopy if reflux disease, colonoscopy if colon cancer suspected.
- Gynaecological referral if post-menopausal bleeding (high incidence of endometrial cancer in women with obesity).
- Transferrin, ferritin, then genetic testing for haemochromatosis in patients with T2DM and abnormal liver function.

Advise on

Risks of obesity, benefits of weight loss and treatment options, and the need for a long-term strategy. Treatment options include:
- Stress management and self-assertiveness training.
- Dietary intervention.
- Physical activity.
- Psychological counselling.
- Anti-obesity medication.
- Bariatric surgery.

Agree on
- Weight loss goals.
- Behavioural goals and health outcomes.
- Management plan.

Assist in

Addressing drivers and barriers to weight management; offering referral to appropriate provider (1° care for diet and lifestyle programmes, psychology services if binge eating disorder or severe depression, 2° care if obesity severe or complex).

General principles

Dietary energy restriction produces greater weight loss than exercise. ↑ physical activity and exercise predict weight loss maintenance.

Patients' expectations frequently exceed realistic goals or need.

A weight loss of 5–10% of the initial body weight reduces many of the health risks associated with obesity and reduces cancer and DM-related mortality; a 5kg loss in adults with prediabetes reduces progression to DM by 60%, maintained even if weight regain occurs. In patients with a BMI >35kg/m², greater weight loss (>10kg or 15%) is likely to be needed to produce a sustained improvement in comorbid diseases.

Diet, physical activity, and behavioural therapy

- Dietary advice should aim to reduce energy intake to produce a 2.5MJ (600kcal)/day deficit (calculated from standard equations of resting energy expenditure and assuming a physical activity level of 1.3). Both low carbohydrate (<30g/day) and low fat (<30% total daily energy) produce equivalent weight loss (4–5kg) at 1 year. High-protein diets may be more satiating.
- Commercial providers (e.g. Weight Watchers, Rosemary Conley) can achieve equivalent, or better, results than GPs or pharmacists.
- Low- (3.4–5MJ; 800–1200kcal/day) and very low-calorie (<3.5MJ; 800kcal/day) diets produce more rapid initial weight loss and, in combination with behavioural therapy and pharmacotherapy, produce sustained weight loss greater than that achieved with conventional diets. There is emerging evidence that a meal replacement approach (aiming for ~800kcal/day for 8–12 weeks with gradual reintroduction of normal food) leads to remission in those with recent-onset T2DM.
- Regular exercise induces cardiorespiratory fitness and leads to a beneficial effect on other risk factors, with a reduction in BP and improvement in lipid profile.
- The Physical Activity Readiness Questionnaire (PAR-Q) provides a quick and validated screening tool to risk-assess patients before they start an exercise programme.
- A total of 225–300min/week of moderate-intensity activity (7.5–10.5MJ; 1800–2500kcal) is recommended for weight loss maintenance.
- Behavioural interventions complement a low-energy diet and ↑ activity; they may include self-monitoring of behaviour and progress, stimulus control, goal-setting, problem-solving and assertiveness training, and relapse prevention and management.
- In most people, lifestyle approaches should be tried before considering drugs or surgery, but the reality is that only about 25–30% will achieve weight loss of at least 5%, and weight regain is common due to changes in appetite regulatory factors and energy conservation that are the normal physiological response to weight loss.
- An obesity MDT might include an endocrinologist or other physician with an interest in obesity, a specialist nurse, a dietician, an exercise physiologist or physiotherapist, a psychologist and a bariatric surgeon.

Anti-obesity drugs

In Europe, orlistat, a combination of naltrexone/bupropion, and the GLP1 receptor agonist liraglutide (at a higher dose than approved for treatment of T2DM) are licensed; elsewhere, phentermine is widely prescribed. Other drugs (e.g. Qnexa®, a combination of phentermine and topiramate) are also available in the USA. Off-label use of drugs is not recommended: the history of anti-obesity pharmacotherapy has seen many adverse effects emerge, even with well-investigated and developed drugs such as sibutramine (withdrawn in 2010 due to adverse cardiovascular outcomes) and rimonabant (withdrawn in 2009 due to depression and suicide risk).

Any medication is best used in those at medical risk of obesity: BMI >30kg/m² or BMI >27kg/m² with established comorbidities (e.g. DM, heart disease, dyslipidaemia). Medication should only be used in combination with lifestyle support. Guidelines and labelling may require stopping treatment if ineffective; this is usually determined after 3 months of treatment at the maximum tolerated dose and most labels suggest stopping if 5% weight loss is not achieved at that point; some guidelines include more stringent stopping rules at later time points.

Orlistat

* Intestinal pancreatic lipase inhibitor; reduces fat absorption.
* Increases dietary fat loss in the stools to 30% (compared to <5% on placebo).
* May have modest insulin-sensitizing effects over and above weight loss (reduced portal TG levels).
* Risk factors, such as lipids, BP, and glucose, all improve with treatment.
* Contraindications: cholestasis, hepatic dysfunction, malabsorption, pregnancy, breastfeeding, concomitant use of fibrate, acarbose, renal impairment (Cr >150micromol/L), anticoagulation (possible ↓ vitamin K absorption with orlistat).
* Consider vitamin supplementation (especially vitamin D) if used beyond 1 year.
* Side effects (must warn patient): flatus (24%), oily rectal discharge, fatty stool (20%), faecal urgency (22%), fat-soluble vitamin deficiency, incontinence (8%). Limited by dietary fat reduction (to <35% of energy).
* Mean weight loss difference from placebo is about 2.6kg after 1 year; 44% of people will achieve and maintain a weight loss of 5% from baseline and about a quarter will achieve 10% weight loss. As with all weight loss drugs, weight regain is likely if treatment is stopped.
* NICE guidelines:
  * At 3 months, stop if <5% weight loss.
  * At 6 months, stop if <10% weight loss (of initial weight).

Naltrexone/bupropion

- A combination of the *mu* opioid antagonist naltrexone with bupropion, an inhibitor of noradrenaline and dopamine reuptake. It is thought to help reduce body weight by enhancing signalling at the MC4R in the hypothalamus, and may also influence extrahypothalamic areas involved in hedonic aspects of eating behaviour.
- In clinical trials, mean weight loss after 1 year of 5kg; 55% of patients achieved a weight loss of at least 5% of starting body weight.
- Adverse effects include dry mouth, dizziness, constipation, and nausea. Bupropion has been associated with ↑ risk of seizures. Because naltrexone is an opioid antagonist, it should not be used in people taking opioids.
- NICE guidelines—reviewed by NICE in 2017; not approved due to insufficient evidence to support cost-effectiveness.

Liraglutide

- GLP-1 receptor agonist. Once-daily SC injection. Approved for treatment of T2DM, and at higher doses for treatment of obesity or overweight (BMI >27kg/m²) with risk factors such as DM, hypertension, or dyslipidaemia.
- Mean weight loss of 5.2kg at 1 year; 63% of patients achieved 5% weight loss and 31% of patients achieved 10% weight loss.
- Weight loss is associated with modest improvements in BP, lipids, and glucose. Those with prediabetes are nearly three times less likely to develop DM than people treated with lifestyle alone.
- Adverse effects: nausea and vomiting are common early during treatment but tend to resolve over a few weeks. Gallstone formation is commoner, but this may be related to greater weight loss. GLP-1 analogues have been associated with pancreatitis, but a direct causal link is uncertain. There was ↑ risk of medullary cell cancer in rodents, but this has not been reported in human studies.
- NICE guidelines—liraglutide was approved for weight management in 2020.

Bariatric surgery

Three types of surgery are commonly performed—all usually done laparoscopically. The most compelling data for the success of bariatric surgery at producing weight loss and improving the clinical outcomes for patients with obesity come from the 20-year follow-up data of the Swedish Obese Subjects study (a case-control study started at a time when surgical techniques were not as advanced as nowadays). The persistent weight loss in the surgical groups was associated with reduced mortality; the unadjusted overall hazard ratio was 0.76 in the surgery group ($P = 0.04$), compared with the control group, and the hazard ratio adjusted for sex, age, and risk factors was 0.71 ($P = 0.01$). Other studies have confirmed that bariatric surgery is associated with reduced all-cause mortality, including deaths from CVD, DM, and cancer.

In patients with T2DM, benefit extends beyond weight loss. Up to 80% of people with T2DM may experience remission of their DM (normoglycaemia without the need for hypoglycaemic medication), the exact remission rate being determined by the type of surgery and the duration of DM prior to surgery.

Hypogonadism may reverse.

Gastric bypass
(See Fig. 17.1.) Patients achieve 30–40% absolute weight loss within 12–18 months of surgery. The large majority (>80%) of patients will have a significant improvement or resolution of their weight-related illnesses, and most patients report dramatic changes to their QoL.

Gastric bypass works in the following way:
- There is restriction in food intake, as the stomach is reduced to the size of a large egg.
- Food bypasses digestive secretions, causing some malabsorption.
- Profound changes are seen in gut hormones that control hunger, satiety, and glucose metabolism (reduced ghrelin, ↑ and earlier release of GLP-1 and PYY).
- Other mechanisms involving changes in gut flora and bile salt metabolism that affect appetite and cardiovascular risk are also postulated.
- Complications include surgical problems such as wound infections, leaks, and strictures. Some patients can develop post-meal symptoms such as dumping and hypoglycaemia. Nutritional deficiencies can develop; routine supplementation of vitamins (B1, B12, D, folic acid) and minerals (iron, zinc, copper, Ca) is required, and lifelong monitoring essential.

(See Box 17.4 for a summary of post-operative monitoring.)

Sleeve gastrectomy
(See Fig. 17.2.) Patients achieve 30–40% absolute weight loss within 12–18 months of surgery. Again, >80% have a significant improvement in weight-related illnesses and improved QoL.

Sleeve gastrectomy works in the following way:
- 75% of the stomach is removed, restricting the volume of food patients are able to eat in one sitting.
- Gastric emptying is faster which alters gut hormone profiles, resulting in satiety (reduced ghrelin, ↑ and earlier release of GLP-1 and PYY).
- Surgical complications can occur, and routine supplementation of vitamins and lifelong monitoring are recommended.

Box 17.4 Post-operative monitoring
- U&E
- LFTs
- Blood count, ferritin, folate, B12
- Ca, vitamin D, PTH
- Fat-soluble vitamins A, E, and K
- Zinc, copper, selenium, Mg
- Thiamine
- Glucose, lipids, HbA1c

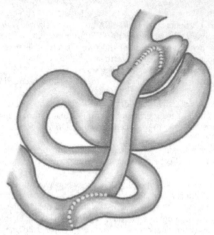

Fig. 17.1 Gastric bypass.

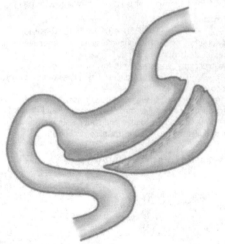

Fig. 17.2 Sleeve gastrectomy.

Adjustable gastric banding
(See Fig. 17.3.) Patients achieve up to 30% absolute weight loss within 2–3 years of surgery. Routine supplementation of vitamins, minerals, and vitamin B12 is not usually needed beyond the 1st year.

Adjustable gastric banding works in the following way:
- Gastric restriction is achieved by placing an adjustable silastic band around the upper gastric cardia that can be tightened or loosened by injecting saline into a tube that connects to a port under the skin. The restriction slows the speed of eating.
- Patients are required to attend clinic for band consultations every 2–3 months until the right degree of band adjustment is achieved.
- Gastric banding is used much less frequently now due to very high rates of revisional surgery (over 30%) as a result of band problems such as slippage and erosion.

For all bariatric surgery, pre- and post-operative care needs to be provided by specialist MDTs, and patients require lifelong vitamin and mineral supplementation, with appropriate monitoring.

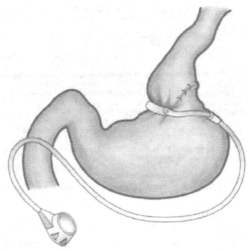

Fig. 17.3 Adjustable gastric banding.

Bariatric surgery and diabetes

In 2011, the International Diabetes Federation recommended that bariatric surgery:

- Constitutes a powerful option to ameliorate DM in severely obese patients, often normalizing blood glucose levels, reducing or avoiding the need for medications, and providing a potentially cost-effective approach to treating the disease.
- Is an appropriate treatment for people with T2DM and obesity not achieving recommended treatment targets with medical therapies.
- Should be an accepted option in people who have T2DM and a BMI >35kg/m², and even an alternative treatment option in patients with a BMI between 30 and 35kg/m² when DM cannot be adequately controlled by an optimal medical regimen, especially in the presence of other major CVD risk factors; this is also reflected in current NICE guidelines.

Further reading

Adams TD, et al. (2017). Weight and metabolic outcomes 12 years after gastric bypass. *N Engl J Med* **377**, 1143–55.

Bray GA, et al. (2016). Seminar: management of obesity. *Lancet* **38**, 1947–56.

Carlsson L, et al. (2020). Life expectancy after bariatric surgery in the Swedish Obese Subjects study. *N Engl J Med* **383**, 1535–43.

Couroulas AP, et al. (2020). Bariatric surgery vs lifestyle intervention for diabetes treatment: 5-year outcomes from a randomized trial. *J Clin Endocrinol Metab* **105**, 866–70.

Farooqi IS (2014). Defining the neural basis of appetite and obesity: from genes to behavior. *Clin Med* **14**, 286–9.

Hall KD, et al. (2011). Quantification of the effect of energy imbalance on bodyweight. *Lancet* **378**, 826–37.

Khera R, et al. (2016). Association of pharmacological treatments for obesity with weight loss and adverse events: a systematic review and meta-analysis. *JAMA* **315**, 2424–34.

Loos RJF (2018). The genetics of adiposity. *Curr Opin Genet Dev* **50**, 86–95.

Mingrone G, et al. (2021). Metabolic surgery versus conventional medical therapy in patients with type 2 diabetes: 10-year follow-up of an open-label, single-centre, randomised controlled trial. *Lancet* **397**, 293–304.

National Institute for Health and Care Excellence (2014). *Obesity: identification, assessment and management.* ॐ https://www.nice.org.uk/guidance/cg189

O'Neil PM, et al. (2018). Efficacy and safety of semaglutide compared with liraglutide and placebo for weight loss in patients with obesity. *Lancet* **392**, 637–49.

Pasquali R, et al. (2020). European Society of Endocrinology clinical practice guideline: endocrine work-up in obesity. *Eur J Endocrinol* **182**, G1–32.

Pi-Sunyer XA, et al. (2015). Randomized, controlled trial of 3.0 mg of liraglutide in weight management. *N Engl J Med* **373**, 11–22.

Sharma AM, Kushner AF (2009). A proposed clinical staging system for obesity. *Int J Obes (Lond)* **33**, 289–95.

Sjöström L, et al. (2012). Bariatric surgery and long-term cardiovascular events. *JAMA* **307**, 56–65.

Sumithran P, et al. (2011). Long-term persistence of hormonal adaptations to weight loss. *N Engl J Med* **365**, 1597–604.

Van Hulsteijn LT, et al. (2020). Prevalence of endocrine disorders in obese patients: systematic review and meta-analysis. *Eur J Endocrinol* **182**, 11–21.

Wilding JPH, et al. (2021). Once-weekly semaglutide in adults with overweight or obesity. *N Engl J Med* **384**, 989–1002.

Pitfalls in laboratory endocrinology

Peter Trainer and *Phillip Monaghan*

Introduction

- The utility of laboratory investigations in endocrinology, as with all biochemical investigations, depends on:
  - Selection of the appropriate test.
  - Careful interpretation.

> Remember, the chemical pathologist, clinical scientist, or other members of the laboratory team will always be happy to help.

- The results from analytical techniques can be altered by many factors.
- These factors may be associated with underlying pathology or may be unrelated.
- Potential confounding factors are outlined in Boxes 18.1 and 18.2.

> ## Box 18.1 Factors influencing laboratory investigations
> *Preanalytical factors*
> - Sample timing—in relation to the dose of any relevant medication, e.g. hydrocortisone when measuring cortisol.
> - Diurnal variation.
> - Collection into the correct tube (e.g. K2EDTA, Li-heparin) and order of draw.
> - Sample handling—rapidity and temperature of transport required to maintain sample stability, the need for centrifugation, and separation of serum or plasma.
> - Biological variation—within-person variation (see Box 18.2).
>
> *Analytical factors*
> - Assay standardization—traceability of calibration, quality control, external quality assessment, and assay methodology.
> - Analytical performance—precision, accuracy, robustness, sensitivity, specificity, and overall assay performance.
> - Hook effect—spuriously low results due to very high concentrations of analyte (e.g. PRL) overwhelming the available assay antibody. Corrected by sample dilution and remeasurement.
> - Sample interference—haemolysis, lipaemia, or elevated bilirubin levels. Most analysers have automated indices of these interferents.
> - Antibody interference—heterophilic antibodies (patient antibodies that cause interference by non-specific binding to assay antibodies) can give rise to spuriously high or low results.
> - Particularly problematic assays—very low concentrations, poor antibody specificity, commonly occurring interferences.
>
> *Post-analytical factors*
> - Reference ranges.
> - Standardization of reporting units, e.g. cortisol—nmol/L or micrograms/dL.
> - Interpretation in the specific clinical setting and dynamic function test—complicated results are often best addressed jointly by the endocrinologist and laboratory.

Box 18.2 Examples of within-person* (biological) variation

- Aldosterone, 36.6%
- Androstenedione, 20.1%
- DHEAS, 6.0%
- PRL, 19.9%
- SHBG, 9.7%
- Testosterone ($\circlearrowleft$), 11.9%
- TSH, 15.9%
- Cortisol, 24%
- IGF-1, 9.4%

Variation expressed as: coefficient of variation (CV, %) = (SD/mean) × 100).

* Data available from the European Federation of Clinical Chemistry and Laboratory Medicine (EFLM) Biological Variation Database (🔗 https://biologicalvariation.eu/).

Common methods of hormone measurement

Immunoassays

The means of routine measurement of most hormones and undertaken on multichannel automated analysers in all clinical biochemistry laboratories.

- Measures the presence of a molecule, known as an analyte or a measurand, using a reagent antibody.
- *Competitive immunoassay:* only one reagent antibody (designed to bind a specific epitope of the hormone to be measured) is immobilized onto a solid phase and in limited quantity. Addition of a labelled analyte, sometimes called the tracer, competes with the endogenous analyte for binding of limited antibody sites; the proportion of antibody-bound tracer (immunoassay signal generated) is inversely proportional to the analyte concentration in the sample. Non-isotopic labels are generally used for safety and ease of use. The catalytic activity of enzymes is often exploited to enhance the analytical sensitivity in immunoassays through signal generation by formation of coloured or fluorescent products from the enzymatic reaction.
- *Immunometric assay:* in this format, the 1st antibody (capture antibody) is immobilized onto a solid support and binds the analyte in the sample; a 2nd labelled antibody that is specific for a different epitope site on the analyte is present in the reaction to form a sandwich complex. The signal generated is directly proportional to the analyte concentration in the sample.
- Choice of competitive vs immunometric immunoassays is analyte-dependent, with larger molecules being more amenable to the two-site immunometric assay format.

Mass spectrometry

Advances in technology have resulted in increasing use of mass spectrometry (MS) in routine laboratories to measure circulating drug concentrations and some hormones, typically steroids. MS has the advantage over immunoassays of being less prone to interference and of lower levels of quantification. Measurement of some peptide hormones (due to size) is too complex for routine reliance on MS.

- Quantifies the analyte based on their mass:charge (or m:z) ratio.
- *Liquid chromatography–tandem mass spectrometry:* the liquid chromatography column eluent undergoes ionization to form charged ions prior to MS. This tandem configuration enables selection of a precursor ion (parent ion) through MS1, and after collision-induced dissociation, the resulting ion fragments enters MS2, tuned to select the product ion (daughter ion) for quantification at the detector.

Analytical factors

Issues with hormone assays

- Often attributed to structurally related molecules that cross-react with the agent antibody (e.g. prednisolone may cross-react in cortisol immunoassays).
- With peptide hormone measurement, post-translational modifications (e.g. glycosylation) can influence antibody binding, e.g. hCG has multiple molecular forms coexisting, which can interfere with accurate test results.
- *Systematic measurement errors:* variation between different assays for the same analyte. Method-specific bias (deviation from the true value) can have major implications for how dynamic function tests are interpreted. For example, bias between different cortisol assays (i.e. the numeric value for a given sample will differ, depending on the choice of assay) means that assay-specific reference ranges should be used when interpretating the results of a random cortisol or SST.
- However, incremental improvements in the design and manufacture of diagnostic tests, including use of monoclonal antibodies, and adoption of recombinant international standard reference materials, particularly for GH and IGF-1 are intended to improve both the clinical performance and the accuracy of assays.
- *The hook effect:* when a very high analyte level saturates the antibody, leading to an artificially low result.
- Biotin, a popular over-the-counter supplement, can interfere with various immunoassays (especially in TFTs), resulting in both artificially high or low readings.

Post-analytical factors

Defining normal

Interpretation of assay results is made in relation to reference ranges provided by the laboratory. These usually represent the 95th centiles of a population of healthy individuals. There is a 1 in 20 chance that a 'normal' result will fall outside of the quoted reference range. The definition of normality is imperfect and often fails to take adequate account of such biological factors, e.g. age, gender, BMI, ethnicity. For some analytes, it is difficult to obtain appropriate samples in health to define reference ranges (e.g. following pharmacological stimulation or samples of CSF).

Timing

- The time of the day or month will be important for some hormone changes.

Units

Literature from the USA and European journals may use different units—beware! SI units use molar or mass (g) and volumes are reported in litres.

- Following stimulation during dynamic function testing, structurally related molecules in a biochemical pathway (e.g. corticosteroid precursors) are also secreted into the circulation at an enhanced rate, compared to baseline, which have different clearance rates and different binding characteristics for the reagent antibodies.

Medicolegal considerations

Confidentiality

- All patient personal information is confidential and should not be shared. Consent to share information within the healthcare team is implied unless the patient specifies.
- All patients should be requested to give explicit consent to disclose identifiable personal information. The patient should be informed about any disclosures.
- Express consent is required for 3rd parties (e.g. insurance, benefits, employer).
- If releasing information, ensure:
  - Written patient consent.
  - Scope and likely consequences understood.
  - Patient offered the opportunity to see the report before sending.

Exceptions where patient consent is not required:
- When required by law.
- Justified in the public interest, e.g. justified to protect individuals or society from risks of serious harm such as from serious communicable diseases or serious crime. In these circumstances, strong consideration of practicality of obtaining consent and the potential harm/distress to the patient or others should be carefully weighed up.
- To prevent abuse/serious harm to others, e.g. DVLA (although if possible, advise patient to release the information with their consent).

Further reading

General Medical Practice (2017, updated 2018). *Confidentiality: good practice in handling patient information.* ℘ https://www.gmc-uk.org/ethical-guidance/ethical-guidance-for-doctors/confidentiality/

DVLA guidance

- A driver is legally required to inform the DVLA about any condition that may affect their fitness to drive. It is the doctor's responsibility to inform a patient if such circumstances arise and also to remind them that they should contact the DVLA. The DVLA medical advisor can provide advice if required. The patient should be reminded that their driving insurance may be invalid if they do not contact the DVLA.
- Patients with visual impairment, e.g. visual field defect, thyroid eye disease causing reduced VA, or diabetes causing hypoglycaemia, should be advised that this may affect their ability to drive and that they should contact the DVLA.
- Diabetes: all drivers must inform the DVLA if they are treated with insulin for over 3 months, demonstrate satisfactory control and recognize hypoglycaemia, with no more than one hypoglycaemic episode in the preceding 12 months, and appropriate blood glucose monitoring. Similar rules apply for tablet-controlled patients with diabetes who are at risk of hypoglycaemia. The other group who may need to contact the DVLA are those with retinopathy causing any impairment to VA (see Box A1.1).
- If a patient refuses/continues to drive against your advice, explain further why they should contact the DVLA, but also explain that you may have to contact the DVLA as there is a public safety issue. This advice should be carefully recorded. A 2nd opinion can be offered, but the patient advised not to drive in the interim. Discussion with the patient's relatives/carers can be helpful if the patient consents.
- Before contacting the DVLA, due to concern about causing serious harm, the doctor should take all reasonable steps to inform the patient and confirm in writing.

Box A1.1 DVLA guidance for diabetes

Insulin-treated diabetes

Group 1 drivers (car and motorcycle)
You need to tell the DVLA if:
- You have had >1 episode of severe hypoglycaemia while awake (needing the assistance of another person) within the last 12 months.
- You develop impaired awareness of hypoglycaemia (difficulty in recognizing the warning symptoms of low blood sugar).

Group 2 drivers (bus and lorry)
You must stop driving Group 2 vehicles and tell the DVLA if:
- You have a single episode of hypoglycaemia requiring the assistance of another person, even if this happened during sleep.
- You have any degree of impaired awareness of hypoglycaemia (difficulty in recognizing the warning symptoms of low blood sugar).

All drivers (Group 1 and Group 2)
You must tell the DVLA if:
- You suffer severe hypoglycaemia while driving.
- You or your medical team feel you are at high risk of developing hypoglycaemia.
- An existing medical condition gets worse or you develop any other condition that may affect your ability to drive safely.

Patients with diabetes treated by tablets and diet

You need to tell the DVLA if:

- You suffer >1 episode of severe hypoglycaemia within the last 12 months while awake. You must also tell the DVLA if you or your medical team feel you are at high risk of developing severe hypoglycaemia. For Group 2 drivers (bus/lorry), one episode of severe hypoglycaemia must be reported immediately.
- You develop impaired awareness of hypoglycaemia (difficulty in recognizing the warning symptoms of low blood sugar).
- You suffer severe hypoglycaemia while driving.
- You need treatment with insulin.
- You need laser treatment to both eyes or in the remaining eye if you have sight in one eye only.
- You have problems with vision in both eyes, or in the remaining eye if you have sight in one eye only. By law, you must be able to read, with glasses or contact lenses if necessary, a car number plate in good daylight at 20m. In addition, the VA (with the aid of glasses or contact lenses if worn) must be at least 6/12 (0.5 decimal) with both eyes open, or in the only eye if monocular.
- You develop any problems with the circulation, or sensation in your legs or feet which makes it necessary for you to drive certain types of vehicles only, e.g. automatic vehicles or vehicles with a hand-operated accelerator or brake. This must be shown on your driving licence.

Patient advice

- If a patient has an accident: *advise to stop and remove the keys from ignition; check blood glucose immediately to demonstrate whether they were/or were not hypoglycaemic.*
- *If a patient has a hypo:* stop the car safely and immediately, and take the keys from ignition and if possible, sit in the passenger seat; do not drive for at least 45–60min after full recovery.
- Keep hypoglycaemic treatment accessible in the car at all times.
- Check glucose no longer than 2h before driving and then every 2h at least during drive.
- If the patient is using CGM, then they should do a finger prick test to meet driving regulations.
- Do not drive if glucose is <5mmol/L, but have a starchy snack and recheck.

Further reading

General Medical Council. *Patients' fitness to drive and reporting concerns to the DVLA or DVA.* ℰ https://www.gmc-uk.org/ethical-guidance/ethical-guidance-for-doctors/confidentiality---patients-fitness-to-drive-and-reporting-concerns-to-the-dvla-or-dva/patients-fitness-to-drive-and-reporting-concerns-to-the-dvla-or-dva

GOV.UK. *Diabetes and driving.* ℰ https://www.gov.uk/diabetes-driving

Consent

Consent is required prior to medical examination, investigation, or treatment. Valid consent must be:
- Voluntary (no influence from medical staff/relatives/friends).
- Informed (having been provided with all relevant information, including risks and benefits, alternative treatments, and outcome if no treatment).
- With capacity to give consent—this is essential, i.e. to understand the information and able to make a decision (usually requires parental consent if aged up to 16 years).

Consent can be written or verbal, or even non-verbal if appropriate. It can also be withdrawn if the person changes their mind.

Drugs
- Explain potential side effects, and document the advice given.
- Consider interaction with other medications and drug allergies.
- Highlight if the drug is being used in an unlicensed indication.
- Ensure appropriate monitoring and clarity of who is responsible for organizing the appropriate safety monitoring and subsequent actions, if any (GP or hospital).

Investigation and treatment
- Ensure *material risk and any possible alternatives* are explained; material risk is defined as 'what is likely to be considered significant by a reasonable person in that particular patient's position, including the nature of the risk, the impact on a person's life, the alternatives (including no investigation or treatment), and the associated risks'.
- Keep a record of the discussion and, if possible, provide the patient with written information.

Principles of information governance and documentation

- All written notes should be legible, comprehensive, dated, and timed, with a signature, name, and status recorded contemporaneously.
- If a retrospective note must be made, the reason and timing should be carefully documented, e.g. emergency management of patient.
- Any alterations should be struck through once, and the amendment signed and dated.
- Protection of confidential patient information is essential and governed by the Caldicott principles:
  - Justify the purpose for use or transfer of confidential information.
  - Do not use personal information unless absolutely necessary.
  - Use the minimum necessary confidential information.
  - Access to confidential information should be strictly restricted.
  - Everyone handling confidential patient information should be aware of their information governance responsibilities.
  - All use of personal information should be lawful.
  - However, the duty to share information can be essential in the best interests of patients.

Further reading

National Data Guardian for Health and Social Care (2020). *The eight Caldicott principles.* ℘ https://www.gov.uk/government/publications/the-caldicott-principles

COVID-19 resources

Arlt W, *et al.* (2020). Endocrinology in the time of COVID-19. *Eur J Endocrinol* **183**, E1–2.

Arlt W, *et al.* (2020). Endocrinology in the time of COVID-19: Management of adrenal insufficiency. *Eur J Endocrinol* **183**, G25–32.

Boelaert K, *et al.* (2020). Endocrinology in the time of COVID-19: Management of hyperthyroidism and hypothyroidism. *Eur J Endocrinol* **183**, G33–9.

Christ-Crain M, *et al.* Endocrinology in the time of COVID-19: Management of diabetes insipidus and hyponatraemia. *Eur J Endocrinol* **183**, G17–23.

Fleseriu M, *et al.* (2020). Endocrinology in the time of COVID-19: Management of pituitary tumours. *Eur J Endocrinol* **183**, G17–23.

Gittoes NJ, *et al.* (2020). Endocrinology in the time of COVID-19: Management of calcium metabolic disorders and osteoporosis. *Eur J Endocrinol* **183**, G57–65.

Newell-Price J, *et al.* (2020). Endocrinology in the time of COVID-19: Management of Cushing's syndrome. *Eur J Endocrinol* **183**, G1–7.

Sharifi N, Ryan C (2020). Androgen hazards with COVID-19. *Endocr Relat Cancer* **27**, E1–3.

Reference intervals

Notes

Reference intervals are variable between analyser platforms and may also be further adjusted, based on locally collected data over time, for specific population demographics. The reference intervals stated here are given as an example, but the analysing laboratory should be consulted for local reference intervals and sample requirements. The following reference intervals apply to adults only, unless stated otherwise. Laboratory UKAS/ISO 15189 accreditation status should be available from the individual website and implies an assured level of analytical processing.

Introduction

(See Box A3.1 for definitions and Box A3.2 for table notes.) (See Table A3.1 for thyroid function; Table A3.2 for adrenal and gonadal function; Table A3.3 for pituitary hormones; Table A3.4 for bone biochemistry; Table A3.5 for plasma gastrointestinal and pancreatic hormones; Table A3.6 for tumour markers; Tables A3.7 and A3.8 for urinary collections; and Table A3.9 for analyses.) All values are for serum unless specified otherwise.

Box A3.1 Definitions
- *Serum.* A serum sample is collected in a plain tube, left to permit clotting, then centrifuged and separated.
- *Plasma.* A plasma specimen is collected in a tube containing EDTA or lithium heparin, centrifuged immediately, and separated.

Box A3.2 Table notes
[a] EDTA tube cold spun immediately and frozen on separation.
[b] Serum, cold spun, flash frozen.
[c] Fasting sample collected into 2 × EDTA tubes, cold spun, and flash frozen.
[d] Acid-containing container (20mL 6M HCl).

Table A3.1 Thyroid function

Analyte	SI units	Traditional units	Conversion factor
TSH	0.38–5.33 mU/L	0.38–5.33 mU/L	1
Free T$_4$	10.5–20 pmol/L	0.8–1.6 ng/dL	12.9
Free T$_3$	3.5–6.2 pmol/L	2.3–4.1 pg/mL	1.54
Thyroid-binding globulin	16–24 mg/L		
Thyroid-stimulating hormone receptor antibodies	0–0.9 IU/L 1.0–1.5 IU/L equivocal >1.5 IU/L +ve		
Antithyroid peroxidase antibodies		<9 IU/mL	

Table A3.2 Adrenal and gonadal function

Analyte		SI units	Traditional units	Conversion factor
Cortisol (9 a.m.)		180–620 nmol/L	6.5–22.5 ng/dL	27.6
Aldosterone	Random	100–800 pmol/L	3.6–28.9 ng/dL	27.7
	Supine	100–450 pmol/L	3.6–16.2 ng/dL	27.7
Plasma renin activity	Random	0.5–3.1 pmol/mL/h	N/A	
	Supine	1.1–2.7 pmol/mL/h	N/A	
	Ambulant (30 min)	2.8–4.5 pmol/mL/h	N/A	
Serum 11-deoxycortisol		24–46 nmol/L		
DHEAS	♀	1.9–9.4 micromol/L	5.1–25.4 ng/dL	0.0027
	♂	2.8–12 micromol/L	7.6–32.4 ng/dL	0.0027
Androstenedione	♀	3.0–8.0 nmol/L	10.5–27.5 micrograms/L	3.49
	♂	3.0–8.0 nmol/L	10.5–27.5 micrograms/L	3.49
17-hydroxy progesterone	♀ Follicular	1–8.7 nmol/L	3.3–28.7 micrograms/L	3.3
	Luteal	<18 nmol/L	<59.4 micrograms/L	
	♂	1–8.7 nmol/L	3.3–28.7 micrograms/L	3.3
	Neonatal	20 nmol/L	<66 micrograms/L	
Oestradiol	♀ Follicular	69–905 pmol/L	248–325 pg/mL	3.6
	Mid cycle	130–2095 pmol/L	468–7542 pg/mL	3.6
	Luteal	82–940 pmol/L	295–3384 pg/mL	3.6
	♂	43–151 pmol/L	155–544 pg/mL	3.6

Analyte		SI units	Traditional units	Conversion factor
Progesterone	♀	0–90 nmol/L	0–288 ng/mL	3.2
	♂	0–10 nmol/L	0–32 ng/mL	3.2
Testosterone	♀	0.5–2.6 nmol/L	1.7–9 ng/mL	3.5
	♂	8.4–28.7 nmol/L	29–100 ng/mL	3.5
DHT	♀	0.1–0.8 nmol/L	2.9–23 ng/dL	0.034
	♂	1–2.9 nmol/L	29–85 ng/dL	0.034
SHBG	♀	18–114 nmol/L	18–114 nmol/L	1
	♂	13–71 nmol/L	13–71 nmol/L	1
Metanephrine (after 30 min resting)		<510 pmol/L		
Normetanephrine (after 30 min resting)		<1180 pmol/L		
3-methoxytyramine		<180 pmol/L		

Table A3.3 Pituitary hormones

Analyte		SI units	Traditional units	Conversion factor
FSH	♀ Follicular	2.5–10.2 U/L	2.5–10.2 mU/mL	1
	Mid cycle	3.4–33.4 U/L	3.4–33.4 mU/mL	1
	Luteal	1.5–9.1 U/L	1.5–9.1 mU/mL	1
	Post-menopausal	23–116 U/L	23–116 mU/mL	1
	♂	1.4–18.1 U/L	1.4–18.1 mU/mL	1
LH	♀ Follicular	1.9–12.5 U/L	1.9–12.5 mU/mL	1
	Mid cycle	8.7–76.3 U/L	8.7–76.3 mU/mL	1
	Luteal	0.5–16.9 U/L	0.5–16.9 mU/mL	1
	Post-menopausal	15.9–54 U/L	15.9–54 mU/mL	1
	♂	1.5–9.3 U/L	1.5–9.3 mU/mL	1
Prolactin	♀	60–620 mU/L	3–31 ng/mL	20
	♂	45–375 mU/L	2.2–19 ng/mL	20

Analyte		SI units	Traditional units	Conversion factor
IGF-1	20 years	16–118 nmol/L	120–885 ng/mL	7.5
	40 years	14–47 nmol/L	105–353 ng/mL	
	60 years	10.5–35 nmol/L	79–263 ng/mL	
	>60 years	7.0–28 nmol/L	52–210 ng/mL	
IGF-1:IGF-2 ratio		>10		
ACTH[a]		2.2–17.6 pmol/L	10–80 ng/L	0.22
Inhibin B		80–150 pg/mL		

[a] EDTA tube cold spun immediately and frozen on separation.

Table A3.4 Bone biochemistry

Analyte	SI units	Traditional units	Conversion factor
Parathyroid hormone[b]	1.3–7.6 pmol/L	13–73 pg/mL	0.1
25-hydroxycalcitriol			
Deficiency	<30 nmol/L	<12.5 ng/mL	2.4
Probable insufficiency	30–49 nmol/L	12.5–20.4 ng/mL	
Probable sufficiency	>50 nmol/L	>20.8 ng/mL	
1,25-dihydroxycolecalciferol[b]	43–144 pmol/L	18–60 pg/mL	2.4
Calcitonin[a]	<0.10 ng/L		
P1NP[b] procollagen extension peptide	20–60 micrograms/L		

[a] EDTA tube cold spun immediately and frozen on separation.

[b] Serum cold spun, flash frozen.

Table A3.5 Plasma gastrointestinal and pancreatic hormones

Analyte	SI units	Traditional units	Conversion factor
Insulin (fasting)	18–77 pmol/L	2.6–11.1 mU/L	6.9
C-peptide (fasting)	0.27–1.28 nmol/L	0.8–3.88 ng/mL	0.33
Gastrin[c]	0–40 pmol/L	0–89 pg/mL	0.45
Glucagon[c]	0–50 pmol/L	0–179 pg/mL	0.28
Vasoactive intestinal polypeptide (VIP)[c]	0–30 pmol/L	0–71 pg/mL	0.42
Pancreatic polypeptide[c]	0–300 pmol/L	0–1250 pg/mL	0.24
Somatostatin[c]	0–150 pmol/L		
Chromogranin A[c]	0–60 pmol/L		
Chromogranin B[c]	0–150 pmol/L		
Neurotensin[c]	0–100 pmol/L		

[c] 2 × EDTA tubes cold spun and flash frozen.

Table A3.6 Tumour markers

Analyte	SI units
β-hCG	0–4 U/L
Carcinoembryonic antigen (CEA)	0–3 U/L
Prostate-specific antigen (PSA)	0–4 micrograms/L
Alpha fetoprotein	0–7 IU/mL

Table A3.7 Urinary collections (1)

Analyte	SI units (micromol/24h)	Same for both genders
Normetadrenaline[d]		
Adult	0–3.0	3.6
Metadrenaline[d]		
Adult	0–1.4	0
3-methoxytyramine[d]		
Adult	0.57–2.4	

[d] Acid-containing container (20mL 6M HCl).

Table A3.8 Urinary collections (2)

Urinary analyte	SI units (mmol/L)	Traditional units	SI units (mmol/ 24h)	Conversion factor
Cortisol			0–560	
Calcium	1.25–3.75	50–150 mg/L	2.5–7.5	0.025
Phosphate	7.5–25	0.2–0.8 mg/L	12.9–42	32.3
Potassium	20–60	20–60 mmol/l	♀: 34–103	1.0
			♂: 37–139	
Sodium	50–125	50–125 mmol/L	♀: 61–214	1.0
			♂: 83–287	
5-hydroxyindoleacetic acid		1.9–7.7 mg/ 24 h	10–40 micromol/L/ 24 h	5.2
Aldosterone			14–53 nmol/L	

[d] Acid-containing container (20mL 6M HCl).

Table A3.9 Table of analyses

Analyte	SI Units	Other Units	Conversion factor
Fasting glucose[1]			0.055
Normal	≤6.0 mmol/L	≤108 mg/dL	
Impaired fasting glycaemia	≥6.1 <7.0 mmol/L	≥11 <126 mg/dL	
Diabetes	≥7.0 mmol/L	≥126 mg/dL	
2-h glucose in 75 g OGTT			
Normal	<7.8 mmol/L	<140 mg/dL	
Impaired glucose tolerance	≥7.8 <11.1 mmol/L	≥140 <200 mg/dL	
Diabetes	≥11.1 mmol/L	≥200 mg/dL	
HbA1c (non-diabetic range)	<48 mmol/mol (IFCC units)	<6.5%	mmol/mol value = (% value × 10.93) − 23.5 % value = (0.0915 × mmol/mol value) + 2.15[2]
Total cholesterol[3]	≤5.2 mmol/L		38.6
HDL-cholesterol[3]	>1.5 mmol/L	>60 mg/dL	38.6
LDL-cholesterol[3]	≤4	115 mg/dL	38.6
Fasting triglycerides	0.55–1.9 mmol/L	49–168 mg/dL	88.5
Adiponectin inversely correlated with % body fat	N/A	♂ 5–25 micrograms/mL ♀ 5–35 micrograms/mL	N/A
Leptin correlated with % body fat	N/A	♂ 1–10 ng/mL ♀ 4–25 ng/mL	N/A

[1] Figures quoted are WHO definitions. The ADA have a lower cut-off for normal fasting glucose of 5.6 mmol/L or 100 mg/dL.

[2] Not straightforward; best to download a converter to your smartphone or print out a chart for the clinic wall.

[3] Suggest to interpret lipid results in light of coronary risk calculator (*British National Formulary*) and NICE guidance CG181. The figures quoted would be appropriate for 1° prevention. (See also ➲ Macrovascular disease, pp. 970–1; ➲ Lipids and coronary heart disease, pp. 982–3.)

Index

Note: Tables, figures, and boxes are indicated by an italic t, f, and b following the page number.